Advanced Pharmacology
Second Edition

Advanced Pharmacology
Second Edition

Bikash Medhi

MBBS, MD (AIIMS), MAMS, FIMSA

Professor,
& Additional Medical Superintendent (AMS),
Founder: Experimental Pharmacology Laboratory and Neurobehavioral Laboratory
(EPL & NBRL Lab: www.epl.pgi.in)
Department of Pharmacology,
Chief Editor, Indian Journal of Pharmacology (IJP),
Coordinator PGIMER Pharmacovigilance and Materiovigilance Centre ,
Regional Coordinator, NADA (North Zone), Ministry of Youth and Sports,Government of India.
Co-Convener India Initiate Programme (IPS)
Ex Secretary Clinical Pharmacology of Indian Pharmacology Society,
Research Block B, 4th Floor, Room no 4043,
Postgraduate Institute of Medical Education & Research, Chandigarh, 160012, India
E-mail: drbikashus@yahoo.com; drbikash11@rediffmail.com; drbikashmedhi@gmail.com

Ajay Prakash

M.Sc (Pharmacology), PhD

Assistant Professor
Associate Editor, Indian Journal of Pharmacology
Co-Founder: Experimental Pharmacology Laboratory and Neurobehavioral Laboratory
(EPL & NBRL Lab: www.epl.pgi.in)
Adjunct Faculty, Department of Physical and Rehabilitation Medicine
Department of Pharmacology, PGIMER, Chandigarh-India-160012
E-mail: ajayprakashpgi@gmail.com, prakash.ajay@pgimer.edu.in

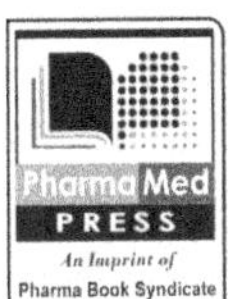

PharmaMed Press

An imprint of Pharma Book Syndicate

A Unit of BSP Books Pvt. Ltd.

4-4-309/316, Giriraj Lane,
Sultan Bazar, Hyderabad - 500 095.

Published by

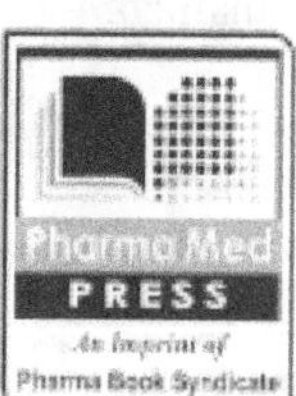

PharmaMed Press

An imprint of Pharma Book Syndicate

A unit of BSP Books Pvt. Ltd.

4-4-309/316, Giriraj Lane, Sultan Bazar, Hyderabad - 500 095.
Phone: 040-23445688, 23445600; Fax: 91+40-23445611
e-mail: info@pharmamedpress.com
www.pharmamedpress.com/pharmamedpress.net

ISBN: 978-93-89354-16-4

Dedicated to

My parents, wife (Dr. Sujata Upadhyay), son "JoJo" (Debayan Medhi) and all my students responsible for constant encouragement during my teaching carrier

- Bikash Medhi

Dedicated to

My respected sir "Dr. Bikash Medhi" who always encouraged and motivated me to do well. Grandma, father and mother for their emotional caring support and My wife "Vishalika" and son "Aarav and Aadvik", for their love, constant support and encouragements

- Ajay Prakash

प्रो. वाई.के. गुप्ता

Dr. Y.K. GUPTA, *MD, FAMS, FNASc, FIPS, FIAN*
Professor and Head
President : Society of Toxicology, India
Co-ordinator : Pharmacovigilance Programme for India
I/c : National Poison Information Centre
Editor (Pharmacology) : I J P P
Member : INSA-ICSU Committee for IUPHAR
Ex-President : Indian Pharmacological Society

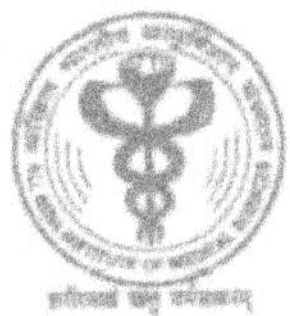

भेषजगुण विज्ञान विभाग
अखिल भारतीय आयुर्विज्ञान संस्थान

DEPARTMENT OF PHARMACOLOGY
ALL INDIA INSTITUTE OF MEDICAL SCIENCES
ANSARI NAGAR, NEW DELHI-110 029

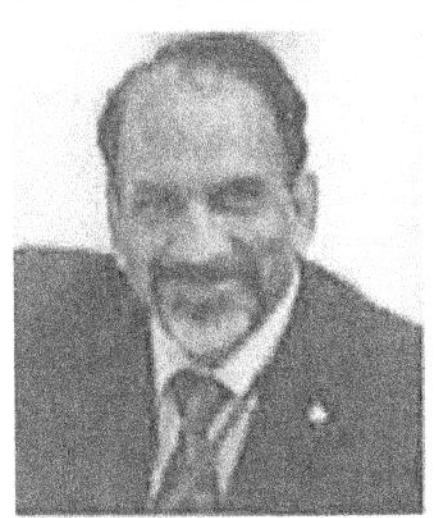

Foreword

Being a Pharmacologist, I know that there was a gap between the academic and industrial prospect of Pharmacology and for a long time we all were waiting to have a book, which could look at the Indian pharmacology from a fresh angle, and I am glad that *"Advanced Pharmacology"* is a good initiative in this direction. I am very happy to know that Dr. Bikash Medhi has expressed his rich experience in this book. This book is very concise, but covers all the vital aspects of drug and pharmacology apart from basic pharmacology. This book also informs about the very recent fields of pharmacovigilance and haemovigilance which sensitizers us about patient care and patient safety in relation to the use of medicines. This is an excellent reference book for medical, pharmacy and nursing undergraduates, postgraduates, doctoral students and other healthcare professionals. This book will facilitate training of pharmacologists who are required to have multidisciplinary knowledge in areas like drug information, clinical implications of drugs, nanomedicines and computer aided drug discovery approach. This book will be an asset for all the biomedical students who have a strong interest in making a major contribution to the understanding of both novel and current disease processes and the development of new therapies and their hurdles.

He deserve our compliments for preparing this easily readable text which I hope will become popular among student, faculties and other healthcare professionals having interest in pharmacology, I wish the book all the success.

Prof. Y.K. Gupta

Phone : (Off.) 91-11-26593282, 26589691, 26593684
Telefax : 91-11-26589691 Fax : 91-11-26588663, 26588641 E-mail : yk.ykgupta@gmail.com

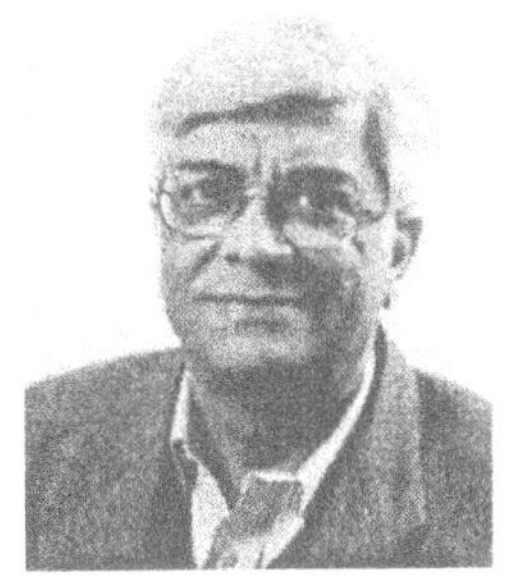

Foreword

I am very happy to write the Foreword Note for the book entitled *"Advanced Pharmacology"* by Dr. Bikash Medhi, Additional Professor, Department of Pharmacology, PGIMER, Chandigarh-160012. Pharmacology is the science of drug action on biological systems and embraces knowledge of the sources, chemical properties, biological effects and therapeutic uses of drugs. It is often described as a bridging science as it incorporates knowledge and skills from a number of basic science disciplines including physiology, biochemistry and cell and molecular biology. The role of Pharmacologist is to 'translate' such knowledge into the rational development of therapeutics. The interdisciplinary nature of pharmacologists has a variety of opportunities and duties to perform to empower the medical field. This book presents the content to enrich medical, pharmacy students and healthcare professionals on the pharmacological aspects of drugs in diverse conditions. The topics covered in the book are important and rarely discussed; hence this book would give the reader a broad horizon of knowledge. I am very happy to extend my best wishes for the book and wish it enlightens the reader about the drug regulatory, drug development and therapeutics.

Prof. Y. K. Chawla
Director, PGIMER

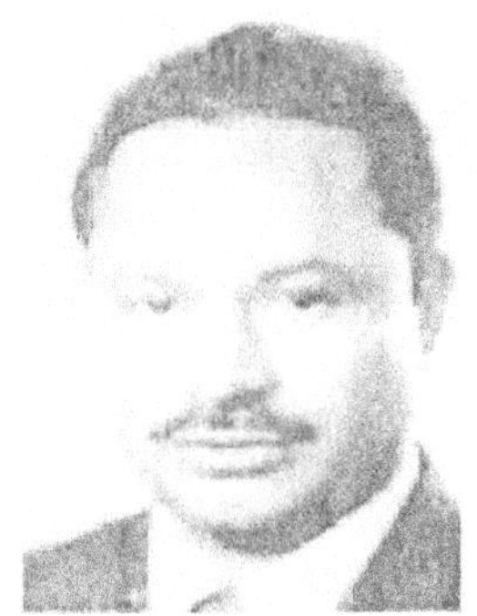

Foreword

Pharmacology is a widely known subject with multi-divisions, which caters the need of every discipline of medical sciences. There are number of reference books available in the market and many of them give only archaic information, which are less informative and relevant in therapeutics. But, topics like essential drugs, orphan drugs, Drug policy, Drug lag are important and need to be known to all health care professionals. The contents of this book include several topics to address the need of modern medicine and have incorporated those topics which are earlier not explored in depth. The importance of pharmacology is rapidly evolving which there was a need to look as it from a fresh angle. This book *"Advanced Pharmacology"* offers fresh angle and new insights into exploring the depths of the drugs and pharmacology.

The format and printing of the book have been of higher quality to preserve the phenotypical presentation. Photographs, lines, drawings, flowcharts and tables in the book are relevant and extremely useful in gaining knowledge on the subject. The language of the book is simple and easy to understand.

I hope that the material in this book by Dr. Bikash Medhi will serve not only as a general therapeutic tutorial, but also as a first step to *"Advanced Pharmacology"* which covers all the aspects of drugs.

I see a bright future for this book….

Dr. A. K. Gupta
Medical Superintendent (MS)

Preface to Second Edition

The issue of the first edition is completely based on topics which were rarely discussed among the healthcare stakeholders and it was important to know the facts regarding these topics. The first edition of *"Advanced Pharmacology"* is being published in 2014 with the objective to familiarize the health professionals and researchers about some important aspects of medicinal use and rare topics. Further, the textbook has been written to update and simulate the pharmacologists and other professionals to keep updated knowledge regarding the *"general topics of pharmacology"*, *"therapeutics pharmacology"*, *"recent advances in pharmacology"* and rare topics in pharmacology. Important topics like drug price, drug policy, orphan drugs, e-prescription, and medication reconciliation, which are under orphanage but possess important stand in the field of drug and other clinical pharmacology of pregnancy, pediatric and geriatric populations to name some of them were included in the chapters.

In the second edition of book we have tried to include the topics which are still very rarely discussed i.e. *Neutraceuticals, Drug Excipients, Forensic Pharmacology, System Pharmacology, and Therapeutic use Exemption for the Sports Person and Virtual Trial.* Each topic described very precisely to make reader understand the topic easily. Therefore, book aimed to designed for those who are eager to know about drug usage and specialized topics in pharmacology. Our aim is to explore our wings in the sky of medical education where we can provide our best efforts to the society and development. We certainly expect that readers will be benefited with the book and feel free to contribute their valuable personal suggestions for the chapters included in the second edition, so that we can improve the future editions.

We are grateful to all the authors and reviewers who aided and supported us in the completion of book throughout the process, especially our students/scholars/residents who always gives us think new for their future and betterment.

Our gratitude is for our institute and faculties who always inspire us to do better and better for the pharmacology. The support is led to establishment of *"Experimental Pharmacology Laboratory (EPL)-www.eplpgi.in and www.eplpgi.res.in"*. We heartedly thanks to the Director, PGIMER and all faculties members who always extend their support and contribution to the laboratory.

- Bikash Medhi
- Ajay Prakash

Preface to First Edition

Over the several decades, the field of pharmacology has evolved greatly and has incorporated the spectacular advances and research and development (R & D) in the field of drugs. Overall pharmacology is concerned with the study of drugs action of any origin and their possible interactions with living organism and chemicals that affect normal or abnormal biochemical and molecular function of body. The first edition of *"Advanced Pharmacology"* is being published this year with the objective to familiarize the health professionals and researchers about some important aspects of medicinal use and topics commonly very few known and discussed elite. Further, the textbook has been written to update and simulate the pharmacologists and other professionals to keep step with these advances and neglected but important topics on drug therapy and other related issues. To make the textbook an invaluable resource for students and health care professionals, we included chapters from *"general topics of pharmacology"*, *"therapeutics pharmacology"*, *"recent advances in pharmacology"* and rare topics in pharmacology. Important topics like drug price, drug policy, orphan drugs, e-prescription, and medication reconciliation, which are under orphanage but possess important stand in the field of drug and other clinical pharmacology of pregnancy, pediatric and geriatric populations to name some of them were included in the chapters. The use of drugs is an art principally underlying the optimal care of the patients. This book is designed for those who are eager to know about drug usage and specialized topics in pharmacology. We certainly expect that readers will be benefited with the book and feel free to contribute their valuable personal suggestions for the chapters included so that we can improve the future editions. We hope that this book will contribute in the field of pharmacology teaching and improve the old approaches of pharmacology teaching.

We are grateful to those who aided and supported us in the journey of completion of book throughout the process, specially our lab mates. Our sincere thanks to students and teachers of pharmacology, from whom we learnt a lot. We sincerely thank and acknowledge the all contributors, without whom the book could not come at conclusive and informative end.

- Bikash Medhi
- Ajay Prakash

List of Contributors

Adeel Malik

School of Biotechnology,
280 Daehak-ro, Gyeongsan, Gyeongbuk 712-749, Republic of Korea.

Amit Raj Sharma

Department of Neurology
Post Graduate Institute of Medical Education and Research (PGIMER),
Nehru Hospital, Sector: 12, Chandigarh, India-160012.

Anand Kamal Sachdeva

Pharmacology, University Institute of Pharmaceutical Sciences (UIPS)
Sector: 14, Panjab University, Chandigarh, India-160014.

Anurag Kuhad

Pharmacology, University Institute of Pharmaceutical Sciences (UIPS)
Sector: 14, Panjab University, Chandigarh, India-160014.

Ashutosh Singh

Department of Pharmacology,
Post Graduate Institute of Medical Education and Research (PGIMER),
Research Block: B, Sector: 12, Chandigarh, India-160012.

Baldeep Kumar

Department of Pharmacology,
Post Graduate Institute of Medical Education and Research (PGIMER),
Research Block: B, Sector: 12, Chandigarh, India-160012.

D. Harikrishna Reddy

Department of Pharmacology,
Post Graduate Institute of Medical Education and Research (PGIMER),
Research Block: B, Sector: 12, Chandigarh, India-160012.

Dhruv Mahendru

Department of Pharmacology,
Post Graduate Institute of Medical Education and Research (PGIMER),
Research Block: B, Sector: 12, Chandigarh, India-160012.

Firoj Ahmad

Biomedical Informatics Centre (BIC),
Post Graduate Institute of Medical Education and Research (PGIMER),
Research Block: B, Sector: 12, Chandigarh, India-160012.

Jyotsna Rani

Department of Obstetrics & Gynaecology
Government Medical College & Hospital, Chandigarh.

Kanwaljit Chopra

Pharmacology, University Institute of Pharmaceutical Sciences (UIPS)
Sector: 14, Panjab University, Chandigarh, India-160014.

Krishan Lal Khanduja

Department of Biophysics,
Post Graduate Institute of Medical Education and Research (PGIMER),
Research Block: B, Sector: 12, Chandigarh, India-160012.

Manisha Prajapat

Department of Pharmacology,
Post Graduate Institute of Medical Education and Research (PGIMER),
Research Block: B, Sector: 12, Chandigarh, India-160012.

Mukesh Nandave

Shobhaben Pratapbhai Patel School of Pharmacy & Technology Management,
SVKM's Narsee Monjee Institute of Management Studies (NMIMS)
V L Mehta Road, Vile Parle (West), Mumbai 400 056.

Navjot Kaur

Department of Pharmacology,
Post Graduate Institute of Medical Education and Research (PGIMER),
Research Block: B, Sector: 12, Chandigarh, India-160012.

Nitika Garg

Department of Pharmacology,
Post Graduate Institute of Medical Education and Research (PGIMER),
Research Block: B, Sector: 12, Chandigarh, India-160012.

Pawan Kumar Singh

Department of Pharmacology,
Post Graduate Institute of Medical Education and Research (PGIMER),
Research Block: B, Sector: 12, Chandigarh, India-160012.

Phulen Sarma

Department of Pharmacology,
Post Graduate Institute of Medical Education and Research (PGIMER),
Research Block: B, Sector: 12, Chandigarh, India-160012.

Pooja Sarotra

Department of Pharmacology,
Post Graduate Institute of Medical Education and Research (PGIMER),
Research Block: B, Sector: 12, Chandigarh, India-160012.

Pramod Avti

Department of Biophysics,
Post Graduate Institute of Medical Education and Research (PGIMER),
Research Block: B, Sector: 12, Chandigarh, India-160012.

Praveen Kumar

Department of Pharmacology,
Post Graduate Institute of Medical Education and Research (PGIMER),
Research Block: B, Sector: 12, Chandigarh, India-160012.

Puneet Dhamija

Department of Pharmacology,
All India Institute of Medical Sciences (AIIMS), Rishikesh, Uttarakhand.

Rahul Singh

Department of Pharmacology,
Post Graduate Institute of Medical Education and Research (PGIMER),
Research Block: B, Sector: 12, Chandigarh, India-160012.

Rakesh Kumar Ruhela

Department of Pharmacology,
Post Graduate Institute of Medical Education and Research (PGIMER),
Research Block: B, Sector: 12, Chandigarh, India-160012.

Rakesh Kumar Sewal

Department of Pharmacology,
Post Graduate Institute of Medical Education and Research (PGIMER),
Research Block: B, Sector: 12, Chandigarh, India-160012.

Razia Adam

Department of Paediatric Medicine,
Advanced Paediatrics Center,
Post Graduate Institute of Medical Education and Research, Chandigarh, India.

Rupa Joshi

Department of Pharmacology,
Post Graduate Institute of Medical Education and Research (PGIMER),
Research Block: B, Sector: 12, Chandigarh, India-160012.

Sanjay Singh

Biomedical Informatics Centre (BIC),
Post Graduate Institute of Medical Education and Research (PGIMER),
Research Block: B, Sector: 12, Chandigarh, India-160012.

Seema Bansal

Pharmacology, University Institute of Pharmaceutical Sciences (UIPS)
Sector: 14, Panjab University, Chandigarh, India-160014.

Shammy Chandel

Department of Neurosurgery,
Post Graduate Institute of Medical Education and Research (PGIMER),
Research Block: B, Sector: 12, Chandigarh, India-160012.

Sharonjeet Kaur

Department of Pharmacology,
Post Graduate Institute of Medical Education and Research (PGIMER),
Research Block: B, Sector: 12, Chandigarh, India-160012.

Shubham Misra

Department of Pharmacology,
Post Graduate Institute of Medical Education and Research (PGIMER),
Research Block: B, Sector: 12, Chandigarh, India-160012.

Shweta Sinha

Department of Medical Parasitology,
Post Graduate Institute of Medical Education and Research (PGIMER),
Research Block: A, Sector: 12, Chandigarh, India-160012.

Sree Lalitha Bojja

Department of Immunopathology,
Post Graduate Institute of Medical Education and Research (PGIMER)
Research Block: A, Sector: 12, Chandigarh, India-160012.

Shringika Soni

Department of Pharmacology,
Post Graduate Institute of Medical Education and Research (PGIMER)
Research Block: A, Sector: 12, Chandigarh, India-160012.

Subodh Kumar

Department of Pharmacology
Post Graduate Institute of Medical Education and Research (PGIMER)
Research Block: A, Sector: 12, Chandigarh, India-160012.

Sudhir C. Sarangi

Department of Pharmacology
All India Institute of Medical Sciences (AIIMS), Raipur, Chattisgarh.

Uttam Saini

Department of Orthopaedics,
Post Graduate Institute of Medical Education and Research (PGIMER)
Nehru Hospital, Sector: 12, Chandigarh, India-160012.

Vidya Mahalmani

Department of Pharmacology
Post Graduate Institute of Medical Education and Research (PGIMER)
Research Block: A, Sector: 12, Chandigarh, India-160012

Vijay Khajuria

Department of Pharmacology,
Government Medical College, Jammu, J & K.

Vipin Arora

Pharmacology, University Institute of Pharmaceutical Sciences (UIPS)
Sector: 14, Panjab University, Chandigarh, India-160014.

Vishal Kumar

Department of Orthopaedics,
Post Graduate Institute of Medical Education and Research (PGIMER)
Nehru Hospital, Sector: 12, Chandigarh, India-160012.

Vishal Tandon

Department of Pharmacology,
Government Medical College, Jammu, J & K.

Zahid Gillani

Department of Pharmacology,
Government Medical College, Jammu, J & K.

CONTENTS

SECTION – I

SECTION – II

SECTION – III

Section – IV

SECTION – I

CHAPTER 1

ESSENTIAL MEDICINES

Introduction

In general, essential medicines are in need of each developed and developing countries to fulfil health care needs of majority of the populations. Essential medicines are defined by the WHO as *"those drugs that satisfy the health care needs of the majority of the population; they should therefore be available at all times in adequate amounts and in appropriate dosage forms, at a price the community can afford"*. In other words, essential medicines are the medicines that address the priority health care requirements of a given population, are life-saving and affordable to the consumer as well as health care professionals (Fig. 1.1). Today $1/3^{rd}$ of world population and 50% population of developing countries are lacking access to essential drugs. Hence, the concept underlying the use of essential medicines is that despite the availability of a humongous number of medicines only a limited number of medicines are very much essential, important, indispensable and necessary with respect to the requirements of a given population. Moreover the careful selection of a limited number of medicines lead to complete and detailed drug information, better management of medicines, better ADR monitoring, rational drug use, better supply of drugs with good quality at affordable costs and ease of storage, distribution and dispensing leading to better health care. The term 'essential drug' was coined by the WHO and currently the term 'essential medicines list' is being used.

Disease Burden

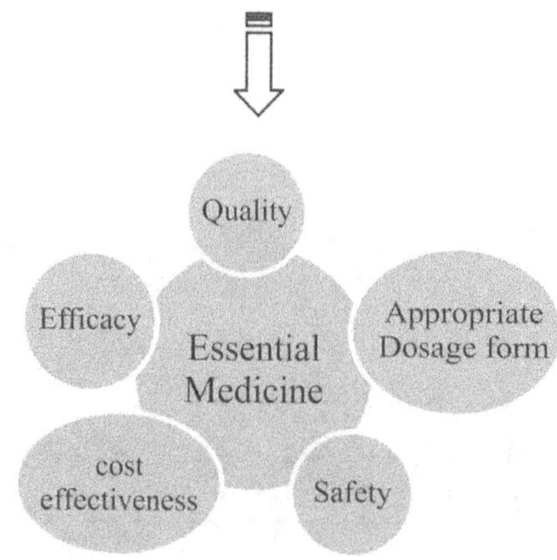

Fig. 1.1 Pre-requisites for essential medicine.

Essential Medicines List (EML)

The first EML of WHO was created in 1977 which included 208 medicines; aimed to provide safe and effective treatment against the global burden of disease at that time. The list is revised by a committee of independent experts every two years to reflect new health challenges, pharmaceutical developments and changing resistance patterns. The current versions are the 18th WHO Essential Medicines List and the 4th WHO Essential Medicines List for Children updated in April 2013 which address most global priority conditions, including malaria, HIV/AIDS, tuberculosis, reproductive health and, increasingly, chronic diseases such as cancer and diabetes. This model list serves as a guide for the developing national and institutional essential medicines lists taking into consideration their local priorities.

The EML published by WHO contains a core list and a complementary list. According to the WHO, core list presents a list of minimum medicine needs for a basic health-care system, listing the most efficacious, safe and cost-effective medicines for priority conditions. Priority conditions are selected on the basis of current and estimated future public health relevance, and potential for safe and cost-effective treatment. While the complementary list presents essential medicines for priority diseases, for which specialized diagnostic or monitoring facilities, and/or specialist medical care, and/or specialist training are needed. In case of doubt, medicines may also be listed as complementary on the basis of consistent higher costs or less attractive cost effectiveness in a variety of settings. The symbol [c] placed next to the complementary list signifies that the medicine(s) require(s) specialist diagnostic or monitoring facilities, and/or specialist medical care, and/or specialist training for their use in children while the [c] symbol placed next to an individual medicine or strength of medicine signifies that there is a specific indication for restricting its use to children. Other symbol used in the list is the square box symbol (□) which primarily intends to indicate similar clinical performance within a pharmacological class. And the symbol [a] indicates that there is an age or weight restriction on use of the medicine.

Aim of Essential Medicines List (EML)

Principally, medicines in EML should cover a range of medical conditions from symptomatic relief, public health care, management of infections as well as for "life threatening" - emergency situations and for critical care. Therefore, categorising EML serves as a valuable tool to determine the drugs which are the most needed for safe and effective treatment. Moreover, it aids in the selection of quality assured pharmaceuticals so as to provide the quality health care and safe use.

EML helps in managing the purchase and distribution of medicines thereby improving the cost-effectiveness of health care. It brings transparency in healthcare system.

Selection Criteria of Essential Medicines

An independent expert committee is held responsible for selection of essential medicines. The main focus of the committee is to make such a list which can cover the large part of the population in terms of economical, safety and efficacy, with due regard to disease prevalence. Selection of essential medicine is a stepwise process and the important steps are as follows:

1. Applications for inclusions, changes or deletions get submitted.
2. Secretary of the expert committee review the application.
3. Assessments are made of the data on comparative economical, safety and efficacy.
4. An expert invited to formulate a draft recommendation for the committee, also summarizes the outcome of the assessments.
5. The relevant departments and experts advisory panels review the draft recommendation and proposed text of the model formulary.
6. The comments get reviewed and expert committee finally get the text for consideration which forward the application as a recommendation to the head of Institution.
7. After the meeting and the final approval by the head of Institution, the recommended changes to the model list, Translations of the report are published as soon as possible for the benefit of the population.

Factors on which the selection of essential medicines depends:

- Disease prevalence
- Benefit/risk ratio in terms of efficacy and safety
- Relative cost-effectiveness of medicines and treatment
- For two or more therapeutically equivalent drugs, priority given to drug with most favourable pharmacokinetic properties or its availability

- Single compounds preferred over fixed dose combinations
- Fixed dose combinations selected if it shows advantage over using different doses individually

However, it is noteworthy that no single factor can govern the selection of a medicine and all factors are equally important while selecting essential medicines. In addition, the choice of essential medicines is a continuous process and requires regular revision due to ever changing priorities of public health activities and continuous development in the field of pharmacology and pharmaceutics. Information on cost and cost-effectiveness should preferably refer to average generic world market prices as listed in the *International Drug Price Indicator Guide*, provided by WHO and maintained by Management Sciences for Health. If this information is not available, other international sources, such as the WHO, UNICEF and *Médecins sans Frontières* price information service, can be used. Always cost analyses should specify the source of the price information selected.

Number of Drugs in EML

The number of drugs present in the EML is maintained in such a fashion that EML should not be bulky enough, so that, it will be impossible for the hospitals to keep all the drugs listed in EML. During the selection process, ideally the best one in each class is selected, so as to avoid confusion originating due to multiplicity. However, in order to achieve flexibility in procurement generally up to 2-3 alternatives are listed.

Advantages of EML

The WHO's model essential medicines list plays a crucial role in placing access to essential drugs as a national and international agenda. In addition, it offers several advantages which are as follows:

- Serve as a tool for countries to identify and choose their drug priorities
- Promote rational drug use
- Development of standard protocols and rational prescribing policies
- Provide latest unbiased clinical information on essential drugs like dosages, usage, contraindications and adverse effects
- Better management of medicines, complete and detailed drug information, better ADR monitoring and ease of storage, distribution and dispensing

Global Status of Essential Medicines

There exists great variation among different countries in terms of prevalence of disease, economy of the country, drug policies etc., so the EML is intended to be flexible and adaptable accordingly. Thus, it is the national responsibility to adapt the model list as per local requirements.

The concept of essential medicines is rising and advanced. EML made it important to frequently update medicine's selection in order to reflect new therapeutic options and changing therapeutic needs which further enhance drug quality. It also incorporates the need for continued development of better medicines with respect to emerging diseases and resistance. In last 30 years period, the EML has led to a world acceptance of the concept by governments and healthcare suppliers worldwide as a robust means that to push health equity even though it was not designed as global standard. Currently, over 150 countries have published their official essential medicines lists. Many major international agencies like UNICEF, UNHCR, UNFPA and IDA as well as non-governmental organizations and international non-profit supply agencies have based their catalogue on the WHO Model List.

It has been estimated that 60-80% of the population in developing nations, specifically in rural areas, still deprived of the essential drugs and WHO highlighted that, about 2,000 million of people do not have even access to essential medicines. Thus, lack of access to essential medicines is a major concern for many developing counties. The current international trade agreement leads to increased prices in these countries which ultimately deprived the population from getting essential medicines. Poor status of research and development (R&D) in the developing economies is another reason for inaccessibility of essential drugs. Other underlying factors for poor accessibility of essential medicines are poor medicine supply and distribution systems and insufficient health facilities and staff. To increase the availability of essential medicines in developing countries an international campaign-The Campaign for Access to Essential Medicines has been started by Medecins Sans Frontieres (MSF)- an international campaign has been started which aim to stimulate and enhance research and development in the field of new diseases that primarily affect the poor, aid in lowering the prices of existing drugs, vaccines and diagnostic tests, and overcome other barriers that prevent patients getting the treatment they need. It is paramount that policies which favour access to essential drugs should be enhanced by promoting research and innovation in areas relevant to developing countries, and those which provide safeguards to ensure affordable access to essential medicines. Effective utilization of all available flexibilities in the TRIPS Agreement, greater integration of traditional medicine systems, building capacity for local manufacture and price control policies are some of the pivotal steps that should be included while making policies. Rebate for generic drug prescribing, appropriate and cost effective prescribing practices and consumer awareness should be the important components of policies for essential medicines. In order to implement the concept of essential medicine, the co-ordination and co-operation at both global and local level is necessary. Local co-operation can widen affordable access to essential drugs. Development of technical expertise on utilizing available flexibilities in trade agreements such as TRIPS; enhancing research and manufacturing capacity of countries in the region; developing technical and infrastructural capability for regulating medicines; and establishing regional procurement systems for pharmaceuticals are the important aspects of local co-operation.

Essential Medicines Library

As the concept of EML is getting strengthen WHO has developed a web based essential medicines library which provide access to the information regarding the evidence for selection such as the reasons for inclusion of a drug, the most important systematic reviews, and important references, summaries of relevant WHO clinical guidelines and price information. WHO model formulary and information on nomenclature and quality assurance standards is also provided (Fig. 1.2). This WHO Essential Medicines Web Library is currently based on the 16th WHO Model List of Essential Medicines and the 2nd WHO Model List of Essential Medicines for Children. Its aim is to facilitate the work of national, hospital and institutional essential medicines selection committees. WHO Essential Medicines internet Library is presently supported the 16th World Health Organization Model List of Essential Medicines and also 2nd World Health Organization Model List of Essential Medicines for children. To facilitate the work of national, hospital and institutional essential medicines choice committees are some of its main objectives.

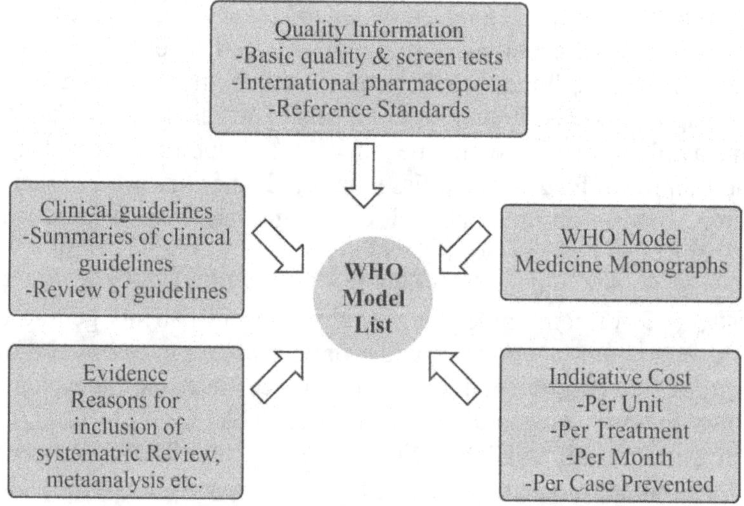

Fig. 1.2 Components of WHO essential medicines list.

Emergency Essential Medicines

To facilitate the emergency response arising from various situations like natural, political and economic disasters, the WHO has designed 'The Interagency Emergency Health Kit 2006' (IEHK 2006). Its aim is to encourage the standardization of medicines and medical supplies needed in emergencies to allow efficient and effective response with medicines and medical devices using standard, pre-packed kits to meet priority health needs in emergencies. IEHK 2006 is the third edition of the WHO Emergency Health Kit which was the first such kit when it was launched in 1990. The second kit, 'The New

Emergency Health Kit 98' was revised and further harmonized by the WHO in collaboration with a large number of international and non-governmental agencies. The next version of the "Interagency Emergency Health Kit" is due in 2010. The updated third edition provides background information on the composition and use of the emergency health kit. It takes into account the global HIV/AIDS epidemic, the increasing parasite resistance to commonly available anti-malarials and the field experience of agencies using the emergency health kit. IEHK 2006 consists of two different sets of medicines and medical devices, named a *basic unit* and a *supplementary unit*. The basic unit contains essential medicines and medical devices to be used by primary health care workers with limited training. It contains oral and topical medicines, none of which is injectable. The supplementary unit contains medicines and medical devices to be used only by professional health workers or physicians. It is noteworthy that no kit can completely meet the requirements because an ideal kit can only be designed with an exact knowledge of the population characteristics, disease prevalence, morbidity patterns and level of training of those using the kit. However, the concept of emergency health kit is being accepted and adopted by many countries so as to cope with the disastrous situations.

Challenges for Essential Medicines Concept

Despite many great developments and achievements in the field, still some pending major obstacles are unfair financing, high prices, unreliable systems for procurement, poor quality and the irrational use of medicines. Thus, to successfully implement the concept of essential medicines following actions should be taken on the priority basis: fair financing, affordable prices, reliable systems for procurement and distribution, effective regulation of quality and rational use of medicine.

Essential Medicine List of India

The National list of essential medicines (NLEM) is the EML of India and made in the objective of WHO i.e., by considering the 3 important aspects i.e., cost, safety and efficacy and also promote prescription by generic names. The list prepared under the Ministry of Health & Family Welfare (MOHFW), Government of India who is responsible to ensure the quality healthcare system by promoting rational use of medicines in India. The first EML was prepared and released in 1996. Further, list was revised in 2003 with 74 bulk drugs and next in 2010 and the list released in 2011. In 2013, MOHFW have direction from the Supreme Court and other alliance to revise 2011 NLEM in the ordnance of new pharmaceutical pricing policy (NPPP). The NLEM is one of the key instruments in Indian healthcare delivery system includes accessible, affordable quality medicine at all the primary, secondary and tertiary levels of healthcare.

Conclusion

Model List of Essential Medicines is a process, model product and public health tool as a limited range of carefully selected medicines which cater for most health care needs especially in developing countries. WHO EML acts as a guideline as well as an outline to select proper advantageous medicine for the targeted population. Sometime, the Essential Medicines Library of WHO serves as an informative database for all member states, international organisations, drugs and therapeutic committees and health insurance organisations. However, despite some promising developments, much work remains to be done to ensure the successful implementation of the concept in different countries, since developing countries still need a good EML for their population.

Suggested Readings

1. Alvarez-Uria G, Thomas D, Zachariah S, Byram R, Kannan S (2014). Cost-analysis of the WHO Essential Medicines List in A Resource-Limited Setting: Experience from A District Hospital in India. *J Clin Diagn Res.* **8(5):** HM01-3.

2. D'arcy PF (1984). Essential medicines in the Third World. *BMJ.* **13:** 289-289.

3. Executive Board WHO. Revised procedures for updating the WHO model list of essential drugs: a summary of proposals and processes. EB108/INF.DOC./2. Geneva: World Health Organization, 2001.

4. Hogerzeil HV (2004). The concept of essential medicines: lessons for rich countries. *BMJ.* **329:**1169-1172.

5. Kindermans JM, Matthys F (2001). Introductory note: The access to Essential Medicines Campaign. *Trop Med Int Health.* **6(11):** 955-956.

6. Laing R, Waning B, Gray A, Ford N, Hoen E (2003). 25 years of the WHO essential medicines lists: progress and Challenges. *Lancet.* **361:** 1723-1729.

7. Laing RO, Hogerzeil HV, Ross-Degnan D (2001). Ten recommendations to improve use of medicines in developing countries. *Health Policy Plann.* **16:** 13-20.

8. Maritoux J, Pinel J. eds. *Essential drugs: practical guidelines intended for physicians, pharmacists, nurses and medical auxillaries.* 3rd edn. Paris: Médecins Sans Frontières, 2002.

9. Martin G, Sorenson C, Faunce T (2007). Balancing intellectual monopoly privileges and the need for essential medicines. *Globalization and Health.* **3:** 4-4.

10. Masuma M, Walker G (2000). Essential drugs in the developing world. *Health Policy and Planning.* **1(3):** 187-201.

11. Reidenberg MM, Walley T (2004). The pros and cons of essential medicines for rich countries. *BMJ.* **329:** 1172-1172.

12. Reidenberg MM (2009). Can the Selection and Use of Essential Medicines Decrease Inappropriate Drug Use? *Clin Pharm & Ther*. **85:** 581-583.

13. Rojo P (2001). Access to essential drugs in developing countries. *Gac Sanit*. **15(6):** 540-545.

14. Sell S (2002). TRIPS and the Access to Medicines Campaign. *Wiscon Internat Law Jour*. **20:**510-510.

15. Smith MK, Tickell S (2003). The essential drugs concept is needed now more than ever. *Trans R Soc Trop Med Hyg*. **97(1):**2-5.

16. Thomas C (2002). Trade Policy and the Politics of Access to Drugs. *Third World Quarterly*. **23:** 251–264.

17. Velasquez G, Boulet P (1999). Globalization and access to drugs: perspectives on the WTO/TRIPS agreement. 2nd ed. Geneva: World Health Organization.

18. WHO. Report of the 17th expert committee on the selection and use of essential medicines. (Tech Rep Ser WHO, 12 February 2010). Geneva: World Health Organization, 2009.

19. WHO. The Interagency Emergency Health Kit 2006. Medicines and medical devices for 10,000 people for approximately 3 months. An interagency document. Geneva: World Health Organization, 2006.

20. WHO. The selection of essential drugs: report of a WHO expert committee. (Tech Rep Ser WHO no 615). Geneva: World Health Organization, 1977.

CHAPTER 2

MEDICATION ERRORS

Introduction

Logically speaking, drug therapy is necessary and important aspect of disease management. But, concurrent complexity of both medication use and the medication management process gives rise to most common, frequently serious problem that is called as *medication errors*. Medication errors can occur at any stage (such as selecting, ordering, transcribing, verifying, dispensing, administering, consumption and monitoring of medication) of medication use process. It is a global public health problem placing considerable economic burden on society and already stretched health care system. Therefore, drug regulatory authorities, the insurance industries, pharmaceutical companies, healthcare professionals doing hard to reduce medication errors and to improve patient safety.

History of Medication Errors

Medication errors is a matter of wide concern and recently it has been received a great attention than any other time. These medication process related problem have a long history. About 40 years ago, in one study Barker and McConnell demonstrated that medication errors are a much bigger problem as demonstrated by comparing the effectiveness of incident reports and voluntary reports to direct observation of nurses as error detection methods. Based on the results of two weeks collected by direct observation method, they extrapolated these results over the same one-year period and indicated that 51,200 errors may have occurred (including 600 wrong time errors) and this figure is 1,422 times the number identified by incident reports. In 1960s, when the unit dose drug distribution system was being developed, researchers were used the medication administration errors for studying the quality of the output of drug distribution systems.

The National Coordinating Council for Medication Error and Prevention (NCC MERP) defines a medication error as *"any preventable event that may cause or lead to inappropriate medication use or patient harm, while the medication is in the control of the healthcare professional, patient, or consumer."* Such events may be related to professional practice, health care products, procedures, and systems, including prescribing; order communication; product labeling, packaging, and nomenclature; compounding; dispensing; distribution; administration; education; monitoring; and use (NCC MERP, 1995). A near miss is a type medication error caught before administering medication and causing any harm to patient.

It is important to distinguish medication errors from adverse drug events. Medication errors are failures in the process of medication use and they have the potential to harm the patient. Adverse drug events, in contrast, related to actual harm caused by medication, rather than solely by the patient's underlying disease state. Medication errors may or may not result in adverse drug event.

Pharmacoepidemiology

A medication error is one of the most common and frequent source of medical misadventures that result in significant morbidity and mortality worldwide. It is difficult to predict the exact incidence of medication errors, but they may occur as frequently as one in every 20 medication orders and 5 per 100 medication administrations. Among these, only 7 in 100 have potential to cause patient injury and only one in 100 actually results in injury. Particularly, in hospital settings, the number on ADEs has been reported to vary from one error per patient per day to about 6.5 events per 100 non-obstetric admissions. Exact incidence rate of medication errors is difficult to access because of following reasons: (1) only small number of errors are detected and even, small numbers of errors are reported, (2) inconsistencies in the way that medication errors are reported and measured, (3) mostly medication errors are reported in the inpatient hospital settings rather than in nursing homes, outpatient and home healthcare settings, and (4) most studies reported errors of commission not the errors of omission, which is also recommended.

Prescription Errors

In general practice, prescription errors account for a significant proportion of overall error. In New Zealand, repeat prescribing occurs commonly and also considered as an important cause of error in practice. In a prospective chart review of 36200 prescription items by wards visiting pharmacist for 4 weeks, around 1.5% prescribing errors were identified. Out of these, 0.4% was serious medication errors. In same type of study, pharmacist reviewed 3540 prescription items and reported around 9.9% prescribing errors. In a prospective chart review of 37821 prescriptions at 23 general practitioners sites and 3 community pharmacies, around 7.46% prescribing errors were reported. Of these, 10.2% and 7.9% prescribing errors were reported for handwritten and computer generated prescriptions respectively.

Dispensing Errors

In case of dispensing errors, there are several studies that examine and report such type errors. It may be due to their low rates of incidence and thereby less concern. In one study, from 1991 to 2001, about 7158 error reports were received from pharmacy departments of 89 hospitals. The prescriptions being dispersed were 34% for inpatient medicines, 28% for discharged medicines, 20% for outpatient medicines and 14% for other uses. The errors were usually detected by nurses (45%), hospital pharmacists (17%), patients (17%) and other hospital staff (21%). As per study results, most common error was due to supply the wrong medicine (23%) and wrong strength of prescribed medicine (23%). The most common causative factor for such error was look alike and sound alike medicines (33%). In a prospective study, pharmacists recorded all type of dispensing errors for 4 weeks in 35 community pharmacies. They reported around 40 errors per 100,000 dispensed items and wrong product selection was the most common error. In United Kingdom, the incidence of dispensing errors is reported as 1% and of that 0.18% are serious errors.

Administration Errors

Administration of medication is the most important and crucial step in the medication use process. A system analysis of ADEs among a sample of hospitalized patients reported that most of the events occurred during ordering (39%) and administration (38%) stages. With consideration of all types of errors, a hospital patient can expect on an average to be subjected to more than one medication error each day. Various studies examined the drug administration errors in hospital settings. They reported the rate of drug preparation and administration errors between 2.5% to 49%. They are most frequent and dangerous, especially when intravenous administration of doses. An analysis of data from the Unites States Pharmacopeia's MEDMARX® program, Hicks and colleagues identified 816 harmful outcomes involving 242 medications over 5-year period in children. During the 5-year period, MEDMARX® received 19,350 pediatric medication errors records, which represented about 3.3% of all records i.e., 580,761. The most commonly reported product associated with harmful pediatric error was morphine sulphate for 5-year. A study investigated the drug treatment of an elderly community in Denmark. This study reported that many patients were administered different drugs (22%), different doses (71%) and using different doses (66%) which were not prescribed in their general practitioners records. The overall rate of medication errors may vary across the various systems (such as inpatient hospital settings, nursing home, and home healthcare settings), types of population (such as elderly and pediatric population) and stages of medication use process. However, the overall incidence rates of prescribing, transcribing and dispensing and administering errors are 39%, 12%, 11% and 38% respectively.

Pharmacoeconomics

Medication error is a concerning threat within the healthcare and medical system. They are undoubtedly harmful and costly to patients and their families, hospitals, healthcare providers and insurance companies. They are most common and frequent drug related problem claiming about 44,000 to 98,000 lives each year in US alone, which is far more than that due to AIDS. It is state that medication errors cause around 7,000 deaths per year. One study found that it cost between $17billion and $29 billion per year in hospitals nationwide. In a report of Institute of the UK Department of Health which estimated that 850,000 ADEs occur annually in hospitals, costing an estimated £2 billion in hospital costs.

The Institute of Medicine (IOM) report also estimated that more than 70,000 lives are lost per year as a result of medication errors, more than the number of Americans injured in the work place each year. In a study conducted by Greene, it is reported that patients have 1 in 200 chance of dying from medical errors occurring during their hospital stay. In addition to these, 2% of patients admitted to the hospital may undergo a preventable ADEs, resulting in an average increase in hospital costs of roughly $4700 per admission. In a study, Phillips and colleagues reported a 2.57 fold increase in medication related deaths from 1983 to 1993.

Several studies estimated the cost of medication errors to patients and healthcare system, but unfortunately these studies not considered the lost earnings such as any compensation for pain and sufferings.

Causes of Medication Errors

As the medication use is a multistep process involving number of individuals, multiple factors are responsible to occur medication errors. However, medication errors mainly occur due to lack of knowledge and or performance deficit. The common causes for errors are as follows:

1. Verbal and/or written miscommunication (due to illegible handwriting, use of abbreviations and non-metric units of measurement)
2. Misinterpretation of the prescription
3. Drug name confusion (look-alike or sound-alike names, use of lettered or numbered prefixes and suffixes in drug names)
4. Improper labeling (Confusing or misleading labels with improper drug name, drug strength, and directions)
5. Lack of knowledge about drug and/or patient
6. Performance deficit
7. Miscalculation of drug dosage
8. Drug preparation error
9. Over workload

10.   Improper transcription
11.   Untrained personnel
12.   Poor lighting
13.   Frequent disturbances and distractions due to noisy work setting
14.   Lack of sufficient staff
15.   Violation of policies and procedures
16.   Lack of availability of health care professionals

Types of Medication Errors

In inpatient hospital setting, there are possible chances of medication errors at every step of the medication use process. Medication errors are broadly classified into 3 groups;

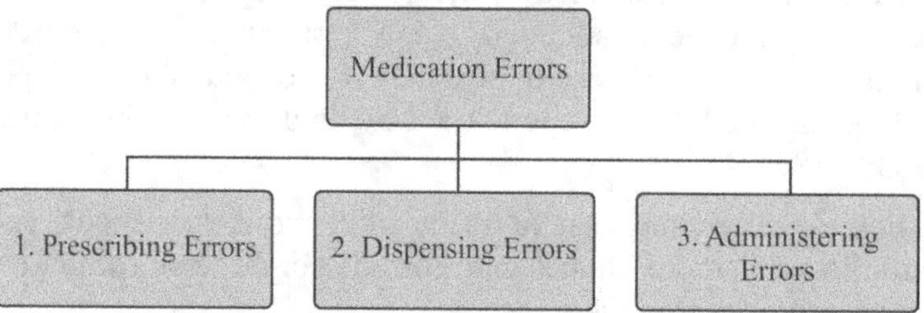

However, errors may occur during procurement, prescribing, transcribing, verifying, dispensing, administering and monitoring of medications.

1. Prescription Errors

Dean and colleagues studied the incidence and clinical significance of prescribing errors in hospital inpatients. Using *Delphi technique*, they defined as, "a clinically meaningful prescribing error occurs when, as a result of a prescribing decision or prescription writing process, there is an unintentional significant reduction in the probability of the treatment being timely and effective or and increased risk of harm when compared to generally accepted practice".

Prescribing errors occurs when

1.   Physician writes a prescription without considering

   Patient's clinical status,

   Age and body weight,

   Comorbid conditions,

   Knowledge of its allergy status and

   Its ability to administer medications properly

   Drug-drug interaction potential

2. Continuing a prescription for longer duration than necessary

3. Writing an ambiguous medication order

4. Continuing a drug in the event of a clinically significant ADR

5. Writing a drug's name using abbreviations or other non-standard nomenclature

6. Not writing a prescription in full if a change has been made to it

7. Overuse of drug without therapeutic benefit

8. Failure to follow system's policies and drug-specific instructions

2. Dispensing Errors

Only few studies examined and studied dispensing errors that might be due to their low incidence rates (10-12%) and less concern. Although, there are few studies, dispensing do occurs and therefore they require further research. Generally, dispensing also includes transcribing and verifying the medication in which mostly nurses and pharmacists are involved. Most of the studies reported that dispensing errors occur due to (1) supply of the wrong medicine, (2) the wrong strength of the prescribed medicine, (3) the wrong directions for use, (4) the wrong quantity of medicine, and (5) wrong calculation of drug dosage.

3. Administration Errors

It is an error having highest incidence rate (about 38%) after prescribing errors. In the analysis of incidence of both actual and potential ADEs, Bates *et al.,* 1995b reported that 26% of preventable ADEs are occurred during the administration stage. This stage of medication use process is very crucial and with high risk. In hospital inpatient setting, nurses are responsible for administration of medicines while in institutions, physicians, dentists, pharmacists, podiatrists, respiratory therapist, radiologist and patients administers medications. In the ambulatory setting, the patients or family members or relatives or caregivers are responsible for medicines administration. The causative factors are similar to that responsible for prescribing and dispensing errors. Administration errors may also includes omission of dose in addition to wrong drug administration at wrong dose, to by wrong route to wrong patient at wrong time. The reasons may be lack of information about patient and drug. The risk of administration error is increased particularly when it is associated with intravenous dosage administration. Sometimes they may occur due to technical problems while administering drug using nebulizer, infusion pump, and metered dose inhalers.

Apart from the above three main types of errors, they may also occur due to patients noncompliance. Patient may omit the dose of drug, may take wrong drug at higher or lower doses. Therefore, patient compliance is also important for safe medication use process.

Detecting and Reporting Medication Errors

Detection and reporting of medication errors is the most important component of their prevention strategies. The study was conducted to assess the ability of pharmacovigilance centers to detect medication errors and to proceed to building patient safety via their information networks and to underline the limits for this challenge. This study results demonstrated that pharmacovigilance centers were able to detect and analyze the medication errors.

There are various methods available for detection and reporting of medication errors depending on the types of systems.

1. Voluntary reporting
2. Direct observation of patient care
3. Chart review
4. Incident reports involving medication errors
5. Attending medical rounds to listen for clues that an error has occurred
6. Doses returned to pharmacy
7. Urine testing as evidence of omitted drugs and unauthorized drug administration
8. Examination of death certificates
9. Attend nurse change of shift report
10. Medication administration record comparison to physician orders
11. Computerized analysis to identify patients receiving target or tracer drugs that may be used to treat a medication error
12. Comparison of drugs removed from an automated drug dispensing device for a patient to physician orders

However, errors are mainly detected by following methods

1. Voluntary Reporting

Person who detects error may voluntarily report it. A healthcare facility that encourages voluntary reporting of all medication errors and provides information that can be used to formulate prevention strategies to prevent future errors. An anonymous reporting program may promote better reporting of errors related to medication use.

2. Direct Observation (Med Pass Observation) Method

Observing directly or video taping of actual patient care in operating rooms, surgical wards, intensive care unit and during medication administration by separate individual may be better way to detect medication errors. This method detects more errors than previous one. But, it has certain methodological and practical demerits. Supervisor or employer may use the data to punish his employees. Confidentiality is another problem related to this method. Direct observation requires time-intensive training of observers to ensure the reliability. This method is also not perfect to detect all types of errors (e.g., errors occurred during purchasing of instrument, errors due to over workload and lack of adequate staffing).

3. Pharmacy Procedures

There are some pharmacy procedures that help to identify and detect the certain errors. These includes attending medical rounds to listen for clues that an error has occurred, doses returned to pharmacy, urine testing as evidence of omitted drugs and unauthorized drug administration, and medication administration record comparison to physician orders.

However, only small percentages of errors are detected and an even small number are reported for many reasons. These includes (1) embarrassment or fear of punishment from colleagues, employer, regulatory agencies, or patients and their families, (2) culture of blaming and litigation among the professionals of healthcare system.

It is well understood that not only individuals, but system failures are also responsible for commission of medication errors. Therefore, there should be a true culture of patient safety and everyone should learn from the mistakes that already happen to avoid future errors and to make the medication process as safe as possible.

There are various organization engaged in tracking the medication errors at national and international level.

1. **The Food and Drug Administration (FDA)**

   Accepts reports from consumers and health care professionals about products regulated by FDA, including drugs and medical devices through MedWatch; the FDA's safety information and adverse event reporting program.

2. **Institute of Safe Medication Practice (ISMP)**

   Accepts reports from healthcare professionals and consumers related to medication and publishes "Safe Medicine" a consumer newsletter on medication errors.

3. **United States Pharmacopeia (USP)**

   MEDMARX® is an anonymous medication errors reporting program used by hospitals. Through this program, USP encourages healthcare professionals to report problems related to medication and collects the reports. Once collected, the reports are shared with the FDA, regulators, product manufacturers and healthcare providers to improve the safety of medication use process.

4. **National Coordinating Council for Medication Error Reporting and Prevention (NCC MERP)**

    The council was founded in 1995 and it contains representation of leading health care and consumer organizations of 16 nations. This council

    1. Examines and evaluates the causes of medication errors;

    2. Increase awareness of medication errors and methods of prevention throughout the healthcare system; and

    3. Recommend strategies relative to system modifications, practice standards, and guidelines.

Measurement of Medication Errors

Over 25 years, various studies measured the medication administration errors and suggested that the incidence of error had been one per patient per day. The NCC MERP index categorizes the medication errors as per severity of patient outcome. The council also categorizes the 'near misses' as potential errors for which a system wide approach is needed for prevention. Some health care and consumer organizations classify errors from NCC MERP risk levels A and B as near misses for categorizing medication errors. Figure 1 shows the NCC MERP index for categorizing medication errors.

Analysis of Medication Errors

Although, there are several methods to analyze medication errors, root cause analysis (RCA) and failure mode and effects analysis (FMEA) are the most commonly used methods.

1. Root Cause Analysis (RCA)

It is a systematic process of investigating a critical incident or an adverse outcome to determine the multiple, underlying contributing factors. The analysis focuses on identifying the latent conditions that underlie variation in performance and, if applicable, developing recommendations for improvements to decrease the likelihood of a similar incident in the future. Root cause analysis is intended to determine three things: *"what happened, why it happened and what can be done to reduce the likelihood of a recurrence"*. It is a technique most commonly used after an incident has occurred in order to identify underlying causes. The process involves data collection, cause charting, root cause identification and recommendation generation and implementation. It needs to involve the "right people" such as leadership representatives, individuals closely involved in process and system under review, consultants/experts (e.g., purchasing), and interdisciplinary individuals. It also needs continue search of root cause, consideration of relevant literature, and time. Before conducting a RCA develop an action plan, define the team (small groups and individuals for consultation, define the problem exactly, study the problem, determine what exactly happened. Moreover, identify proximate and underlying causes, confirm the causes through consultation, explore and identify risk reduction strategies, formulate recommendations/actions, and consider human factors and failure mode and effects analysis (FMEA) before changes.

2. Failure Mode and Effects Analysis

FMEA provides a way to examine the use of new products and the design of new services and processes, so that points of potential failure and their effects can be determined before any error actually occurs. FMEA differs from root cause analysis (RCA). Root cause analysis is a reactive process that is used after an error occurs in order to identify the error's underlying causes. In contrast to this method, FMEA is a proactive process that is used to examine vulnerable areas or practices more carefully and systematically. Moreover, its structured approach makes it easy to use and even for non-specialist a powerful quality method.

Prevention of Medication Errors

Medication use is multistep process that includes selecting, ordering, transcribing, verifying, dispensing, administering, consumption and monitoring of medication. The chances of errors are present at every step and systems; therefore the prevention strategies should cover the whole process and various systems. An understanding of the reasons of preventable adverse drug events may help to formulate the effective countermeasures to the events or their effects. The medication error prevention strategies includes

(i) Strategies focusing on various stages of medication use process

(ii) Strategies focusing on various health care systems

In addition to prevention strategies we should allow and encourage the patients to take more and more active role in their own medical care. Patients should be well aware about their medications, purpose of medications, expected outcome and probable ADRs from medications. For these, a strong partnership between the patients and the healthcare professional is needed.

A. Strategies Focusing on Various Stages of Medication use Process

1. Prevention of errors during ordering/prescribing medications

As the high proportion of injuries occurs at this stage of medication use, most effective and preventive strategies are warranted. Most of the times, orders and prescription are transmitted orally or in written orders. Although, information technology automated the prescribing process, manual methods are still in use in many hospitals. Therefore, to avoid medication errors associated with verbal orders and written prescriptions, NCC MERP provided elements that should be included in a verbal order (Table 2.1) and recommendations to enhance accuracy of prescription writing (NCC MERP, 1995).

Table 2.1 Elements that should be included in a verbal order

Name, age and weight of patient
Drug name and dosage form (e.g., tablets, capsules, inhalants)
Exact strength or concentration
Dose, frequency, and route
Quantity and/or duration
Purpose or indication (unless disclosure is considered inappropriate by the prescriber)
Specific instructions for use
Name of prescriber, and telephone number when appropriate
Name of individual transmitting the order, if different from the prescriber

Source: From NCC MERP recommendations to enhance accuracy of prescription writing. Elements that should be included in a verbal order. Revised February 24, 2006. Available at www.nccmerp.org, accessed April 6, 2007.

1. All prescription documents should be legible. Verbal orders should be minimized.

2. Prescription orders must include a brief notation of purpose (e.g., for cough), for an extra safety check in the process of prescribing and dispensing a medication.

3. All prescription orders should be written in the metric system except for therapies that use standard units such as insulin, vitamins, etc. Units should be spelled out rather than writing "U."

4. Prescribers must include age and, when appropriate, weight of the patient on the medication order which can help dispensing health care professionals in their double check of the appropriate drug and dose.

5. Medication orders should be complete with drug name, exact metric weight or concentration, and dosage form. Strength should be expressed in metric amounts and concentration should be specified. The pharmacist should check with the prescriber if any, information is missing or questionable.

6. A leading zero should always precede a decimal expression of less than one and a terminal or trailing zero should never be used after a decimal to avoid ten-fold errors in drug strength and dosage.

7. Prescriber should avoid the use of abbreviations including those for drug names (e.g., MOM, HCTZ) and Latin directions for use.

8. Prescriber should avoid vague instructions such as "Take as directed" or "Take/Use as needed" as the sole direction for use. Specific directions to the patient are useful to help reinforce proper medication use, particularly if therapy is to be interrupted for a time. Clear directions are a necessity for the dispenser to: (1) check the proper dose for the patient; and, (2) enable effective patient counseling.

The NCC MERP council provides list of error prone abbreviations, their intended meaning and misinterpretation (Table 2.2).

Table 2.2 Dangerous abbreviations

Abbreviation	Intended meaning	Common error
U	Units	Mistaken as a zero or a four (4) resulting in overdose. Also mistaken for "cc" (cubic centimeters) when poorly written.
μg	Micrograms	Mistaken for "mg" (milligrams) resulting in an overdose.
Q.D.	Latin abbreviation for every day	The period after the "Q" has sometimes been mistaken for an " I", and the drug has been given "QID" (four times daily) rather than daily.
Q.O.D.	Latin abbreviation for every other day	Misinterpreted as "QD" (daily) or "QID" (four times daily). If the "O" is poorly written, it looks like a period or "I".
SC or SQ	Subcutaneous	Mistaken as "SL" (sublingual) when poorly written.
T I W	Three times a week	Misinterpreted as "three times a day" or "twice a week".
D/C	Discharge; also discontinue	Patient's medications have been prematurely discontinued when D/C, (intended to mean "discharge") was misinterpreted as "discontinue", because it was followed by a list of drugs.
HS	Half strength	Misinterpreted as the Latin abbreviation "HS" (hour of sleep).
cc	Cubic centimeters	Mistaken as "U" (units) when poorly written.
AU, AS, AD	Latin abbreviation for both ears; left ear; right ear	Misinterpreted as the Latin abbreviation "OU" (both eyes); "OS" (left eye); "OD" (right eye)
IU	International Unit	Mistaken as IV (intravenous) or 10 (ten)
MS, MSO$_4$, MgSO$_4$	Confused for one another	Can mean morphine sulfate or magnesium sulphate

Source: From NCC MERP recommendations to enhance accuracy of prescription writing.

Dangerous abbreviations. Revised February 24, 2006. Available at www.nccmerp.org, accessed April 6, 2007.

2. **Prevention of errors during dispensing medications**

At this stage several successful developments has been occurred such as dispensing of medications in a single unit or a unit dose in a ready to administer format. It is most common, useful and time saving strategy to eradicate errors during dispensing of medications. As per the strategy, no more than 24 hours of medications are dispensed at once to patients.

Another strategy having promising role in prevention of medical misadventures is pharmacy control systems. NCC MERP council provides recommendations to enhance accuracy of dispensing medications (NCC MERP, 1995).

1. Prescriptions/orders always be reviewed by a pharmacist prior to dispensing. Any orders that are incomplete, illegible, or of any other concern should be clarified using an established process for resolving questions.

2. Patient profiles be current and contain adequate information that allows the pharmacist to assess the appropriateness of a prescription/order.

3. The dispensing area should be properly designed to prevent errors. Design should address fatigue-reducing environmental conditions (e.g., adequate lighting, air conditioning, noise level abatement, ergonomic fixtures); minimize distractions (e.g., telephone and personnel interruptions, clutter, unrelated tasks); and provide sufficient staffing and other resources for workload.

4. Product inventory be arranged to help differentiate medications from one another. This may include the use of visual discriminators such as signs or markers. This is particularly important when confusion exists between or among strengths, similar looking labels, and names that sound or appear similar.

5. Whenever possible, an independent check by a second individual should be used to assess the accuracy of the dispensing process prior to the medication being provided to the patient. Other methods of checking include the use of automation (e.g., bar coding systems), computer systems, and patient profiles.

6. Labels should be read at least three times (e.g., when selecting the product, when packaging the product, and when returning the product to the shelf).

7. Pharmacy staff should triple check replenishment of regular medication stock or automated dispensing machines/cabinets (e.g., Pyxis, etc.) to ensure accuracy of product and precision of placement (e.g., when selecting the product, before the product leaves the pharmacy, and prior to placing the product in the automated dispensing machine/cabinet).

8. Pharmacists should counsel patients at the time of dispensing to verify the accuracy of dispensing and the patient's understanding of proper medication use. Counseling should include indications, precautions, warnings, expected outcome, potential adverse reactions and interactions with food or other medications, actions to take when adverse reactions or interactions occur, and storage requirements of medication.

9. Pharmacies should collect and analyze data regarding actual and potential errors for the purpose of continuous quality improvement (e.g., provide feedback to local prescribers, provide error information to national reporting programs/databases).

10. Both initial and ongoing training of pharmacy staff on accepted standards of practice related to accurate dispensing processes with the ultimate goal of medication error reduction are needed.

11. Each pharmacy should establish policies and procedures for the medication dispensing process to ensure that all personnel, including pharmacists, support staff, and relief staff, are informed of expectations related to the dispensing process.

3. **Prevention of errors during administering medications**

In hospitals, institutions and ambulatory settings, different health care providers are responsible for administration of medications, therefore prevention program should be designed to cover all healthcare professionals. In all health care system, medication administering individual must be aware about indications, precautions, warnings, expected outcomes, potential adverse reactions and interactions with food or other medications, actions to take when adverse reactions or interactions occur, and storage requirements of medication. The NCC MERP council provides following recommendations to enhance accuracy of administration of medications (NCC MERP, 1995).

1. Any order that is incomplete, illegible, or of any other concern should be clarified prior to administration using an established process for resolving questions.

2. The following checks should be performed immediately prior to the medication administration: the right medication, in the right dose, to the right person, by the right route using the right dosage form, at the right time, with the right documentation.

3. Organizations/companies should provide employees with adequate training regarding medication administration devices and routinely monitor or verify that users of such devices demonstrate competency regarding the device, its operation, and its limitations.

4. When electronic infusion control devices are employed, only those that prevent free-flow upon removal of the administration set should be used.

5. The use of integrated automated systems (e.g., direct order entry, computerized medication administration record, bar coding) to facilitate review of prescriptions, increase the accuracy of administration, and reduce transcription errors.

6. All persons who administer medications should have adequate and/or appropriate access to patient information, as close to the point of use as possible, including medical history, known allergies, diagnoses, list of current medications, and treatment plan, to assess the appropriateness of administering the medication.

7. All persons who administer medications should have easily accessible product information as close to the point of use as possible, and are knowledgeable about indications, precautions, warnings, expected outcome, potential adverse reactions and interactions with food or other medications, actions to take when adverse reactions or interactions occur, and storage requirements of medication.

8. Healthcare professionals administer only medications that are properly labeled and that during the administration process, labels be read three times: when reaching for or preparing the medication, immediately prior to administering the medication, and when discarding the container or replacing it into its storage location.

9. At the time of administration, the name, purpose and effects of the medication be discussed with the patient and/or caregiver, especially upon first time administration and reviewed upon subsequent administrations.

10. Ongoing patient monitoring for therapeutic and/or adverse medication effects.

11. To assess safety of the drug administration process, factors such as lighting, temperature control, noise-level, occurrence of distractions (e.g., telephone and personal interruptions, performance of unrelated tasks, etc.) should be examined. Sufficient staffing and other resources must be provided for the given workload. The science of ergonomics should be employed in the design of safe systems.

12. Data should be collected and analyzed regarding the actual and potential errors of administration for the purpose of continuous quality improvement.

13. Both initial and ongoing training of staff, including licensed staff, support staff or non-licensed staff, and relief staff on accepted standards of practice related to accurate medication administration with the ultimate goal of medication error reduction.

14. Every organization should establish policies and procedures for the medication administration process. This will ensure that all personnel, including licensed staff, support staff or non-licensed staff, and relief staff are informed of expectations related to the medication administration process.

B. Strategies Focusing on Various Healthcare Systems to Prevent Medication Errors

It is demonstrated that the majority of medication errors reflect system failures, not individuals. Such as, lack of standard policies, staffing and work distribution, medication order tracking, communication network among various departments, device use, standardization of doses and frequencies, drug distribution system within unit, procedures for medication preparation, and transfer/transition problems. Any healthcare system comprised of healthcare professionals, patients, and various regulatory authorities, therefore it is everyone's responsibility to medication safety. With collaboration amongst healthcare providers including physicians, pharmacists, nurses, routine monitoring of medication use process can give positive outcomes in patient care. This approach is quite effective particularly at the transitions from one setting to another. Development of reporting system in a health care facility is another closely related strategy. The collected reports and information can be used to prevent future errors in any part of facility's medication process. The success of reporting system is mainly depends on the facility's culture. It is demonstrated that non-punitive and non-blaming culture encourages the active reporting of medication errors.

The understanding and preventing medication errors, a training program created by the United States Pharmacopeia (USP), uses a multidisciplinary, systems-based approach to help identify and prevent future errors. It includes lecture/slide materials, videotape, case studies, role-playing exercises, discussion topics, calculation quizzes, patient education guidance, supplemental resources, and a bibliography.

Role of Information Technologies in Prevention of Medication Errors

In recent years, there is increasing trend of using information technologies (Table 2.3) to prevent medication errors, which includes computerized or electronic medical record, computerized physician order entry, automated prospective drug utilization review systems, automated drug dispensing systems, bar coding, and clinical pharmacy information systems. These emerging technologies provide patient care with high accuracy, efficiency and promising advancement.

Table 2.3 Benefits and barriers to using information technology to improve medication administration

Information technology	Benefits Medication prescribing	Barriers
Computerized or electronic medical record	Provides patient information to guide drug selection and regimen Reduces errors related to order transcription Reduces errors related to use of abbreviations and name confusion	Not widely available or used Systems may be incompatible outside an organization or institution
Computerized provider order entry	Legible prescription Integrates drug formularies Provides clinical decision-making support with alerts and reminders as prescriber enters an order Requires verification of drugs that may be confused with similar sounding or potentially misspelled medications Double checks an order before it goes forward Assists with converting oral to IV doses	Patient data not up to date High cost of implementation Not widely available
Automated prospective drug utilization review systems	Gives alerts to ensure accurate prescription	Alerts can be overridden Too many alerts cause frustration False-positive alerts
Medication dispensing		
Automated dispensing devices	Holds medications at a specific location and allows dispensing only to a specific patient Helps assess the full range of medications a patient is receiving Assesses drug allergies Identifies inappropriate drug therapies, averting hospitalizations resulting from adverse drug events	Not linked with bar coding and electronic information systems No communication with the prescriber Doesn't fully assess potential interactions because of limited data

Table 2.3 Contd…

Information technology	Benefits	Barriers
Medication administration		
Physical packaging changes	Changes appearance of medications to avoid errors associated with similar looking or similarly spelled drugs Uses only one name and one look for each drug, or uses standardized labels	Cost of repackaging New packaging may not be in stock Is not mandated
Bar coding	Verifies medications and patients Automated record of medication administration to specific patients Used in dispensing and verification process Counters the misreading of drug names and dosages	Has not been widely used, but is now required by the U.S. Food and Drug Administration on most drugs Cost of scanners Can introduce human error by requiring manual loading of equipment and bar-code verification Limited number of portable scanners Complex bar-coding systems lead to errors Lack of universal bar codes Packaging changes needed for bar codes on unit doses Problematic for doses such as half a tablet Requires costly relabeling using a standard that needs to be defined

Source: Hughes R.G. and Ortiz E. 2005. Medication errors: why they happen, and how they can be prevented. *Am. J. Nurs*, supplement, 14-24.

1. Computerized or Electronic Medical Records or Smart Cards

It is just credit card like device containing all medical information about the patient. Due to its portability, patient can virtually carry his all upto date medical records at all times. Also, healthcare providers involved in treatment of patient can easily access this information whenever it is required. This card can be operated with almost any computer system. Updated medical records of patients in smart cards eliminate the use of multiple charts, dependency on memory and redundancy in treatment. However, standardization of data, privacy and confidentiality agreements, and its widespread compliance are the serious issues in using smart cards.

2. Computerized Physician Order Entry (CPOE)

It is simply entering medication orders online rather than on paper or verbally. These orders are instantly transmitted to nursing units and pharmacies. Computerized physician order entry integrated with clinical decision support systems (CDSS) provides computerized advice on drug doses, routes of administration and doses frequencies. This combined system can check drug allergy and drug-drug interaction as well as prompt for corollary orders (such as glucose levels after insulin have been ordered). Additionally, this system eliminates the need of transcription, thereby holds great promise in reducing errors. Despite these advantages, this system faces challenges due to their high cost, physician and organizational resistance and product/vendor immaturity.

3. Computerized Pharmacy Systems

This system is designed to alert the pharmacist to potential problems associated with prescription. Generally in absence of this technology, pharmacists manually review the medication orders. Whenever there is any discrepancy, in the prescription, this electronic system alerts the pharmacist. However, effectiveness of this system may get limited due to ignorance of alert by pharmacist.

4. Automated Dispensing Devices

This system ensures that medication is only dispensed to patients to whom it is prescribed. This system maintains a record of which drug, to whom and at what time is dispensed. Systems linked with inventory are able to reduce medication errors significantly. However, high cost this system is the challenge for majority of systems to adopt this system.

5. Bar Code-Enabled Point of Care Technology (BPOC)

This system ensures that the right drug is administered to the right patient at a right dose by right route at right time. The BPOC system combines bar code scanners (similar to that used in supermarkets) with sophisticated medication administration software. Other input devices that used by nurses are hand held computers, mobile laptops or bedside computers equipped with bar code scanner/reader.

When patient enter the hospital, they get a bar coded identification wristband that can transmits information to the hospital's computer. Bar codes are also printed on staff identification badges and medication packages. To administer a medication, nurses scan his or her name badge, patient's identification wristband

and the medication to be given. Then software checks the data of patient, medication and prescription. If there is a match, the medication is given and automatically documented on the electronic medication administration record. If there is any discrepancy, a warning box pops up on the screen and asks the nurse for more information or warns of an impending error.

This can prevent the most types of medication errors. It also assists to medication administering individual by providing instructions for reconstitution, dilution, administration and handling of medications. Major challenges in using BPOC systems are high cost, therefore limited use, lack of universal bar codes, and inability to confirm the right dose particularly when unit doses are not available.

Conclusions

The medication use process is complex and multistep process involving selecting, ordering, transcribing, verifying, dispensing, administering, consumption and monitoring of medications. Medication error potential is prevalent at each step. For medication errors not only healthcare professionals but failure of health care system in which they work is also responsible. These medication errors are most common and frequently harmful to patients, their caregivers, health care system and insurance companies. Therefore, this serious problem related to medications need to be addressed. However, due to adoption of new standards, policies and technologies across all areas of medication use process, very soon healthcare system will see improvements that will translate into enhanced patient care with safe use of medications.

Suggested Readings

1. Anderson D.J. and C.S. Webster (2001). A systems approach to the reduction of medication errors on the hospital ward. *J. Adv. Nurs.* **35:** 34-41.

2. Barat I., F. Andreasen and E.M. Damsgaard (2001). Drug therapy in elderly: what doctors believe and patients actually do. *Br. J. Clin. Pharmacol.* **51:** 615-622.

3. Barker K.N. and W.E. McConnell (1962). The problems of detecting medication errors in hospitals. *Am. J. Hosp. Pharm.* **19:** 360-369.

4. Bates D.W (1996). Medication errors: how common are they and what can be done to prevent them. *Drug Safety.* **15:** 303-310.

5. Bates D.W, N. Spell, D.J.Cullen, E. Burdick, N. Laird, L.A. Petersen, S.D. Small, B.J. Sweitzer and L.L. Leape (1997). The costs of adverse drug events in hospitalized patients. *JAMA.* **277:** 307-311.

6. Bates D.W., D.J. Cullen, N. Laird, L.A. Petersen, S.D. Small, D. Servi, G. Laffel, B.J. Sweitzer, B.F Shea and R. Hallisey (1995). Incidence of adverse drug events and potential adverse drug events: implications for prevention. ADE Prevention Study Group. *JAMA.* **274:** 29-34.

7.   Bates D.W, D.L. Boyle, M.B. Vander Vliet, J. Schneider and L. Leape (1995). Relationship between medication errors and adverse drug events. *J. Gen. Intern. Med.* **10:** 199-205.

8.   Becker S. (1999). Common causes for medication errors identified. *Int. J. Trauma Nurs.* **5:** 113-115.

9.   Benabdallah G, R Benkirane, A Khattabi, IR Edwards, RS Bencheikh (2011). The involvement of Pharmacovigilance Centres in medication errors detection: a questionnaire-based analysis. *Int J Risk Saf Med.* **23(1):** 17-29.

10.   Cohen M.R., N.M. Davis and J. Senders (1994). Failure mode and effects analysis: A novel approach to avoiding dangerous medication errors and accidents. *Hosp. Pharm.* **29:** 319-324.

11.   Cousins D (2005). Medication practice: what we know. Available at www.saferhealthcare.org.uk/IHI/topics/medicationpractice/whatweknow, accessed April 6, 2007.

12.   Dean B., M. Barbera and M. Schachter (2000). What is prescribing error? *Qual. Health Care.* **9:** 232-237.

13.   Dean B, M. Schachter, C. Vincent, and M Barber (2002). Prescribing errors in hospital inpatients: their incidence and clinical significance. *Qual. Saf. Health Care.* **11:** 340-344.

14.   Expert Group on Learning from Adverse Events in the NHS (EGLAE). An organization with a memory. London, UK: Stationery Office; 2000.

15.   Flynn E.A. and K.N. Barker (1999). Medication error research. *In:* Cohen, M.R., *ed., Medication Errors: Causes and Prevention.* Washington, DC: American Pharmaceutical Association.

16.   Greene J. (1999). From whodunit to what happened. *Hosp. Health Netw.* **73:** 50-54.

17.   Gurwitz J.H. and P. Rochon (2002). Improving the quality of medication use in elderly patients: A not-so-simple prescription. *Arch. Intern. Med.* **162:** 1670-1672.

18.   Hughes R.G. and Ortiz E (2005). Mediation errors: why they happen, and how they can be prevented. *Am. J. Nurs. supplement* 14-24.

19.   Joanna Briggs Institute (2005). Strategies to reduce medication errors with reference to older adults, *Best Practice.* **9:** 1-6.

20.   Kaynes S (1996). Negligence and the pharmacist: dispensing errors and prescribing errors. *Pharm. J.* **257:** 32-35.

21.   Kienle P.C (2004). Medication errors. *In:* Peterson, A.M., *ed., Managing pharmacy practice: principles, strategies and systems,* CRC Press, New York, pp. 261-278.

22. Kohn LT, Corrigan JM, Donaldson MS, ed. (1999). *To Err is Human: Building a Safer Health System.* Washington, DC: National Academy Press.

23. Kohn L.T, J.M. Corrigan and M.S. Donaldson (2000). To Err is Human: Building a Safer Health System. National Academy Press, Washington.

24. Leape L.L, D.W. Bates, D.J. Cullen, J. Cooper, H.J. Demonaco, T. Gallivan, R. Hallisey, J. Ives, N. Laird and G. Laffel (1995). Systems analysis of adverse drug events. ADE Prevention Study Group. *JAMA.* **274:** 35-43.

25. Lillis S, H. Lord (2011). Repeat prescribing - reducing errors. *J Prim Health Care.* **3(2):** 153-8.

26. Mahajan RP (2011). Medication errors: can we prevent them? *Br J Anaesth.* **107(1):** 3-5.

27. Merry AF and BJ Anderson (2011). Medication errors - new approaches to prevention. *Paediatr Anaesth.* **21(7):** 743-53.

28. National Coordinating Council for Medication Error Reporting and Prevention (NCC MERP), 1995. Available at www.nccmerp.org, accessed April 6, 2007.

29. NCC MERP. 1995. Recommendations to enhance accuracy of prescription writing. Revised June 2, 2005. Available at www.nccmerp.org, accessed April 6, 2007.

30. NCC MERP. 1995. Recommendations to enhance accuracy of dispensing medications. Revised June 2, 2005. Available at www.nccmerp.org, accessed April 6, 2007.

31. NCC MERP. 1995. Recommendations to enhance accuracy of administration of medications. Revised June 2, 2005. Available at www.nccmerp.org, accessed April 6, 2007.

32. Oren, E., E.R. Shaffer and B.J. Guglielmo (2003). Impact of emerging technologies on medication errors and adverse drug events. *Am. J. Health-Syst. Pharm.* **60:** 1447-1458.

33. Phillips, D.P., N. Christenfeld and L.M. Glynn. (1998). Increase in US medication error deaths between 1983 and 1993. *Lancet* **351:** 643-644.

34. Roberts, D.E., M.G. Spencer, R. Burfield and S. Bowden (2002). An analysis of dispensing errors in UK hospitals [abstract]. *Int. J. Pharm. Pract* **10** (Suppl): R6.

35. Rodney, W.H., S.C. Becker and D.D. Cousins (2006). Harmful Medication Errors in Children: A 5-Year Analysis of Data from the USP's MEDMARXR Program. *J. Pediatric Nurs.* **21:** 290-298.

36. Shah S.N., M. Aslam and A.J. Avery (2001). A survey of prescription errors in general practice. *Pharm. J.* **267:** 860-862.

37. Skiba, M (2006). Strategies for identifying and minimizing medication errors in health care settings. *The Health Care Manager.* **25:** 70-77.

38. Stokowski L.A (2001). Using technology to improve medication safety in the newborn intensive care unit. *Adv. Neonatal Care.* **2:** 70-83.

39. Stolarz S.A, N. Hartnell and N.J. MacKinnon (2005). Approaches to improving the safety of the medication use system. *Healthcare Quarterly.* **8:** 59-64.

40. Taxis K. and N. Barber (2003). Ethnographic study of incidence and severity of intravenous drug errors. *BMJ.* **326:** 684.

41. Thomas E.J. and L.A. Petersen (2003). Measuring errors and adverse events in healthcare. *J. Gen. Intern. Med* **18:** 61-67.

42. Van den Bemt P.M, M.J. Postma, E.N. Van Roon, M.C. Chow, R. Fijn and J.R. Brouwers (2002). Cost-benefit analysis of the detection of prescribing error by hospital pharmacy staff. *Drug Saf.* **25:** 135-143.

43. Wichman K. and J. Greenall (2006). Using root cause analysis to determine the system-based causes of error. *CPJ/RPC.* **139:** 63-65.

44. Yang M, M.M. Brown, B. Trohimovich, M. Dana and J. Kelly (2005). The effect of barcode-enabled point of care technology on medication administration errors. Available at: *http://www.mederrors.com/* resource_main set.html. Accessed April 6, 2007.

CHAPTER 3

CHRONOPHARMACOLOGY: DIURNAL VARIATION OF DRUG ACTION

Introduction

To regulate the homeostasis within the body, certain reversible periodic changes occur at the cellular, organ and system level and analysis of these frequently occurring temporal changes is called chronobiology. This analysis involves collection of observations and measurement of physiologic reproducible changes existing at different intervals also referred to as rhythmatic phenomenon within the biological system. These rhythmic changes are mainly due to external environmental factors or cues, in addition to these, living organisms also possess internal biological clock which contributes to maintain the rhythmicity in biological system. When the rhythmatic changes are exactly for a day and get affected by both external cues and internal biological system is called diurnal (varying with time of day) rhythm, but when observed for approximately a day and independent of external factors is called circadian rhythm. If the organism is placed in an environment devoid of time cues, for constant light or constant darkness, diurnal rhythms may persist. So, diurnal variations can be either light-or clock-driven. Cues often referred to as synchronizers, zeitgebers, and entraining factors that are responsible for alteration of light-dark, heat-cold, noise-silence, and electromagnetic field. Oscillator is an internal pacemaker coupled to variety of physiological processes and unaffected by temperature.

Table 3.1 Various terms related to rhythms with their duration

Rhythms	Duration
Ultradian	12 hours
Circadian	24 hours
Circatrigintan	30 days
Circannual	1 year

Circadian Clocks

Cells have internal oscillators that operate independently of light stimulus (free-running). Circadian clock consists of 3 components: inputs, oscillator, and outputs (Fig. 3.1).

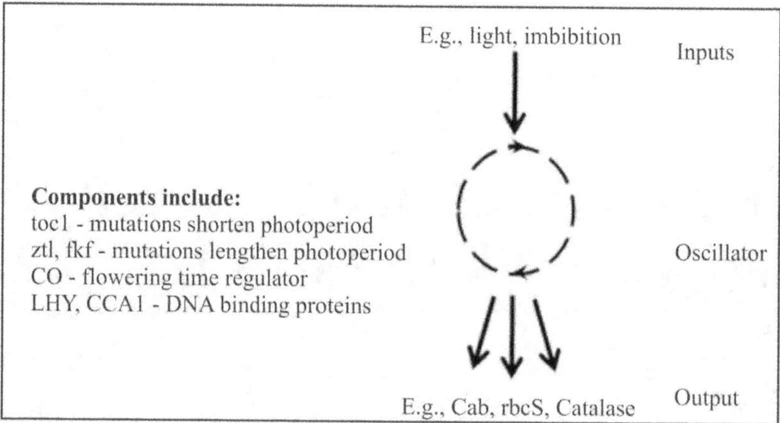

Fig. 3.1 Circadian clock. Oscillator must be entrained by input. A complete mechanistic model for the oscillator does not yet exist, but genes encoding some of the component have been identified. Various metabolic processes (oxygen evolution, respiration) cycle alternately through high and low activity phases with a regular periodicity of ~ 24 hours.

Circadian Rhythms

They arise from cyclic phenomena that are defined by three parameters (Fig. 3.2):

1. *Period of a rhythm* = time between comparable points in the repeating cycle - measured as the time between consecutive maxima (peaks) or minima (troughs).

2. *Phase* = any point in the cycle that is recognizable by its relationship to the rest of the cycle - most obvious phase points are the peak and trough positions.

3. *Amplitude* = distance between peak and trough - can vary while period remains unchanged.

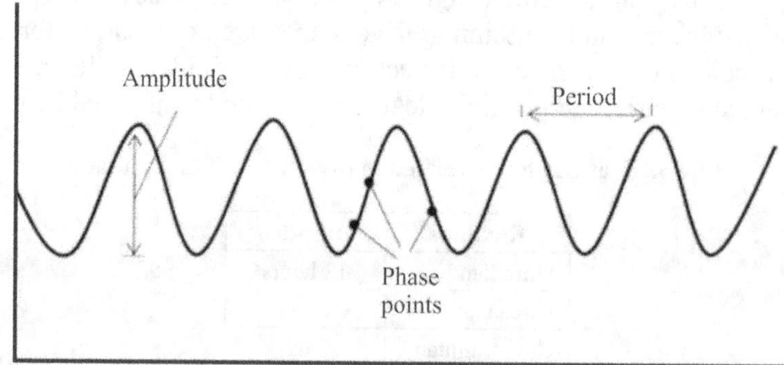

Fig. 3.2 Circadian rhythms.

In *chronopharmaceutics*, the approach is to link between existing concepts of *chronobiology, chronopharmacology, chronopharmacokinetics*, and *chronotoxicology*. *Chronophysiology* is the investigation of temporal features in the physiological factors underlying biological temporal characteristics. When, there is a change in biological temporal functions due to disease, the study of this alteration is called *chronopathology*. Drugs following administration itself affect the biologic rhythm or biological rhythm can affect the action of drug and the investigation of this science is known as *chronopharmacology*. Administration of drug according to biological rhythm helps in optimization and quantification of the drug effect thus, study of *chronopharmacology* aids in potentiation of desired effects while minimizing the undesired effects. The harmful and undesired effect of any chemical physical and other agents including poisons, pollutant and overdoses of drug on biological temporal characteristics is explained by the concept of *chronotoxicology*. Time dependent variation in the onset of several acute medical diseases is known as *chronoepidemiology*. To achieve the desired action enough concentration is desired at the site of action and ultimately in the blood. Circadian timing system may affect the action if, free active drug at desired site of action. *Chronopharmaceutics* is the branch of pharmaceutics which designs and develops a drug delivery system in accordance with biological rhythm to optimize the treatment of disease. *Chronotherapeutics* is the science which involves the administration of the medication using modern technology in accordance with biological rhythm.

Underlying mechanism responsible for circadian rhythms

The mechanism for the maintenance of these biological rhythms involves the control as well as coordination of inherit pacemaker clocks present in different parts of the body. Among these all internal biological clocks arranged at different levels of body, the one which is located within the brain believed to be most important. Within brain the master clocks resides in the supra chiasmatic nucleus (SCN) of hypothalamus which controls or drives the message of time to the peripheral cells through autonomic neuronal and humoral signals (involves the coordination of ANS).

The factors that are mainly responsible in resetting the rhythmic signals by directly or indirectly affecting SCN are the light perceived by visual pathway, enzyme activities governed by local circadian clocks in peripheral cells, secretion of melatonin - a hormone released by the pineal gland during darkness (melatonin is endogenous sedative) and gene expression. The genes maintaining the biological rhythmicity are *per1, per2, per3, cry1, cry2, frq, clock* and *tau*. These genes code for the synthesis of proteins which regulate the positive and negative loop in the SCN.

The molecular basis for protein synthesis is multistep process. The basic helix loop helix transcription factor BMAL1, CLOCK, NPAS2 form heterodimer. BMAL1 forms heterodimers with CLOCK and its paralog NPAS2. These heterodimers bind E-box *cis*-regulatory enhancer sequences and activate the transcription of genes such as Per1–3, Cry1 and 2, Rev-erbα, and Rorα. PER and CRY proteins heterodimerize, translocate to the nucleus, and interact with BMAL1: CLOCK/NPAS2 heterodimers to inhibit their transcriptional activity. After a certain period of time, the PER:CRY complex degrades and BMAL1:CLOCK/NPAS2 heterodimers start a new cycle of transcription. Additional feedback strengthens the robustness of the circadian clock. REV-ERBα and RORα compete for the same ROR response elements in the BMAL1 promoter. REV-ERBα inhibits, whereas RORα activates, the transcription of BMAL1. Posttranslational modification and degradation of clock proteins are crucial steps in circadian period. Phosphorylation of the PER:CRY heterodimer by CK1ε/δ is critical for the nuclear translocation of the complex. The FBXL3 targets CRY proteins for degradation.

Chronobiology, Health and Associated Diseases

All the physiological and behavioral functions in humans occur on a rhythmic basis, which in turn leads to dramatic diurnal rhythms in human performance capabilities. Regardless of whether it results from voluntary or involuntary (e.g., illness or advanced age) circumstances, a disturbed circadian rhythmicity in humans has been associated with a variety of mental and physical disorders and may negatively impact safety, performance, and productivity. Many adverse effects of disrupted circadian rhythmicity may be linked to disturbances in the sleep-wake cycle whereas some rhythmic processes are more affected by the circadian clock than by the sleep-wake state, whereas other rhythms are more dependent on the sleep-wake state (Fig. 3.3).

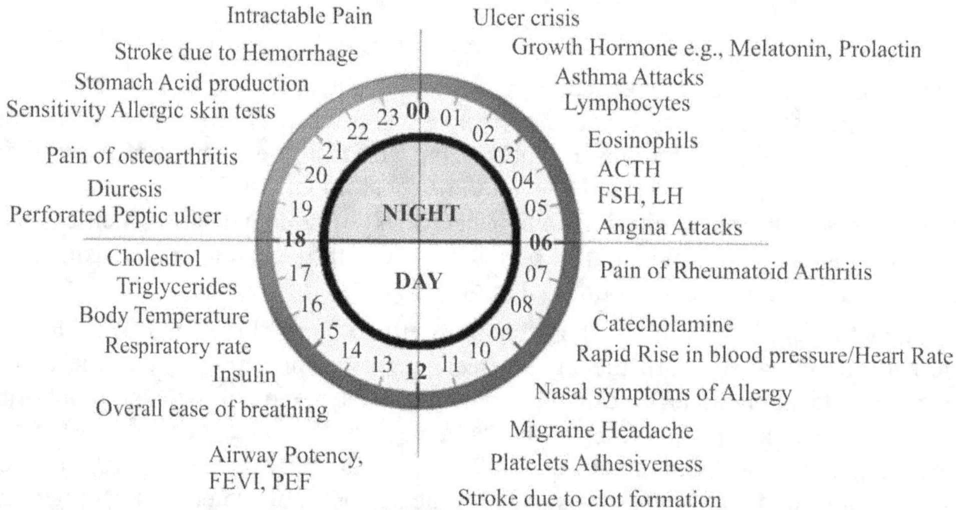

Fig. 3.3 Circadian rhythm of human; common physiological and disease status changes.

Hence, the disease pattern changes according to physiological changes like asthma attacks precipitate in midnight and heart/angina attacks are very likely at morning just within few hours of awakening. Hormones secretion in the women causes menstrual cycles to start in the early morning. Likely, many disease pattern changes as per the time of events and the treatment guidelines follow at the time of highest risk to alleviate the disease.

1. Hypertension

Blood pressure profile in normotensive as well as in hypertensive individual shows different circadian patterns during 24 hours period. In normotensive and person suffering from primary hypertension there is nightly drop in blood pressure and thus they are called dippers, while in secondary hypertension (due to diabetes mellitus, Cushing's syndrome, renal diseases etc.) elevated values are seen mostly at night and thus, they are called risers.

The reason for different blood pressure profile in primary hypertension may be due to increased level of noradrenaline and cAMP during day, while in secondary hypertension there are increased level of renin, aldosterone and corticosterone at night. This help in setting proper chronotherapy for primary and secondary hypertension. Antihypertensive treatment mainly involves β-blockers, Ca^{2+}-channel blockers, ACE inhibitors and diuretics.

β-blockers are sympathomimetic and thus they help in improving blood pressure profile during day time, while they are less effective in night. Ca^{2+}-channel blockers differ in their pharmacokinetic profile so their effect also varies during 24 hours period. A single morning dose of sustained release verapamil showed a good 24 hours blood pressure control. Dihydropyridine derivative differing in pharmacokinetic profile seem to reduce blood pressure to varying degree during day and night time. ACE inhibitors for sustained day time reduction in blood pressure.

2. Asthma

Asthma a chronic inflammatory disease of airway shows circadian rhythm in its manifestation and intensity. The increased risk of asthmatic attack is in the early morning nearly at 4 a.m. as compared to afternoon. This is due to increase in diameter of bronchi during day time while decrease in diameter of bronchi at night. At night, there is a blockade of β-adrenergic receptor, dominance of α-adrenergic pathway, cholinergic dominance, smallest concentration of cortisol, IgE and highest concentration of histamine in early morning.

Chronotherapy of asthma with β_2 agonist (Terbutalin) shows circadian dependent changes in peak expiratory airflow. Theophylline showed improved results when given as evening dose i.e., $1/3^{rd}$ dosing of regimen in morning and $2/3^{rd}$ dosing of regimen in evening, along with this the pharmacokinetic profile of theophylline also shows circadian dependent variations i.e., C_{max} was lower and/or t_{max} was longer after evening when after morning dosing.

3. Depression

There are no primary disturbances of circadian system in depression but, diurnal and nocturnal variations are observed as a part of multiple manifestations of the primary pathophysiology of depression. These include changes of both intrinsic rhythms of circadian oscillators and in the sensitivity of retinal light, which is the only photo receptor for circadian entrainment. Dysregulation of hypothalamic – pituitary – adrenal as well as gonadal axis have been documented in depressed patients. Along with it there are also abnormalities in circulating melatonin have been found with affective disorders.

Chronopharmacology of selective serotonin reuptake inhibitors (SSRIs) was observed in some animal models, that they are more active in dark phase than in light phase. This is due to increased mRNA expression for serotonin transporter in dark phase. Some SSRIs like fluvoxamine shows increased plasma concentration when administered at 9 a.m. than that at to 9 p.m. as fluvoxamine metabolizing enzyme secretion shows time dependent variation.

4. Cancer

Toxicity of cancer chemotherapy is major hurdle in treating cancers; however, these cytotoxic drugs can be made more effective and less toxic if they are given at right time. The biological clock was shown to exert negative control on the transcriptional activity of some key genes involved in cell cycle regulation. Thereby suggesting that, the circadian clock could regulate cell proliferation. Many other cell cycle related genes display 24 hours rhythm in mRNA and/or protein expression, this is special in case of gene's expression patterns which control cell cycle check points such as *cdlk2* cyclines *a, b, c, d, e* or *mdm2* or which regulate apoptosis.

From animal studies it has been found that cytotoxic drugs like cisplatin, carboplatin and oxaliplatin are well tolerated near the middle of nocturnal activity span of animals whereas, in case of antimetabolites like 5-flurouracil and floxuridine are best effective exactly at opposite circadian patter than platinum compounds. The least toxic dosing time is indicated for each cytostatic or immunologic agent as a function of the rest activity cycle.

Principles of Chronobiology in Drug Therapy

The mammalians circadian pacemaker resides in the paired suprachiasmatic nuclei (SCN) and influences a multitude of biological processes, including the sleep-wake rhythm. Clock genes are the genes that control the circadian rhythms in physiology and behavior. The effectiveness and toxicity of many drugs vary depending on dosing time associated with 24 hours rhythms of biochemical, physiological and behavioral processes under the control of circadian clock. Such chronopharmacological phenomena are influenced by pharmacokinetics and pharmacodynamics of medications. Identification of an appropriate rhythmic marker for selecting dosing time leads to improved progress of chronopharmacotherapy. Several drugs have an effect on circadian clock. Chronopharmacology is the investigative science that elucidates the biological rhythm dependencies of medications. Chronopharmacokinetic studies of many drugs attempt to explain chronopharmacological phenomenan and demonstrate that the time of administration is a possible factor of variation in the pharmacokinetics of a drug. Time-dependent changes in pharmacokinetics may proceed from 24 hours rhythms in each process, e.g., absorption, distribution, metabolism and elimination. Hence the quantitative response (duration or intensity of the action) of an organism, as well as the qualitative response (i.e., inhibition or induction, increase or decrease of its effect), varies with time of administration. Thus, pharmacokinetic parameters [including the peak drug plasma concentration (C_{max}), time to reach C_{max} (t_{max}), the area under the concentration-time curve (AUC), volume of distribution (Vd), protein binding, elimination half-life ($t_{1/2}$) and clearance (CL)] which are conventionally considered to be constant in time are circadian time-dependent.

Table 3.2 Possible physiological factors influencing circadian
stage dependent pharmacokinetics of drugs

Absorption	*Oral:* Gastric pH, gastric motility, gastric emptying time, gastrointestinal blood flow, transporter
	Parental: Transdermal permeability, ocular permeability, pulmonary permeability
Distribution	Blood flow, albumin, alpha1-acid glycoprotein, red blood cells, transporter
Metabolism	Liver enzyme activity, hepatic blood flow, gastrointestinal enzymes
Elimination	*Renal, biliary, intestinal:* Glomerular filtration, renal blood flow, urinary pH, electrolytes, tubular reabsorption, transporter

1. Circadian Rhythms and Drug Absorption

The 24 hours rhythms of physiology and behavior are influenced by various environmental factors such as feeding schedules, genetic factors and social interactions as well as lighting conditions and several drugs. The period of the central circadian pacemaker in humans is slightly longer than 24 hours, synchronization of the circadian system with the light-dark cycle occurs by daily phase-advances of the circadian clock. Morning light advances the central circadian pacemaker, late afternoon and evening light delays the pacemaker, and light at midday is without phase-shifting effects. The phase-shifting agents (zeitgebers) such as melatonin, 5-hydroxytryptamine (5-HT, serotonin), and behavioral arousal have a Phase Response Curve distinct from light. Phase advances occur between midday and early evening. Phase delays occur between late night and midday. Photic and nonphotic (i.e., extrinsic timekeeping) effects on intrinsic time keeping may be important components of disordered timekeeping in depressive illness.

Circadian changes in the absorption of drugs depends upon various factors like gastric acid secretion, pH, motility, gastric emptying time, and gastrointestinal blood flow which vary along the 24 hours scale. These changes may be implicated in variability of drug absorption and are differently implicated according to time of administration. For instance, circadian changes of pH may induce circadian modifications of drug ionization according to its physicochemical properties. Increased gastric acidity reduces the absorption of lipophilic drugs, and the diurnal variation in gastric acidity contributes to differences in drug absorption over different times of the day. Also, a faster gastric emptying time and a higher gastrointestinal perfusion in the morning were demonstrated in humans. This may participate to usual better drug bioavailability often observed in man after morning administration compared to evening administration. Chemical properties like lipophilicity and hydrophilicity of drug may also affect the chronokinetics of drugs. Marked circadian changes in drug absorption are significant for lipophilic drugs while such changes are not documented for hydrophilic drugs. Such variations may be predicted by physico-chemical properties of a drug since most of the lipophilic drugs seem to be absorbed faster when the drug is taken in the morning as compared to evening dosing. At the opposite, the absorption processes of highly water-soluble drugs were not demonstrated to change according to time of day. Posture and feeding conditions (e.g., possible influence of food), even if indirectly imposed, are known to be involved in drug absorption variability. A variety of physiological rhythmic variables are influenced by the cyclic variation of environmental factors. One of those factors is feeding schedule. The change in glucocorticoid rhythmicity appears to play an important role in physiological rhythmicity by the manipulation of the feeding schedule, because plasma corticosterone levels show anticipatory increases before the time of feeding, and the continuous administration of corticosterone disturbed the rhythmicity of behavior, physiological function and cyclic gene expression. Obviously, these factors are circadian time-dependent, in usual resting/activity conditions, but they must be controlled to avoid a masking effect since they may be superimposed to circadian variations. As an illustrative example, chronokinetic changes of carbamazepine, an antiepileptic drug, were documented in rats with a significant higher absorption when the drug was given orally during the night active period. This circadian variation was confirmed and amplified in fasting conditions, demonstrating that food may influence but not create the rhythm. Drug absorption by other than oral route of administration may also be influenced by biological rhythms. For instance, skin permeability is circadian time-dependent and may be implicated in temporal variation in drugs penetration as previously documented for local anesthetic agents in animals as well as in man. Specific drug penetration through the skin when using patches must take in account these phenomena since these transdermal devices are applied for at least 24 hours day long. Ocular absorption of topically applied beta-blockers was also documented to be circadian time-dependent. Thus, all factors including route of administration, feeding conditions, posture, and formulation need to be controlled, taking into account the concerned biological rhythms.

2. Circadian Rhythms and Drug Distribution

Circadian changes in biological fluids and tissues have been found to vary along the 24 hours scale; such changes may obviously be affecting drug distribution. Underlying factors involved are perfusion, blood distribution, peripheral distribution, blood cells, serum protein, and sleep-awake cycle. Blood flow depends on several regulatory factors including sympathetic and parasympathetic systems whose activities are known to be circadian time-dependent with a predominant diurnal effect of the sympathetic system in man. Thus, diurnal increase and nocturnal decrease of blood flow and local tissular blood flows may explain a possible difference in drug distribution according to time of administration. Plasma proteins such as albumin or orosomucoid (e.g., alpha 1 glycoprotein acid) have been documented to be circadian time-dependent in man despite a low amplitude rhythm. Maximum albumin and orosomucoid plasma concentrations in man are located around noon. As a consequence, daily variations for drug protein binding have been reported both in animals and in human. These changes may also depend on factors such as temperature, pH, and physicochemical properties of the concerned drug which may possibly be subject to temporal variations. More recently, diurnal variations of P-glycoprotein (P-gp), a multidrug transporter which contributes to renal, biliary, and intestinal elimination of drugs have been reported. Clinically significant consequences of such temporal changes in drug binding are relevant only for drugs which are highly bound (e.g., 80%). Thus, temporal variations in plasma drug binding may have clinical implications only for drugs characterized by a high protein binding and a small volume of distribution. Nevertheless, to our knowledge, clinical consequences due to circadian variations in plasma proteins have not yet been demonstrated.

3. Circadian Rhythms and Drug Metabolism

Drug metabolism depends on enzyme activities and blood flow; both are described to change with 24 hours scale. First-pass effect and protein binding may also affect metabolism. Enzyme activities to endogenous substrates are time dependent in perfused tissues such as brain, kidney and liver and the chronokinetic and chronodynamic changes are dependent on such variations. Various oxidative reactions catalyzed by the microsomal mono-oxygenases systems have been shown to vary along the 24 hours scale as well as reduction, hydrolysis, and conjugation. The cytochrome P450 monooxygenase enzyme system is mainly responsible for drug oxidation. Cytochrome P450 oxidoreductase provides electrons for all P450 mediated monooxygenase reactions and hence variations of P450 oxidoreductase cause a circadian rhythm in all the activities of cytochrome P450 enzymes. Molecular mechanisms of circadian rhythm and rhythmic transcription of clock output regulators such as an enzyme of the cytochrome P-450 super family in liver have recently shown. Circadian PAR-domain basic leucine zipper transcription factors DBP, TEF, and HLF modulate basal and inducible xenobiotic detoxification. Temporal variations in hepatic glucuronidation and sulphonation reactions which are the two major pathways for the elimination of the drugs, example of temporal variation in conjugation reactions comes from those that use glutathione as a substrate. Reduced glutathione forms adduct with reactive intermediates of drugs produced by the cytochrome P450 monooxygenase system and promote their detoxification. The hepatic concentrations of glutathione change with time, and this variation determines the diurnal changes in conjugation elimination of several drugs. When considering metabolism of drugs with a high hepatic extraction ratio, hepatic blood flow is of particular importance: any significant variation in hepatic blood flow may induce changes in drug metabolism. It is reported on daily variations in hepatic blood flow as measured by indocyanine green clearance in clinical studies with highest values in the early morning. Such temporal changes are of particular interest to explain mechanisms for circadian rhythms of drugs with a high hepatic extraction ratio.

4. Circadian Rhythms and Drug Elimination

Rhythmic variations in the functions of glomerular filtration, renal blood flow, effective renal plasma flow, tubular secretion, urine output, and urinary excretion of electrolytes and other endogenous substances may result different excretion rates for drugs at different intervals of day time. It is more likely that diurnal variations in systemic blood pressure, the renin-angiotensin system, and renal blood flow are responsible for time-dependent changes in renal hemodynamic. Urinary pH is an important factor in the urinary excretion of drugs that shows diurnal variations. Passive reabsorption of drugs depends on urinary pH, because renal tubular cells are less permeable to the ionized form of weak acids, alkalis. Temporal changes in urinary pH modify drug ionization and may explain that acidic drugs are excreted faster after an evening administration as documented for sodium salicylate and sulphonamide; such variations are obviously more pronounced for hydrophilic drugs. Amphetamine is more strongly ionized at lower pH, and it is readily excreted in the urine. When the urinary pH is more basic, the non-ionized fraction is increased, and its urinary excretion is decreased markedly, urinary pH is lower during the night and higher in the day. The pH difference over the 24 hours span could also be important in explaining the renal toxicity of drugs such as the aminoglycoside. Food appears to influence the diurnal variation of urinary pH, which in turn modifies the binding or the excretion of drugs.

5. Circadian Rhythms and Drug Dynamics

Circadian changes involves a major interactions between the active forms of the drug and its molecular targets which includes rhythmicity in membrane viscosity or permeability, receptor density or binding enzymatic activities and transport or repair proteins and ion channels that are the major determinants of molecular and cellular responses. Drug interaction with its target is a specific time dependent variation that attributes to the specific effects of drugs. Evidence of diurnal effect in pharmacodynamic effect depends on the affinity of the drug for its target, the amount of the drug present in the tissue and the baseline activity of the target system determine the response of drug.

Biological rhythms at the cellular and subcellular level can give rise to significant dosing-time differences in the pharmacodynamics of medications that are unrelated to their pharmacokinetics. This phenomenon is termed chronesthesy. A rhythm in receptor number or conformation, second messengers, metabolic pathways, and/or free-to-bound fraction of medications is responsible for this phenomenon.

Renin Angiotensin System: Homeostasis of the blood pressure depends on the renin angiotensin system. Two proteolytic enzymes, renin that cleaves angiotensinogen to angiotensin-I and angiotensin converting enzyme leads to the conversion of the inactive angiotensin-I into the formation of an active agonist angiotensin-II that has a multiple effects on vasculature, adrenal glands, kidneys and brain resulting in the regulation of systemic blood pressure and fluid homeostasis. Human plasma renin activity is low in the afternoon and increases during the night as reported in several clinical studies such as diurnal variation in the plasma renin activity potentially influences blood pressure circadian rhythm and hence, inhibitors of the renin angiotensin system are more effective during the rest period that is when both blood pressure and plasma renin activity are at highest. This concludes that rhythms in the plasma renin activity leading to the diurnal variations in the formation angiotensin peptides, largely depends on the clinical effects of the inhibitors of the renin angiotensin system.

Nitric Oxide-Cyclic GMP System: Endothelium derived nitric oxide (NO) is an important regulation of vascular toe and loses of this endogenous NO synthesis in hypertension leads to cardiovascular applications. In hypertension, NO is synthesized by the endothelial cells by passive diffusion and once synthesized enters the adjacent smooth muscle cells and activates the cGMP generating enzymes. In normotensives, the NO oxidation end products is higher during the night than in daytime, showed pronounced 24 hours rhythmicity with the peak values at the end of the day and trough values in the second half of the night whereas rhythmic changes in the NO-cGMP pathway was lost in hypertensive individuals. Hence, rhythmic changes in the NO oxidation end products and the cGMP excretion during the day time have possible implications in the treatment of patients receiving drugs that are NO donors.

Table 3.3 Drugs for which daily variation in their effects were
reported in clinical studies

Class of Drug	Examples
β-blockers	Atenolol, metoprolol, carvidilol, lobetalol
β-agonists	Terbutaline, adrenaline
Calcium channel blocker	Amlodipine, nifedipin, verapamil, diltiazem
ACE inhibitors	Captopril, enalpril, lisinopril
AT1-receptor antagonists	Losartan, irbesartan
Diuretics	Hydrochlorthiazide, furosemide, indapamide
Organic nitrates	Glyceryl-trinitrate, isosorbide-dinitrate
Other cardiovascular drugs	Clonidine, prazosin
Anti-cancer	Cisplatin, doxorubicin, busulphan

Table 3.3 *Contd...*

Class of Drug	Examples
Psychotropic	Diazepam, haloperidol
H_1 blocker	Clemastine, terfinadine
H_2 blocker	Cimetidine, famotidine, ranitidine
Anti-asthmatic	Theophylline, terbutaline, dexamethasone
Ophthalmology	Terbutaline, timolol
NSAID and opiods	Aspirin, ibuprofen, paracetamol, fentanyl, morphine
General and local anaesthetics	Halothane, lidocaine
Endocrinology	Insulin, tolbutamide, prednisolone

Table 3.4 Drugs for which daily variations in their pharmacokinetics were reported in clinical studies

Class of Drug	Examples
β-blockers	Atenolol, propranolol
ACE-inhibitors	Enalpril
Organic nitrates	Isosorbide dinitrate
Calcium channel blocker	Diltiazem, verapamil
Psychotropic drugs	Diazepam, levodopa, valproic acid
Anti-asthmatic drugs	Aminophylline, theophylline
NSAIDs, local anaesthetics	Aspirin, indomethacin
Opioids	Dihydrocodeine, tramadol
Anticancer drugs	Cisplatin, doxorubicin
Antibacterial agents	Ampicillin, amikasin,
Gastroenterology	Cimetidine, omeprazole

Table 3.5 Chronopharmacological recommendations of some drugs used in treatment of various conditions

Disease	Class of Drug	Recommendations
Asthma	Glucocorticoids	When given as morning dose shows 24 hours mean in FEV_1 with more pronounced effect at night and reduced amplitude of the rhythm of FEV_1.
	Theophylline	Due to high prevalence of asthma at night and chronokinetic profile of the drug it is administered at evening.
	$β_2$ agonist	Chronokinetic profile of $β_2$ agonist leads to its administration at evening.
Hypertension	Primary hypertension	Due to increased level of noradrenaline and cyclic AMP during day, drugs are given as morning dosing
	Secondary hypertension	Due to Increased level of renin, aldosterone and corticosterone at night, evening dosing is beneficial.
Ulcers	H_2 blockers	Evening or night dosing is beneficial because of increased gastric acid secretion at late afternoon and early night.
Addison's diseases	Corticosteroids	ACTH levels are increased in afternoon and at early evening, so splitting of dose in afternoon and evening will give more improved results.

Source: Arzneimittelkommission der deutschen Arzteschaft ed. *Arzneiverordnungen*, 17th edn. Ko¨ln: Deutscher Arzte, 1992.

Future Directions in Chronopharmacology

Modern chronopharmacology is moving toward applying the current understanding of circadian rhythms to predict the circadian variability in drug effectiveness and toxicity. One of the major challenges in this effort is the identification of circadian oscillations at the protein level. Although information about circadian changes in gene expression for a number of different tissues is available but the circadian variation of proteins is still largely unknown. Desired effects of drugs can be maximized by timing drug administration according to hours of changing response. To treat according to arbitrarily fixed schedules is to ignore the implications of circadian functions in both health and disease. A drug should be administered when or where it is needed in the minimum required dose. Time controlled and site specific drug delivery system should be conducted irrespective of the route of administration.

Conclusions

Today safety measures for any new medication are the predominant requirement for the regulatory bodies. Understanding the concepts of chronobiology along with chronopharmacology may help in minimizing the all drug toxicity as well as efficacy related issues. Drug show their different pharmacokinetic and pharmacodynamic profile thus, their effect are dependent on circadian variation and these circadian variation ultimately under the influence of zeitgebers on inherent pacemaker clocks. Now, due to influence of external and internal factor these pacemakers show periodic difference in drug action. Timely administration of drugs in many diseases like asthma, hypertension, depression, cancer and many more disease has shown many improvements in their effectiveness compared to normal conventional therapy. Thus, inclusion of chronopharmacological concept in prescribing medicine will be helpful to decrease drug related toxicity and to enhance the effectiveness.

Suggested Readings

1. Arzneimittelkommission der deutschen Arzteschaft ed. (1992). *Arzneiverordnungen*, 17th edn. Ko"ln: Deutscher Arzte.

2. Bae K, Jin X, Maywood ES, Hastings MH, Reppert SM, Weaver DR (2001). Differential functions of mPer1, mPer2, and mPer3 in the SCN circadian clock. *Neuron.* **30:** 525-536.

3. Bruguerolle B, Boulamery A, Simon N (2008). Biological rhythms: a neglected factor of variability in pharmacokinetic studies. *Journal of Pharmaceutical sciences* **25(1):** 1-15.

4. Evans RM, Marain C (1996). Taking your medication: A question of timing. *Am Med Assoc.* 3-8.

5. Godfrey K.R (1989). Chronopharmacology and its Application to the Development of Theophylline Treatment Schedules for Asthma. *European Journal of Clinical Pharmacology* **36:** 103-109.

6. Gollapudi R, Javvaji H, Arpineni V, Tadikonda RR (2011). Chronopharmacokinetics – administration, time dependent effects of drugs with different diseases. *An international journal of advances in pharmaceutical sciences* **2(1):** 68-72.

7. Halberg F, *Chronobiology. Annu. Rev.Physiol.* **31:** 675-726.

8. Isadora Stehlin (1997). A time to heal: Chronotherapy tunes in to body's rhythms. *FDA Consumer* **31:** 16-20.

9. Jones PJ, Schoeller DA (1990). Evidence for diurnal periodicity in human cholesterol synthesis. *J Lipid Res.* **31:** 667-673.

10. Khasawneh SM, Affarah HB (1992). Morning versus evening dose: A comparison of three H2-receptor blockers in duodenal ulcer healing. *Am J Gastroenterol.* **87:** 1180-1182.

11. Kume K, Zylka MJ, Sriram S, Shearman LP, Weaver DR, *et al.,* (1999). mCRY1 and mCRY2 are essential components of the negative limb of the circadian clock feedback loop. *Cell.* **98:** 193-205

12. Lemmer B (2007). Chronobiology, Drug delivery and Chronotherapeutics. *Advanced Drug Delivery Review.* **59:** 825-827.

13. Lemmer B (1994). Chronopharmacology: Time, a key in drug treatment. *Ann Biol Clin.* **52:** 1-7.

14. Lemmer B (2009). Discoveries of Rhythms in Humans Biological Functions: A Historical Review. *Chronobiological International.* **26(6):** 1019-1068.

15. Lemmer B (2000). Relevance of Chronopharmacology in Practical Medicine. *Seminars in Perinatology.* **24(4):** 280-290.

16. Lemmer B (2005). Chronopharmacology and controlled drug release. *Expert Opinion on Drug Delivery.* **2(4):** 667-681.

17. Lemmer B (2007). Chronopharmacology of cardiovascular medications. *Biological Rhythm Research.* **38(3):** 247-258.

18. Lévi F, Okyar A, Dulong S, Innominato PF, Clairambault J (2010). Circadian timing in cancer treatments. *Annu Rev Pharmacol Toxicol.* **50:** 377-421.

19. Levi F, Schibler U (2007). Circadian rhythms: mechanisms and therapeutic implications. *Annu Rev Pharmacol Toxicol.* **47:** 593-628.

20. Lévi F (2006). Chronotherapeutics: the relevance of timing in cancer therapy. *Cancer Causes and Control.* **17(4):** 611-621.

21. Micheal, Hastings (1998). The brain, circadian rhythms and clock genes. *Br Med J.* **317:** 1704-1708.

22. Moore R.Y (1997). Circadian rhythms: basic neurobiology and clinical applications. *Annu Rev Medicine.* **48:** 253-266.

23. Moore-Ede MC, Sulzman FM, Fuller CA. *The Clocks That Time Us.* Cambridge, MA: Harvard Univ. Press. 1982, 448.

24. Paschos G.K, Baggs J.E., Hogenesch J.B, FitzGerald G.A (2010). The role of clock genes in pharmacology. *Annu Rev Pharmacol Toxicol.* **50:** 187-214.

25. Prasanthi NL, Swathi G, Manikiran SS (2011). Chronotherapeutics: a new vista in novel drug delivery systems. *International Journal of Pharmaceutical Sciences Review and Research.* **6(2):** 66-74.

26. Preitner N, Damiola F, Luis Lopez M, Zakany J, Duboule D, *et al.,* (2002). The orphan nuclear receptor REV-ERB alpha controls circadian transcription within the positive limb of the mammalian circadian oscillator. *Cell.* **110:** 251-260.

27. Radzialowski F. M., Bousquet W. F (1968). Daily rhythmic variations in hepatic drug metabolism in the rat and mouse. *J. Pharmacol. Exp. Ther.* **163:** 229-238.

28. Reinberg A., Halberg F (1971). Circadian chronopharmacology. *Annu. Rev. Pharmacol.* **11:** 455-492.

29. Sarasija Suresh, Stutie Pathak (2005). Chronotherapeutics: Emerging role of biorhythms in optimizing drug therapy. *Indian J Pharm Sci.* **67:** 135-140.

30. Smolensky M.H (1996). Chronobiology and chronotherapeutics applications to cardiovascular medicine. *American Journal of Hypertension.* **9:** 11-21.

31. Ushijima K, Sakaguchi H, Sato Y, To H, Koyanagi S, Higuchi S, Ohdo S (2005). Chronopharmacological study of antidepressants in forced swimming test of mice. *J Pharmacol Exp Ther.* **315(2):** 764-770.

32. Vitaterna MH, Takahashi JS, Turek FW (2001). Overview of circadian rhythm. *Alcohol Research and Health.* **5(2):** 83-95.

33. Youan B. B. C (2004). Chronopharmaceutics: gimmick or clinically relevant approach to drug delivery? *Journal of Controlled Release.* **98:** 337-353.

34. Zheng B, Albrecht U, Kaasik K, Sage M, Lu W, *et al.,* (2001). Nonredundant roles of the mPer1 and mPer2 genes in the mammalian circadian clock. *Cell.* **105:** 683-694.

CHAPTER 4

OVER THE COUNTER (OTC) DRUGS

Introduction

Over-the-counter (OTC) drugs are those drugs/substances/products available without a prescription to consumer. In 2000, it was estimated that the consumers of USA spent approximately \$19.1 billion on OTC drugs on over 1 in 25,000 products to medicate themselves for ailments ranging from acne to warts.

Generally, drugs are available by two ways in most countries either by access with a prescription provided by a licensed doctor/healthcare professional or access without a prescription i.e., by over the counter purchase, called OTC agents. In addition, there is third one in which sales of certain drugs without a prescription requires consultation with a pharmacist known as restricted OTC products/substances. The number of OTC drugs is increasing because some prescription drugs those were previously available only by prescription is released by the regulatory bodies according to their safety and efficacy parameters. The role of regulatory bodies is vital in the selection of OTC products, since it is taken without the supervision of qualified doctors.

Regulation of OTC drugs is as per their ingredients, not as final products which make the manufacturer freedom to formulate ingredients, or combinations of ingredients, into their proprietary mixture and give regulatory guidelines for their sell without a pharmacy like general confectionary shops, gas stations, supermarkets, etc., and who is authorized to dispense them, and whether a prescription is required varies principally country to country. OTC drugs enable people to relieve many annoying symptoms and to cure some diseases simply and without the cost of seeing a doctor. However, safe use of these drugs requires knowledge, common sense, and responsibility.

Prescription drugs, after several years of safe use in clinics under prescription regulation, drugs may be approved by the regulatory bodies for OTC sale such as ibuprofen (analgesic) and famotidine (indigestion). There are several OTC drugs which are not always better tolerated than similar prescription drugs e.g., diphenhydramine is neither effective nor as safe as many prescription sleep aids.

History

Before the establishment of regulatory bodies such as FDA-USA, EMA-Europe, DCGI-India; practice of drugs in market was in pathetic condition and could be sold anything in bottle for a sure-fire cure such as alcohol, cocaine, marijuana, and opium were few of them. The Food, Drug and Cosmetic Act of 1938 established the requirement that new drugs must be proved safe and must be properly labelled before being marketed.

Although, this act had provisions regarding adulterated products, misbranding and new drugs; no criteria were provided for use in distinguishing between prescription and OTC drugs. Durham-Humphrey Amendment (1951) provided a statutory basis and specific criteria for differentiating prescription from OTC drugs which includes three considerations:

(i)   Habit forming drugs must be available only by prescription.

(ii) Drugs that can be used safely only under supervision of a licensed health care practitioner also require prescription.

Several factors must be assessed, like potential of toxicity or other harmful effects, methods of use, any requirement for collateral measures for its use, such as laboratory or clinical monitoring, etc.

(iii) If a drug has been approved as the result of a new-drug application for use under professional supervision, then its purchase requires a prescription.

Kefauver-Harris Amendments of 1962 require the FDA to assess the efficacy as well as safety of new drugs. These amendments require the review of both prescription and OTC drugs, thus, mandating evidence that an OTC product is effective and safe when used without supervision by a healthcare practitioner. Since 1972, FDA has been engaged in a methodical review of OTC ingredients for both safety and efficacy.

Two major outcomes of this review are:

(i)   Ingredients designated as ineffective or unsafe for their claimed therapeutic uses are being eliminated from OTC product formulation (e.g., antimuscarinic agents have been eliminated from OTC because of combination with benzodiazepine).

(ii) Agents have been switched from prescription only to OTC drugs because they were judged by the review panel to be generally safe and effective for consumer use without medical supervision.

OTC and Safety

Safety is the major concern and challenges for regulatory bodies when re-classification of prescription drug as OTC drugs. However, all drugs have known and unknown benefits and risks. As noted by an amendment to the FD&C Act of 1962, OTC drugs were required to be both effective and safe. However, determining effectiveness and safety can be difficult. What is effective for one person may not be for another, and any drug may cause unwanted side effects. Always safety concern is at the stake of these drugs may be due to nature of drugs or multiple OTC drugs containing the same active ingredient, which could lead to an overdose or increased side-effects. Logically, sometimes it is noted that patients may take more than the recommended dose of a drug, believing higher dose will be more effective or not read or understand the directions. Therapeutic ranges of OTC drugs are wide, but some drugs may produce greater risks, if not used as recommended, e.g., acetaminophen is an OTC drug, widely used as antipyretic and believed as safe if used as directed, but it may induce acute liver failure if, recommended doses are exceeded and/or when combined with alcohol. Further, these problems may be precipitated with the combination with other drugs like Acetaminophen + Ibuprofen/Chlorpheniramine/Pseudoephedrine/Chlorzoxazone.

Criteria for Evaluating a Drug for OTC Marketing

FDA is using criteria for evaluating for OTC drug marketing. These criteria include components distinct from those for prescription drugs

(i) Ability of patients to recognize and diagnose them self the condition specified in proposed medication.

  Alternatively, a health care professional might make the diagnosis, particularly if it is a chronic condition and patients can avail the required medications over the counter.

(ii) Ability of patients to extract key information by reading a product label necessary for using the drug properly.

(iii) Effectiveness of the OTC drug when used as recommended.

(iv) Safety of the drug when used as instructed.

The trend among manufactures of seeking an approval of a wide variety of drugs for OTC use poses challenges for the evaluation process.

Although studies indicate that 96% of consumers read the label before the first use; this doesn't mean they can extract and comprehend critical information if not prompted. Study conducted in PGIMER, Chandigarh among medical personal, nursing and patients concluded majority of the respondents believed to know the importance of package inserts. General agreement for relevance of information and opinion was against adequate mentioning of negative points, references quoting and regular updating. Small font of letters was a common problem. A lot needs to be done to make package inserts more reader friendly and enhance their utility. With more stringent rules for regulating the contents and references, their quality can be improved. Henceforth, people should take the caution to use these products and should take precautions in following manners;

(a) Should read and follow the instructions carefully, because formulation may be immediate-release and controlled-release (slow-release) formulations

(b) Should be checked every time for product name and dosage

(c) Should read the insert label carefully (Labels on OTC drugs, which are required by the regulatory bodies)

(d) Should ask a registered pharmacist if they have any questions about an OTC product.

(e) Should determine and confirm the administration oral or parenteral and duration properly, since long term use of NSAIDs may cause liver damage.

Restricted OTC Substance

Few OTC products needs close observation of use, and not legally classified as OTC drugs. These types of OTC drug are available without the prescription and stored behind the pharmacy counter and are only sold by a registered pharmacist. Further, such items may be unavailable in confectionary or grocery stores that stock other non-restricted OTC medications. For example, many U.S. drug stores have moved products containing pseudoephedrine and emergency contraception, an OTC product, into locations where customers must ask a pharmacist for them and must obtain counselling and education and seller must record the identity of the purchaser and enforce quantity restrictions. In other example Viagra sold in UK as restricted OTC drug to 30-65 years of male and restricted to take only 4 tablets under the guidance of registered pharmacist.

Another survey data suggests that 1/3 of consumers using on OTC drug exceeds the doses recommended on labels in an effort to obtain a benefit. However, the package label on OTC drug does not address all relevant issues surrounding co-morbidities and polypharmacy. The inadequacy of labelling is confounded by the functional illiteracy rate, which is approximately 20% in USA.

Reasons why it is Essential for Clinicians to be Familiar with OTC Drugs

(i) Many OTC medications are effective in treating common ailments, and it is important to be able to help the patients to select a safe, effective product.

(ii) Many of the ingredients of OTC drugs may worsen existing medical conditions or interact with prescription medications.

(iii) Misuse or abuse of OTC products may actually produce significant medical complications e.g., phenylpropanolamine used in many cold, allergy and weight control products causing haemorrhagic strokes.

Potential Effect on Health Care of Switching the Status of Prescription Drugs to Over-the-Counter Drugs

Possible Benefits

1. **Greater access to effective therapy**

   Due to financial, transportation or scheduling limitation, many patients can't visit medical professional. By switching, there will be increased access to effective drugs. To estimate patients access to drugs, sales volume can be used as a surrogate marker. In a study in Sweden, 16 drugs when switched from prescription only to OTC status showed 36% increase in sales of drugs. In USA, when 0.5% hydrocortisone was made available as OTC drug, there was an increase in sales from $12 million to $88 million. Likewise, sales of diphenylhydramine quintupled after its status was changed to OTC drug.

2. **Lower health care cost by decreasing frequency of visits to physicians**

   Carlsten and colleagues studied 16 products, and they estimated saving of $30 million to the Swedish health care system on the basis of number of provider visits required to generate the prescription subsequently represented in over the counter sales. In the analysis done by the Consumer Health Care Products Association, there was saving of $20 billion in 1996 in USA due to sale of OTC drugs.

3. **Increased in autonomy and education of patients**

   Because of several cultural and social trends, there is increased interest among patients in self-care and in control over their medical treatment. According to survey data, consumers think that some prescriptions should be made available OTC and it will results in cost saving. They also believe that OTC drugs that were previously available only by prescription are more effective than products that have always been available OTC. The educational material and support services that were provided by manufacturers may improve patient's knowledge and leads to increase compliance as in nicotine products for smoking cessation.

Possible Risks

1. **Self-diagnosis-inaccurate**

   OTC drug administration relies on patient's judgement, supplemented by the information on the label, for correct diagnosis of the disorder or symptom. But, an incorrect diagnosis may cause treating the disorder with OTC drugs which has no efficacy in the present condition e.g., inability to distinguish fungal vaginitis from other similar condition. Complication of misdiagnosis involve not only the risks associated with lack of treatment but also the potential of drug causing adverse effects.

2. **Issue of suboptional or delayed treatment of serious conditions**

This is of particular concern in treating some chronic asymptomatic conditions, such as hypercholesterolemia. Generally, the drugs available as OTC which is inferior to standard drug or which is 2nd line therapy may distort pattern of care away from superior treatment available by prescription only. Some manufacturers have now sought to merge the marketing of OTC drugs with the recommendation that patients seek professional assistance before and during the therapy.

In actual use trials for approval to market, a statin without a prescription, it was observed that large number of patients thought that the drug was approved for them, even though, they were not included in the definition of qualified users provided on the label. Similar issues are involved in antihypertensive drugs for OTC availability and other chronic disorders.

3. **Inappropriate use of drugs and associated risks**

Safety data submitted to switch a drug from prescription to OTC status come from clinical trials and post-marketing studies. In the case of OTC drugs, more patients at high risks will be exposed to drugs with unknown consequences than would be exposed if the drug required a prescription. Post Marketing Surveillance (PMS) data can provide only limited reassurance concerning such risk because of limitations of such non-systematically collected data. Some classes of drugs are at particular risk when made widely available e.g., increased use of not prescribed antimicrobial agents may increase the problem of drug resistance.

Though such issues are of more concern with public health importance than the risk associated with individual patterns, it has contributed to non-approval of acyclovir as OTC drug.

4. **Change in physician's role in supervising care**

Certain types of encounter between patients and physician may cease, and expectation on part of patients may change by increasing availability of OTC drugs. Patients might not present early in the course of illness. Also tracking of all the drugs used by patients may be highly difficult. Although some physicians support OTC availability as a means of removing barriers to care, they are often concerned when drugs used in their own specialty are proposed for OTC status.

How You can Select and use OTC Drugs?

If people want to use the OTC drugs for their common problems such as cold, fever, body ache, headache, spasm or any acute pain etc., they should be clear and confident enough regarding:

Diagnosis:

- Self-diagnosis should be as accurate as possible

Selection of OTC Drug

- Always choose the products as per their ingredients and not because the product has a familiar brand name.
- Always try to choose monotherapy instead of polytherapy (multiple ingredients in a formulation).
- Always read the insert label before use carefully to determine the appropriate dose, duration and precautions if any.

Administering CAUTIONS

- If case of doubt, ask a registered pharmacist or doctor for their ingredients, use and precautions.
- Always ask a registered pharmacist to check for potential interactions with other concomitant use of drugs and their side effects.
- Never take more than the recommended standard dose.
- Duration of OTC drug should be checked with registered pharmacist either one or two dose or need to take longer.
- Always vigilant for any side effects and stop taking the drug if symptoms worsen or any ADR occurs.

Switches between Prescription and OTC

After the approval of drugs for the marketing, drugs are available for prescription drugs. After its safe use in clinics for 3-5 to 10 years, drugs have been proven safe and effective. If regulatory bodies accept its safety profile then, may be switched from prescription to OTC. As a golden rule, OTC drugs are considered safe as compared to prescription drugs and do not require the direct supervision of a doctor. E.g., diphenhydramine (Antihistamine), cimetidine and loratadine (H_2-receptor antagonists), ibuprofen and paracetamol (NSAIDs) etc. Among the different properties OTC drugs may also have little or no abuse or habit forming potential but in some areas drugs such as codeine are available as OTC.

The rate of switches from prescription to OTC status has accelerated. Indeed, more than 700 OTC products contain ingredients and dosages that were available only by prescription less than 30 years ago.

Considerations in Reclassifying a Drug as OTC

Safety

- Has the drug been used for a long enough time so that any harmful effects are fully understood?
- What harmful effects (including those from misuse) may the drug produce?
- Is the drug habit forming?
- Do the benefits of OTC status outweigh the risks?

Ease of diagnosis and treatment

- Can the average person self-diagnose the condition that calls for the drug?
- Can the average person treat the condition without the help of a doctor or other health care practitioner?

Labelling

- Can adequate directions for use be written?
- Can warnings against unsafe use be written?
- Can the average person understand the information on the label?

Drugs Previously available by Prescription and now available on OTC

1. H_1-receptor antagonist

    Diphenhydramine

2. H_2-receptor antagonists

    Cimetidine

    Ranitidine

    Famotidine

3. NSAIDs

    Acetaminophen

    Ibuprofen

    Naproxen

    Ketoprofen

4. Smoking-cessation aids

    Nicotine (gum and patches)

5. Hair-growth stimulants

    Minoxidil (2% and 5%)

6. Antifungal drugs

    Clotrimazole

    Ketoconazole

7. Antidiarrheal drugs

    Loperamide

8. Decongestants

    Pseudo ephedrine

Other prescription drugs, currently under consideration for OTC reclassification include cyclobenzaprine, sucralfate, non-sedating antihistamines (cetrizine, fexofenadine) and topical penciclovir. OTC drugs are found comparatively safe but unusually withdrawn from the market as a result of safety concerns e.g., phenylpropanolamine was removed from sale in the United States over concern regarding strokes in young women. In other incidence chemist tried to sell Viagra as OTC in chemist stores in Manchester, England, in United Kingdom as restricted OTC substances.

OTC Drugs and Drug Interactions

OTC Drug	Prescription Drug	Adverse Effect
Acetaminophen	Antibiotics rifampin and isoniazid (INH)	Increased risk of liver damage
Aspirin	Diabetes medicines such as chlorpropamide, insulin and others	Aspirin increases the blood-sugar-lowering effects
	Anti-seizure drugs such as phenytoin and valproic acid.	Increased anti-seizure drug levels in blood
NSAIDs, including: Aspirin Ibuprofen Ketoprofen Naproxen	Anti-cancer drug methotrexate drugs to suppress the immune system, such as cyclosporine, heart medicines such as digoxin	NSAIDs reduce clearance of methotrexate, cyclosporine and digoxin and increase their blood level
	Beta –blockers such as propranolol, metoprolol and atenolol	NSAIDS reduce the blood-pressure-lowering effects
	Diuretics	NSAIDS decrease effectiveness of diuretics
Acetaminophen Ibuprofen Naproxen sodium	Oral anticoagulants such as warfarin	Acetaminophen and NSAIDs increase the effect
	Lithium	Ibuprofen and naproxen reduce renal clearance of lithium
Antihistamines Brompheniramine Chlorpheniramine Dimenhydrinate Diphenhydramine Doxylamine	Sleeping pills, sedatives, muscle relaxants, anti-anxiety drugs, including alprazolam diazepam, lorazepam, temazepam and others	These antihistamines increase the depressant effects (for example, sleepiness) of sleeping pills, sedatives, muscle relaxants or anti-anxiety drugs on the central nervous system (brain)
Decongestants Pseudoephedrine	Monoamine oxidase inhibitors including isocarboxazid, phenelzine, selegiline and tranylcypromine.	Pseudoephedrine can cause dangerous increases in blood pressure and heart rhythm problems when taken with MAOIs
Cough Medicines Dextromethorphan	Monoamine oxidase inhibitors	Dextromethorphan, when taken with MAOIs, can cause "serotonin syndrome" with symptoms such as agitation, high body temperature, sweating, rapid heart rate, and trouble moving
	Sedatives or tranquilizers	Dextromethorphan increases the sedative effects of the sedatives or tranquilizers

Conclusions

The increased availability of drugs as OTC is a two-edged sword which has both potential benefits and risks associated with them. In one hand, they improve the access to effective therapies, saves the time of both physician and patient and they are generally cost-saving, but on the other hand, there is concern about patient's self-diagnosis, possible drug interaction, delay in seeking appropriate treatment or inappropriate use with associated adverse effects. Advances in technology may facilitate the growth of OTC drug therapy. In future, more drugs will be available as OTC and for varieties of new indications for their use. A nation cannot afford the luxury of having consumers and health professionals trivializing or undervaluing non-prescription drug therapy as a critical component of health care.

Suggested Readings

1. Alastair J.J. Wood (2001). Changing The Status of Drugs From Prescription to Over-the-Counter Availability. *N Eng J Med* **345:** 810-816.

2. Bansal V, Dhamija P, Medhi B, Pandhi P (2006). Package inserts-do they have any role? *JK- Practitioner* **13(3):** 152-154.

3. Bradley B, McCusker E, Scott E, Li Wan Po A (1995). Patient information leaflets on over-the-counter (OTC) medicines: the manufacturer's perspective. *J Clin Pharm Ther* **20:** 37-40.

4. Brewer T, Colditz GA (1999). Postmarketing surveillance and adverse drug reactions: current perspective and future needs. *JAMA* **281:** 824-829.

5. Consumer survey on self-medication. Washington D.C.: Consumer Healthcare Products Assosiation 2001.www.chpa-info.org.

6. Gossel TA (1991). Implication of the reclassification of drugs from prescription only to over the counter status. *Clin Ther* **13:** 200-215.

7. Juhl RP (1998). Prescription to over-the-counter switch: a regulatory perspective. *Clin Ther* **20:** Suppl C: C111-C117.

8. OTC facts and figures. Washington, DC: Consumer Healthcare Products Association 2001. www.chpa-info.org.

9. OTC sales by Category. Washington D.C.; Consumer Healthcare Products Association, 2001 [www.chpa-info.org].

10. Robin L. Corelli (2007). Therapeutic and Toxic Potential of Over-the-Counter Agents. In, Basic and Clinical Pharmacology. [Bertran G Katzung, ed.], Mc Graw Hill, Asia, 1041-1049.

11. Rosenau PV (1994). Rx to OTC switch movement. *Med Care Rev* **51:** 429-466.

12. Sande MA, Armstrong D, CoreyL (1998). Perspective on switching oral acyclovir from prescription to over the counter status: report of a consensus panel. *Clin Infect Dis* **26:** 659-663.

13. Schulke DG (1998). American Pharmaceutical Association review of literature on prescription to over the counter drug switches. *Clin Ther* **20:** Suppl C: C124-C133.

14. Wedgeworth R (2003). The number of functionally illiterate adults in U.S. is growing. National Assessment of Adults Literacy Proliteracy Worldwide, 2003.

CHAPTER 5

RATIONAL USE OF DRUGS

Introduction

Rational Use of Drugs (RUD), convened by the World Health Organization (WHO) in Nairobi in 1985 as follows: Rational use of drugs require that patients receive medicines appropriate to their clinical needs, in doses that meet their own individual requirements, for an adequate period of time, and at the lowest cost to them and their community (Fig. 5.1).

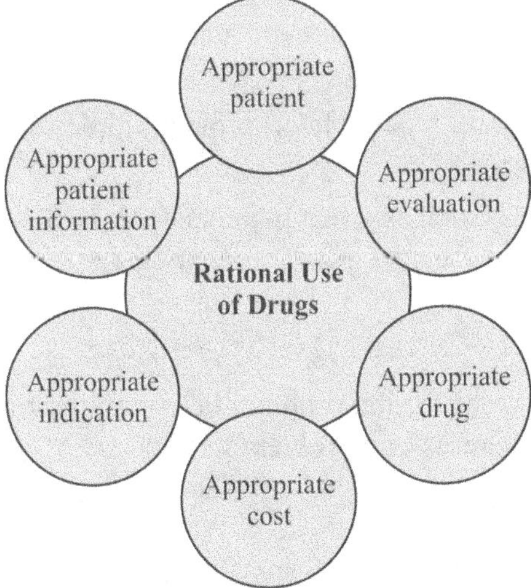

Fig. 5.1 Principle components of rational drug use.

Prescribing patterns do not always conform to these criteria and can be classified as inappropriate or irrational prescribing.

Status of Drug Use

Global sales of medicines in 2004 amounted to about US$ 550 000 million and 10% to 40% of health budgets are spent on medicines. Evidence suggests that more than half of all medicines in developing countries and a substantial proportion of medicines, particularly antibiotics, in developed countries are prescribed, dispensed and consumed inappropriately, leading to wastage of resources and widespread health hazards. Examples of irrational use of medicines include: use of too many medicines per patient ("poly-pharmacy"); inappropriate use of antimicrobials, often in inadequate dosage, for non-bacterial infections; over-use of injections when oral formulations would be more appropriate; failure to prescribe in accordance with clinical guidelines; inappropriate self-medication, often of prescription-only medicines; non-adherence to dosing regimes.

Disadvantages of Irrationality

The impact of this irrational use of drugs can be seen in many ways:

- *Morbidity and mortality:* Reduction in the quality of drug therapy leading to poor patient outcomes, increased morbidity and mortality.

- *Financial hardship:* Waste of resources leading to reduced availability of other vital drugs and increased costs. It has been estimated to cost annually US$ 4000-5000 million in the United States of America and $ 9000 million in Europe according to WHO 2007 data.

- *Harm to patients:* Increased risk of unwanted effects such as adverse drug reactions.

- *Drug resistance emergence:* Malaria or multiple drug resistant tuberculosis, antimicrobial resistance.

- Psychosocial impacts, such as when patients come to believe that there is "a pill for every ill". This may cause an apparent increased demand for drugs.

Cause of Irrational use-Different Stakeholders

Always understand the reasons for the problem behaviour before starting an intervention. Following are the possible causes of a problem in drug use.

Health Care Professionals

- Lack of knowledge about diagnosis, therapeutics, or the efficacy and risks of particular drugs
- Acquired habits in diagnosis and treatment that may not reflect what providers actually know, but are patterns of behavior they have come to adopt
- Polypharmacy (prescribing multiple drugs)
- Patient driven prescribing

- Over prescribing of antibiotics
- Lack of specific standard treatment protocols
- Incomplete prescription
- Beliefs about illness and drugs, such as increased power of injections over oral drugs, which do not always reflect their level of scientific knowledge
- Personal economic motivations for prescribing or dispensing particular drugs, such as drug company incentives, dispensing fees, and referrals to private practice

Patients and Providers Interactions

- Socio-cultural attitudes and beliefs, including social distance and cultural barriers between patient and provider, beliefs about illness, or provider beliefs about patient expectations
- Quality of communication, which may be influenced by the setting, underlying beliefs and attitudes, language barriers, or a number of other factors
- Patient demand for specific drugs or forms of treatment (like injections)

Work Environment of HealthCare Professionals

- Authority and power relationships such as relationships with supervisors, criteria for performance evaluation, and practices of opinion leaders
- Influence of drug availability, due to purchase restrictions, irregular supply, overstocked products
- Availability of diagnostic services, such as diagnostic equipment or laboratory facilities
- Limitations of the physical environment, such as lack of privacy for consultation during examination or dispensing
- Workload, which may limit the ability of providers to spend an adequate amount of time with each patient
- Institutional economic motivations, such as the need to sell drugs to generate recurrent revenues or to capitalize revolving drug funds

Drug Information and Marketing

- Poor availability of scientific information about drugs provided by neutral scientific or professional organizations
- Availability of potentially biased information about drugs provided by drug companies
- Marketing pressure by industry, including media advertising, sales visits by industry representatives, and industry-sponsored "educational" meetings

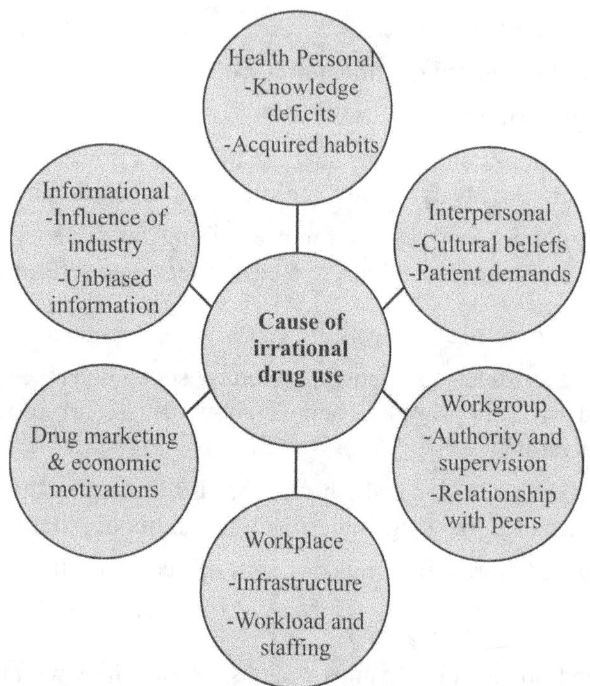

Description of Drug use Practices by Drug Use Indicators (DUI)

Experience from many countries has encouraged the development of a standard method of measuring drug use practices, based on drug use indicators. These indicators include the processes of making a diagnosis, prescribing, dispensing, and using of drugs by the patient. DUI indicators are divided into three groups: Prescribing Indicators; Patient Care Indicators; and Facility Indicators. The list of the indicators follows:

Prescribing Indicators

1. Average number of drugs per prescription
2. Percentage of drugs prescribed by generic name
3. Percentage of prescriptions with an antibiotic prescribed
4. Percentage of prescriptions with an injection prescribed
5. Percentage of drugs prescribed from Essential Drugs List or Formulary

Patient Care Indicators

1. Average consultation time
2. Average dispensing time
3. Percentage of drugs actually dispensed

4. Percentage of drugs adequately labeled

5. Patient's knowledge of correct dosage

Facility Indicators

1. Availability of Copy of Essential Drugs List or Formulary

2. Availability of key drugs

DIUs are used to measure drug use in a representative group, to compare facilities, providers, or groups at a single time, to identify whether a facility is above or below a set norm of practice, to assess the impact of an intervention in an intervention group and a control group, by measuring indicators before and after. The basic design of an indicators study carried out to characterize drug use practices in a region would call for a sample of at least 20 health facilities, with at least 30 prescriptions being recorded in each facility.

Strategies to make Drug use Rational

Ideally, therapeutically sound and cost-effective use of medicines by health professionals and consumers is achieved at all levels of the health system, and in both the public and the private sectors. A sound rational drug use program in any country has three elements:

Rational medicine use strategy and monitoring: Support countries in implementing and monitoring a national strategy to promote rational use of medicines by health professionals and consumers.

Rational medicine use by health professionals: Develop national standard treatment guidelines, essential medicine lists, educational programs and other effective mechanisms to promote medicine use by health professionals.

Rational medicine use by consumers: Establishing effective medication information systems to provide independent and unbiased medicine information including on traditional medicine – to the general public and to improve medicine use by consumers.

The above elements were developed in close collaboration with the regional and country offices.

Examples of Strategies to Improve Drug Use

1. Knowledge enhancement of health professional

Training

- Medical curriculum (Pre-service Training)
- Short term Training (In-service Training)

Face-to-Face Interactive Discussion/Persuasion

- Symposium/Seminar/Lectures
- Panel or Small Group Discussion
- Clinical Supervision or Consultation
- Influence by Opinion Leaders
- Demonstration of Patient Counseling

Printed Educational Materials

- Drug Formulary and Standard Treatment Guidelines
- Newsletters, Drug Bulletins, Clinical Literature
- Illustrated Persuasive Materials (Flyers, Posters)

Media-oriented Approaches

- Public Health Spots in Newspapers, Radio, Television
- Audiovisual aids
- Direct mailing
- Internet

2. Role of dispensers/pharmacists

- The dispenser should receive the correct prescription, verify origin, validity, relevant instructions, information on patient, therapeutic appropriateness, economic consideration of the prescription. Communicates with prescribers for dubious or unclear instructions.
- Correctly interprets the prescription or instructions on the prescription: name of drugs, dosages, administration, and duration
- The medicine should not expired or damaged
- Communicates the correct way to take the medication to the patient through good labeling so that patient understands the instructions
- Keeps accurate records of operations.

3. Managerial: Structure or guide decisions

Selection and Procurement

- Essential Drug Lists/Drug Formularies
- Morbidity-Based Quantification to Guide Drug Supply
- Pack/Kit System Distribution

Prescribing and Dispensing

- Structured Drug Prescribing Forms
- Standardized Diagnostic and Treatment Protocols
- Prescription Audits plus "Feedback" to Prescribers
- Effective Clinical Supervision
- Improvements in Packaging or Labeling
- Pharmacovigilance system

Drug Pricing

- Low price of essential drugs
- Manpower Development
- Rational Drug Use Team
- Central Drug Committee
- Hospital Drug and Therapeutics Committees
- Tutors in Training Institutions

4. Regulatory: Restrict decisions

Market Controls

- Drug Registration or Ban of Certain Drugs based on medical need
- Changes in Product Registration/labeling

Prescribing and Dispensing Controls

- Level of use distribution/prescribing restrictions
- Limits on which drugs are supplied in public sector
- Restrictions for specific drugs to higher levels of care
- Requirements for generic prescribing
- Allowing generic substitution of branded drugs
- Limits on number or quantity of drugs per patient

The most effective interventions often combine different aspects of knowledge enhancement, managerial, and regulatory strategies to achieve maximum impact.

Decision Making for Rational Drug Use Interventions

Problem of irrational drug use is by and largely persists all over the world in various parts of health care set up. After identification of a drug use problem in an institution, an area, or a country, action to remedy the problem usually follows. To decide which intervention(s) will be most effective, preliminary study is required.

First, the drug use problem should be clearly defined, along with identification of its all contributing, motivating factors. Then the possible interventions are assessed. Once these possibilities have been listed, the difficult task of choosing one or two interventions should occur. When more than one intervention is selected, each should be of a different type (regulatory, managerial, and knowledge enhancement).

When the intervention is undertaken, it is important that there should be a control group and the sample sizes must be adequate to detect differences if they exist.

After completion of the control study, the results should be assessed and follow-up decided. In a few cases, the intervention may be clearly effective, and such interventions can then be translated into national programs.

Standard Treatment Guidelines

Because of differing decisions about drug choices and the patterns of illness within a country, even in presence of essential drug lists, there exists ample opportunity for ineffective, unsafe, or wasteful prescribing. This problem can be settled by *Standard Treatment Guidelines* - also known as Standard Treatment Schedules (STS); standard treatment protocols; therapeutic guidelines; and so forth list the preferred drug and non-drug treatments for common health problems experienced by people in a specific health system. Each drug treatment should include for each health problem the name, dosage form, strength, average dose (pediatric and adult), number of doses per day, and number of days of treatment. Potential benefits of introducing standard treatments include:

For Patients

- Treatment efficacy
- Increased compliance
- Good availability of economic drugs/treatment due to improved supply

For Health Professional

- Provider can concentrate on correct diagnosis
- Provide a standard to assess quality of care
- Simplification of monitoring and supervision
- Reduced confusion in prescribing.

For Drug Suppliers

- Improved drug supply/production
- Pre-packaging facilitated for course-of-therapy

For Health Policy Makers

- Method for drug price control
- Facilitate integration of special programs (diarrhea disease control, acute respiratory infection, tuberculosis control, malaria, and so on) at the primary health care facilities.

In the development of standard treatments, following are the important considerations.

1. Target priority conditions
2. Base on local disease factors
3. Coordinate with special programs
4. Use fewest drugs necessary
5. Choose cost-effective treatments
6. Use essential drug list drugs only
7. Involve respected clinicians
8. Consider patient perspective

Role of WHO

In the world health assembly held in April 2009, provisional agenda was prepared for WHO's leadership in promoting rational use of medicines which include:

1. Undertaking evidence-based information on patterns of medicines use and on the impact of interventions on medicines use;
2. Strengthening coordination of international support;
3. Promoting research on sustainable interventions;
4. Promoting discussion among health authorities, professionals and patients.
5. Technical support to countries on various aspects of promoting rational use of medicines which includes review of essential medicines lists, development and implementation of clinical guidelines, monitoring of medicines use practices, interventions to correct drug-use problems, and training of health professionals and consumers.

The suggestions on behalf of WHO for governments, the health professions, civil society, the private sector and the international community for rational use of medicines include:

1. Establishing and/or strengthening, as appropriate, a national drug regulatory authority and a full national program and/or multidisciplinary body, involving civil society and professional bodies, to monitor and promote the rational use of medicine.

2. Application of an essential medicines list into the benefit package of the existing or new insurance funds.

3. Training programs on rational use of medicines, to be incorporated in the curricula for all health professionals and medical students, including their continuing education, where appropriate, and to promote programs of public education in rational use of medicines.

4. To enact new, or enforce existing, legislation to ban inaccurate, misleading or unethical promotion of medicines, to monitor promotion of medicines, and to develop and implement programs that will provide independent, non-promotional information about medicines.

5. To consider developing, and strengthening where appropriate, the capacity of hospital drug and therapeutic committees to promote the rational use of medicines.

6. To expand to national level sustainable interventions successfully implemented at local level.

Role of other Organizations

Several international organizations are playing actively for implementation of rational use of medicines worldwide. International Conferences on Improving Use of Medicines (ICIUM) was held twice in 1997 and 2004, as part of a global effort for improvement of medicines use in non-industrialized countries. The objectives are to reach consensus on the past and ongoing programs, long term strategies for improving the use of medicines worldwide, to define evidence-based recommendations for program implementation, and to generate global research agendas to fill gaps in knowledge. These conferences assembled leading national and international policy makers, program managers, researchers, clinicians, and other stakeholders to produce up to date harmony for achievement of rational use of medicines. The ICIUM 2004 Conference was collaboratively organized by the following organizations:

- Boston University School of Public Health Center for International Health and Development

- Harvard Medical School Department of Ambulatory Care & Prevention

- International Network for Rational Use of Drugs

- Rational Pharmaceutical Management Plus (RPM Plus)

- Strategies for Enhancing Access to Medicines (SEAM)

- Thai Network for Rational Use of Drugs

- World Health Organization Department of Essential Drugs and Medicines Policy

The **International Network for Rational Use of Drugs (INRUD)** was established in 1989 to design, test, and disseminate effective strategies to improve the way drugs are prescribed, dispensed, and used, with a particular emphasis on resource poor countries. The network comprises 24 groups - 20 from Africa, Asia, Latin America, and Eastern Europe, and other groups from the World Health Organization/Medicines Policy and Standards, the Harvard Medical School Department of Ambulatory Care, the Karolinska Institute in Sweden, and a secretariat based in Management Sciences for Health in the United States.

Conclusion

Hence, for the success of rational use of drugs, there should be an improved communication with professional (doctor) and population (patients); is needed. There should be better planning (diagnosis), objective-setting (drug treatment) and materials (availability and cost of drugs). Overall public education in rational drug use is needed and can work better as compared to other practices.

Suggested Readings

1. Daphne A. Fresle, Cathy Wolfheim. Public Education in Rational Drug Use: a Global Survey. World Health Organization, Geneva, March 1997.

2. Grimshaw JG, Russell IT (1993). Effect of Clinical Guidelines on Medical Practice: A Systematic Review of Rigorous Evaluations. *Lancet.* **342:** 1317.

3. Hogerzeil HV (1995). Promoting Rational Prescribing: An International Perspective. *Br J Clin Pharmacol.* **39:** 1-6.

4. Hogerzeil HV, *et al.,* (1993). Field Tests for Rational Drug Use in Twelve Developing Countries. *Lancet.* **342:** 1408-1410.

5. International Conferences on Improving Use of Medicines (ICIUM 2004)

6. Laing R, Hogerzeil HV, Ross-Degnan D (2001). Ten Recommendations to Improve the Use of Medicines in Developing Countries. *Health Policy Plan.* **16(1):** 13-20.

7. Progress in the rational use of medicines. Report by the Secretariat. 16 World Health Assembly A60/24. Provisional agenda item 12.17 22 March 2007.

8. Progress reports on technical and health matters. Report by the Secretariat. Rational Use of Medicines (resolution WHA60.16). Sixty-Second World Health Assembly A62/23. Provisional agenda item 12.18 9 April 2009

9. Promoting Rational Drug Use. Course Materials (Year 2000). http://archives.who.int/PRDUC2004/RDUCD/TOC.htm

10. Rational Drug Use. Sultanate of Oman. Ministry of Health. The Directorate General of Pharmaceutical Affairs and Drug Control. May 2000.

11. S.D. Seth (2004). Essential drugs and Rational Therapeutics Text book of Pharmacology 2nd Ed. 907-916.

12. Ten recommendations to improve use of medicines in developing countries. Health Policy and planning; **16(1):** 13-20, Oxford University Press 2001.

13. The International Network for Rational Use of Drugs (INRUD); http://www1.msh.org/global-presence/INRUD.cfm

CHAPTER 6

SELF-MEDICATION

Introduction

Self-medication is the use of non-prescription medicines (such as OTC drugs) by people on their own initiative. It is the process of treatment of common health problems with medicines especially designed and labelled for use without medical supervision and approved as safe and effective for such use.

Paracelsus (1493-1541), the alchemist-physician, in the 16th century observed that *"all drugs are poisons"*. The availability of potent and dangerous drugs has increased considerably since the close of the 19th century. At the same time expanding availability of medical care, exposes a large population of people to drugs, leading to a greater number of risks. This situation is further worsened in our country by the slack implementation of *"Drug Control"*. Even certain prescription drugs are available to the lay person without the physician's advice. As people vary greatly in their sensitivity to drugs, an appropriate dose for one person can be an overdose for another. Even skilled physicians sometimes fail to avoid such reactions. Thus, the lay person is ill-advised in subjecting himself to potentially dangerous self-medication.

Self-medication usually involves common drugs which are freely available as OTC. A study carried out in the United States showed that nearly 2 billion dollars per year spent on such remedies. It is questionable whether the benefits outweigh the potential hazards and further, account for poisonings, allergy, habituation, addiction, and other adverse reactions. Above all their use often delays proper treatment of the disease.

Great English philosopher-physician Sir William Osler (1849-1919) who said, *"One of the first duties of the physician is to educate the masses when not to take medicines"*.

It has been estimated that between 70% to 90% of all illness episodes are handled by some form of self-treatment and are not brought to the attention of a health professional. While most people apparently rely on self-care as the predominant mode of treatment for daily symptoms, the ways in which they actually experience specific symptoms and decide on appropriate therapeutic actions are not readily apparent.

Laypersons do indeed carry on extensive medication activities as a regular aspect of family life. For example, Knapp & Knapp studied decision making and self-medication and found that, on average, families deal with an illness episode every four days. Similarly, a number of other studies have reported that self-medication (using prescription and/or non-prescription drugs) is the most frequent daily response to symptoms. According to Roghmann and Haggerty, 93% of adult are self-medicated. Studies in both Great Britain and the United States have demonstrated that household stocking of drugs is common. The evidence indicates that families have greater access to non-prescribed drugs and their use exceeds that of prescribed drugs. However, it is important to realize that self-treatment does not only involve the use of non-prescribed medications. The use of prescribed drugs can also be included within the rubric of self-care if, it is based on lay decision making. Obviously, the actual consumption of medicines (including prescribed ones) is clearly under the direct control of the lay individual/consumers.

Altering the way in which medically prescribed drugs are used may be interpreted as a form of self-care. This type of behavior may involve getting the prescription filled but not taking the medication, changing the prescribed dosage level or length of use, sharing prescribed medications with other household members, or simply saving un-used drugs for long periods of time and taking them for subsequent self-diagnosed illness episodes. Thus, prescribed drugs may be a significant element in self-medication activities.

"Irrational" use of pharmaceuticals, in particular self-medication with antibiotics, has been widely reported leading the World Health Organization to call attention to the dangers of self-medication as a cause of antibiotic resistance. In addition to the problem of resistant microbial strains resulting from the inappropriate use of antibiotics, drug side-effects, allergic reactions and toxicity have become a cause of alarm.

The rising tendency for people in developing countries to self-medicate with commercial medicines has been associated with marked decreases in thresholds of tolerance for symptoms, greater familiarity with drugs and medicine vendors, changing health concerns related to defective modernization (e.g., environmental degradation, adulteration of food), dramatic increases in the number of products available in the marketplace and changes in the purchasing power of consumers. Now a days, health is becoming increasingly pharmaceuticalized and commoditised as more and more people conveniently *"reach for the pill"* at the first sign of ill health or malaise.

Health is being treated as a state which one can obtain (or maintain) through the consumption of medicines, even under adverse conditions, if one has the capital to invest. In India, for example, environmental degradation and a rising concern for food adulteration has been accompanied by the proliferation of pharmaceuticals marketed to purify and protect the body. Attention has also been called to the role played by pharmacists and shop attendants in fostering self-medication and medicine experimentation among the public. Studies in several local chemists and dispensaries have reported that these are not only sites where medicines are bought and sold, they are also places where information and advice on health problems and treatment is sought.

Some studies have found that it is fairly routine for people to seek the advice of pharmacists and medicine shop attendants for common ailments. Such consultations are convenient: it save time, money and the opportunity cost of waiting to be seen by a doctor. Clients who directly consult pharmacy personnel for medications often have unrealistic expectations. They expect immediate demonstration effects from the medicines they purchase. Therefore, it has been suggested that pharmacy personnel tend to recommend medicines which have dramatic effects as well as lucrative profit margins.

Drugs are often stored for long periods at the patient's home, and leftover medication may later be considered for self-medication, especially when only manufacturer's standard package sizes are used and drug repackaging to tailored amounts is not allowed. The readability of package inserts (i.e., drug information for patients provided by the manufacturer and enclosed in the drug package) is suboptimal and package inserts are thought to be read by only one-third of patients.

Finally, even when instructions on use are given by healthcare professionals at the time of prescription or delivery, this information may have faded from memory when self-initiated treatment is started. Numerous drug utilization reviews have been published in recent years. Few of them discriminate, however, between prescribed and self-initiated use of drugs, and even fewer provide documentation on the general intention to self-medicate or on the nature and size of drug reserves at people's homes. The regular lack of a safe storage space for medicines and the frequent occurrence of drug containers without a package insert raise concern. Although the intention for self-treatment was mostly acceptable in terms of indication and dosage, high rates of intended self-medication with prescription drugs and a significantly higher intention to self-medicate by younger people represent potential health threats.

Thus, to avoid or minimize the dangers of self-medication, *firstly,* the lay person should be educated about the dangers of indiscriminate use of drugs. *Secondly,* the physicians should be more judicious in prescribing, and must insist on drugs being supplied by the chemist only on a valid prescription. *Thirdly,* a proper statutory "Drug Control" must be implemented, rationally restricting the availability of drugs to the public. These *three* measures would definitely reduce the incidence of drug-related mishaps, and help in maintaining good health of the individual and society.

The World Medical Association (WMA) has developed this statement to provide guidance to physicians and their patients regarding responsible self-medication.

1. Distinction between Self-Medication and Prescription Medicine

(a) Medicinal products can generally be divided into two separate categories: prescription and non-prescription medicines. This classification may differ from country to country. The National Regulatory Authorities must assure that medicines, categorized as non-prescription medicines or OTC medicine *(for details see chapter 4 Over the Counter (OTC) drugs)*.

(b) Prescription medicines are those which are only available to individuals on prescription from a physician following a consultation. Prescription medicines are not safe for use except under the supervision of a physician because of toxicity, other potential or harmful effects (e.g., addictiveness), the method of use, or the collateral measures necessary for use.

(c) Responsible self-medication, as used in this document, is the use of a registered or monographed medicine legally available without a physician's prescription, either on an individual's own initiative or following advice of a healthcare professional. The use of prescription medicines without a prior medical prescription is not part of responsible self-medication.

(d) The safety, efficacy and quality of non-prescription medicines must be proved according to the same principles as prescription medicines.

2. Use of Self-Medication in Conjunction with Prescription Medication

A course of treatment may combine self-medication and prescription medication, either concurrently or sequentially. The patient must be informed about possible interactions between prescription medicines and non-prescription medicines. For this reason, the patient should be encouraged to inform the physician about his/her self-medication.

3. Roles & Responsibilities in Self-Medication

(a) In self-medication, the individual bears primary responsibility for the use of self-medication products. Special caution must be exercised when vulnerable groups such as children, elderly people or pregnant women use self-medication.

(b) If individuals choose to use self-medication, they should be able:

    (i)   to recognize the symptoms they are treating;

    (ii) to determine that their condition is suitable for self-medication;

    (iii) to choose an appropriate self-medication product;

    (iv) to follow the directions for use of the product as provided in the product labelling.

(c) In order to limit, the potential risks involved in self-medication it is important that all health professionals who look after patients should provide:

    (i) Education regarding the non-prescription medicine and its appropriate use, and instructions to seek further advice from a physician if they are unsure. This is particularly important where self-medication is inappropriate for certain conditions the patient may suffer from;

    (ii) Encouragement to read carefully a product's label and leaflet (if provided), to seek further advice if necessary, and to recognize circumstances in which self-medication is not, or is no longer, appropriate.

(d) Individuals involved in self-medication should be aware of the benefits and risks of any self-medication product. The benefit-risk balance should be communicated in a fair, rational manner without overemphasizing either the risks or the benefits.

(e) Manufacturers in particular are obliged to follow the various codes or regulations already in place to ensure that information provided to consumers is appropriate in style and content. This refers in particular to the labelling, advertising and all notices concerning non-prescription medicines.

(f) The pharmacist has a professional responsibility to recommend, in appropriate circumstances, that medical advice be sought.

4. Role of Governments in Self-Medication

Governments should recognize and enforce the distinction between prescription and non-prescription medicines, and ensure that the users of self-medication are well informed and protected from possible harm or negative long-term effects.

5. The Promotion and Marketing of Self-Medication Products

(a) Advertising and marketing of non-prescription medicines should be responsible, provide clear and accurate information and exhibit a fair balance between benefit and risk information. Promotion and marketing should not encourage irresponsible self-medication, purchase of medicines that are inappropriate, or purchases of larger quantities of medicines than are necessary.

(b) People must be encouraged to treat medicines (prescription and non-prescription) as special products and that standard instructions should be followed in terms of safe storage and usage, in accordance with professional advice.

The trend towards increased self care and, with it, self medication with ever more powerful drugs seems unstoppable. The potential benefits of this trend, with the increasing empowerment of patients, are many. Nevertheless, developments in self medication will need to be carefully managed if these benefits are to be maximised and the potential risks kept to a minimum. Greater collaboration between doctors and pharmacists will be critical and joint training on OTC medicines is helpful. In addition, professional bodies and consumer and patient groups need to look closely at how they can build stronger alliances.

The increasing scope for self medication and its likely consequences can be seen as a shift from "primary care" of both minor and stable health care problems to "self care". Whether this transition occurs smoothly or not depends to a large extent on the attitudes and responses of the primary health care professionals involved, and whether they view this as a positive or negative development. It will also depend on how well informed and equipped the consumers are to take on the burden of self care.

Conclusion

Self-medication is a double edged sword which will only counter if we able to bring together the health care professionals (doctors, nurses, and pharmacists) into a new and more constructive interaction with each other.   Further, the public interest will best be served when pharmacists and the non-prescription medicines industry work together to ensure that self-medication is responsible, is only undertaken when it is appropriate to do so and advice is always given to seek a consultation from a physician when that is necessary.

Suggested Readings

1. Barnett CW, Nykamp D, Ellington AM (2000). Patient-guided counseling in the community pharmacy setting. *J Am PharmAssoc (Wash)*. **40:** 765-772.

2. Bjerrum L, Foged A (2003). Patient information leaflets-helpful guidance or a source of confusion? *Pharmaco epidemiol Drug Saf.* **12:** 55-59.

3. Bradley B, McCusker E, Scott E, Li Wan Po A (1995). Patient information leaflets on over-the-counter (OTC) medicines: the manufacturer's perspective. *J Clin Pharm Ther.* **20:** 37-40.

4. Etkin N (1992). Side effects: cultural construction and reinterpretation of Western pharmaceuticals. *Medical Anthropology Quarterly.* **6(2):** 99-113.

5. Jayaraman K (1986). Drug policy: playing down main issues. *Economic and Political Weekly.* **26(25-26):** 1129-1132.

6. Knapp D, Knapp D (1972). Decision-making and self- medication. *American Journal of Hospital Pharmacy.* **29:**1004.

7. Kunin C. M, Helene L, Tupasi T, Sacks T, Scheckler W. E, Jivani A, Goic A, Martin R. R, Guerrant R. L and Thamlikikul V (1987). Social behavioral, and practical factors affecting antibiotic use worldwide: report of Task Force 4. *Reviews of Infectious Disease.* 9 Suppl. **3:** S270 ± S283.

8. Lader S (1965). A survey of the incidence of self-medication. *Practitioner.* **194:** 132.

9. Nichter M. Pharmaceuticals, the commodication of health care Medicine use transition. In Anthropology and International Health, 1996 ed. M. Nichter, 2nd ed., Gordon and Breach Publishers, Amsterdam. pp. 265-326.

10. Roghmann KJ, Haggerty RJ (1972). The diary as a research instrument in the study of health and illness behavior. *Med Care.* **10:** 143.

11. Roghmann KJ, Haggerty RJ (1972). The diary as a research instrument in the study of health and illness behavior. *Med Care.* **10(2):** 143-163.

12. Verbrugge LM, Ascione FJ (1987). Exploring the iceberg of common symptoms and how people care for them. *Med Care.* **25(6):** 539-69.

13. Wilkinson IF, Darby DN, Mant A (1987). Self-care and self-medication: an evaluation of individual health care decisions. *Med Care.* **25:** 965.

CHAPTER 7

DRUG INFORMATION UNIT (DIU)

Introduction

Drug Information Unit/Center (DIU) may play an indispensable role in the promotion of rational usage of drug (RUD), essential drug concept and improvement of therapeutic outcomes by dissemination of unbiased and evidence based scientific drug information to a community and doctors. Historically, the first DIU was opened at the University of Kentucky Medical Center, USA in 1962 to promote information and updates related to drug to their doctors and nurses.

In India, more than 100,000 drug formulations are available in market but lack in a proper information center/media to consumers to reduce the unwanted effects or improve safety concern of consumers. DIU shall help clinicians to get updated, discuss problem related to drugs can be worked out in comprehensive way in the interest of best patient care.

Definition

Drug Information is the provision of written or verbal information or advice about drugs and drug therapy in response to a request from healthcare providers, doctors, organizations, committees, patients or members of the public societies.

Objectives to set up DIU

- Lack of awareness regarding drugs.
- Availability of huge number of (>100,000) formulations/Drugs which has created state of Therapeutic Jungle.
- Lack of awareness of Rational Drug Use among doctors.
- Most of the doctors predominantly depend on drug information being provided by Pharmaceutical companies, which at many times are incomplete and biased projecting positive aspects and hiding negative aspects of the drug marketed.

- Legally, pharmaceutical companies cannot provide drug information directly by most common medias i.e., print and electronic (TVs, Radios, Newspapers).
- Widespread availability of OTC drugs.
- High level illiteracy, poverty among patients, > 40,000 biomedical journals & 6,000 articles/day still lack of unbiased drug information.
- Recent advances in research and clinical experiences keep on changing the drug therapy for many diseases. Therefore, recent scientific information on new drugs and therapeutics is undoubtedly of paramount importance.
- Industry drug advertisements are intended to be persuasive rather than educational and it is not meant for educating the physicians in the use of drugs. However, a busy doctor unable to find time to update himself may start relying on drug advertisements. The drug advertisements in journals usually give inadequate and substandard information.
- This discrepancy in the drug information provided by drug advertisements in national and international journals might possibly be due to different regulatory requirements of various countries.

"The Drug and Magic Remedies Act 1954" of India with amendment in 1992, is to control drug advertisements which are false/misleading and objectionable. However, this Act is silent on ensuring the adequacy of drug information in new drug advertisements in journals; as a result the industry has learnt to take advantage of the loopholes in the law. We also have an organization of pharmaceutical manufacturers in India (OPPI), which is bound to follow a self-regulatory code of pharmaceutical marketing suggested by the International Federation of Pharmaceutical Manufacturers Association (IFPMA). Regulatory requirements are different even in the various developed countries.

The US-FDA under the authority of the Federal Food, Drug and Cosmetic Act lay down guidelines for "product claim" advertisements to provide basic pharmacological information, including the name of product, uses, side-effects, contraindications, drug benefits with regard to safety and effectiveness, risk information, limitation of efficacy, limitation to use, product hazards, and management of over dosage. Further, these drug advertisements cannot be false or misleading and cannot omit material facts. Whereas the UK legislation (The Medicines, Monitoring of Advertising, Amendment Regulations, 1999) requires the license number, supply classifications, name and address of the marketing authorization holder, name of the product, list of its active ingredients, indications, side-effects, precautions, contraindications, dosage form, method of use, warnings and cost to be included in the advertisements meant for persons qualified to prescribe or supply. Moreover, there are agencies like the MCA (Medicine Control Agency) in the UK to ensure these regulations are followed strictly.

However, how far these guidelines are followed by various national/international journals is still a matter of concern across the world. These days DIUs are fully electronic with Electronic library as backbone to retrieve drug information beside other conventional print medical library which makes DIUs more prompt and efficient.

Primary Role of DIU

- To give clear and definite information on drugs and promote their rational use.
- To promote Essential Drugs/P-drugs Concept.
- To run drug information OPDs.
- To provide drug information services to inpatients.
- To hold awareness lecture for medical/paramedical staff for safe handling of drugs.
- To conduct CME for Community for providing drug awareness and upgrading the knowledge regarding recent advances of doctors working in community.

Secondary Role

- To keep up to date with pharmacological and therapeutic literature and disseminate relevant information when it becomes available.
- Publishing drug information bulletin or newsletter/electronic or print.
- Participate in clinical activities, assisting developing formulary.
- Organize continuing professional development program for healthcare professionals.

Approach/Working of DIU

Step I. Secure demographics of request: There are three common ways of drug information through DIU.

1. Personal Query by doctor within institution or outside institution working in community/person from community
2. By e-mail
3. By Telephone
4. Through website

Thus, detail of the drug information query demographics need to be secured to develop database of request seeking drug information, which can be studied in future to make necessary improvisation and make functioning of the DIU more efficient and prompt.

Step II. Obtain background information: This is basic preliminary step to follow before actual information is retrieved. This step helps to categorize type of drug information and helps in narrowing the domain of literature review subsequently.

Step III. Categorize ultimate question: This is an essential step before an actual reviewing of the literature. The request most commonly pertains to one or other category mentioned below.

1. General information regarding drug
   - An account of the disease and reasons for prescribing
   - Objective of drug to treat disease or symptoms
   - How and when to take the medicine
   - When benefits are expected to occur
   - Whether it matters if a dose missed
   - What to do about it
   - How long the medicine needed
   - How to recognize ADR
   - What is needed to be done
   - Effect on routine working/driving of vehicle
   - Any interaction with food, alcohol, smoking, drugs and herbal
2. Pharmacokinetic Information
3. Pharmacodynamic Information
4. Drug of choice queries
5. Drug interaction queries
6. ADR queries
7. Drug disease query- Drug best suitable in co-morbid condition
8. Newer treatment/Best treatment option over the current conventional drugs prescribed to information seeker
9. Poison/Toxic product information
10. Banned drug information
11. Updated advances in treatment guidelines in the treatment of a disease

Step IV. Conduct search: The following principle need to be adopted and follow while reviewing the literature
   - How far similar problems/queries have been addressed
   - Wide to Narrow to specific
   - Understand /Make provisional reply to query

- Get Critically assessed by peer reviewing
- Get input from your senior faculty member
- Make necessary Modifications
- Make Final reply

(a) **Common agencies/mean used to review literature in DIU are Books-**

- Pharmacology
- Medicine and allied subjects
- Surgery and allied subjects
- Gynecology and Obstetrics and allied subjects
- Others as per need

(b) **Pharmacopoeias (Print & Electronic)**

- British Pharmacopoeias (BP)
- United State Pharmacopoeias (USP)
- Indian Pharmacopoeias (IP)
- European Pharmacopoeias (Ph. Eur.)
- Russian Pharmacopoeias
- WHO - International Pharmacopoeias (Ph. Int.)

(c) **Formulary**

- Pharmaceutical Codex
- National formulary of India
- National Formulary of American Pharmaceutical Association
- Printed Journals in Institutional library

(d) **Monographs, patents, thesis, reports, MIMS, CIMS etc.**

(e) **e-Library forms back bone that include free information retrieving agencies and paid agencies like**

- Pubmed central
- Pubmed
- DOAJ
- Cochrane database
- NLM
- Science Free Medical Journals List
- Biology & Medicine Online Journals

- EMBASE
- Index copernicus
- Google
- Google scholar
- Yahoo search
- IndMed

(f) **e-Library: Shall Include**

- All journals from India

    http://www.medknow.com/journals.asp

    http://medind.nic.in/

    http://openmed.nic.in/

    http://www.openj-gate.com/Browse/ByJournal.aspx?alpha=ALL

- Free Full text Journals -Scopus/Elsevier's
- Free Full text Journals-DOAJ

    http://www.doaj.org/

- Free Full text Journals-PubMed Central

    http://www.ncbi.nlm.nih.gov/pmc/

    http://www.nml.nic.in/

- Many Paid Journals more than 10,000-Pubmed/Elsevier's - Annual Subscription Required

    http://www.elsevier.com/wps/find/journal_ browse.cws_home

    http://www.ncbi.nlm.nih.gov/projects/linkout/journals/jourlists.fcgi?typeid=1&type=journals&operation=Show

Step V. Perform evaluation, analysis; evaluate the information available at various sources

This is an important step in the sequence, which composed of evaluation of shortlisted data and analysis will be done as per requirement of the DIUs objectives.

Step VI. Formulate and provide the relevant necessary, unbiased, evidence based scientific information/ response to the information seeker by

1. Telephone

    Initially within time frame like 24 hr of time of seeking drug information, which can be tailored subsequently to prompt immediately reply with experience and with development of database of request entertained under DIU.

2. Email

3. Through Website
4. Written format
5. Verbal communication

At the same time a feedback form on functioning of DIU may be asked to be filled for improvisation in future.

Drug Information OPDs

These types of OPDs are mainly to support clinical OPDs in a similar way as that of diet/nutrition clinics or physiotherapy clinics preferably be cited & located in the same OPD Complex or in the Department of Pharmacology. The role of OPD should be defined by administration of the hospital to only provide relevant scientific evidence based drug information on being asked and to make contents of prescription more understandable by the patients in their own local language. Role of OPD should be restricted not to make any comment/Advise on Prescription which contradicts the prescriber to avoid conflict with clinicians. If any difference of opinion gets generated, can be worked out separately and communicated to the prescribers first for his response and with his consent only and if clinical situation demands may be corrected. In no way DIU OPDs should deny privilege or which prescribers are entitled officially. In no way working of OPD should interfere with clinical OPDs.

Drug information OPD- Working Domain
DIU for Community

- An account of the disease and reasons for prescribing
- Objective of drug to treat disease or symptoms
- How and when to take the medicine
- When benefits are expected to occur
- Whether it matters if a dose missed
- What to do about it
- How long the medicine needed
- How to recognize ADRs
- What is needed to be done
- Effect on routine working/driving of vehicle
- Any interaction with Food, Alcohol, Smoking, Drugs and Herbal
- Compliance motivated, ensured evaluated
- Consequences of under dosing/missed dose/overdosing can be explained
- Anxiety/inappropriate health beliefs can be addressed
- Frequency and complexity of drug regimen

- Helping hand to prescribers in preventing
    - Generic Substitutions
    - Therapeutic Substitutions
    - Relevant/Irrelevant/Specific/Non specific queries of general public which many times are irritants to a busy prescriber
- Essential Drugs and P-Drug program–Sensitization of Doctors
- Rational therapeutics sensitization of doctors
- Pharmacoeconomics sensitization of the doctors
- Treatment options in regards to below mentioned points can be ensured
    - **S**- Safety
    - **T**-Tolerability
    - **E**-Efficacy
    - **P**-Price

DIU for Doctors

- Any new drug development
- Drugs related to pharmaco-dynamic/kinetic query
- Drug-Safety in pregnancy
- Drug-Safety in geriatrics/pediatric population
- Problem based query can be addressed
- Consensus Treatment International Guidelines can be made available to prescribers.

Connecting/Interlinking e-Library with DIU and with community and Doctors

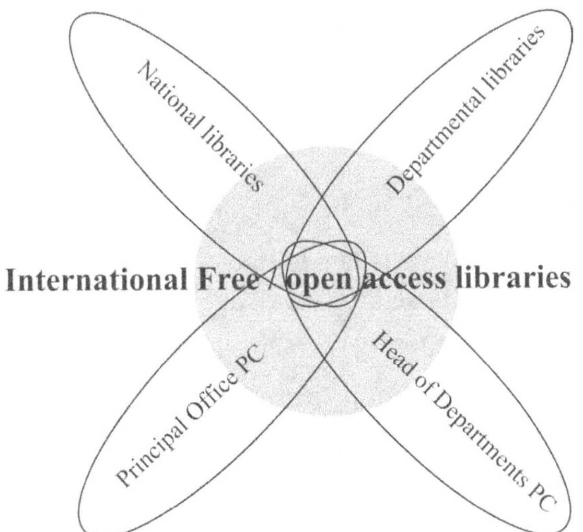

Connecting/Interlinking e-Library and DIU

- International Free/open access libraries
- National libraries
    http://www.nml.nic.in/
- Departmental libraries
- Office computer

Connecting/Interlinking e-Library and DIU to Information Seekers

Mobile Alerts to Faculty, PGs, UGs, Other Doctors from the community in a state
(mobile database)

Email Alerts to Faculty, PGs, UGs, Other Doctors from the community in a state
(email database)

Email alerts to all contacts of Institution by developing a e mail database

DIU & e-Library: Improves research citation of institute

DIU and e-Library can also help institutions to develop thesis/projects/research publication database and can help then for converting it into Self Archive Database which help make the work of institution more citable and thus helping to increase impact factor of research generated by any institution.

National

- Open Med

International

- DOAJ
- Index copernicus Library
- Google Scholar
- Yahoo

Advantages of running a DIU and e-library

- Interlinking of faculty/registrars/postgraduates/undergraduates with national/ international library and medical knowledge updating agencies
- Regular Updating of faculty/registrars/postgraduates/undergraduates
- Help to improve health care of patients indirectly
- Work of institution shall be available for citation /referral across the world

- Thesis/dissertation/research work database can be developed, which can help us in planning treatment guidelines as per research findings generated from our own population
- It shall help in converting research into knowledge and then knowledge into education
- Shall help in self indexing and archiving of thesis research work and publications and conference proceedings
- Busy doctors also can receive regular medical updates on mobile and e-mail
- Larger number of Journals can be made available which otherwise is very costly affair
- Thought, academically interaction shall be possible at very cost effective manner
- No need of maintaining stocks
- No fear of theft

Spreading information to community

- Drug (connecting to Pharmacology) information
- Center for general public
- Current medical problem (PSM/Medicine Dept.)
- Information center to general public
- Information about facilities–Department Wise
- Medical College is providing
- General Public Grievance –connecting to PMC through Control Room and
- Connecting to PMC & CM Grievance cell

Post graduate guide-service jointly by pharmacology and PSM departments which shall help in research scholars to choose

- Choosing Research Question
- Advise on Ethical issues- both preclinical and Clinical studies
- Designing Research Protocol for descriptive/interventional preclinical or clinical studies (Phase 1-4) for your research and thesis of PGs
- Scientific editing
- Medical writing
- Statistical advise before, during and after submitting research protocol

Community teaching is possible

- Drug information to community
- Disease information to community
- Database developed from hospitals shall go long way in helping us to formulate health policy and strategies and frame guidelines at hospital and state level as per need of our population

Minimum Requirement to Set up DIU and e-Library, which may vary in different DIUs

S. No.	Particulars
1.	Laptop
2.	Desktop
3.	2.5 inch portable HDD with USB interface for backup software
4.	Tablet Pen to annotate
5.	Laser jet printer basic
6.	Colour Laser jet printer
7.	Document scanner A4 size
8.	Photostat/Xerox machine
9.	Fax machine plain paper
10.	Pen drive 4/8/16 GB
11.	Multimedia projector
12.	Projection screen big size
13.	Server for database management
14.	Internet facility with extensive usage plan annually
15.	Phone (Landline/Mobile)
16.	White board (1200mmx2400mm)
17.	Office table
18.	Computer chairs
19.	Computer table
20.	DVD writer external for preventive maintenance of infrastructure
21.	AC window type 2 TON with emergency power supply

Conclusion and future direction

DIUs are a useful communication media and source of information about drugs for both healthcare professionals and consumers. It will be really helpful for the healthcare professionals, offering complete information on different aspects of drugs. In future,

DIUs will play an important role in healthcare system and will improve the rational usage of drugs in clinics.

Suggested Readings

1. Amerson AB, Wallingford Dm (1983). Twenty Years Experience With Drug Information Centers. *Am J Hosp Pharm.* **40:** 1172-1178.

2. Clauson KA, Polen HH, Marsh WA (2007). Clinical Decision Support Tools: Performance Of Personal Digital Assistant Versus Online Drug Information Databases. *Pharmacotherapy.* **27(12):** 1651-1658.

3. Clauson KA, Polen HH, Peak AS, Marsh WA, Discala SL. Clinical Decision Support Tools: Personal Digital Assistant *Versus* Online Dietary Supplement Databases. *Ann Pharmacother.* **42(11):** 1592-1599.

4. Hazra A, Sen A, Roy S (2001). One Year Experience Of Drug Information Service In The Ngo Sector. *Indian J Pharmacol.* **33:** 44-45.

5. Joshi MP (1997). University Hospital-Based Drug Information Service In A Developing Country. *Eur J Clin Pharmacol.* **53:** 89-94.

6. Kasilo OJ, Nhachi CF (1991). Recommendations For Establishing A Drug And Toxicology Information Center In A Developing Country. *Dicp.* **25(12):** 1379-1383.

7. Kasilo OJ, Nhachi CF (1993). How To Establish A Drug And Toxicology Information Centre In A Developing Country. *Essent Drugs Monit.* **(16):** 8-9.

8. Kevin A Clauson, Wallace A Marsh, Hyla H Polen, Matthew J Seamon and Blanca I Ortiz (2007). Clinical Decision Support Tools: Analysis of Online Drug Information Databases. *BMC Medical Informatics and Decision Making.* **7:**7.

9. Parker PF (1965). The University of Kentucky Drug Information Center. *Am J Hosp Pharm.* **22:** 42-47.

10. R. D. Hunashal, B. Kudagi, M. Kamadod & S. Biradar (2008). Drug Information Center. *The Internet Journal Of Medical Informatics.* Volume 4 Number1.

11. Rosenberg JM (1983). Drug Information Centers: Future Trends. *Am J Hosp Pharm.* **40:** 1213-1215.

12. Suresh C. Pradhan (2002). The Performance of Drug Information Center At The University of Kansas Medical Center, Kansas City, USA - Experiences And Evaluations. *Ind J Pharmacol.* **34:** 123-129

13. Tatro DS (1983). Computer-Assisted Drug Literature Retrieval. *Am J Hosp Pharm.* **40:** 220.

CHAPTER 8

DRUG COMPLIANCE

Introduction

Drug compliance is an extent to which the patient's behavior matches the prescriber's recommendations and in other words patient's adherence to drug/treatment. However, it is a challenging issue since Hippocrates era. Although the term compliance is commonly used in the medical and pharmaceutical literature, adherence has been preferred over compliance as compliance implies an element of fault or blame on the part of the patient. The term adherence has been adopted as an alternative to compliance, in an attempt to emphasize that the patient is free to decide whether to follow the prescriber's recommendations and that failure to do so should not be a reason to blame the patient. It refers to as till how much extent a patients follows the instructions regarding medication, given to him by the clinical practitioners/health care workers. It also denotes how much a person's behavior coincides with medical advice. In clinical practice, when drug are prescribed it is referred to as the degree of correspondence of the actual dosing history with prescribed regimen. About 1 in 4 people show non-compliance to drug therapy. Individually if taken, rates of drug adherence are the percentage of the prescribed doses of the medication actually taken up by the patient over a specified period of time. Drug compliance is more problematic with elderly due to multiple drug regimens they are already taking and also an issue in pediatric populations.

Importance of Drug Compliance

The ultimate aim of the drug therapy is to improve the symptomatology of the patient disease or the cure his disease. This is relevant in case certain disease like HIV, in which high compliance is essential to extend the life expectancy of the individual. Similarly, drug compliance has shown to reduce the mortality in patients with organ transplantation.

Variations in Drug Compliance

A patient follows a prescribed drug as per scheduled depending upon the illness, he/she is suffering from. The various examples are like when a person is motivated to lose weight or smoking, it has been seen that compliance is less than 10%. Similarly, better compliance is seen mainly with acute diseases as compared to chronic disease e.g., hypertension. It has been observed that compliance drops substantially after six months of therapy. Even compliance is remarkably high in individuals in clinical trials due to the attention they receive, but it may still vary from 43% to 78%. Adherence to drug therapy has shown to reduce the risk of mortality not only to drugs but, also to placebo. Adherence data indicate that it can vary from 0% to 100% since, a person can take more than prescribed doses. Different methods have been adopted to measure compliance/adherence but inconsistent results, along with complexity associated with them and the cost factors of these interventions is also a limiting factor.

Consequences of Poor Compliance

A great impact due to non-compliance is numerous which includes hospital admissions, economic burden, worsening of the disease and death. A recent meta-analysis by Simpson (2006) from 21 studies regarding drug compliance evaluated association between adherence to drug therapy and mortality demonstrated that a good adherence to drug therapy is associated with positive health outcomes and also adherence to drug therapy may be a surrogate marker for overall healthy behavior.

Factors Contributing to Non-Compliance

Compliance/Adherence is a behavior with biomedical, psychological and anthropological explanations competing for attention. Non-adherence to medication has profound implications on the patient as well as on doctor-patient relationships and interactions, plans of care, and the healthcare system and it is multi-factorial (Fig. 8.1).

1. **Socio-economic factors**

   Several types of support including practical, emotional, and uni-dimensional social support; family cohesiveness and conflict; marital status; and living arrangements of adults can influence the adherence. Gender, personality, and cultural factors may influence adherence-compliance rates. For instance, women may be better at adhering to their medication regimens than men. This may be particularly so for drugs that treats behavioral health conditions, such as antidepressant medication. People who have social support from family, friends, or caregivers to assist with medication regimens have better adherence to treatment. Unstable living environments, limited access to health care, lack of financial resources, cost of medication, and burdensome work schedules have all been associated with decreased adherence rates. Cost and access barriers are identified as important influences on the uptake of prescriptions and repeat medicines are of particular significance in healthcare systems with a high cost of co-payments and deductibles. It has a particular influence on medicines use among more disadvantaged groups in situations where charges are levied.

2. Provider-patient/health care system

The relationship of the doctor-patient is one of the most important health care system-related factors impacting adherence. A good relationship between the patient and health care provider, which features encouragement and reinforcement from the provider, has a positive impact on adherence poor or lack of communication concerning the benefits, instructions for use, and side effects of medications can also contribute to non-adherence, especially in older adults with memory problems.

3. Condition-related

Long term drugs administration for many chronic illnesses and adherence to such treatment regimens often declines significantly over time. This often happens when patient have few or no symptoms and the absence of them is a barrier for people to take their medication. It is important for the patient to understand the illness and what will happen, if it is not treated.

4. Therapy-related

The complexity and demands of the treatment regimen are potential causes of non-adherence. The complexity of the medication regimen, which includes the number of medications and number of daily doses required; duration of therapy; therapies that are inconvenient or interfere with a person's lifestyle and side effects have been associated with decreased adherence. For example, the elderly patient with multiple medical problems requiring complex drug regimens may find it difficult to take numerous medications multiple times each day. Moreover, patients often find it difficult, how to take medication (such as orally, twice daily, with food, etc.).

Original prescription not filled: Approximately, 20 per cent of primary care patients fail to present the prescription for dispensing in the first place and this has been termed primary noncompliance.

Sub-optimal dosing: Most of the published studies in the adherence area have focused on what the patient does with the medication once it has been dispensed. In this context, adherence may be categorical or incremental. In categorical definitions, patients are judged to be adherent or non-adherent based on the amount of medication taken in relation to a defined 'cut-off' point.

5. Patient-related factors

Physical impairments and cognitive limitations may increase the risk for non-adherence in older adults. Memory performance has been found to correlate with reduced adherence in patients with HIV infection, chronic obstructive pulmonary disease, elderly patients with type 2 diabetes, and generally among elderly patients. Accurate recall of instructions for medicine taking is a pre-requisite for adherence.

Patients are often not forthcoming about non-adherence because of lack of knowledge about the disease or understanding about the importance of adherence, the reasons medication is needed, lack of motivation, low self-efficacy, substance abuse, guilt, embarrassment about their inability to manage an overwhelmingly complex drug regimen or about their financial limitations, or fear of angering their physicians.

6. Miscellaneous

Patient's beliefs, concerns about potential adverse effects, perceptions of prescribed medicines, presence of depression or anxiety etc can also affect adherence.

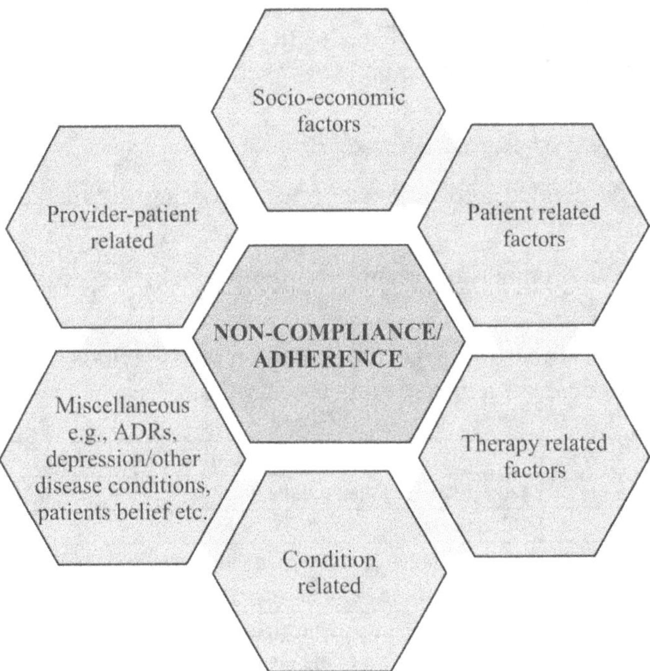

Fig. 8.1 Factors affecting Non-adherence.

Identifying and Measuring Non-Compliance

Types of Non-Compliance to Medication

Three broad categories of medication non-compliance have been described in the literature:

Original Prescription not Followed

Approximately, 20% of primary care patients fail to present the prescription for dispensing in the first place and this has been termed primary non-compliance.

Refills not Obtained

This problem was illustrated in a study in which only 10% of a sample of over 7000 patients with chronic heart failure filled enough prescriptions to ensure a regular daily supply of medication.

Suboptimal Dosing

Most of the published studies in the adherence area have focused on what the patient does with the medication once it has been dispensed. In this context, adherence may be categorical or incremental. In categorical definitions, patients are judged to be adherent or non-adherent based on the amount of medication taken in relation to a defined 'cut-off' point. Incremental definitions conceptualized adherence as a continuum.

Methods to Improve Compliance

Compliance can be divided into two categories according to whether the assessment is direct or indirect.

Direct measurement: entails observing the ingestion of the drug or by detecting its presence in body fluids.

Indirect measurement: assume ingestion based on proxy-evidence, such as the patient's report or number of dosages removed from a container.

S. No.	Type of method
1	Questionnaire to the patient
2	Pill count
3	Supervening drug intake: Directly observed therapy
4	Detecting the tracer
5	Assaying the drug in the biological fluid • Measurement of the medicine or metabolite in blood • Measurement of the biological marker in blood
6	Automatic recoding of daily activities

Table *Contd...*

S. No.	Type of method
7	Rate of prescription refills
8	Assessment of patients clinical response
9	Electronic medication monitors
10	Patients dairies
11	Measurement of physiological markers (heart rate in patient taking beta blockers)
12	Simultaneous use of the these procedures

Different methods have been adopted as seen above for improving the compliance of the patients, but no method is yet a gold standard.

Questioning a patient or self reporting by the patient is one of the simplest method to know compliance and the best way to do it is by asking the patients how many times a person has forgotten to take the medicine. But, sometimes this method is overestimated. Similarly, using patient's dairies and assessment of clinical responses are relatively easy to use with clinical assessment of response to drug therapy confounded by many factors. We mean that subjects is asked to return any drug that is left over at each follow up visit, and by this the unused drug can be determined. This method is associated with flaws that patient can switch medicines between the bottles and may discard before visit in order to appear to be following the regimen. Hence, it may not be good measure of drug adherence. Apart from this pill count may not give information about timing of drug intake and drug holidays.

Supervising drug intake also refers to as directly observed therapy is said to be most accurate method in which the nursing staff may be asked to supervise patients, by asking patients to take the drug in her presence. This method too has lacunae that the patient might hide pill in his mouth and in psychiatric setting the patient may vomit the drug out.

Tracers like phenol red, trace amounts of isoniazid, fluorescein, riboflavin, bromide and phenobarbitone are used. The tracer should possess the property of being inert and chemically un-reactive. The major drawback of this procedure is that most recent dose taken is traced by this method. Rate of refilling prescription is also close to accurate method of adherence, but requires a closed pharmacy system.

Apart from these measuring the concentration of a drug or its metabolite in blood, urine and also using biological markers are also the other methods of measuring drug compliance. The disadvantage is that these methods are expensive and burdensome. Measuring drug concentration is important in certain regimens such as antiepileptic drugs like phenytoin, carbamazepine or valproic acid and psychiatric drugs like lithium. Again while using this method, variation in metabolism and white coat adherence can give a false impression of adherence.

Electronic methods are being used since approximately 30 yr, which are capable of recording and stamping the time of opening of the bottles, dispensing drops or activating canister on multiple occasions. These methods also measure compliance between two visits along with regularity over time but with the disadvantage that no doubt this system have been activated, the drug could have been discard instead of ingesting it.

An advanced electronic device have been developed with two components which constitutes a plastic vial (pill container) with a closure that contains a micro-electronic circuit which registers time when closure is opened and when it is closed. The events of electronically stored medication events are transferred to computer, and then time series data are subsequently processed with the potential of being illustrating the data graphically.

Different Methods to Enhance Drug Compliance

- Better and improved communication skills between physician and patients with emphasises on value of regimen and effect on adherence.
- Provide simple and clear instructions about the regimen as much as possible.
- Listen to patient and try to negotiate the regimen along with determination of cost and other barriers that hinders with compliance.
- Evaluate any lacunaes in poor adherence like if patient had missed any appointments, or there is lack of response.
- Provide motivation of use of a medication taking system.
- Alternate medication regimens like medication with long half lives and depot (extended release medications, transdermal medications) if adherence is unlikely.
- For short term treatment, reminder packages like calendars packs to be provided.

Conclusion

Conclusively, we can say that compliance/adherence is necessary and important for a successful treatment outcome for a patient. Worldwide, non-compliant is a vast problem in delivering successful healthcare services. Compliance in all respect i.e., drug dosage, time interval and duration of treatment is necessary. More importantly, compliance should be monitored for the each patients, but more concern must be paid to geriatric and chronic disease patients; patients suffering from life threatening diseases like HIV, cancer, stroke etc. The only way out to improve the compliance is education to the patients and caregivers, self-motivation and routinely follow up by healthcare professionals play an important role.

Suggested Readings

1. Bernstein GA, Anderson LK, Hektner JM, Realmuto GM (2000) Imipramine compliance in adolscents. *J Am Acad Child Adolesc psychiatry.* **39(3):** 284-291.

2. Cramer JA, Mattson RH, Preveem Z, Scheyer RD, Ouellette VL (1989). How often is medication taken as prescribed? A novel assessment technique. *JAMA.* **261:** 3273-3277.

3. Cromer BA, Steinberg K, Gardner L, Thornton D, Shannon B (1989). Psychosocial determinants of compliance in adolscents with iron deficiency. *Am J Dis Child.* **143:** 55-58.

4. De Geest S. et al., (1995). Incidence, determinants and consequences of subclinical noncompliance with immunosuppressive therapy in renal transplant recipients. *Transplantation.* **59:** 340-347.

5. De Geest S. *et al.,* (1998). Late acute rejections and subclinical noncompliance with cyclosporine therapy in heart transplant patients. *Journal of heart and lung transplantation.* S54-63

6. Di Matteo MR (2004). Variations in patient's adherence to medical recommendations: a quantitative review of 50 yr of research. *Med Care.* **42:** 200-209.

7. Dolgin MJ, Katz ER, Doctors SR, Siegl SE (1986). Caregivers perception of medical compliance in adolscents with cancer. *J Adolesc Health Care.* **7:** 22-27.

8. Eisen SA, Miller DK, Woodward RS, Spintznagel E, Przybeck TR (1990). The effect of prescribed daily dose frequency on patient medication compliance. *Arch Intern Med.* **150(9):** 1881-1884.

9. Evans L, Spelman M (1983). The problem of non compliance with drug therapy. *Drugs.* **25(1):** 63-76.

10. Gordis L. Methodologic varies in the measurement of patient compliance. In: Sackett DL, Haynes RB eds. Complaince with therapeutic regimens. Baltimore: Johns Hopkins University Press 1976: 51-66.

11. Haynes RB (2001). Improving patient adherence state of the art with special focus on medication taking for cardiovascular disorders. In: Burke LE, Okene IS eds. Patient compliance in health care search: American heart association monograph series. Armonk NY: Futura Publishing Co; 3-21.

12. Hodgson I (1999). HIV and combination therapy: Meeting the challenge of a new era. *British journal of nursing.* **8(1):** 39-43.

13. Hulka BS, Kuppler LL, Cassel JC, Efird RL, Burdette JA (1975). Medication use and misuse: Physician-patient discrepancies. *J Chron Dis.* **28:** 7-21.

14. Isenalumhe AE, Oviame O (1988). Polypharmacy its cost burden and barriers to medication, a drug oriented health care system. *Health serv.* **18:** 335-342.

15. Kass MA, Meltzer DW, Gordon M (1984). A miniature   compliance monitor for eyedrop medication. *Arch Ophthalmol.* **102:** 1550-1554.

16. Liptak GS (1996). Enhancing patient compliance in paediatrics. *Pediatr Rev.* **17:** 128-134.

    monetary reinforcement: pilot study of an antiretroviral adherence intervention. *J Gen Intern Med.* **15:** 841-847.

17. Norell SE (1981). Monitoring compliance with pilocarpine therapy. *Am J ophthalmol.* **92:** 727-731.

18. Osterberg L, Blaschke T (2005). Adherence to Medication. *N Engl J Med.* **353:** 487-497.

19. Patient compliance and discontinuation of treatment. In: Spriet A, Spriet D T, Simon P. eds. Methology of clinical drug trials. 2nd ed.

20. Rigsby MO, Rosen MI, Beauvais JE, *et al.,* (2000). Cue-dose training with

21. Rudd P, Byyny RL, Zachary V, *et al.,* (1989). Pill count measure of comlaince in drug trial: variability and suitability. *Am J hypertens.* **11:** 309-312.

22. Rullar T, Kumar S, Tindall H, Felly M (1989). Time to stop counting tablets ? *Clin Pharmacol Ther.* **46:** 63-68.

23. Schroeder K, Fahey T, Ebrahim S (2004). How can we improve adherence to blood pressure lowering medication in ambulatory care? Systematic review of randomized controlled trials. *Arch Intern Med.* **164:** 722-732.

24. Simoni JM, Frick PA, Pantalone DW, Turner BJ (2003). Antiretroviral adherence interventions: a review of current literature and ongoing studies. *Top HIV Med.* **11:** 185-98.

25. Simpson SH. *et al.,* (2006). A meta-analysis of the association between adherence to drug therapy and mortality. *BMJ.* **333:** 15-20.

26. Sorensen C (1998). Medication adherence strategies for drug abusers with HIV/ AIDS. *AIDS care.* **10(3):** 297-312.

27. Spector SL, Kinsman R, Mawhinney H, *et al.,* (1986). Compliance of patients with asthma with an experimental aerosolized medication: implications for controlled clinical trials. *J Allergy Clin Immunol.* **77:** 65-70.

28. Urquhardt J (1994). Role of patient compliance in clinical pharmacokinetics: review of recent. *Clin Pharmacokinet.* **27:** 202-215.

29. W and start TL, Kaplan B (1997). Pharmacoeconomic impact of factors affecting compliance with antibiotic regimens in the treatment of otitis media. *Pediatr Infect Dis J.* **16:** S27-29.

30. Winnick S, Lucas DO, Hartman AL, Toll D (2005). How to improve your compliance? *Pediatrics.* **115:** 718-724.

CHAPTER 9

DIRECT-TO-CONSUMER ADVERTISING: BENEFACTION OR AFFLICTION

Introduction

Before 1997, pharmaceutical companies were allowed to advertise with their brand name, however they have to provide "brief summary", of side effects, contraindications and effectiveness. For the proper check, FDA issued guidance in 1997 and formally adopted in 1999 which allowed TV ads to name a pharmaceutical brand and the condition it treated, thereafter Direct-to-Consumer (DTC) advertising made easy to reach at population. Direct-to-Consumer Advertising (DTCA) is a promotional effort by a pharmaceutical company or other provider of medical services to present information about medications or medical services to the public in the lay media as television, radio, internet, newspaper and magazine advertisements, billboards, and direct mailings. DTCA is legal only in the United States and New Zealand and has been linked with drug overutilization, public health concerns, and higher costs. Despite global proscriptions, DTCA is the most rapidly increasing form of pharmaceutical marketing. The first direct-to-consumer advertisement for a prescription drug appeared in *Reader's Digest* in 1981 in USA, held the revolution in the field of DTCA of prescription drug, this is well seen with approximately 4 folds rise in the spending for DTCA from $1.2 billion in 1998 to $4.7 billion in 2009. In light of these trends it is important to understand the impact of DTCA on its target audience. All advertising for medications, including DTCA, is regulated by the Food and Drug Administration (FDA). The history of advertising of medicines directly to consumers coincides with the history of mass media advertising in the early 18th and 19th centuries when patent medicines with 'colorful' names were directly marketed to people. In fact, patent medicine advertisements accounted for almost 50% of newspaper advertising revenue by the beginning of the twentieth century, an activity that occurred with no regulation. The lack of regulation allowed companies to make exaggerated claims about the efficacy of their 'drugs' - compelling the US Government to take steps to regulate such claims, starting in 1906 with the Pure Food and Drug Act. Successive steps for the next few decades in the United States included major legislative and regulatory efforts in 1938, 1951 and 1962, when jurisdiction over prescription advertising was transferred to the US-FDA from the US Federal Trade Commission (FTC). To ensure that advertisements for medications provide public health benefits without creating health risks, the FDA determined more than 30 years ago that under the 1962 Kefauver-Harris Amendments to the Federal Food, Drug, and Cosmetic Act, advertisements must have 4 basic attributes:

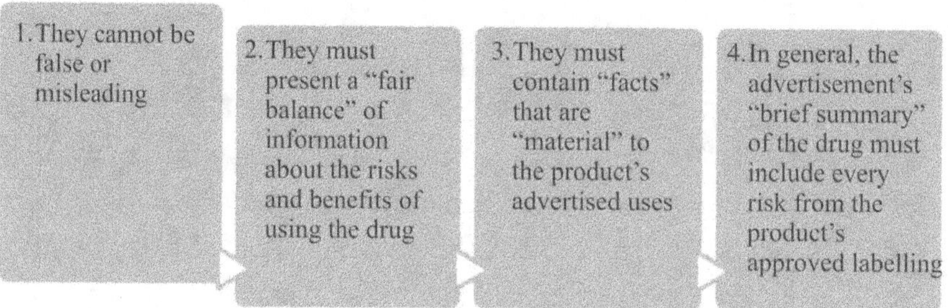

A succession of changes by the FDA to regulate the efforts of advertising by drug companies resulted in the release of more liberal regulation in 1999. This allowed drug companies to use broadcast media, especially television, to provide information only on major risks instead of more detailed information on risks and side effects. The 1999 regulation allowed for a great increase in DTCA.

Since the first DTC prescription drug advertisements appeared in the early 1980s, researchers began to question whether pharmaceutical advertisements could "serve two masters: the promotional interest of the pharmaceutical industry and the public's health needs". From the drug industry perspective that they respond to consumer's right to information and informed health care choices, and increase awareness for new, more effective drugs. Other perceived benefits of DTCA include patient education about new medication, an empowerment to seek medical care for a yet undiagnosed condition, and potentially improved patient-to-provider communication. For this to happen, the DTCA must address important health concerns, focus on patients likely to benefit from diagnosis and treatment, and steer them towards appropriate care. For the individual patient, drug treatment is worth pursuing if potential benefits outweigh potential harm. But as healthier people are targeted, the added benefit of drug treatment can become increasingly elusive. However, there is little evidence to support that DTCA indeed leads to earlier diagnosis of serious conditions, better treatment adherence, or improved health outcomes.

Impact of DTCA

Impact on Patient-Physician Relationship

Recent studies have shown beyond a doubt that DTCA motivates discussions between patients and their physicians about pharmaceutical products. What could be wrong with that? These complicated issues raised by DTCA can be illustrated by an example. Imagine a patient who sees a magazine advertisement for an antidepressant and decides that her symptoms are suggestive of major depression. She reveals her symptoms to a physician, who performs a careful history and physical exam and decides that hypothyroidism could be responsible. After testing confirms the diagnosis, the patient is successfully treated with thyroid hormone replacement therapy. In a different scenario, the patient waves the same advertisement in front of another physician and demands the drug. After taking a cursory history that suggests depressive symptoms, the second physician writes the prescription. Six months later, the patient is hospitalized for severe hypothyroidism. What should physicians do with patients who make advertisement-induced requests? Indeed, one study found that as many as half of patients would register disappointment, and 15% would consider switching physicians, if their physician refused a request for an advertised prescription medication, implies that DTCA may erode public trust in physicians when advertising messages conflicts with the professional advice. Physicians also share concern for the effect of DTCA on their patient population, as many believe that the advertising erodes the fragile patient-provider relationship. Studies of physicians regarding DTCA suggest that physicians are growing dissatisfied with their encounters with patients as they increasingly use valuable clinic time to discuss information that a patient may have garnered from a DTCA. Physicians and other medical experts are also wary of the potential of DTCA to affect over-prescribing behaviors when providers try to meet the demands of their patients.

Is DTCA Deceptive?

To understand the potential impact of DTCA, it is essential to determine how widespread it is and what types of claims are being made. Perhaps the most common criticism of DTCA is that it is misleading and deceptive, overstating product benefits and understating product risks. Additionally, the information that is provided has not been shown to be 'fair and balanced', in which both risks and benefits are equally reviewed. Content analyses suggest that DTCA tend to allot more space to the positive features of the product, relegating information about risks and adverse effects to the small print. This issue raised by DTCA can be illustrated by an example - Pfizer, the manufacturer of Lipitor (atorvastatin), ran a campaign in France and Canada in 2003 with print advertisements that used images of a tagged toe of a corpse (the Canadian campaign was in association with the Canadian Lipid Nurse Network and the Canadian Diabetes Association). On television, a youthful, healthy man died suddenly of a heart attack, leaving his family devastated with grief. The message of these two advertisements was that cholesterol testing and treatment could prevent premature death from heart attacks in healthy people. This was at odds with existing scientific evidence: a meta-analysis (2003) of cholesterol lowering drugs in primary prevention found no difference in mortality between drug and placebo. This impression of inappropriately minimizing risks (e.g., downplaying or omitting information on side effects), and exaggerating effectiveness (e.g., portraying the indication too broadly or making unsubstantiated claims) are the two major reasons for the FDA issuing regulatory letters to the advertisers.

Second point on this issue is based on the fact that the DTCA campaigns generally begin within a year after the introduction of a pharmaceutical product, which raises questions about the extent to which advertising increases the use of drugs with unknown safety profiles. They frequently focus on blockbuster and lifestyle drugs that have limited drug patient safety experience and post market surveillance. This could be well exemplified by the Merck's (Whitehouse Station, NJ, USA) Vioxx (rofecoxib) illustrates the risk of how aggressive DTCA can increase the likelihood of a drug being prescribed beyond that drug's labeled indication and against a background where information about that drug's safety profile is limited at best. Merck had launched rofecoxib in the U.S.A. in May 1999. In 2001, Merck's spending on direct to consumer advertising of the drug was the highest in industry at $161 million. By April 2001, rofecoxib, along with the other approved cyclo-oxygenase-2 (COX-2) at that time, celecoxib, accounted for 38% of all NSAID prescriptions according to a study conducted in Alabama. Merck voluntarily withdrew rofecoxib, on a global basis on September 30th, 2004. Public statements by Merck that it made the decision to withdraw rofecoxib on the basis of a trial results that indicate an increased risk of cardiovascular events in patients treated with 25 mg daily of rofecoxib compared to placebo. Rofecoxib was an important drug for Merck, as it sold $2.5 billion in 2003, or 11% of the company's revenue following the news of rofecoxib's withdrawal, Merck's stock plummeted 27%, reducing Merck's market capitalization by $25 billion. In response to these concerns, the drug industry association Pharmaceutical Research and Manufacturers of America adopted voluntary guidelines encouraging companies to educate physicians and patients before they commence their first DTCA campaigns. In a recent study of drug safety, the Institute of Medicine recommended that the FDA restrict advertising for newer prescription drugs and at least one pharmaceutical manufacturer (Bristol-Myers Squibb) recently announced a voluntary moratorium on DTCA for drugs in the first year after FDA approval. The European community code on medicinal products for human use states that advertising of medicinal products "must encourage the rational use of the product and may not be misleading". Canada's Food and Drugs Act prohibits advertising of a drug that is "false, misleading or deceptive or is likely to create an erroneous impression regarding its character, value, quantity, merit or safety". The World Health Organization's Ethical Criteria for Medicinal Drug Promotion states that advertisements "should not take undue advantage of people's concern for their health".

Impact of DTCA on Cost of Drugs

Spending on DTCA has continued to increase recently in absolute terms and as a percentage of pharmaceutical sales. Driven by increases in DTCA, total promotion as a percentage of sales has increased substantially during the past 5 years, leading to worry that consumers must bear these increased costs in the form of higher prices. In 2004, Astra-Zeneca spent $216 million promoting Crestor, almost matching the $212 million spent on Pepsi for that year. In the same year, Bayer, Schering-Plough and GlaxoSmithKline spent $157 million on advertising Levitra, a treatment for erectile dysfunction. Advertising spending positively correlates with increases in the number of prescriptions written for DTC drugs. A study reviewed by the GAO found a median increase in sales of more than $2 for every $1 spent on advertising. Another study found that each dollar spent on advertising in 2000 generated additional sales of $4.20. So, the critics maintain that there is a direct correlation of the higher drug prices with the amount pharmaceutical companies spend on DTCA. The implication is that the pharmaceutical companies raise the price of their product in order to recover the advertising cost. In the recent study done by Law and co-workers on clopidogrel, a commonly used and heavily marketed antiplatelet agent, which was first sold in 1998 and first direct-to-consumer advertised in 2001; from 2001 through 2005 DTCA spending exceeded $350 million. It was concluded that DTCA was not associated with an increase in clopidogrel use over and above pre-existing trends. However, Medicaid pharmacy expenditures increased substantially after the initiation of DTCA because of a concomitant increase in the cost per unit. The 10 most common conditions (Fig. 9.1) identified from DTCA (DTCA were defined as physician visits in which the patient initiated discussion about a prescription drug that had been advertised on broadcast media).

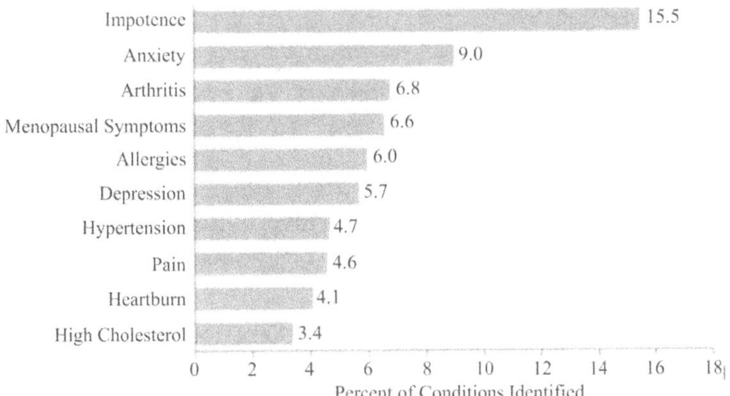

Fig. 9.1 Ten most common conditions identified from DTCA.

Discussion

Whether a reduction in DTCA would be desirable or undesirable from a public health perspective is a question that continues to be debated by proponents or opponents. Proponents assert that DTCA: (a) provides educational information; (b) enhances the physician-patient relationship; (c) stimulates competition and (d) results in lower prices for pharmaceuticals. Opponents counter that: (a) the promotional aspect of advertising will not communicate risk information effectively; (b) it will harm the physician-patient relationship; (c) it will lead to increased drug prices; (d) it will encourage overuse of medications. But the net public health impact of DTCA is a function of 3 factors: the current prevalence of under treatment of conditions that could be treated with advertised pharmaceuticals, the amount of appropriate and inappropriate prescribing that might be stimulated by DTCA, and the amount of benefit or harm accruing to under treat and over treated patients.

The liberalization in regulatory efforts and a tremendous increase in information delivery platforms the DTCA represent the fastest growing form of pharmaceutical marketing and have a global reach. Currently, New Zealand is the only other developed country, besides the United States, where DTCA is legal. However, the drug industry is mounting major lobbying campaigns to have DTCA allowed in Europe and Canada. In addition, as more drugs, are becoming available over the internet, the implications of DTCA go well beyond national and geographic boundaries means that it will be difficult to limit the flow of information across international borders. Given the limited effectiveness of current FDA efforts regarding US DTCA and the legal difficulty of implementing a DTCA ban, a different approach may be more fruitful. This requires a coordination and dialogue among consumer, regulatory and pharmaceutical groups and strong regulatory regimes to protect consumer interests.

Suggested Readings

1. Abel GA, Lee SJ, Weeks JC (2007). Direct-to-consumer advertising in oncology: a content analysis of print media. *J Clin Oncol.* **25:** 1267-1271.

2. Abel GA, Penson RT, Joffe S, *et al.,* (2006). Direct-to consumer advertising in oncology. *Oncologist.* **11:** 217-226.

3. Bell RA, Wilkes MS, Kravitz RL (1999). Advertisement-induced prescription drug requests: patients' anticipated reactions to a physician who refuses. *J Fam Pract.* **48:** 446-452.

4. Bell R. A., Kravitz R. L. & Wilkes M. S (2000). Direct-to-consumer prescription drug advertising, 1989-1998 - A content analysis of conditions, targets, inducements, and appeals. *J Fam Pratc.* **49:** 329-335.

5. Bell R. A., Wilkes M. S. & Kravitz R. L (2000). The educational value of consumer-targeted prescription drug print advertising. *J Fam Pract.* **49:** 1092-1098.

6. Berndt ER (2002). Pharmaceuticals in U.S. health care: determinants of quantity and price. *J Econ Perspect.* **16:** 45-66.

7. Bradley LR, Zito JM (1997). Direct-to-consumer prescription drug advertising. *Med Care.* **35:** 86-92.

8. Brown H (2007). Advertising prescription drugs: Sweetening the pill. *Br Med J.* **334:** 664-666.

9. Cassels A (2006). Canada may be forced to allow direct to consumer advertising. *Br Med J.* **332:** 1469.

10. Committee on the Assessment of the US Drug Safety System, Baciu A, Stratton K, Burke SP, eds (2006). The future of drug safety: promoting and protecting the health of the public. Washington, DC: National Academies Press.

11. Department of Justice [Canada]. Food and Drugs Act. Chapter F-27. Ottawa (Ontario). Available: http://laws.justice.gc.ca/en/ F-27/191368.html. Accessed 7 March 2006.

12. Donohue J.M., Cevasco M. & Rosenthal M.B (2007). *N Engl J Med.* **357:** 673-681.

13. Drug firms back-pedal on direct advertising (2005). *Nature.* **436(7053):** 910-911.

14. European Commission (2003) Community code relating to medicinal products for human use. Brussels: European Commission. Available: http://europa.eu.int/scadplus/leg/en/lvb/l21230.htm. Accessed 7 March 2006.

15. Felix M. Arellano (2005). The withdrawal of rofecoxib. *Pharmacoepidemiology and drug safety.* **14:** 213-217.

16. Frosch DL, Grande D, Tarn DM, Kravitz RL (2010). A decade of controversy: balancing policy with evidence in the regulation of prescription drug advertising. *Am J Public Health.* **100(1):** 24-32.

17. Gagnon M. A. and Lexchin J (2008). The Cost of Pushing Pills: A New Estimate of Pharmaceutical Promotion Expenditures in the United States. *PloS Medicine.* **5(1):**e1.

18. Gardner DM, Mintzes B, Ostry A (2003). Direct-to-consumer prescription drug advertising in Canada: permission by default? *CMAJ.* **169:** 425-427.

19. Huh J, DeLorme DE, Reid LN, An S (2010). Direct-to-consumer prescription drug advertising: history, regulation, and issues. *Minn Med.* **93(3):** 50-52.

20. Huh J. & Langteau R (2007). Presumed influence of DTC prescription drug advertising. *Commun Res.* **34:** 25-52.

21. Kefauver-Harris Act 21. Code of Regulations. 2.2.1 (1962).

22. Kolata G (2004). Awidely used arthritis drug is withdrawn. New York Times.

23. Kuehn BM (2010). FDA weighs limits for online ads. *JAMA*. **303(4):** 311- 313.

24. Law MR, Soumerai SB, Adams AS, Majumdar SR (2009). Costs and consequences of direct-to-consumer advertising for clopidogrel in Medicaid. *Arch Intern Med.* **169(21):** 1969-1974.

25. Lexchin J, Mintzes B (2002). Direct-to-consumer advertising of prescription drugs: the evidence says no. *J Publ Pol Market.* **21:** 194- 201.

26. Liang BA, Mackey T (2009). Searching for safety: addressing search engine, Website, and provider accountability for illicit online drug sales. *Am J Law Med.* **35(1):** 125-184.

27. Lipsky M. S. & Taylor C. A (1997). The opinions and experiences of family physicians regarding direct-to-consumer advertising. *J Fam. Pract.* **45:** 495- 499.

28. Lyles A (2002): Direct marketing of pharmaceuticals to consumers. *Annu Rev Public Health.* **23:** 73-91.

29. Maguire P (2004). How direct to consumer advertising is putting the squeeze on physicians. *ACP/ASIM Observer.* **1999:** 1-25.

30. Mueller C, Schur C, O'Connell J (1997). Prescription drug spending: the impact of age and chronic disease status. *Am J Public Health.* **87:** 1626-1629.

31. Patino FG, Allison J, Olivieri J, *et al.,* (2003). The effects of physician specialty and patient comorbidities on the use and discontinuation of Coxibs. *Arthr Rheum.* **49:** 293-299.

32. Perri M III, Shinde S, Banavali R (1999). The past, present, and future of direct-to-consumer prescription drug advertising. *Clin Ther.* **21:** 1798-1811.

33. Pharmaceutical Research and Manufacturers of America (2005). PhRMA guiding principles: direct-to-consumer advertising about prescription medicines. Washington, DC: PhRMA.

34. Pines WL (1999). A history and perspective on direct-to-consumer promotion. *Food Drug Law J.* **54:** 489-518.

35. Rosenthal MB, Berndt ER, Donohue JM, Frank RG, Epstein AM (2002). Promotion of prescription drugs to consumers. *N Engl J Med.* **346:** 498-505.

36. Spake D.F. and Mathew J. (2007). Consumer opinion and effectiveness of direct-to-consumer advertising. *Journal of Consumer Marketing.* **24(5):** 283-292.

37. Strange K. C. (2007). Time to ban direct to consumer prescription drug marketing. *Annals of Family Medicine.* **5(2):** 101-104.

38. The Henry J. *Kaiser Family Foundation.* Impact of Direct-to-Consumer Advertising on Prescription Drug Spending. (2003, June). http://kaiserfamily foundation.files.

wordpress.com/2003/06/6084-demand-effects-of-recent-changes-in-prescription-drug-promotion-report.pdf

39. Therapeutics Initiative (2003). Do statins have a role in primary prevention? *Ther Lett.* **48:** 1-2.

40. United States Congress (1984), House of Representatives, subcommittee on oversight and investigations of the committee on energy and commerce. Staff report on prescription drug advertising to consumers. Washington: Government Printing Office.

41. United States Government Accountability Office (2006). Prescription Drugs: Improvements Needed in FDA's Oversight of Direct-to-Consumer. PP: ii-47.

42. Vastag B. US aims to tighten rules on direct-to-consumer drug ads (2007). *Nat Biotechnol.* **25(3):** 267.

43. Watson R (2003). EU health ministers reject proposal for limited direct to consumer advertising. *BMJ.* **326:** 1284.

44. Wilkes MS, Bell RA, Kravitz RL (2000). Direct-to-consumer prescription drug advertising: trends, impact, and implications. *Health Aff (Millwood).* **19:** 110-128.

45. World Health Organization (1988). Ethical criteria for medicinal drug promotion. Geneva: World Health Organization. Available: http://mednet2.who.int/tbs/promo/whozip08e.pdf. Accessed 7 March 2006.

CHAPTER 10

ORPHAN DRUGS: FROM DEVELOPMENT TO MARKET

Introduction

Rare diseases and their diagnosis, and management are rarely discussed in scientific forums. Discussion about such disorders is as rare as the disorder itself. Except for few societies, specialist physicians and patient groups, not many are interested in discussions and research about such disorders. However, in last few years, there are increased attention is being paid currently to various issues dealing with rare diseases. This chapter intends to provide the reader with updated information on various aspects dealing with these diseases, issues plaguing research in rare diseases and the means and incentives being offered by various regulatory bodies for promotion of research in such conditions. In the end, the misuse of these provisions by pharmaceutical industry will also be discussed briefly.

Rare Diseases and Orphan Status

Rare diseases are called 'rare' on the basis of prevalence of disease. European standards call a disease to be rare if the prevalence is < 1 case per 2000 population, while the same is < 1 case per 1250 population in United States of America. The definition (according to prevalence) of rare disease in different regions of world is given in Table 10.1.

Table 10.1 Definitions of orphan diseases in major regions of world

Country	No. of Affected Individuals	Prevalence (per 10,000)
United States	< 200,000	7.5
European Union	< 2,15,000	5.0
United Kingdom	< 1000	0.18
Japan	< 50,000	4.0
India	?????	??

Reproduced in part from, Christopher McCabe, Karl Claxton, Aki Tsuchiya. Orphan drugs and the NHS: should we value rarity? British Medical Journal 2005; 331: 1016–1019.

As per World Health Organization > 5000 such diseases are known currently. According to one estimate, the number of people affected by rare diseases could be 25 million in North America and 30 million in Europe. The count is increasing day by day with more and rarer diseases being identified and notified.

These diseases are often called '*health orphans*' for being neglected for many years by medical community and pharmaceutical industry. The high cost of drug development, coupled with the low return on investment, discourage the pharmaceutical industry from developing products for extremely small patient populations.

Designation as Orphan Disease/Drug

Several jurisdictions have established regulations for orphan drugs. The United States was the first country to do so, through the 1983 United States Orphan Drugs Act. The European Union did not establish orphan drugs status until 2000.

From regulatory perspective, a drug or biologic becomes an "orphan drug" when it receives orphan-drug designation from the Office of Orphan Products Development at the US-FDA. Orphan-drug designation qualifies the sponsor to receive certain benefits from the Government in exchange for developing the drug for a rare disease or condition.

According to European Regulations, a medicinal product can be designated as an orphan medicinal product if the sponsor can establish

(a) That, it is intended for the diagnosis, prevention or treatment of a life-threatening or chronically debilitating condition affecting not more than 5 in 10,000 persons in the community when application is made or it is intended for the diagnosis, prevention or treatment of a life-threatening, seriously debilitating or serious and chronic condition in the community and without incentives, it is unlikely that the marketing of the medicinal product in the community would generate sufficient return to justify the necessary investment.

(b) And, that there exists no satisfactory method of diagnosis, prevention or treatment of the condition in question that has been authorized in the community or, if such method exists, that the medicinal product will be of significant benefit to those affected by that condition.

The designation of disease as rare does not remain forever. With changing epidemiological status of disease, it may be de-categorized to a common disease. Let's take the example of Achondroplasia. It is the most frequent type of chondrodysplasias with prevalence of 1:15,000 in Europe. An autosomal dominant disorder, it is characterized by short limbs, hyperlordosis and macrocephaly with normal mental development and functions. Most patients are born to unaffected parents following new mutation in fibroblast growth factor receptor-3 (FGFR3) gene. Pre-natal diagnostic techniques are available as preventive measure and no pharmacotherapy is effective in prevention or management of primary condition. This is one extreme of rare disease with minimal functional impairment where timely diagnosis is the only means of prevention. It is quite unlikely that the incidence of mutation will ever change leading to increase or decrease in the prevalence of condition in general public.

At the other extreme is Acquired Immune Deficiency Syndrome (AIDS), which was considered an extremely rare in early 1980's and with gradual increase in prevalence, the category of disease is changing frequently and may reach epidemic if not controlled with adequate preventive measures. Presently, a lot of research is going on in this field which does not qualify for being labeled as a rare disease. The number of drugs available for treatment of AIDS and diagnostic modalities is also increasing day by day.

These two diseases represent the extreme ends of spectrum of rare diseases. Almost all other diseases fall somewhere in between these two ends. With many potentially treatable conditions without any specific therapy but with some research going on into their management and others with no research just because there will not be any commercial gains from it.

Research in Rare Diseases

1. Lack of Clear Diagnostic Criteria

There is absence of universally recognized coding system for reliable registration of patients suffering from these diseases in various health care registries and databases. International Classification of Diseases (ICD) used in most countries is not convenient for rare diseases. Even though ICD is the international standard diagnostic classification for all general epidemiological, many health management purposes and clinical use, its use in general public by physicians is hampered either by lack of clear diagnostic and clinical criteria or lack of knowledge of physician about the disease. Additionally, all rare diseases are presently not classified in this system and major revisions are under consideration. The proposals can be accessed at the website www.orpha.net.

2. Lack of Knowledge in Medical Community

Among members of medical community, information about rare disorders is significantly less. During the days spent in medical schools most of the physicians rarely encounter patients with rare disorders. Lack of information affects diagnosis of such disorders leaving aside research and management of such patients. Patients with these disorders suffer from incorrect diagnosis, diagnostic delays and futile medical interventions. Number of patients dies from complications of such diseases, undiagnosed by physicians in primary or secondary care settings. In tertiary care centers, the knowledgeable physicians consider such diseases in their differential diagnosis, but for a definitive diagnosis, the patients might not be able to afford the cost of diagnostic tests in case such means do exist.

3. Lack of Diagnostic and Treatment Facilities

Most of these disorders are disabling, affect mental and physical capabilities, life expectancy and quality of life significantly. Very few centers are equipped to diagnose such disorders definitively. Even if, diagnosed, available treatment modalities do not offer significant improvement in clinical outcomes. With many diseases leading to shorter life-spans, the time period available for research into diagnosis and treatment is short enough to provide a meaningful answer.

4. Inadequate Sample Size and Effect Size for Clinical Trials

These diseases being rare, the sample size required for conducting clinical trials in such diseases is a difficult task. To arrive at a meaningful conclusion in times of evidence-based medicine, randomized controlled clinical trials offer the best evidence. With small sample size the strength of evidence decreases. Additionally, since very less is known about the course of rare diseases, the effect size might not be defined adequately for meaningful clinical or statistical significance.

5. Lack of Comparators and Standardization

Since not many drugs or therapies which can affect the course of disease are known, choice of control group becomes more and more difficult in such disorders. Moreover, with variety of treatment options being practiced across different countries, standardization of groups for comparison also becomes difficult.

A lot of research is still required in field of known rare diseases. With all these and many more issues plaguing research in orphan diseases, these conditions will remain as *'health orphans'* and drugs used to treat these condition\s will be called *'orphan drugs'*.

Promotion of Research in Rare Diseases

Pharmaceutical companies practically develop almost all medicinal products. They aim to recover their drug research and development outlay by market sales. Therefore, when a company is deciding, whether or not to develop a given drug, it may well opt out on economic and commercial grounds, if it thinks that market sales will not cover the research and development costs due to a low incidence of the disease in question. It is because of this concept of abandonment that these types of drugs with no commercial interests are called 'orphan drugs'.

In recent past, a number of new initiatives had been taken to promote research and improve outcomes and in the field of rare diseases. US Orphan Drug Act was passed in 1983 and has promoted development and marketing of drugs for rare diseases in United States of America. The European Platform for Patient, Organizations, Science and Industry is a partnership between patients, industry, and scientists, set up in 1994 to exchange information and discuss policies on healthcare promotion. The International Conference on Rare Diseases and Orphan Drugs was first held in 2005 in Stockholm, Sweden, covering a range of issues related to rare diseases and orphan drugs. A lot more needs to be done in the field of rare diseases and their management.

A number of incentives for promotion of research in orphan diseases have been proposed and implemented in Orphan Disease Act of United States of America. The incentives include new drug applications fee waiver, tax credits for clinical research on orphan products, grant funding for the investigation of rare disease treatment and market exclusivity. Market exclusivity is the most powerful incentive. It assures that no other sponsor will receive FDA marketing approval for the same drug for the same indication for 7 years after marketing approval of the innovators product. Also, it is a more comprehensive incentive than a patent because product approval and orphan designation by the FDA are essentially the only requirements for orphan market exclusivity.

Drug Development and Issues

Orphan drugs vary from chemicals, complex enzymes and biologics, specific antidotes for poisoning for diagnosis to preventive vaccines for rare infections. With clouds of chemical warfare looming large on mankind, the development of antidotes for such situations has gained significant importance. Such scenarios will affect the mankind rarely and is likely to affect few subjects as compared to the world population. Antidotes to such agents enjoy orphan drug status from the drug regulatory bodies of the world. Most of research on antidotes is concentrated in institutes affiliated with armed forces of various countries.

The development of biologics and other agents for rare genetic disorders is done by very few pharmaceutical industries. Major regulatory bodies in the world provide incentives for promotion of research and development activities in such disorders. The cost of drug development seems to over-shadow the benefit gained out of such incentives.

Incentives for Drug Development for Rare Diseases

Economics of drug discovery, development and research and revenues generated from marketing do not favor investment in research and development of new molecules for rare disorders unless incentives for such an endeavor are provided to the pharmaceutical industry. Governments and regulatory bodies across the developed world have understood the importance of such methods and have devised a number of such activities. Broadly, incentives can be divided into three major areas: setting up of tax credits and research aids, simplification of and advantages in drug authorization process, and marketing exclusivity of orphan drugs. Special stress is laid on marketing exclusivity with periods varying in different regulatory regions.

1. United States of America

In 1983, the Congress passed the Orphan drug Act, which was signed into law by President Reagan. This act provided tax relief for companies investing in clinical research for orphan drugs, and it provided for seven years of exclusivity for a product approved for an orphan disease, even though the product might be otherwise in common use. This means that no other company could advertise or market a drug (whether already available) for this particular indication during this period. Additionally, marketing application for a prescription drug product that has been designated as a drug for a rare disease or condition is not subject to a prescription drug user fee unless the application includes an indication for other than a rare disease or condition.

The law also provides for a waiver from user fee paid by the sponsor to FDA for the reviewing the application. A human drug application for a prescription drug product that has been designated as a drug for a rare disease or condition shall not be subject to a fee unless the human drug application includes an indication for other than a rare disease or condition.

To expedite the marketing of new molecules for rare diseases, the approval time for orphan products as a group has been considerably shortened than the approval time for other drugs. This reduced approval time is often due to the fact that many orphan products receive expedited review or accelerated approval because they are for serious or life-threatening disease.

2. European Union

As a counterpart to the United States Orphan Drug Act, 1983, European Union Regulation on Orphan Medicinal Products came into force year 2000. As per the law, a number of provisions have been made to promote research in orphan drugs. The provisions include protocol assistance, community-marketing authorization, market exclusivity and other incentives. Protocol assistance provides for advice from regulatory body on the conduct of various tests and trials to demonstrate quality, efficacy and safety of medicinal product. Special contribution from community shall be provided to the regulatory agency to waive off fee charged for conduct of studies. A marketing exclusivity for a period of 10 years is granted to the marketing authorization holder for orphan drug with a rider that the period can be reduced to 6 years in case the criteria defining the rarity of disease changes at the end of 5 years. Other incentives include support for research into and development and availability of drug in community. More details about European Union Regulations can be obtained from Regulation (EC) N 141/2000 of the European Parliament and of the Council of 16 December 1999 on Orphan medicinal products. Official Journal 2018, 22 January 2000; 0001–0005.

	USA	EU	Japan	Australia	India
Marketing Exclusivity	7 years	10 years	10 years	5 years	NA
Tax Credits (variable)	Yes	No	Yes	No	NA
Protocol Assistance	Yes	Yes	No	No	NA
Regulatory Body Fee Waiver	Yes	Yes	No	Yes	NA
Financial Grants	Yes	Yes	Yes	No	NA

Clinical Trials on Orphan Medicines

Conducting clinical trials in orphan diseases to generate appropriate evidence for safe and effective use of new medicine requires special mention. Such clinical studies are special in many aspects. The problems encountered include the source of funding (government body or private pharmaceutical industry) and recruitment of competitive and trained physicians for the job, finding laboratories having expertise in conducting diagnostic and prognostic tests. The biggest hurdle is finding the adequate number of patients at a similar state of illness. The prevalence of disease constrains the conduct, analysis and interpretation of study results. Patient population becomes too less for extrapolation of results of this study to general population. The choice of trial designs other than randomized, double-blind, placebo controlled design for disease with low prevalence is required. Use of Bayesian approaches, N-of-1, crossover, sequential and adaptive designs are being explored more and more for rare diseases. Regulatory bodies have not specified any trial design requirements for conducting clinical studies in patients suffering from rare diseases. They are open to new and scientifically rational clinical trial designs.

Orphan Disease status: *In Indian Scenario*

India have joined the hand with U.S. NORD (National Organization for Rare Disorders, a NGO) to create the awareness in country and to promote the drug development in the area of treatment of orphan disease. According to the Office of the Registrar and Census Commissioner, Government of India the current rare disease reached to the population about 72,611,605 in India.

However, they have organized Rare Disease Day in the last day of February in 2010, 2011 and 2012. But, there was no tangible effect of the programme to Indian government and still we are waiting for the policy regarding the control of orphan diseases in the country.

Suggested Readings

1. Drummond M, Towse A (2014). Orphan drugs policies: a suitable case for treatment. *Eur J Health Econ*. [Epub ahead of print].

2. Fellows GK, Hollis A (2013). Funding innovation for treatment for rare diseases: adopting a cost-based yardstick approach. *Orphanet J Rare Dis*. **8:** 180.

3. Food and Drug Administration, HHS (2013). Orphan drug regulations. Final rule. *Fed Regist.* **78(113):** 35117-35135.

4. Health Resources and Services Administration (HRSA), Department of Health and Human Services (HHS) (2013). Exclusion of orphan drugs for certain covered entities under 340B Program. Final rule. *Fed Regist.* **78(141):** 44016-44028.

5. Hyry HI, Roos JC, Manuel J, Cox TM (2013). The legal imperative for treating rare disorders. *Orphanet J Rare Dis.* **8:** 135.

6. Kanters TA, de Sonneville-Koedoot C, Redekop WK, Hakkaart L (2013). Systematic review of available evidence on 11 high-priced inpatient orphan drugs. *Orphanet J Rare Dis.* **8(1):** 124.

7. O'Sullivan BP, Orenstein DM, Milla CE (2013). Pricing for orphan drugs: will the market bear what society cannot? *JAMA.* **310(13):** 1343-1344.

8. Pastores GM, Gupta P (2013). Orphan drug development. *Pediatr Endocrinol Rev.* **11(1):** 64-67.

9. Putzeist M, Mantel-Teeuwisse AK, Llinares J, Gispen-De Wied CC, Hoes AW, Leufkens HG (2013). EU marketing authorization review of orphan and non-orphan drugs does not differ. *Drug Discov Today.* **18(19-20):** 1001-1006.

10. Shani S, Yahalom Z (2013). Legal and regulatory aspects of orphan drugs. *Pediatr Endocrinol Rev.* **11(1):** 110-115.

CHAPTER 11

DRUG LABEL

Introduction

Label is the face of any product. Apart from providing an identity to the product it also serves several other purposes like source of information to different stakeholders, fulfillment of regulatory requirements etc. Labeling is defined as all labels and other written, printed, or graphic matter upon any article or any of its containers or wrappers, or accompanying such article. The term 'accompanying' is interpreted liberally to mean more than physical adherence with the product. It extends to posters, tags, pamphlets, circulars, booklets, brochures, instructions, websites, etc. Regulatory body of every country has a set of requirements for labeling of drugs. Keeping those requirements under consideration, labels are designed by the manufacturers. Some important aspects of the labeling are discussed in this chapter.

Types of Drug Label

Depending upon the physical association of label with the container or package of the drug there are three type of label which are described as under:

Inner Label: Inner label is a type of label in which there is a physical association of the label with the immediate container or packing of the drug. This type of labeling is found on the smallest packed unit of the drug .The label on the container e.g., ampoule or the bottle should show Proper name, Contents in millilitres or doses, Potency, if any, Batch number, Expiry date of the formulation.

Outer label: Outer label belongs to the label on the package having small packages of the drug formulation e.g., cardboard cartons carrying the syrups bottles or strips of the tablets.

SmPC & PIL: Summary of Product Characteristics (SmPC) is a document of information pertaining to the drug which is submitted to the regulatory bodies along with the approval application by the company seeking market authorization. Patient information leaflet is prepared in accordance with the SmPC. SmPC is the basis of information for healthcare professionals on how to use the medicinal product safely and effectively. The guidelines on excipients in the label and package leaflet of medicinal products for human use are also applicable to the SmPC.

Components of Drug Label

In Indian context, Labeling Rule 96 of the DCR ('Manner of Labeling') mandates the minimum information which needs to be put on the label of all medicines other than ISM medicines (*ayurveda, siddha and unani*). The minimum information required to be put on label includes;

(a)   Proper (generic) and trade (brand) name

(b)   Net contents and content of active ingredients

(c)   Name and address of manufacturer including manufacturing license number

(d)   Distinctive batch number, manufacturing and expiry date etc.

(e)   Maximum Retail Price (inclusive of all taxes)

Various segments of drug labels are described briefly here as below;

Name of Drug/Drugs

In India, *Rule 96 of Drugs and cosmetics Rules, 1945* describes the manner of labeling. Proper name should be printed or written more prominent than the trade name of the drug. Trade name of the product should be written after the proper name.

In USA, labeling and advertising regulations (21 CFR 201.10 (g) and (h); 202.1(b), (c) and (d)) Title 21 is the portion of the Code of Federal Regulations which specifies the placement, size, prominence, and frequency of the proprietary and official names for prescription human drugs, including biological drug products, and prescription animal drugs. These regulations are applicable to prescription human and animal drug products that contain one or more active ingredient(s). The regulation states that where the official name is required to accompany or to be used in association with the proprietary name or designation, the official name should be placed in direct conjunction with the proprietary name or designation, and the relationship between the proprietary name or designation and the official name should be made clear by use of a phrase such as "Brand of" preceding the official name, by brackets surrounding the official name, or by other suitable means. Symbols of intellectual property rights like trademark are allowed after proprietary name of the product. USFDA recommends that the official name should be presented with equal prominence as that of proprietary name.

As far as it is concerned with the size of proprietary name and official name it is recommended as per regulation (21 CFR 201.10(g)(1) and (2); 202.1(b)(1) and (2)) that size of smallest font of official name should be at least half in size to the size of largest letter in the proprietary name. Such requirement is applicable when proprietary name is to be mentioned outside the running text otherwise both the name should carry the same size usually in practice.

Net Contents and Content of Active Ingredients

Content is a very important part of information on label as dosage is to be ascertained on the basis of this vital component of the label.

USFDA has set guidelines on "How to mention the ingredients". In case of products with two or more active ingredients the regulations 21 CFR 201.10(h) (1) and 202.1(c) describes the way to declare content information on label of drug products.

The quantitative ingredient information required on the label by section 502(e) of the act [or in the advertisement by section 502(n) of the act] should be placed in direct conjunction with the most prominent display of the proprietary name or designation. The prominence of the quantitative ingredient information should bear a reasonable relationship to the prominence of the proprietary name. Similarly, a product with one proprietary name might refer to a combination of active ingredients present in more than one preparation. Different products may be produced by varying the quantities of active ingredients and/or the form of the finished preparation, and there might not be an established/official name corresponding to the proprietary name. In such instances, the advertising regulations (21 CFR 202.1(d)(1)) requires that a lists showing the established names of the active ingredients should be placed in direct conjunction with the most prominent display of such proprietary name or designation. The prominence of this listing of active ingredients should bear a reasonable relationship to the prominence of the proprietary name and the relationship between such proprietary name or designation, and also the listing of active ingredients should be made clear by use of such phrase as "brand of", preceding the listing of active ingredients.

In India, ingredients information is to be included in the label of drug products. The requirements are summarized in the table shown below:

Table 11.1 Methods of mentioning the active ingredients in different type formulations

Formulation	Way to mention ingredients
Oral liquid preparations	Indicated in 5 millilitres or lower volume. E.g., each 5 ml of syrup contains
Liquid parenteral preparations ready for administration	1 millilitre or percentage by volume or per dose in the case of single dose container contains
Solid form intended for parenteral administration	Units or weight per milligram or gram
Tablets, Capsules, Pills	Content in each tablet, capsule, pill or other unit
Other preparations	Percentage by weight or volume or in terms of unit per gram or millilitre

Name and Address of the Manufacturer

Name of the manufacturer and address of the manufacturing site is required to be mentioned on label. However, it may be relaxed in the case of small packing like ampoules to put the name of manufacturer along with place of the manufacturing but not the full address.

Drug License Number under which Drug has been Manufactured

Every drug manufactured in India bears on its label, the number of the license under which the drug is manufactured, words "Manufacturing License Number" or "Mfg. Lic. No." or "M.L." is written before the figure representing the manufacturing license number.

Batch Number/Lot Number

Batch number is an identity of the bulk of substance from which the packings are done. The figure representing the batch number is being preceded by the words 'Batch No.' or 'B. No.' or 'Batch' or 'Lot No.' or 'Lot'.

Batch number is crucial for drug control authorities, when there is some quality issue is raised for a particular set of products.

Date of Expiry

Date of expiry is information that healthcare professionals and consumer always look for the assurance of safety and efficacy of the product. According to regulatory agencies requirements; Date of expiry must be on the inner and outer labels of all drug products. The date of expiry should be in terms of month and year and it would mean that the drug is recommended for use till the last day of the month. The date of expiry should be preceded by the words 'Expiry date'. In Canada however, for guidance, some acceptable terms include "Expiration" or "Expiration date" in English, and "Expiration" or "Date d'expiration" in French. The term "Expiration" or its abbreviation "EXP". is acceptable as a bilingual expression. In case of cosmetics and nutritional supplements, some of the regulatory agencies like MHRA also relax the manufacturers by allowing them to state the life of product in the form of "Best before".

Precautions and Warnings

The "Warnings and Precautions" section of a label is of paramount importance because this section describes a discrete set of adverse reactions and other potential safety hazards that are possible with the use of drugs and may be sometimes serious or are otherwise clinically significant and plays an important role in patient care.

Caution statements on label are required for different drug schedules under the rule 97 of drugs and cosmetics rules in India. For example, drugs falling under Schedule G require "Caution: it is dangerous to take this preparation except under medical supervision". Schedule H drugs need the symbol "Rx" as well as "Schedule H – Warning: To be sold by retail on the prescription of a Registered Medical Practitioner only".

The same requirements are also applicable for Over The Counter (OTC) drugs.

For the drugs specified in Schedule H, symbol Rx should be displayed on the left top corner of the label and be also labeled with the following words: 'Schedule H drug-Warning: To be sold by retail on the prescription of a Registered Medical Practitioner only'.

If a drug product contains a substance specified in Schedule X, it should be labeled with the symbol XRx which should be in red color conspicuously displayed on the left top corner of the label and be also labeled with the following words

'Schedule X drug -Warning: To be sold by retail on the prescription of a Registered Medical Practitioner only'.

The container of an embrocation, liniment, lotion, ointment, antiseptic cream, liquid antiseptic or other liquid medicine for external application should be labeled with the words: *"For External Use only"*.

According to MHRA in United Kingdom, only those warnings, specifically required by the terms of the marketing authorization to be stated on the labeling, will form part of the critical labeling. Many medicines will not need the addition of any warnings on the front of the pack. This section is intended to convey only those critical warnings which are necessary immediately, prior to administering the product.

Black boxed warning is a type of special warning given for certain prescription drugs. The United States Food and Drug Administration (USFDA) can require a pharmaceutical company to place a boxed warning on the labeling of a prescription drug, or in literature describing it. It is the strongest warning that the FDA requires for any drug and it implies that the drug may pose a significant risk of serious or even life-threatening adverse effects. For example, antidepressant drugs require their suicidal tendency as a possible adverse effect to be placed black box warning.

Possible Adverse Drug Reactions

According to USFDA requirements, the "ADVERSE REACTIONS" section is required to list the adverse reactions that occur with the drug and with drugs in the same pharmacologically active and chemically related class. Adverse reactions identified from clinical trials (§ 201.57(c)(7)(ii)(A)) and those identified from post marketing surveillance should be listed separately (§ 201.57(c)(7)(ii)(B)). This section of the guidance provides recommendations for ensuring that information about the most clinically important adverse reactions is readily accessible (see III.A), and for organizing the information on adverse reactions from clinical trials (see III.B) and from post-marketing safety reports (see III.C).

Dose and Administration of Drug

According to USFDA requirements a concise summary of the information required under paragraph (c)(3) of 21CFR201.57 should be incorporated in the labeling material. The recommended dosage regimen, starting dose, dose range, critical differences among population subsets, monitoring recommendations, and other clinically significant clinical pharmacological information are required contents of this segment of label.

Dosages information for different age groups is mentioned on the label under Indian requirements of labeling. This is suggestible to specify the phrase "As directed by Registered medical Practitioner" in absence of concrete information available on the dosage and administration of the drug.

Indications

After a rigorous testing of the drug through clinical trials, drug is approved by regulatory authorities for specific use *viz* indications. Every time, if the market authorization holder wants to add some additional indications for use of the drug then it is required to get fresh approval for the drug for new indications and under such instances drugs are treated as new drugs. Use of drug beyond the indications mentioned in labeled or approved by the regulators is termed as off label use.

Contraindications

Information on the restricted use in particular population e.g., pregnant or lactating women is declared in this section of the label. For example, thalidomide is known for its teratogenic properties so, it should be clearly displayed on the label that this drug should not be taken by pregnant women or women planning to conceive.

Directions for use

This segment of the label is important for intended use of the drug as, it instructs the consumers or healthcare professionals regarding the method of using the drug product for its best outcomes. E.g., SHAKE WELL BEFORE USE, is printed on the containers of suspension which is very important for uniform drug delivery in each dosage of such formulations because drug content settle down in the container with the course of time.

Clinical Pharmacology

Clinical pharmacology section of labels informs the practicing healthcare professionals regarding the various pharmacological descriptions of the drug product. Components of this section are tabulated in the Table 11.2.

Table 11.2 Subsections of clinical pharmacology section of drug label

Clinical pharmacology in label				
Pharmacokinetics	Pharmacodynamics	Mechanism of action	Pharmacogenomics	Microbiology in case of antimicrobials

Such information is usually supplied in the SmPC not in the adhered label of the pharmaceutical product. SmPC is a reference document accompanying the product.

Price

Under The "Standards of Weights & Measures (Packaged Commodities) Rules", most packaged consumer products including, Indian System of Medicine (ISM) drugs are required to have the Maximum Retail Price (MRP) printed on the label. The maximum retail sale price of scheduled and non-scheduled drugs is as per the provisions of Drugs Price Control Order (DPCO) 1995. The trade margins (wholesale and retail) are also restricted under DPCO. The selling of any product at a price higher than the MRP is not permitted.

Labeling of Professional Samples

Every drug intended for distribution to the medical profession as a free sample labeling should comply with the labeling provisions under clauses (i) to (viii) of rule 96 of the drugs and cosmetics act, 1940. In addition to these requirements, the words 'Physician's Sample-Not to be sold' on the label of the container is overprinted.

Calendar Packs Labeling

Calendar packs are only appropriate for tablets or capsules that are taken as a single dose once (or twice) daily. The packs must be supplied in multiples of 7 and all blister pockets must be labeled with the days of the week.

Functions of Label

Identity of products: Label accompanying the drug product serves as an identity as it contains both proprietary and generic name. It helps in proper inventory management and distribution of the drugs.

Information: Label serves as an information tool for various stakeholders *viz* professionals and patients. Different areas of interest of the stakeholders in a label are summarized as under.

For healthcare professionals, various information regarding the indications, storage, contraindications are available in the label.

For many patients this is the only written information they will have about the medicines which they are taking.

Good information helps patients to participate fully in concordant decision-making about medicines prescribed for or recommended to them by healthcare professionals. Self-care, a key government objective relies heavily on patients having sufficient high quality information on which to base their decision-making. For medicine purchase OTC interaction between the patient and a healthcare professional may be limited or unavailable. In this latter case written information has an increased importance for safe use of the medicine.

Economics: Price of the product is also a part of label which guides the buyer for purchasing the drug. To curb the problem of disproportionate profit reaping, drug price policies have been drafted and are being revised periodically by the various drug regulating agencies.

Attraction: Drug label can render the product attractive to the physician and customer of the drug product.

Regulatory compliance: If a drug product is not labeled in a prescribed format and it is somehow, presents the false claims then, such drugs are categorized as misbranded, spurious and attracts the legal actions.

Prescription Labels

When drug is dispensed by the pharmacist by formulating the preparation or repackaging the drugs in pharmacy then following information is needed on label:

Pharmacy's name, address and telephone number

Unique prescription number assigned only to that very prescription

Date of filling the prescription

Name and address of the patient

Instructions for taking the medication

Number of refills allowed or required

Expiry date

Name of physician who prescribed medication

Bar Codes

Bar codes may be used on a drug label for appropriate purposes e.g., retail inventory, tracking, confirmation of identity, potency, etc. provided that all regulatory requirements concerning the label are met and the bar code information does not change the terms of market authorization for the product; and the bar code does not obscure or displace the required and approved information on the label, especially on small product labels. Bar coding proves to be helpful in reducing the medication errors in healthcare settings.

International Regulations

In India, Drugs and cosmetics rules, 1945 (amended up to June 2012) rule 94-97 describes the labeling requirements. The labeling provisions of Indian system of medicines are covered by Rule 161 of Indian Drugs and cosmetics rule.

In United Kingdom, according to MHRA article 54 of Council Directive 2001/83/EEC speaks about labeling and defines the essential content of a label. It must contain all elements required by article 54 of Council Directive 2001/83/EEC. Nevertheless, certain items of information are deemed critical for the safe use of the medicine. These items are name of the medicine, expression of strength, route of administration, posology and warnings.

In United States of America, USFDA has issued the guidance for industry regarding various components of label of drugs and biological products. Federal Food, Drug, and Cosmetic Act details the requirements of the manner of labeling.

Drug labeling by pharmaceutical companies, selling their products internationally are influenced by the following factors:

1. Home country: Regulations of the country in which the parent company is headquartered e.g., the United States, in the case of U.S. based MNCs affect the labeling of the drugs. For example, a drug manufactured in US but exported to some other country for sale should comply with the US standards of drug labeling with minor changes required by the importer.
2. Host country: The laws and policies of the foreign country in which the MNC is manufacturing or importing or marketing the drug also sometimes asks for the specific formats and contents of the drug label.
3. International organizations.
4. Self regulation: Internal company policies and national and international codes of conduct developed to standardize certain practices worldwide.
5. Public interest groups and consumer activists: political and media pressure.

Labeling of Ayurvedic and other Alternative Systems of Medicines in India

Labeling requirements of Ayurvedic, Siddha, Unani drugs is governed by the Drugs and Cosmetics act 1940 and rules 1945 in India.

The label of the container or package of an Ayurvedic (including Siddha) or Unani drug should display the true list of all the ingredients along with the quantities their-of used in the manufacture and a reference to the method of preparation thereof as detailed in the standard text. In case of large list of ingredients contained in the medicine which cannot be accommodated on the label, it may then be printed separately and enclosed with packing and its reference should be made on the label.

The container of a medicine for internal use made up ready for the treatment of human ailments should, if it is made up from a substance specified in Schedule E(1), be labeled conspicuously with the words 'Caution: To be taken under medical supervision' both in English and Hindi language.

The following particulars should be either printed or written in indelible ink and should appear in a conspicuous manner on the label of the innermost container of any Ayurvedic (including Siddha) or Unani drug and on any other covering in which the container is packed:

1. The name of the drug as mentioned in the authoritative books included in the first schedule of the Drugs and Cosmetics Act.

2. A correct statement of the net content of the ingredients expressed in terms of weight, measure or number as the case may be.

3. The name and address of the manufacturer.

4. Licence number under which the drug is manufactured, the figure representing the manufacturing licence number should be preceded by the words 'Manufacturing Licence Number' or 'Mfg. Lic. No.' or 'M.L.'.

5. Batch number and the figure representing the batch number should be preceded by the words "Batch No." or "Batch" or "Lot Number" or "Lot No." or "Lot" or any distinguishing prefix.

6. Manufacturing date which is the date of completion of the final products, or the date of bottling or packing for release.

7. The words "Ayurvedic medicine" or "Siddha medicine" or "Unani medicine" as the case may be.

8. The words "FOR EXTERNAL USE ONLY" if the medicine is for external application.

9. Every drug product intended for distribution as a free sample should while complying with the labeling provisions listed above should additionally bear the words "Physicians sample. Not to be sold" which should be over-printed.

Labeling of Cosmetics

Rule 148 of Drugs and Cosmetics Rules, 1945 explains the manner of labeling applicable on cosmetics. According to these rules; subject to other provisions of the rules, a cosmetic should carry on:

1. **Both the inner and outer labels**

    (a) The name of the cosmetic,

    (b) The name of the manufacturer and complete address of the premises of the manufacturer where the cosmetic has been manufactured.

If the cosmetic is contained in a very small size container where the address of the manufacturer cannot be given, the name of the manufacturer and his principal place of manufacture should be given along with pin code.

2. **On the outer label**

A declaration of the net contents expressed in terms of weight for solids, fluid measure for liquids, weight for semi-solids, combined with numerical count if the content is sub-divided.

Provided that this statement need not appear in case of a package of perfume, toilet water or the like the net content of which does not exceed 60 ml or any package of solid or semi-solid cosmetic the net content of which does not exceed 30 grams.

3. **On the inner label, where a hazard exists**

   (a)   Adequate direction for safe use.

   (b)   Any warning, caution or special direction required to be observed by the consumer.

   (c)   A statement of the names and quantities of the ingredients those are hazardous or poisonous.

4. A distinctive batch number, that is to say, the number by reference to which details of manufacture of the particular batch from which the substance in the container is taken; are recorded and are available for inspection, the figures representing the batch number being preceded by the letter "B", provided that this clause should not apply to any cosmetic containing 10 grams or less if the cosmetic is in solid or semi-solid state, and 25 milliliters or less if, the cosmetic is in a liquid state:

   Provided, further that in the case of soaps, instead of the batch number, the month and year of manufacture of soap should be given on the label.

5. Manufacturing license number, the number being preceded by the letter 'M'.

6. Where a package of a cosmetic has only one label, such label should contain all the information required to be shown on both the inner and the outer labels, under Drugs and cosmetics Rules.

The cosmetics distributed in the United States of America must be in accordance with the labeling regulations published by the USFDA under the authority of the FD&C Act and the FP&L Act. The label statements required under the authority of the FD&C Act must appear on the inside as well as any outside container or wrapper. FP&L Act requirements, e.g., ingredient labeling and statement of the net quantity of contents on the principal display panel, only apply to the label of the outer container. The labeling requirements are codified at 21 CFR 701 and 740. The principal display panel, i.e., the part of the label most likely displayed or examined under customary conditions of display for sale (21 CFR 701.10), must state the name of the product, identify by descriptive name or illustration of the nature or use of the product, and bear an accurate statement of the net quantity of contents of the cosmetic in the package in terms of weight, measure, numerical count, or a combination of numerical count and weight or measure.

Labeling of Hair Dyes Containing Dyes, Colors and Pigments

Hair dyes containing Para-Phenylenediamine or other Dyes, Colors and Pigments should be labeled with the following legend in English and local languages and these should appear on both the inner and the outer labels.

"Caution—this product contains ingredients which may cause skin irritation in certain cases and so, a preliminary test according to the accompanying direction should first be made. This product should not be used for dyeing the eye-lashes or eye-brows; as such a use may cause blindness".

Each package should also contain instructions in English and local languages on the following lines for carrying out the test:

"This preparation may cause serious inflammation of the skin in some cases and so, a preliminary test should always be carried out to determine whether or not special sensitivity exists. To make the test, cleanse a small area of skin behind the ear or upon the inner surface of the forearm, using either soap and water or alcohol. Apply a small quantity of the hair dye as prepared for use to the area and allow it to dry. After twenty-four hours, wash the area gently with soap and water. If no irritation or inflammation is apparent, it may be assumed that no hypersensitivity to the dye exists. The test should, however, be carried out before each and every application. This preparation should on no account be used for dyeing eye-brows or eye-lashes as severe inflammation of the eye or even blindness may result.

Special provisions relating to toothpaste containing fluoride:

 (i)   *Fluoride content in tooth paste should not be more than 1000 ppm and the content of fluoride in terms of ppm should be mentioned on the tube and carton.*

 (ii) *Date of expiry should be mentioned on tube and carton.*

Labeling of Medical Devices

In India, Rule 109A of Drugs and Cosmetics Act, states that the labeling of Medical Devices should also comply with the specifications laid down from time to time by the Bureau of Indian Standards (BIS) in addition to any other requirement prescribed under the rules.

Conclusive Remarks

Label of drug products serve several purposes apart from being the primary source of identity. Every country has a set of requirements for the labeling of drug being marketed in their territory. Drug label carries various segments of information useful for different stakeholders *viz* healthcare professionals, patients, regulatory agencies. Label should be in compliance with the acts or guidelines explain the requirements and it should also carry the maximum useful information. Readers of the label are encouraged to follow the instruction, cautions given in this piece of information.

Suggested Readings

1. Best practice guidance on the labelling and packaging of medicines. [Internet] 2003 Jun[Cited on 2014 Jan 18] Available from http://www.mhra.gov.uk/home/ groups/ commsic/documents/publication/con007554.pdf.

2. Drug Labeling in Developing Countries February. [Internet]1993 Feb [Cited on 2014 Jan 21] 1993. Available from http://www.princeton.edu/~ota/disk1/1993/ 9321/ 9321.PDF.

3. Government of India. Ministry of Health and Family Welfare. The Drugs and Cosmetic Act 1940 and the Rules 1945; Amended up to the 30 June, 2005 India..

4. Release of Draft Guidance Document for Consultation: Labelling of Pharmaceutical Drugs for Human Use, Health Canada. [Internet]2014 Jan [Cited on 2014 Jan 21] Available from http://www.hc-sc.gc.ca/dhp-mps/prodpharma/applic-demande/guide-ld/label_guide_ld-eng.php.

5. United States of America (2006). Department of Health and Human Services. Food and Drug Administration Center for Drug Evaluation and Research (CDER) Center for Biologics Evaluation and Research (CBER). Guidance for Industry Clinical Pharmacology Section of Labelling for Human Prescription Drug and Biological Products-Content and Format.

6. United States of America (2010). Department of Health and Human Services. Food and Drug Administration Center for Drug Evaluation and Research (CDER) Center for Biologics Evaluation and Research (CBER). Guidance for Industry Dosage and Administration Section of labelling for Human Prescription Drug and Biological Products-Content and Format.

7. United States of America (2011). Department of Health and Human Services. Food and Drug Administration. Code of Federal Regulations Title 21.

8. United States of America (2011). Department of Health and Human Services. Food and Drug Administration Center for Drug Evaluation and Research (CDER) Center for Biologics Evaluation and Research (CBER). Guidance for Industry Warnings and precautions, contraindication, boxed warning section of labelling for human prescription drug and biological product- Content and Format.

9. United States of America (2012). Department of Health and Human Services. Food and Drug Administration Center for Drug Evaluation and Research (CDER) Center for Biologics Evaluation and Research (CBER). Guidance for Industry Product Name Placement, Size, and Prominence in Advertising and Promotional Labelling.

CHAPTER 12

P-DRUG

Introduction

In the present scenario, a doctor may examine more than 50 patients per day or even more in government hospital in India. Therefore, he has to choose the right drug for each patient in a relatively short time. Hence, bound to use *P-drugs* which refer to *Preferred or Personal or Priority choice of drugs*.

These drugs are the most familiar for clinicians/practitioners which are based on priority base which may includes name of a drug, dosage form, dosage schedule and duration of a treatment for a specified condition (Fig. 12.1). The choice of P-drugs may differ from country to country, company to company and even doctor to doctor, due to varying availability and cost of drugs, different national formularies and essential drug lists, medical culture and individual interpretation of information. However, the basic principle of P-drug choice is same universally.

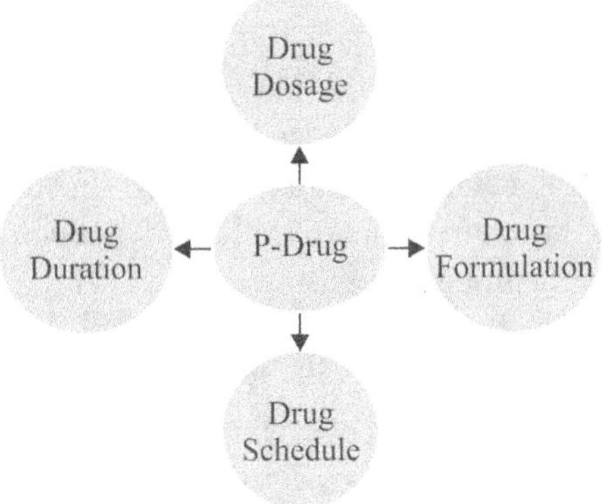

Fig. 12.1 Choice of P-drug in rational way.

In daily practice, clinicians/physicians have very small time for a selection of drug for particular disease, therefore, choice of P-drugs enable the clinicians/physicians to avoid repeated searches for a good drug and save time. Regular use of a drug enables to get their pharmacological effects and side effects thoroughly, with obvious benefits to the patient.

In general, the list of drugs registered for use in the country and the national list of essential drugs contain many more drugs than one is likely to use regularly. Practically, if we see most clinicians/physicians use only 40-60 drugs routinely. It is, therefore, useful to make your own selection from these lists in a rational way. In fact, in doing so, the physician prepares his own essential drugs list. A physician should compile his own list of P-drugs from existing national or local treatment guidelines or formularies.

There are four reasons for this:

1. One has the final responsibility for his/her patient's well-being which he/she cannot pass on to others.

2. By developing one's own set of P-drugs one can learn, how to handle pharmacological concepts and data.

3. By compiling one's own set of P drugs, one can prescribe alternatives when P-drug cannot be used.

4. It is not necessary that latest and most expensive drug is always good to prescribe; drug should be safe and cost effective.

How do you go about the process of selecting a P-drug? P-drugs are for a particular disease and not for a particular patient. After selecting a P-drug for particular disease, the treatment can be tailored for a particular patient.

The steps for choosing a P-drug is divided in five steps:

Step I: Define the diagnosis

To be able to select the best drug for a given condition, it is necessary to study the pathophysiology of the disease. More the knowledge, easier it is to choose a P-drug. Sometimes the physiology of the disease is unknown, while treatment is possible and necessary. Treating symptoms without really treating the underlying disease is called symptomatic treatment and when treating an individual patient, it should start by carefully defining the patient's problem and diagnosis.

Step II: Specify the therapeutic objective

It is very useful to define exactly what we want to achieve with a drug, for example, to decrease the diastolic blood pressure to a certain level, to cure an infectious disease, or to suppress feelings of anxiety.

Step III: Make an inventory of effective groups of drugs

In this step we have to link the therapeutic objective with various drugs. Drugs that are not effective are not worth examining any further, so efficacy is the first criterion for selection. Initially, you should look at group of drugs rather than individual drugs. As the active substances in a drug group have the same working mechanism, their effects, side effects, contraindications and interactions are also similar. The benzodiazepines, beta-blockers and penicillins are examples of drug groups. Most active substances in a group share a common stem in their generic name, such as diazepam, lorazepam and temazepam for benzodiazepines, and propranolol and atenolol for beta-blockers.

There are two ways to identify effective groups of drugs. First is to look at formularies or guidelines that exist in your hospital or health system, or at national and international guidelines, such as the FDA/NIH/WHO/ICMR treatment guidelines for certain common disease groups, or the WHO Model List of Essential Drugs. Another way is to check the index of a good pharmacology reference book and determine which groups are listed for confirmed diagnosis or therapeutic objectives.

Step IV: Choose an effective group according to criteria

Efficacy: When considering the term efficacy, it is not based on pharmacodynamics alone. The therapeutic objective is that the drug should work as soon as possible therefore, pharmacokinetic properties are also important.

Safety: When considering the safety of a drug, it is important to consider the incidence as well as the severity of adverse reactions. It is also important to appreciate special groups who may be particularly at risk of adverse reactions e.g., the incidence of adverse reactions with serotonin reuptake inhibitors is only slightly less than that of tricyclic antidepressants. However, whereas the former tends to cause predominantly mild gastrointestinal and CNS side-effects, the adverse reactions with the latter are more serious including postural hypotension, sedation, seizures, and cardiac effects. These reactions can also be particularly troublesome in elderly patients. Similarly, tricyclic antidepressants are more dangerous in over dose, hence they are less safe than SSRI's in patients at risk.

Convenience: Although the final check will only be made with the individual patient, some general aspects of suitability can be considered when selecting P-drugs. Contraindications are related to patient conditions, such as other illnesses which make it impossible to use a P-drug that is otherwise, effective and safe. A change in the physiology of the patient may influence the dynamics or kinetics of the P-drug: the required plasma levels may not be reached, or toxic side effects may occur at normal plasma concentrations. In pregnancy or lactation, the well-being of the child has to be considered. Interactions with food or other drugs can also strengthen or diminishes the effect of a drug. A convenient dosage form or dosage schedule can have a strong impact on patient adherence to the treatment.

All these aspects should be taken into account when choosing a P-drug. For example, in the elderly and children, drugs should be in convenient dosage forms, such as tablets or liquid formulations that are easy to handle. For urinary tract infections, some of the patients will be pregnant women in whom sulfonamides-a possible P-drug - are contraindicated in the third trimester. Anticipate this by choosing a second P-drug for urinary tract infections in this group of patients.

Cost: The cost of the treatment is always an important criterion, in both developed and developing countries, and whether it is covered by the state, an insurance company or directly by the patient. Cost is sometimes difficult to determine for a group of drugs, but it should always be kept in mind. Certain groups are definitely more expensive than others. Always look at the total cost of treatment rather than the cost per unit. The cost arguments really start counting, when you choose between individual drugs.

The final choice between drug groups needs practice, but making this choice on the basis of efficacy, safety, suitability and cost of treatment makes it easier.

Step V: Choose a P-drug

Choose an Active Substance and a Dosage Form

Choosing an active substance is like choosing a drug group, and the information can be listed in a similar way. In practice, it is almost impossible to choose an active substance without considering the dosage form as well; so consider them together. First, the active substance and its dosage form have to be effective, as per pharmacokinetics and pharmacodynamic differences.

Although, active substances within one drug group share the same working mechanism, differences may exist in safety and suitability because of differences in kinetics. Large differences may exist in convenience to the patient and these will have a strong influence on adherence to treatment. Different dosage forms will usually lead to different dosage schedules, and this should be taken into account when choosing your P-drug. Last, but not least, cost of treatment should always be considered.

Keep in mind that drugs sold under generic (non-proprietary) names are usually cheaper than patented brand-name products. If two drugs from the same group appear equal we could consider which drug has been safe longest on the market (indicating wide experience and probably safety), or which drug is manufactured in the country. When two drugs from two different groups appear equal we can choose both. This will give us an alternative, if one is not suitable for a particular patient. As a final check, we have to compare our selection with existing treatment guidelines, the national list of essential drugs, and with the WHO Model List of Essential Drugs, which is reviewed every two years.

Choose a Standard Dosage Schedule

A recommended dosage schedule is based on clinical investigations in a group of patients. However, this statistical average is not necessarily the optimal schedule for individual patient. If age, metabolism, absorption and excretion in patient are all average, and if no other diseases or other drugs are involved, the average dosage is probably adequate. More the patient varies from this average, the more likely the need for an individualized dosage schedule.

Recommended dosage schedules for all P-drugs can be found in formularies, desk references or pharmacology textbooks. In most of these references we found, vague statements such as '2-4 times 30-90 mg per day', the best solution is to copy the different dosage schedules into our own formulary. This will indicate the minimum and maximum limits of the dosage. When dealing with an individual patient we can make our definitive choice. Some drugs need an initial loading dose to quickly reach steady state plasma concentration. Others require a slowly rising dosage schedule, usually to let the patient adapt to the side effects.

Choose a Standard Duration of the Treatment

By knowing the pathophysiology and the prognosis of the disease you will usually have a good idea of how long the treatment should be continued. Some diseases require life-long treatment (E.g., diabetes mellitus, congestive cardiac failure, Parkinson's disease).

The total amount of a drug to be prescribed depends on the dosage schedule and the duration of the treatment. It can easily be calculated. For example, in a patient with bronchitis we may prescribe penicillin for seven days. There is a need to see the patient again if there is no improvement and so we can prescribe the total amount at once.

If the duration of treatment is not known, the monitoring interval becomes important. For example, we may request a patient with newly diagnosed hypertension to come back in two weeks so that, we can monitor blood pressure and any side effects of the treatment. In this case, only prescribe the drugs for 2-week period. As we get to know better health of the patient, we could extend the monitoring interval, say, to one month. Three months should be about the maximum monitoring interval for drug treatment of a chronic disease.

Personal formulary of P-drugs

On the basis of the above criteria, choose drugs that you would prescribe for different indications, and these together make up your Personal Formulary. These represent drugs that you will prescribe commonly and become most familiar with.

Case no. 1:

Selecting a P-drug for angina pectoris

Angina pectoris is one of the common cardiovascular disorders, and it is relatively easy to understand the pathophysiology as well as treatment of angina. Therefore, we have selected the example of angina pectoris.

A 70-year old man, with no previous medical history, during the last month he had several attacks of suffocating chest pain, which began during physical labor and disappeared quickly after he stopped. He has not smoked for six years. His father and brother died of a heart attack. Apart from occasionally taking some aspirin he has not used any medication in the past year. Auscultation reveals a murmur over the right carotid artery and the right femoral artery. Physical examination reveals no other abnormalities. Blood pressure, pulse, and body weight is normal.

Table 12.1 The steps for selection of P-drug

i.	**Define the diagnosis:** Stable angina pectoris, caused by a partial occlusion of coronary artery			
ii.	**Specify therapeutic objective:** Stop an attack as soon as possible, reduce myocardial oxygen need by decreasing preload, contractility, heart rate or after load			
iii.	Make inventory of effective groups Nitrates β-blockers Calcium channel blockers			
iv.	Choose a group according to criteria: efficacy safety suitability cost			
	Nitrates (tablet)　+　±　++　+			
v.	**Choose a P-drug:**	efficacy safety	suitability cost	
	Glyceryl trinitrate -tablet	+	±	+　+
	Glyceryl trinitrate -spray	+	±	(+)　-
	Isosorbide dinitrate -tablet	+	±	+　±
	Isosorbide mononitrate -tablet	+	±	+　±
Conclusion				
Active substance, dosage form: Glyceryl trinitrate, sublingual tablet 1 mg				
Dosage schedule: 1 tablet as needed; second tablet if pain persists				
Duration: length of monitoring interval				

Flow chart to select a P-drug

Identify the pathophysiology (Diagnosis)

↓

Target the therapeutic benefit

↓

Make a list of effective drug groups

↓

Summaries the drugs into important criteria namely, *efficacy, safety of drugs, their suitability and comparable cost*

↓

Finally, choose a P-drug based on above parameters

Conclusion

At present, we have more than a thousand drugs in our therapeutic armamentarium. The concept of P-drug helps in the rational use of drugs. These are the drugs that we prescribe regularly, and are priority choice for given indication. Doctor must not be overconfident that he/she is the only person the patient is consulting. Proper choice and use of drugs will be a great help in ensuring appropriate and affordable care and should be incorporated, into daily clinical practice.

P-Drug should not misunderstand as *"personalized drug or medicine"*!

Personalized drug is the invention of genetic science *"pharmacogenomics"* and technology to pharmaceutical therapy. Principally, it is based on individual *genetic makeup* which means that doctors can adjust a standard drug or dose to patients which limits the adverse drug reaction/toxicity of drug. Hence, it is aimed to maximize the therapeutic efficacy and safety to an individual patient. The other advanced diagnostic and prognostic tools such as genetic mapping and sequencing increased the diagnostic ability to predict the outcomes of drug therapy with the help of *"bio-markers"*; biological/physiological molecules which directly associated with pathological changes of disease. Currently, genetics database, voluntarily made by FDA's office of clinical pharmacology and biopharmaceutics to record the genetic pattern among worldwide population through clinical trials will give a guide to the clinicians/physicians to select more appropriate drugs in their classes to treat a disease.

Suggested Readings

1. De Vries TP, Henning RH, Hogerzeil HV, Fresle DA (1994). Guide to Good Prescribing: A Practical Manual. Geneva: WHO.

2. Parmar DM, Jadav SP (2007). The concept of personal drugs in the undergraduate pharmacology practical curriculum. *Indian J Pharmacol.* **39:** 165-7.

3. Wilke RA, Lin DW, Roden DM, *et al.,* (2007). Identifying genetic risk factors for serious adverse drug reactions: current progress and challenges. *Nature Reviews Drug Discovery.* **6(11):** 904-917.

CHAPTER 13

DRUG PRICE

Introduction

Indian pharmaceutical industry is one of the largest and most advanced industries among the developing countries. Drug prices are under the insight of Department of Pharmaceuticals, Ministry of Chemicals and Fertilizers. The World Health Organization (WHO) reported that one third of the world's population lacks reliable access to required medicines and the situation is even more worse in developing countries, which are finding it increasingly difficult to finance medicines as expenditure on medicines has been growing steadily (World Health Report, WHO). Over the last several years, various pharmaceutical policies and control inputs have been directed in order to promote the growth of the industry. In brief, the development of Indian pharmaceutical industry from 70's to 90's is mostly due to the drug policy in which the report of the Hathi Committee (1975) is an important milestone. The Hathi Committee in particular emphasized the need for achieving self-sufficiency in medicines and ensuring the availability of essential medicines to the people at reasonable and affordable prices. The drug prices in India are regulated ever since, the Drug Price Control Order (DPCO) came into force. The order has been revised several times since then. The prices of bulk drugs and the formulations included in the schedules categories were being fixed by the Government of India as per the Drugs (Prices Control) Order, issued and amended from time to time. Earlier, the drug prices of controlled formulations were decided by applying the method based on MAPE[*] (Maximum Allowable Post manufacturing Expenses) which was a mark-up on ex-factory

---

[*] MAPE (Maximum Allowable Post-manufacturing Expenses) means all costs incurred by a manufacturer from the stage of ex-factory cost to retailing and includes trade margin and margin for the manufacturer and it shall not exceed one hundred per cent for indigenously manufactured Scheduled formulations (Source: Drug Price Control Order 1995)

costs, provided to cover selling and distribution costs, including retail and wholesale trade margins. But according to the latest notification (not published yet), the final price of the drug will be calculated by adding the average of the prices of all the brands that have at least 1% market share plus local taxes and a 16% retailer's profit margin (DPCO 2013). Ideally, drug price is composed of several variable factors which influence the costing of drugs to consumers (Fig. 13.1).

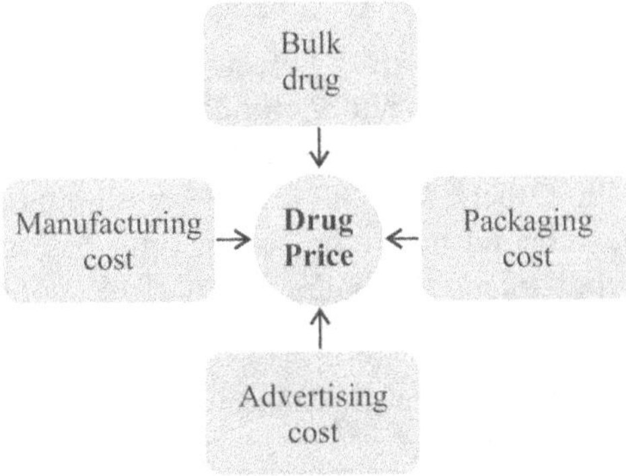

Fig. 13.1 Composition of drug price.

DPCO identifies Active Pharmaceutical Ingredients (APIs) for which a pricing formula is used to set the MRP. Earlier, there were only 74 bulk drugs under price control (DPCO, 1995) whereas, the current DPCO (2013) will regulate prices of as many as 348 medicines and are called scheduled[†] medicines. For all other medicines called "non-scheduled medicines". The manufacturer sets the price and registers that price with the National Pharmaceutical Pricing Authority (NPPA) under Department of Pharmaceuticals (NPPA).

History of Regulation of Drug Price

Price controls for drugs and formulations have a long history in India. The first price control order was issued under the Defence of India Act in 1963. Price control orders have been issued under the Essential Commodities Act, from 1970 onwards. The DPCO in 1970 was a measure to safeguard the interests of the consumer, while providing for a restricted but reasonable return to the producers. Simultaneously, with the negation of

---

[†]Scheduled formulation means a formulation containing any bulk drug specified in the First Schedule either individually or in combination with other drugs, including one or more than one drug or drugs not specified in the First Schedule except single ingredient formulation based on bulk drugs specified in the First Schedule and sold under the generic name (Source: DPCO 1995)

product patents in 1970, the measure brought about an era of economical medicines in India, albeit at the expense of diluting intellectual property rights. The DPCO was then revised in 1979, 1987, 1995 and recently in 2013 (Table 13.1).

Individual as well as comparative analysis of all the DPCOs illustrates that there has been a measured but sturdy decontrol of drug prices in India. This analysis has been given below:

Before 1970

At the time of independence, the bulk drug industry in India was in the infancy stage with a meager investment of Rs. 10 Crores and a production worth just Rs. 26 Crores. Most of the bulk drugs and formulations were imported. Till 1962, the drug industry was deprived of any price control. In 1962, there was Chinese aggression on India and Emergency was declared. The Government feared that, as a result, drug prices might rise. Accordingly, for the first time, under the Defense of India Act of 1915, statutory control was imposed on the prices of drugs and pharmaceuticals.

Table 13.1 List of regulations for drug price control in India

Drug Regulations	Issuing Year
Drug (display of prices) Order	1962
Drug (control of prices) Order	1963
Drug Prices (Control) Order	1966
Drug (Price Control) Order	1970
The Hathi Committee	1974
Drug (Price Control) Order	1979
The Kelkar Committee	1984
Drug (Price Control) Order	1987
Drug Policy	1994
Drug (Price Control) Order	**1995**
Pharmaceutical Policy	2002
National Pharmaceutical Pricing Policy	2011
Drug Price Control Order	2013

The Drugs (Display of Prices) Order, 1962 and the Drugs (Control of Prices) Order, 1963 were formally declared in public. Under the Drugs Prices (Display and Control) Order of 1966, it was made mandatory for the manufacturers to obtain prior approval from the government before increasing the prices of any formulation.

DPCO, 1970

A comprehensive order was promulgated on 16th May, 1970, under Section 3 of the Essential Commodities Act and authorizing it to fix and regulate the prices of essential bulk drugs and their respective formulations. It was called "The Drugs (Prices Control)

Order, 1970". In its introductory form, DPCO was a direct control on the profitability of a pharmaceutical business, and an indirect control on the prices of pharmaceuticals. The order contains a list of bulk drugs whose prices are to be controlled, the procedure for fixation and revision of prices, the procedure for implementation, the procedure for recovery, the penalties for contravention, and various other guidelines and directions. The order was subject to the guidelines of drug policy and aims to ensure unbiased distribution, increased supply, and economical availability of bulk drugs. The government stipulated that a company's pre-tax profit should not exceed 15% of its pharmaceutical sales   (net of excise duty and sales tax). In case profits exceeded this sum, the surplus was deposited with the government. So, a pharmaceutical company had the freedom to decide the prices of its products. Product-wise margins were also flexible, so as long as the overall margin did not exceed the set norms. DPCO (1970) effectively put a ceiling on prices of all mass-usage bulk drugs and their formulations. Its primary objective was to protect the interests of consumers, and ensure a restricted but reasonable return to manufacturers. The order was a landmark regulation and has had several implications in shaping the Indian pharmaceutical industry. At that time, the Indian pharmaceutical industry was largely dominated by MNC affiliates and subsidiaries. These MNCs were hardly affected by the relatively mild form of DPCO and continued operating in the domestic market. However, Foreign Exchange Regulation Act (FERA) which came in mid 70's did curtail the operations of these MNCs. Overall, the Indian pharmaceutical industry prospered from 1970 to the next DPCO in 1979.

The Hathi Committee, 1974

In 1974, the Government of India (GoI) appointed a Committee under the chairmanship of Rajya Sabha MP, Jaisukhlal Hathi to enquire into the conditions prevailing in the sphere of pharmaceuticals in the country. The Committee submitted its report in 1975 which is widely known as the Hathi Committee report. The report strongly emphasized the achievement of self-sufficiency and abundant availability at reasonable prices of essential medicines. The DPCO, 1979 was loosely based on the recommendations of the Hathi Committee but many a provisions were not implemented.

DPCO, 1979

The Drug Prices Control Order was issued on 31st March 1979. In its revised version, the DPCO stipulated ceiling prices for controlled categories (Appendix I) of bulk drugs and their formulations. In fixing the price, the government continued to advocate the profitability ceiling and an upper limit was put on the return on net worth or capital employed for pharmaceutical companies. [‡]The retail prices of controlled formulations were decided by applying the concept of MAPE (Maximum Allowable Post manufacturing Expenses). It was a mark-up on ex-factory costs, provided to cover selling

---

[‡]Detailed list of different categories is given in Appendix I

and distribution costs including retail and wholesale trade margins. The pricing formula was retail price = (MC + CC + PM + PC) x (1 + MAPE/100) + excise duty, where MC was the material cost including cost of bulk drugs/excipients, CC was the conversion cost as per the dosage form, PM was the cost of packing material suitable to dosage form and PC was the packaging charge worked out in accordance with established costing procedures.

The DPCO 1979 put 370 drugs under price control. According to this, these drugs were classified into four categories: I - Life-saving, II - Essential, III - Less essential, and IV - Non-essential/simple remedies. These categories have different MAPE (Table 13.2). The most important drugs, including life saving drugs were put in Category I which had the least MAPE.

Table 13.2 Segregation of drugs as per DPCO, 1979

Category *	MAPE
I	40%
II	55%
III	100%
IV	60%

However, Transnational Corporations (TNCs) challenged the order and succeeded in obtaining a stay on the DPCO, 1979, from High Courts and ignored the prices fixed under this.

Ultimately the Government of India had to appeal to the Supreme Court, which upheld the validity of its action and directed the Government to assess and recover the amounts. By this DPCO, around 80% of the Indian pharmaceutical industry (in value terms) was brought under strict price control. The MNCs were the worst hit. With profitability falling steeply, they discontinued many products, especially the life saving products in Category I. In addition, the industrial licensing requirements made it impossible for MNCs to introduce new products. The local players were, nonetheless, in a better position. They could obtain licenses much easily than MNCs could. They were also able to speedily introduce new drugs. The local players, as a result, were able to keep the coverage of DPCO low and fight the might of established MNCs. However, profitability wise, the Indian pharmaceutical sector went through its worst phase from 1979 to 1987.

The Kelkar Committee, 1984

In 1984, the Kelkar Committee came out with its report in which, it recommended the exclusion of a number of drugs from the horizon of price control. Various suggestions were made for determining the criteria for inclusion and exclusion. The committee stressed the need to liberalize the strict profitability curbs that were acting as a hurdle to the growth of the pharmaceutical sector.

DPCO, 1987

The DPCO, 1987 was promulgated on 26th August on the basis of the Drug Policy of 1986 and the Kelkar Committee Report. In DPCO, 1987 the number of bulk drugs under price control was significantly reduced from 370 to 142. Twenty drugs were taken off from Category I and 122 from Category II. In addition, the categories of control were reduced to two and higher MAPE was provided for each category of controlled drugs (Table 13.2). The MAPE for Category I and Category II was increased from 40% and 55% respectively to 75%. The MAPE for Category IV was increased from 60% to 100%. Even the new drugs that were brought under price control got a liberal 75% MAPE.

Furthermore, industrial licensing norms were made softer thereby, improving the situation of MNCs desirous of amending their product mix. As a result of all these factors, profitability improved. However, around 75% of the pharmaceutical industry was still under price control.

The Drug Policy, 1994

In September 1994, the new drug policy was announced. It is the Drug Policy of the government that decides the criteria for selecting bulk drugs or formulations for price control. The New Drug Policy liberalized these criteria. In addition, industrial licensing was abolished for all bulk drugs. All hindrances to capacity expansions were removed and it was expected that, as a result, supply would rise resulting in higher competitive pressures. Foreign investment up to 51% was also permitted in case of all bulk drugs, their intermediates and formulations. FDI above 51% was to be considered on a case to case basis.

DPCO, 1995

The latest Drug Price Control Order was passed on 6th January 1995. The basic structure of this DPCO is the same as that of the earlier two orders. Nevertheless, the span of price control under DPCO 1995 has been liberalized considerably from 142 drugs to just 76. The prices of which are controlled under DPCO 1995, have been enlisted in the First Schedule of Drugs and Cosmetics Act 1940. The methodology through which prices of DPCO-controlled bulk drugs are fixed is as follows. While fixing the maximum sale price of a bulk drug, the government has to provide either a post-tax return of 14% on net worth or a return of 22% on capital employed. Each company can choose one of the two methods mentioned above as per its own free will. So, the choice of method is company-specific and not product-specific. Then based on the chosen method, each company submits to the government, a detailed working of the prices of various bulk drugs that it requires. The prices submitted by the companies are such that the allowed profitability parameters are achieved. The government subsequently studies the applications made by the major players for every bulk drug and cost audits reports of manufacturers, before arriving at the final price. The price so decided will be binding on all manufacturers, irrespective of their actual cost of production.

The DPCO covers all the formulations that utilize the bulk drugs listed in the First Schedule*[§].

The methodology through which prices of formulations are fixed is as follows: Under DPCO 1995, a uniform MAPE of 100% is given on all formulations under price control. This is in contrast to the earlier practice of giving a MAPE of 75% on some formulations. In the new system, the retail price of a DPCO formulation is fixed equal to (MC + CC + PM + PC) x 2 + excise duty. It is this price that is printed on the pack of a DPCO controlled formulation. This price is not the Maximum Retail Price (MRP). Local taxes are additional. In order for the government to decide the price of a controlled formulation, each manufacturer is supposed to submit to the government details of material cost, manufacturing process cost etc. The ceiling prices, once decided, are notified in the Official Gazette.

For imported drugs and formulations, the landed cost including customs duty and clearing charges is the benchmark to fix prices. The margin allowed to the importer is such that selling and distribution expenses including interest and profit are covered. However, the margin allowed cannot exceed 50% of the landed cost.

Pharmaceutical Policy 2002

A new pharmaceutical policy was approved by Government in 2002 wherein the number of drugs under price control and span of price control was sought to be reduced.

The main objectives of this policy are:

- Ensuring abundant availability at reasonable prices within the country of good quality essential pharmaceuticals of mass consumption.

- Strengthening the indigenous capability for cost effective quality production and exports of pharmaceuticals by reducing barriers to trade in the pharmaceutical sector.

- Strengthening the system of quality control over drug and pharmaceutical production and distribution to make quality an essential attribute of the Indian pharmaceutical industry and promoting rational use of pharmaceuticals.

- Encouraging R&D in the pharmaceutical sector in a manner compatible with the country's needs and with particular focus on diseases endemic or relevant to India by creating an environment conducive to channelizing a higher level of investment into R&D in pharmaceuticals in India.

- Creating an incentive framework for the pharmaceutical industry which promotes new investment into pharmaceutical industry and encourages the introduction of new technologies and new drugs.

However, before this policy could be implemented it was stayed by the Karnataka High Court in a PIL filed before the Court on the ground that a large number of essential

---

[§] Provides the list of Bulk Drugs (including salts, derivatives and esters, if any) used in Categories I and II formulations appearing in Third Schedule of DPCO, 1979.

drugs would go out of price control. An SLP was filed by Government in the Supreme Court against the order of the Karnataka High Court. The Supreme Court vide its interim order on 10th March, 2003, stayed the order of the Karnataka High Court. However, it also ordered that "the petitioner shall consider and formulate appropriate criteria for ensuring essential and life saving drugs not to fall out of price control, and to review the drugs which are essential and life saving in nature till 2nd May, 2003". After consideration, the government announced a new pharmaceutical policy in 2005, wherein it was proposed to bring an additional 354 drugs under a National List of Essential Medicines (NLEM) under price control. It is also proposed that patented drugs would be subject to price negotiations, prior to grant of marketing approvals. A system of reference pricing is to be evolved for these, based on prevailing practices in other 'comparable' countries. Drug pricing mechanism in India is still based on DPCO 1995. The table 13.3 shows number of drugs and percentage of market under price control.

Table 13.3 Number of drugs under price control order

DPCO Year	No. of drugs	Percentage of controlled market
1970	All	100
1979	347	90
1987	142	70
1995	76	50

National Pharmaceuticals Pricing Policy 2011

Department of Pharmaceuticals has prepared a draft National Pharmaceutical Pricing Policy (NPPP) 2011. The draft policy envisages bringing the National List of Essential Medicines 2011 and associated medicines under price control. The proposed National Pharmaceutical Pricing Policy of 2011 is structured around three key principles of (i) Essentiality of drugs; (ii) Market-based pricing and (iii) Control of formulations only.

Salient Features of NPPP 2011

- The pricing mechanism of the NPPP 2011 is based on regulating the prices of formulations through Market Based Pricing (MBP), instead of Cost Based Pricing (CBP) under the Drug Policy 1994.
- The regulation of prices of drugs in the NPPP 2011 is on the basis of regulating the prices of formulations only. This is different from regulating the prices of specified Bulk Drugs and their formulations adopted in the Drug Policy 1994.
- The regulation of prices of drugs in the NPPP 2011 is based on essentiality of drugs than the economic criteria/market share principle adopted in the Drug Policy of 1994.
- The new policy proposes that the non-essential drugs should not be under a controlled regime and their prices should be fixed by market forces. The new

policy aims to keep a check on overall drug prices and the price hike should not be at a rate of 15% per annum or the increase in the wholesale price index (WPI), whichever is higher.

- In case of imported drugs, there will be no separate determination of ceiling prices for imported drugs falling under the span of control.

- Streamlining of the system of procurement of drugs by the Government for ensuring procurement of quality drugs at reasonable prices. This would apply for all Government procurement, both by the Central Government, States and PSUs.

National Pharmaceutical Pricing Authority (NPPA)

The NPPA is an organization of the government of India established to fix or revise prices of controlled bulk drugs and formulations. Companies must keep drug prices affordable to the general public. To keep medicines within reach of the poor population, the government has covered 76 scheduled drugs. The prices and the margins of drugs for the wholesaler and retailers are largely decided by NPPA, which varies depending on whether the active constituent of the product is a scheduled drug or a non-scheduled drug (Scheduled drugs are price controlled whereas non-scheduled drugs are not).

NPPA was established on 29th August 1997 as an independent body of experts as per the decision taken by the Cabinet Committee in September 1994 while reviewing Drug Policy. The Authority, *inter alia*, has been entrusted with the task of fixation/revision of prices of pharmaceutical products (bulk drugs and formulations), enforcement of provisions of DPCO and monitoring of the prices of controlled and decontrolled drugs in the country. The organization is also entrusted with the task of recovering the amounts overcharged by the manufacturers for the controlled drugs. The main functions of NPPA are to:

- Implement and enforce the provisions of the DPCO in accordance with the powers delegated to it.

- Deal with all legal matters arising out of the decisions of the Authority.

- Monitor the availability of drugs, identify shortages, if any, and to take remedial steps.

- Collect/maintain data on production, exports and imports, market share of individual companies, profitability of companies etc., for bulk drugs and formulations.

- Undertake and/or sponsor relevant studies in respect of pricing of drugs/ pharmaceuticals.

- Recruit/appoint the officers and other staff members of the authority, as per rules and procedures laid down by the government.

- Render advice to the central government on changes/revisions in the drug policy.
- Render assistance to the central government in the parliamentary matters relating to the drug pricing.

NPPA during the last two years has tried to perform its main task of fixing/revising the prices of scheduled formulations and making the drugs available at reasonable prices in the country. As part of its regular interaction with consumers and to gain understanding about the availability and prices of drugs in select regions, it appointed *voluntary organisation in interest of consumer education* (VOICE) to undertake market survey on the prices and availability of essential life saving and prophylactic medicines of good quality in India.

Effects of Patents on Prices of Drugs/Medicines

Under the TRIPS agreement, finalized in 1995, the countries need to recognize and enforce product patents in all fields of technology. There has been much debate and controversy regarding the merits of the new patent regime for pharmaceuticals, particularly from the point of view of developing countries. The unqualified patent protection of pharmaceutical products will lead to substantially higher prices for medicine, not good for health and welfare of the developing countries. An opposite view is that the introduction of pharmaceutical product patents is unlikely to give a significant rise in the prices of drugs because of the presence of many therapeutic substitutes of patented products.

Very less information is available about the increase in the prices of pharmaceutical products as a result of production patents. Various previous studies on the impact of patents on prices have been conducted only for developed countries and not or less for developing countries.

Generic versus Patented Medicines

Some findings have also revealed that there are huge markups for retailer on branded-generic medicines. The retailer margin for five branded medicines studied was in the range of 25-30%, but for their branded-generics version manufactured by the same company it was in the range of 201-1016%. There exists a widespread belief among people and dispensing chemists that a branded product is better in terms of quality and safety than the generic. Unlike developed countries, people in developing countries pay the cost of medicines out-of-pocket. In India, more than 80% health financing is borne by patients. India is known to export medicines to various countries at low cost, but faces the challenge of access to affordable and quality medicines for its own population. Hence, the government should have a policy whereby, the prices of branded-generic drugs can be made realistic and affordable to common man. We need to have legislation to that effect.

The profit margins presently being shared by traders must be passed to consumer. Suitable changes in the drug price policy may be made to have lower prices for branded-generic versions. Transparency in fixing the MRP by the manufacturer and clear guidelines for mark-ups at least for branded-generics is required in pharmaceutical trade. The government must take up generic promotional schemes, general awareness programs on quality of generics to build confidence among prescribers, pharmacists, and consumers. Availability of generics or branded-generics in the market with lower price tag and assured quality is essential to make the medicines affordable.

Drug Price Calculation

On a regular basis the list of drugs whose prices are controlled and the methodology of fixing prices is issued, referred to as the Drug Price Control Order (DPCO).

Procedure for Price Fixation of Bulk Drugs

As per paragraph 3 of DPCO, 1995 prices of scheduled bulk drugs are fixed by the NPPA to make them available at a fair price from different manufacturers. These prices are fixed from time to time by notification in official gazette.

Following steps are involved in fixation/revision of bulk drug prices:

Step 1: Identification of bulk drugs

Bulk Drugs are taken up for study on following basis:

- Whose validity period is due to expire.
- Request from the concerned manufacturer/company.
- Drug produced in the country for which no price has been notified under DPCO, 1995.

Step 2: Collection of data

Data is collected by issuing questionnaire/Form I (Appendix II) of DPCO, 1995/cost-audit report etc., and verification by plant visits, if required.

Step 3: Preparation of actual cost statement

Actual cost for the year for which data is submitted is prepared based on data submitted/collected & verified during plant visit.

Step 4: Preparation of Technical Parameters

Technical parameters are prepared based on data submitted, collected and verified during plant visits. Plant capacity is assessed considering 330 working days for normal operation of plant leaving 35 days for scheduled maintenance of plant. The achievable production level is considered at 90% utilisation of assessed capacity allowing 10% production loss on account of unforeseen break down and non-scheduled maintenance.

Step 5: Preparation of Estimated Cost

The estimated cost for the pricing period are then prepared based on actual cost and the technical parameters. While projecting the future cost, an increment is recognised at 5% per annum in respect of salaries and wages. Wage agreement, if any, which has been finalized and signed is also recognised while preparing the estimates. In respect of other overheads of fixed/semi variable nature, increase at 2.5% per annum is made to cover the normal incremental effects. The customs duty and other taxes as per the current budget are considered.

Step 6: Calculation of Fair price of bulk drug

Fair price is calculated by providing returns as specified in sub paragraph (2), 3 of DPCO, 1995. While fixing the maximum sale price of the bulk drug, a post tax return of 14% on net worth or a return of 22% of capital employed or in respect of a new plant an internal rate of return of 12% based on long term marginal costing is considered depending upon the option exercised by the manufacturer of the bulk drug. In case, the production is from basic stage, additional 4% return is considered on net worth/capital employed.

Step 7: Fixation of maximum sale price of the drug

When the number of manufacturers of the said drug is more than one, the maximum sale price is fixed at $2/3^{rd}$ cut off level or weighted average price, depending upon the situation.

Step 8: Notification of bulk drug price in official Gazette

Note: The fair price may be further revised, if asked by the manufacturers, based on escalation formula for change in major raw materials and utilities rates.

Procedure for Price Fixation of Formulations

Prices of formulations based on scheduled bulk drugs are fixed in two ways viz.

   (i) Based on applications of the manufacturers and

   (ii) Suo-motu basis[**].

As per paragraph 8(2) of DPCO 1995, a manufacturer using scheduled bulk drug in his formulation is required to apply for fixation of price of formulation within 30 days of fixation of price of such bulk drug (s).

[**] The NPPA also fixes/revises prices of both bulk drugs and formulations on suo-motu basis, where it is felt that manufacturers are not filing their applications as per the provisions of the DPCO, 1995 after the decrease in bulk drug prices and statutory duties, etc. Hence, with a view to passing on the benefits of such decreases to the consumers, suo-motu price is fixed.

Applications received in NPPA from manufacturers in Form III (Appendix III) and importers in Form IV (Appendix IV) of DPCO are considered for price fixation. The time frame for granting price approval on formulation is 2 months from the date of receipt of the complete information from the company.

Procedure

(a) **Examination of Technical Parameters:** Checking the quantity of bulk drug as per label claim. The overage claim is allowed as per batch production record or norms fixed by Govt.

(b) **Examination of Prices of Bulk Drug:** When notified price of bulk drug exists, the notified price or actual price is considered. In the case of imported bulk drug used in the formulation, weighted average import price is considered vis-à-vis the price submitted by the applicant. For non-scheduled bulk drug used, the available information on prices is applied.

(c) **Examination of Excipient Claims:** Excipient claims given in the application are examined and allowed after referring to information available in NPPA.

(d) **Examination of PL, CC, PC and PM cost:** The process loss (PL), conversion cost (CC) and packing charges (PC) are considered as per the norms notified in the Gazette vide S.O. 578(E) dated 13.07.99. The packaging material (PM) cost is allowed as per the actual claim supported by invoices and after referring to information available with NPPA.

(e) **Application of MAPE:** Maximum allowable post manufacturing expenses (MAPE) is given at 100% on the ex-factory cost for indigenous formulation, while MAPE up to 50% of the landed cost is allowed for imported formulation.

(f) **Working out the retail price:** The retail price of formulations is worked out as per the formula given in paragraph 7 of DPCO, 1995 *viz.*

"R.P. = [M.C. + C.C. + P.M. + P.C.] x [1 + MAPE/100] + E.D."

Where "R.P." means retail price;

"M.C." means material cost and includes the cost of drugs and other pharmaceutical aids used including overages, if any, plus process loss thereon, specified as a norm from time to time by notification in the Official Gazette in this behalf.

"C.C." means conversion cost worked out in accordance with established procedures of costing and shall be fixed as a norm every year by notification in the Official Gazette in this behalf.

"P.M." means cost of the packing material used in the packing of concerned formulation, including process loss, and shall be fixed as a norm every year by, notification in the Official Gazette in this behalf.

"P.C." means packing charges worked out in accordance with established procedures of costing and shall be fixed as a norm every year by notification in the Official Gazette in this behalf.

"MAPE" (Maximum Allowable Post-manufacturing Expenses) means all costs incurred by a manufacturer from the stage of ex-factory cost to retailing and includes trade margin and margin for the manufacturer and it shall not exceed one hundred per cent for indigenously manufactured Scheduled formulations.

"E.D." means excise duty.

(a) **Treatment of Taxes:** For bulk drugs used in formulation, all the statutory taxes are considered at the actual and net of MODVAT. Allowance upto 8% on the notified price of scheduled bulk drugs is considered on this account. The excise duty element is worked out in NPPA based on companies claim. Allowance is made for 16% margin on price to retailer (as per DPCO, 1995) and 8% margin to wholesaler as per practice, both on the ex-factory price, which is the assessable value.

    (i) The prevailing excise duty rate is applied to the said assessable value. For ceiling packs, notified prices are exclusive of excise duty. Manufacturers are required to work out the excise duty.

    (ii) **Suo-Motu Basis:** If the manufacturers or companies do not apply for revision of formulation prices as required under paragraph 8(2) of DPCO, 1995 within a period of 30 days of price reduction of bulk drug or fall in other statutory levies, steps are taken for suo-motu basis. Broadly, the procedure given above is followed.

    (iii) **Notification of ceiling prices in the Gazette of India:** Ceiling prices are fixed or revised under paragraph 9 of DPCO, 1995 for commonly marketed standard pack sizes of price control formulations. It is obligatory for all, including small scale units, to follow the ceiling prices which are notified in the Gazette of India (Extraordinary).The ceiling prices are usually notified as exclusive of excise duty, local tax etc., but maximum retail price (MRP) printed includes excise duty.

    (iv) **Pro-rata Price:** NPPA has issued notification no. S.O.83 (E) on pro-rata pricing. As per this notification, the manufactures of all the scheduled formulation pack sizes different from the notified pack sizes under sub-paragraph (1) and (2) of the paragraph 9 of the DPCO, 1995, shall have to work out the price for such pack sizes, in respect of tablets and capsules of the same strength or composition packed in different strips or blisters, on pro-rata basis of the latest ceiling price fixed for such formulations.

    (v) **Non-ceiling Price Order:** Non-ceiling Prices are fixed under paragraph 8 (1), (2) and (4) and paragraph 11 of the DPCO, 1995. They are specific to particular pack size and dosage form of scheduled formulation of a particular company. Hence they are pack specific and company specific. The prices fixed for non-ceiling packs are communicated to the respective firms by issuing office orders. In such order, usually excise duty element is shown separately. However, local taxes are not included in Non-ceiling price.

Implications of Drug Price Regulation for the Pharmaceutical Industry

The impact of drug price regulations on the Indian pharmaceutical industry can be analysed on the following three factors:

Profitability

The profitability is the most important factor amongst all the factors which can be useful to judge the impact of drug price regulations on pharmaceutical industry. Till 1987, 90% of all drugs produced in India were controlled as regards their prices. This put severe strain on the profit margin of the industry. There might have been other factors as well but drug price control was certainly a major factor responsible for the decline in industry profits in the pre-1990 period. The post-1987 period saw the DPCO being revised twice - first in 1987 and then in 1995. In the first revision, price control on drugs was eased and made applicable to 65% of all drugs as opposed to 90% earlier. In the second revision, this came down to 40%. With the strain on profit margin being eased, the industry's profits sky rocketed. As the industry became more profitable and viable, capital investment into the Indian Pharmaceutical Industry increased.

Manufacturing

In the DPCO 1979 which stayed enforced till 1987, 90% of all drugs were under strict price control. With such massive regulation on the prices of most drugs and thereby on the profitability of the manufacturing companies, the production of scheduled drugs became unfeasible. For instance, no export orders were taken on controlled drugs since their supply had to be under certain parameters. As a result, the level of manufacture by the pharmaceutical industry declined.

In the DPCO 1987 and then in the DPCO 1995, the proportion of drugs under price control declined to 65% and to 40% respectively. With a large number of drugs being taken out of price control, the production of these drugs became feasible again. As a result, the manufacture of these drugs increased.

Research and Development (R&D)

Until around the 1990s, the drug prices were strictly controlled and further stifled expenditure on R&D in more ways than one. First of all, the profit margin of the industry came down. With an inadequate profit margin, the industry never ventured out in the field of R&D. Secondly, it dissuaded foreign players and MNCs from entering the market. In fact, the share of foreign companies in the domestic drug market has continuously declined. Also, the imports and exports were meager. With the local players hardly getting any competition from foreign drug manufacturers, they never felt the need of investment in R&D. There were also reasons other than the control of drug prices for the slack R&D expenditure. For instance, process patents had been granted to the industry under the Indian Patent Act of 1970 and the domestic manufacturers simply had to reverse engineer 22 drugs made abroad. They were able to foray into various therapeutic segments and there was no need to indulge in any R&D.

However, things changed in the 1990s, when controls on drug prices were eased. First of all, profit margin for the domestic drug manufacturers increased thereby, enabling local players to provide for R&D. Secondly, foreign trade in drugs increased thereby raising the level of competition in the domestic and international market and necessitating greater R&D. However, there were factors other than the decontrol of drug prices which propelled R&D. For instance, under the TRIPS agreement, process patents were replaced with product patents. This shut the door on reverse engineering and made expenditure on R&D inevitability for the local players.

DPCO 2013

After the implementation of DPCO 1995, the prices of bulk drugs are fixed and revised as per given in this order. Recently, the Department of Pharmaceuticals in the Union Ministry of Chemicals and Fertilizers has notified the Drugs (Prices Control) Order 2013.

The new order will bring 652 drugs under price control and will enable the National Pharmaceutical Pricing Policy 2012 to regulate prices of 348 drugs which are covered under National List of Essential Medicines (NLEM) 2011 thus, effectively replacing the earlier DPCO 1995. Previous DPCO 1995 order regulated drug prices based on the manufacturing costs stated by their manufacturers. However in the current order, ceiling prices would be calculated by taking simple average of all the drug brands having a market share of more than 1% in their segment. This shifts the ceiling price calculation from a cost based to a market based method. The DPCO 2013 will come into effect somewhere around July 1st i.e., 45 days from the date of issue of the order.

Summary and Conclusion

From the historical analysis, it is cleared that the Indian Government has successfully controlled the drug prices steadily. Previously, the regulations on drug prices were not very strict but by time to time changes in the drug price control order made the precise guidelines for pharmaceutical industries. With the implementation of drug price control order, the drug formulations are now available to people at economical prices. It is also clear from the above discussion that the Indian pharmaceutical industry has heavily benefited from deregulation. The production capacity and the research and development expenditure of Indian companies have also witnessed a significant increase in the drug market.

NPPA is mainly responsible for fixing/revising the prices of scheduled formulations and making the drugs available at reasonable prices to public. Recently, the department of pharmaceuticals notified the latest Drug Price Control Order in July 2013. The new order authorises the NPPA to regulate prices of essential medicines as listed in the National List of Essential Medicines (NLEM) 2011. The Indian consumer will be benefited under the new Drug Price Control Order 2013.

Suggested Readings

1. Drug Price Control Order (DPCO), Pharmaceutical Industry, published by India Info line Limited.

2. Goldar B, Gupta I (2010). Effects of New Patents Regime on Consumers and Producers of Drugs/Medicines in India, Report submitted to UNCTAD, Institute of Economic Growth, New Delhi.

3. History of Drugs Price Control, Role of NPPA in Drug Pricing, published by National Pharmaceutical Pricing Authority. [http://nppaindia.nic.in/index1.html], Government of India (1975). Hathi Committee Report on Drugs and Pharmaceuticals. Department of Chemicals and Fertilizers, New Delhi.

4. Kjoenniksen I, Morten Lindbaek M, Granas AG (2006). Patients' attitudes towards and experiences of generic drug substitution in Norway. *Pharm World Sci.* **28:** 284-9.

5. Kotwani A, Ewen M, Dey D, Iyer S, Lakshmi PK, Patel A, Raman K, Singhal GL, Thawani V, Tripathi S, Laing R (2007). Prices & availability of common medicines at six sites in India using a standard methodology. *Indian J Med Res.* **125(5):** 645-54.

6. Narayan S. Price controls on Pharmaceutical products in India. Institute of South Asian Studies. Working Paper No. 20: March 19, 2007.

7. Shafie AA, Hassali MA (2008). Price comparison between innovator and generic medicines sold by community pharmacies in the state of Penang, Malaysia. *J Gen Med.* **6:** 35-42.

8. Singal GL, Nanda A, Kotwani A (2011). A comparative evaluation of price and quality of some branded versus branded-generic medicines of the same manufacturer in India. *Indian J Pharmacol.* **43(2):** 131-6.

9. The Decontrol of Drug Prices in India - Implications for the Indian Pharma Industry. Available at: http://www.ccsindia.org/ccsindia/interns2002/27.pdf.

CHAPTER 14

CLINICAL RELEVANCE OF DRUG ISOMERISM (ENANTIOPURE DRUGS)

Introduction

Drug discovery is a multidivisional and multitasking approach to search a new medicine for clinical use. However, it's diversified approach gives us tremendous useful targets. Since long time, drugs are available in the market to ameliorate the diseases. As the new technologies evolved into the drug development process and many new methods have been named for the selection of new compounds. Racemic drugs have been available since long but been extensively recognized in the last two decades. Selection and isolation of single enantiomers drug is well studied. Recently in pharmaceutical industries, 56% of the drugs currently in use are chiral products and 88% of the last ones are marketed as racemates (±) consisting of an equimolar mixture of two enantiomers. Such new compounds/stereoisomers are significantly differing in terms of their pharmacodynamic and pharmacokinetic profiles and the use of such mixtures may contribute to the adverse effects of the drugs due to nonselectivity, so, isomers play an important role in clinical pharmacology and pharmacotherapeutics. Therefore, isomerism has given us introducing safer and more effective drug alternatives of the newer as well as old drugs with more selectivity towards receptor. Overall, enantiomers of an active drug can be differ in selectivity, potency, toxicity, and behavior in biological systems. Viewing, its demands and safety profile regulatory bodies of U.S.A. (FDA), Europe, China, and Japan have provided a separate guidelines indicating that preferably only the active enantiomer of a chiral drug should be brought to market, hence it need to be separated and tested before clinical uses thoroughly.

Bioisosteres and Enantiopure/Chiral Drugs

The interaction of ligands with the receptor of interest is based on their pharmacophoric groups/properties. Hence, their structural pattern is responsible for their affinity for the pharmacophore and pharmacological effect. Replacement or modification of any functional groups may alter their physiochemical properties, affinity for pharmacophore /receptor, bioavailability etc. and finally results in different pharmacological action. Hence, pharmacophore is *'hypothetical electronic features derived to ensure the specific supramolecular interactions with present biological ligands and show or block the effect'*. It is very difficult to integrate and quantitate the relationship between the biological properties and physico-chemical properties of individual atoms, functional groups or entire molecules because many physical and chemical parameters are depend on conformation of atoms in molecules. Most common example of these types of interactions is of isosteric or bioisosteric molecules. Friedman introduced the term "bioisosterism" and defined it as *"Bioisosteres are (functional) groups or molecules that have similar chemical structure and physical similarities, and proposed to have similar pharmacological properties"* (Fig. 14.1).

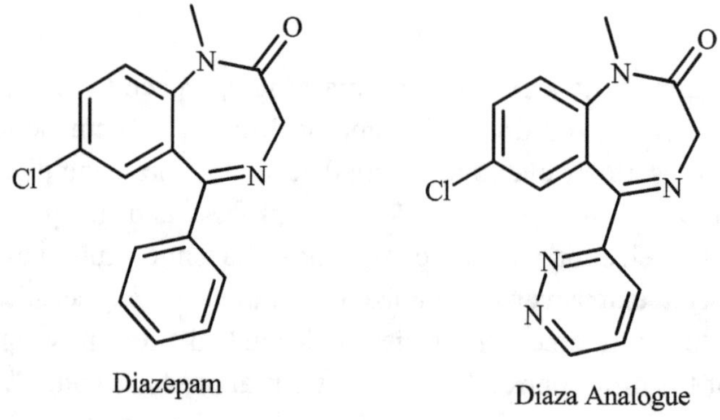

Diazepam   Diaza Analogue

Fig. 14.1 Bioisosters of diazepam.

Recently, Burger expanded this definition to take into account biochemical views of biological activity. "Bioisosteres are compounds or groups that possess nearly equal molecular shapes and volumes, approximately the same distribution of electrons and which exhibit similar physical properties such as hydrophobicity. The search for bioisosteres is very old and dates back to 1900 where Langmuir (1919), Grimm (1925), Erlenmeyer (1932) and Freidmann (1951) tried to identify the substances possessing atoms or groups with the same number of electrons, their arrangement, same physical properties". Bioisosteric compounds affect the same biochemically associated systems as agonist or antagonists and thereby produce biological properties that are related to each other. The key point is that the same pharmacological target is influenced by bioisoteres as agonists or antagonists. What may work as a bioisosteric group in one biological system (or receptor) may not have similar effects on another. There might be various advantages of using the phenomenon of bioisosterism (Fig. 14.2).

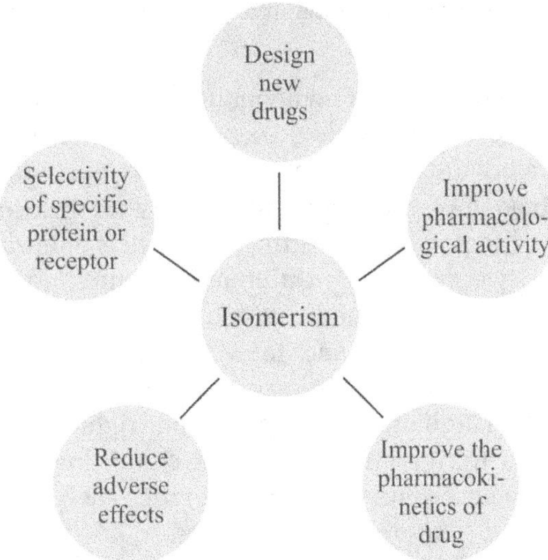

Fig. 14.2 Advances of bioisosterism/isomerism.

Bioisosteres were classified and subdivided into two main categories in 1970 by Alfred Burger namely, *(a) Classic and (b) Non-classic.* The atoms or molecular subunits or functional groups of the same valence and rings equivalents as classic bioisosteres, while non-classic are those which do not fit into the above classification. The main aim of the present classification is to give an umbrella type covers to all the chemical atoms to form a valid and active compound whether it is monovalent atoms or groups (-OH, -CH3, -OR, -F –Cl, -Br, -I, -SH etc.), Divalent atoms or groups (-CH2-, -O-, -S-, -Se-, -Te-), Trivalent atoms or groups (=CH-, =N-, =P-, =As-, =Sb-), Tetra substituted atoms (=C=, =Si=, =N$^+$=, =P$^+$= etc.) or it is cyclic/non cyclic.

Mainly, bioisosteres are used to modify the pharmacological activity of the old or lead drugs like to reduce toxicity or to modify selectivity, or metabolism. The correct use of the strategy of molecular modification also allows the identification of new classes of lead compounds with attractive pharmacotherapeutic activity, minimizing the efforts of synthetic work and, consequently, maximizing the chances for success in discovering medications both more efficient and of safer use.

Further, Isomers are the product of optical rotation of atoms (amino acids) during bioisosterism. Hence, isomers are with identical atomic compositions, but having different orientations of their atoms in space means the molecules/compound with two or more different form with the same molecular formula e.g., Glucose and fructose.

Logically speaking, if compounds have similar biological activities, it means have similar molecules/atoms/formula. Hence, during the drug development there is concept of modifying the structures of biologically active compounds and formulates several bioisosteres. However, surprising structure-activity relationships (SAR) suggested that organically/chemically similar compounds may have significantly different biological actions and activities.

Chemical similarity and diversity of compounds/molecules depend on the binding site and 3D structural properties of the biological targets. The most of drug and receptors interactions are illustrated in 3D format, resulting the role of stereochemistry. *Stereochemistry* is the branch of chemistry concerned with the 3 dimensional natures of molecules. The activity of molecules can differ as per their optical activity and form two diverse identity. Hence, two physically different structures/ identity may treat as the optical isomers of the parent compounds. A molecule is optically active, if it is not superimposable on its mirror image and these molecules/compounds are commonly known as enantiopure/*chiral compounds or drugs*. Chiral is a Greek word means *"cheir"*, which means 'handedness. These drugs are just like our right and left hand, looking same but non-superimposable as mirror image. Further, chiral drugs/compounds are divided into three broad categories according to optical activities such as *Constitutional isomers, Configurational isomers* and *Conformational isomers*.

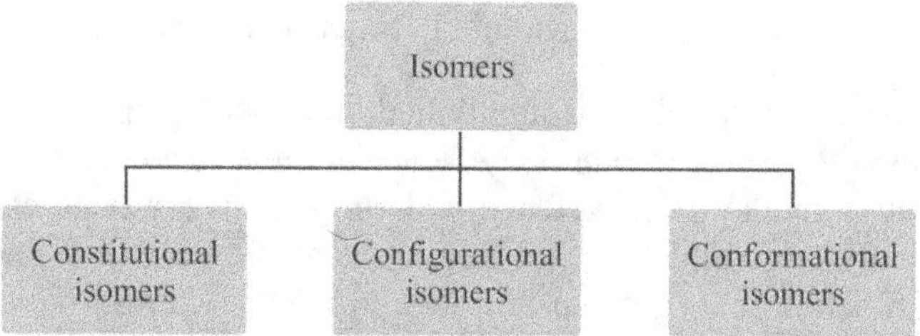

Constitutional or structural or positional isomers are molecules having same atomic composition but bonding arrangements between atoms are different, e.g., propanol can exhibit in two forms propan-1-ol and propan-2-ol (Fig. 14.3). All of these compounds have the same atomic composition (C_3H_8O), but different bonding arrangements of atoms and are thus distinct chemical entities with different chemical and physical properties.

(a) Propan-1-ol   (b) Propan-2-ol

Fig. 14.3 Constitutional isomers of propanol.

Configurational isomers are stereoisomers and defined as identical atomic composition and bonding arrangements, but different orientations of atoms in space and cannot interconvert freely by bond rotation. Further, it is subcategorized as optical isomers (*enantiomers*) or geometric isomers (*diastereomers)* (Fig. 14.4). *Enantiomers* are drugs/molecules which are related to each other as its mirror image but are not-superimposable, Hence, enantiomers are most commonly formed when a carbon atom contains four different substituents (asymmetric carbon atom or stereogenic carbon or also called *chiral center*). A chiral molecule is a molecule having at least one asymmetric carbon, whereas, *diastereomers* are drugs which have identical molecules, but are not related through the mirror image. The chirality of drugs depends on their bond length, bond polarity, hydrophobicity, rotation angle and importantly chirality of the amino acid. Hence, optical enantiomers most often have different biological activities, a sophisticated consideration of "chemical similarity" and "activity diversity".

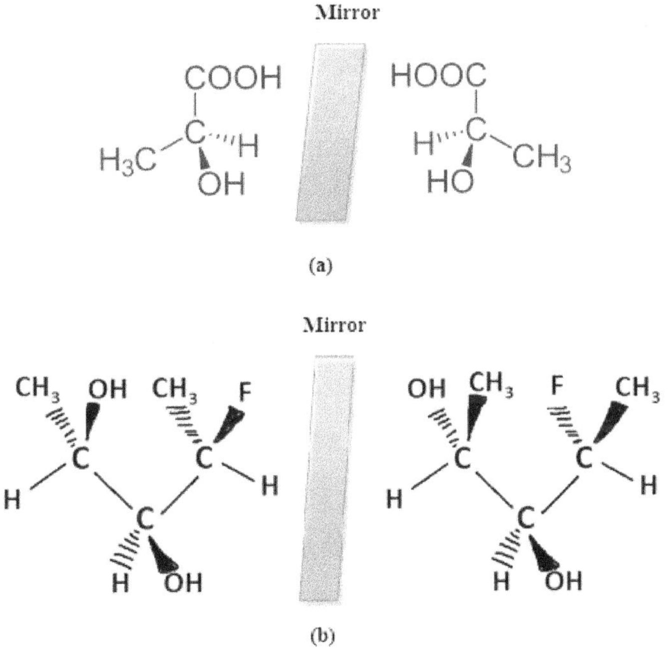

Fig. 14.4 (a) Enantiomers and (b) Diastereomers.

Whereas, *conformational isomers* (conformers) are stereoisomeric forms of molecules which may be characterized by different relative spatial arrangements of atoms that result from rotation about sigma bonds. Thus, unlike configurational isomers, conformers are interconverting stereochemical forms of a single compound.

Nomenclature of Chiral Compounds

We are always confused with the terminology like, (R), (S), (l) and (d). What does it means? Actually, enantiopure drugs are molecule having at least one asymmetric atom like carbon as with most of drugs. In some drugs nitrogen may act as asymmetric atom for example omeprazole, cyclophosphamide and methaqualone.

These compounds may be classified according to the movement or conformation changes in plane polarized light. The molecules are levorotary (l)-isomer when it move anticlockwise or sinister (S) or left (−) and dextrorotary (d)-isomer, when it rotate plane-polarized light in clockwise or rectus (R) or right (+). Further, equimolar mixture (1:1) of the two enantiomers of a chiral compound is known as *racemic mixture (racemate)*, designated with sign (±) or (d, l) and does not exhibit any optical activity.

Golden Rules to Name Isomers as per Optical Activity

1. Atom with the higher atomic mass receives higher priority and numbered first than others

2. If two substituents with equal rank, you must proceed along the two substituent chains until you find a point of difference

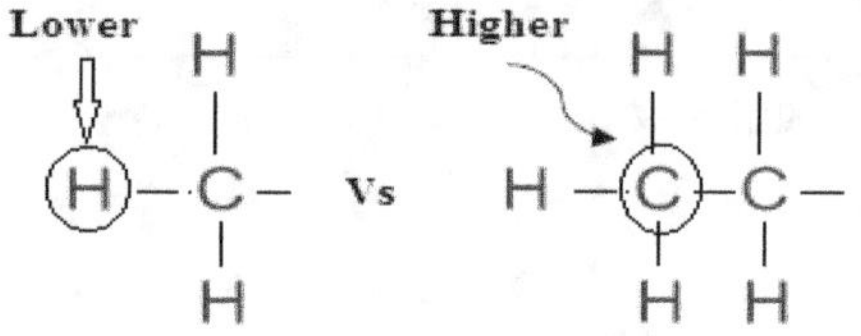

3. If a chain is connected to the same kind of atom twice or three times

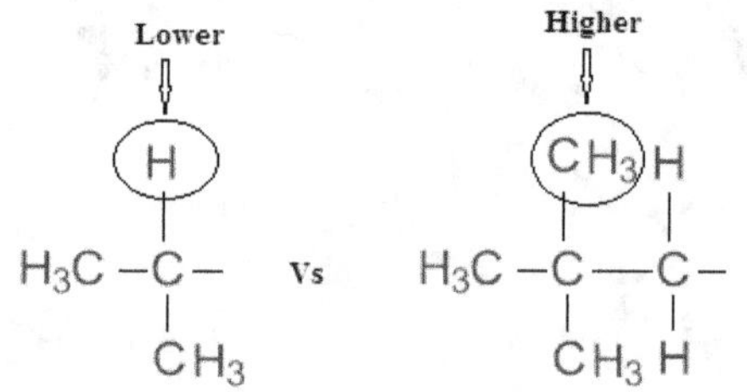

4. When all the substituents have been prioritized correctly, you will easily make out the name/label the molecule as **R** or **S.**

5. Try to make the arcing arrow from 1, 2, 3, 4 and more in such manner, that it will give out clockwise (R) or anti-clockwise (S)

Pharmacological Aspects of Racemate/Enantiopure Drugs

In the current scenario, enantiomers of a racemate drugs are considered distinctly different drug/molecules due to their distinct biological interactions, consequently different pharmacological, pharmacokinetic, or toxicological activities. The differences nature of the molecules may be due to its different selectivity profile and separate pathway for metabolism. One isomer may thus produce the desired therapeutic activities, while the other may be inactive or produce unwanted side effects. Patients safety is a prime concern and hence investigating single stereoisomers have advantages over their racemic mixture, for example, Penicillamine has two isomers *S*(-)-penicillamine, and *R*(+) penicillamine. The (S) isomer is used to treat Wilson's disease, (a defect in the body's ability to metabolize copper), acts as a strong copper chelating agent, whereas its (R) isomer is toxic and can cause blindness (Fig. 14.5).

(l) or (S) Penicillamine **(d) or (R) Penicillamine**

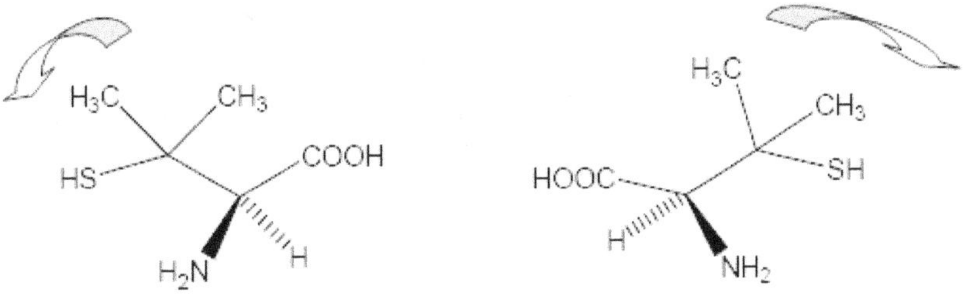

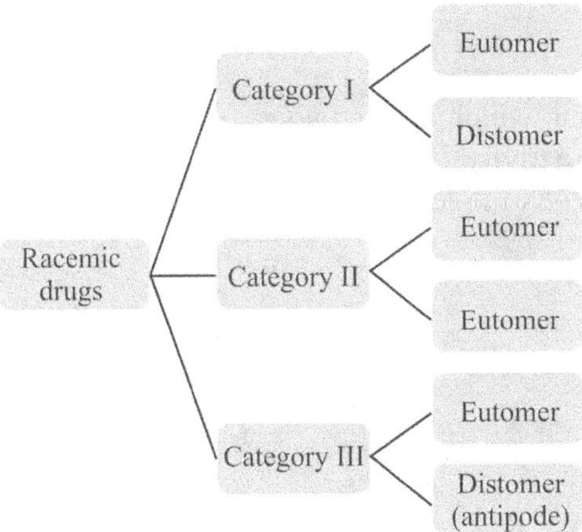

Fig. 14.5 Different role of penicillamine isomers (R,S).

As per mechanism, enantiopure drugs are more selective than the racemic drugs/mixtures. Most of the drugs sold as racemate drugs, however in last two decades market value of enantiopure drugs were increased significantly. The racemic mixture/drugs are of different properties and depend on the conjunction of their mixture of isomers. As per their enantiomers properties, it is divided into three main groups (Fig. 14.6).

Fig. 14.6 Classification of racemic drugs.

Category I are drugs, which have one main effective enantiomer known as *eutomer*, and the other is inactive or less active or can exert other desired or undesired pharmacological properties known as *distomer* e.g., Thalidomide and Citalopram (Fig. 14.7).

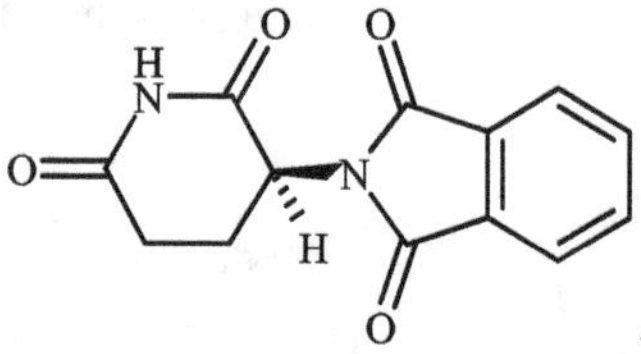

(S)-Thalidomide
(Teratogen)

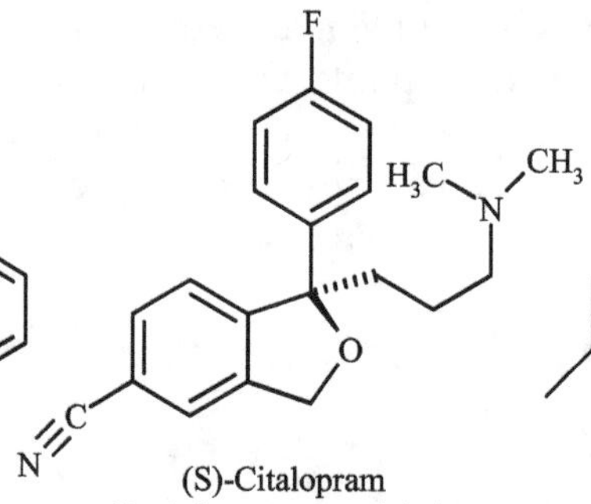

(S)-Citalopram
(Anti-depressant activity)

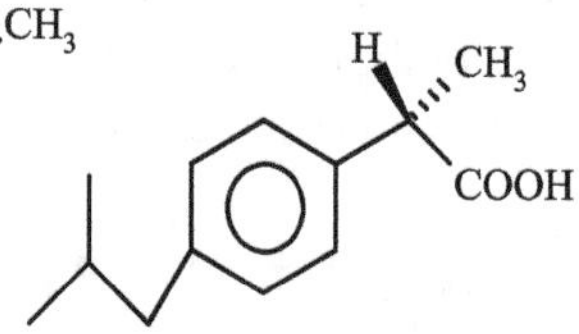

(S)-Ibuprofen
(NSAID)

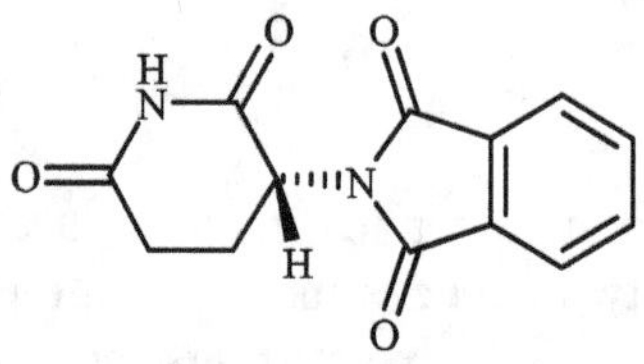

(R)-Thalidomide
(Sedative)

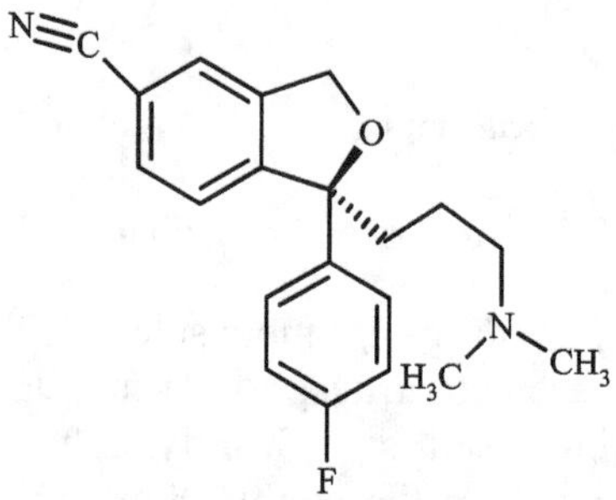

(R)-Citalopram
(Antagonist of (S)-Citalopram)

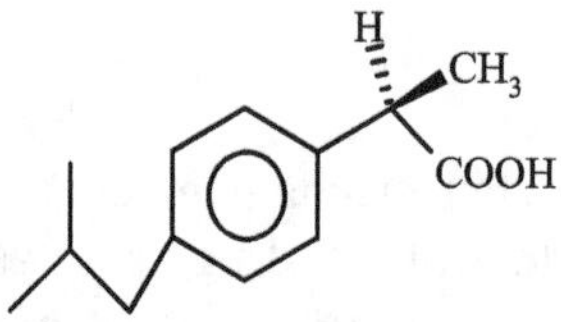

(R)-Ibuprofen
(Less active NSAID)

Fig. 14.7 Category I racemic drugs.

Category II are drugs in which all the two enantiomers are equally active and have the same pharmacological activity. E.g., cyclophosphamide (antineoplastic), flecainide (antiarrhythmic), fluoxetine (antidepressant) (Fig. 14.8).

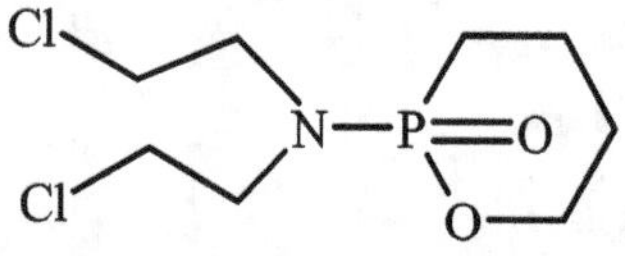

Cyclosporamide

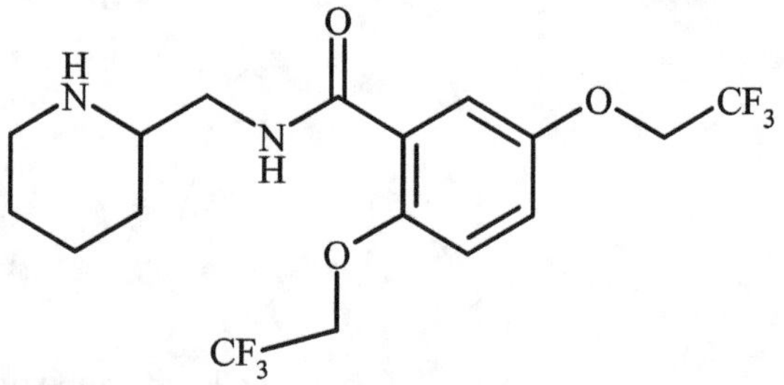

Flecainide

Fig. 14.8 Category II racemic drugs.

Category III are the combinations of enantiomers which is having only one active eutomer, but the distomer could be transformed in body into its bioactive antipode by chiral inversion. E.g., oxazepam, lorazepam, temazepam (Antianxiety drugs) (Fig. 14.9)

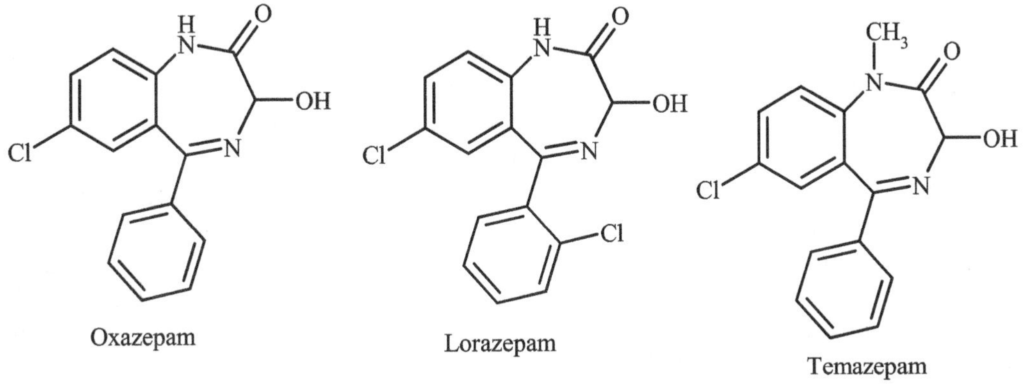

Oxazepam

Lorazepam

Temazepam

Fig. 14.9 Category III racemic drugs.

Advantages of Enantiopure Drugs over Racemic Drugs

1. More selective pharmacodynamic profile and less complex in nature
2. Less complex pharmacokinetic profile
3. Fewer or diminished side effects, which may result from the unwanted isomeric form.
4. Potential for an improved therapeutic index
5. Lower the dosage for a patient.
6. Enantiopure drugs are less potential for drug interactions
7. Easy to study plasma concentration and effect relationship
8. As per Pharmaceuticals points of view, useful for extending
9. Patent protection
10. Decreased waste due to decrease in manufacturing of unwanted isomer

Enantiopure Drugs and Side Effects

A designed drug is said to be more effective, if it has maximum therapeutic potential, bioavailability, less toxic or adverse reactions. While, designing new drugs one should consider the adverse drug reactions (ADR) which these new molecules might impart. Understanding the different types of ADRs might help in better structural modifications from the lead structures and minimize them. The ADRs can be broadly classified into 7 categories (*detailed in chapter 38; Tools of patients safety*).

Many drugs which are introduced into the market are withdrawn soon, because of the organ toxicity, they induce due to adverse reactions that are mediated during their metabolism. These days awareness is increasing for the consideration of the adverse reactions mediated organ toxicity in order to improve and design new safer drugs for the future. Thus, it is very essential to have the understanding of the possible toxicity and the metabolic fate of designed drugs physiologically. Therefore, some of the important features essential to be considered during metabolism which can be helpful in drug designing and to reduce toxicity are – the enzyme involved, the site of metabolism in the molecule, the resulting metabolites, the stability and the inhibition or it induction of drug metabolism which can result in drug-drug interactions. The drugs/xenobiotics in the body undergo phase-I and phase-II metabolism brought about by the Cytochrome p450 family and phase-II family of enzymes predominantly present in liver including other organs. The substrate selectivity of human CYPs is related to both the substrate structure and the key features of the active sites: namely, the disposition of certain amino acid residues within the haem environment. In the absence of three-dimensional (3D) structures for many of these enzymes, the prediction of whether a molecule binds to them rests with our limited knowledge of specificity and selectivity of the binding sites derived from *in vivo* and *in vitro* data. The metabolizing enzymes have affinity for the structurally diverse hydrophobic molecules that are used as pharmacological and toxicological models. Thus, the metabolic transformations of the drug/xenobiotics have profound impact on their bioavailability, efficacy, chronic toxicity, excretion rate and route. Therefore, the parent molecule and the products of metabolic transformations may interfere with the endogenous metabolism or the metabolism of other co-administered molecules. The understanding of these processes is very complex to evaluate the new molecule. The initial behavior is traditionally studies *in vitro*, but due to advances in computational chemistry software and the rapid accumulation of empirical data on drug-drug interactions, it can also be predicted to some degree computationally. These computational quantitative structure-activity-relationship (QSAR) models enable the selection of the most promising compounds (Table 14.1).

It is utmost important during drug designing using theoretical principles to consider the structural effects which govern the pharmacokinetic factors, such as absorption, biotransformation and elimination to predict the expected bioavailability of the newly designed drug-candidate for its clinical success or failure. Therefore, it is now understood that selection of a specific drug molecule requires a balance between efficacy, safety, metabolism and pharmacokinetic properties and screening of these characteristics should be carried out as early as possible in the discovery process. With the advent of the non-classic bioisosteres have been predominantly useful over the classic forms in designing the new drugs according to their therapeutic potential, selective receptor agonist antagonist drugs, enzymatic inhibitors or anti-metabolites in cardiac diseases (Demetri, 2007), platelet aggregation inhibitors. The use of this phenomenon demands physical, chemical, electronic and conformational parameters involved in the substitutions, theoretical prediction, alterations in the pharmacodynamic and pharmacokinetic properties which the designed compounds presents. These substitutions should be carefully analyzed by considering the following parameters.

(a) size, volume and electronic distribution of the atoms or the considerations on the degree of hybridization, polarizability, bonding angles and inductive and mesomeric effects when fitting

(b) Degree of lipidic and aqueous solubility, so as to allow prediction of alteration of the physicochemical properties such as logP and pKa;

Conclusion and Future Trend

There are newer and faster technologies in the areas of molecular and cellular biology, structural, computational and chemical biology. The pharmacological, pharmacokinetics and toxicological activities are important to consider for the better and safe development of drugs.

The enantiomers of racemates/chiral drugs may vary due to their interactions with chiral environments such as enzymes, proteins, receptors, etc of the body. Further, several studies have shown that stereoisomers of a chiral drug/racemates often exhibits pronounced differences in their pharmacokinetic and metabolic profiles both quantitatively and qualitatively. The more and more information is needed for the ADME properties which should be increased.

The main objective of enantiopure drugs is to protect the patent expiration of drugs. When patent is nears expiration, pharmaceutical manufacturers come out with its single stereoisomer as a new drug with the claim of higher activity and safe.

But, surely stereospecific enantiopure drugs are more safe and potent for the patients and have improved pharmacodynamic and pharmacokinetics profile, but on the other hand pharmaceutical companies introduce these drugs in higher price, hence regulatory bodies should have some regulations on enantiopure drugs.

Table 14.1 Some examples of racemic and enantiomeric form of drug have clinical relevance

Racemic drug (Therapeutic Class)	Enantiopure drug	Comments
Asparagine	(S)- Asparagine	Bitter in taste
	(R)- Asparagine	Sweet in Taste
Atracurium	(S)-Atracurium	Inactive
	(R)- Atracurium (Cisatracurium)	Neuromuscular blocker , three fold more potent than the racemate

Table 14.1 *Contd...*

Racemic drug (Therapeutic Class)	Enantiopure drug	Comments	
Albuterol	(S)-Albuterol	Bronchodilator	
	(R)-Albuterol	Antagonist activity of (S) form	
Bupivacaine	(S)-Bupivacaine (Levobupivacaine)	Local anaesthesia	
	(R)-Bupivacaine	More potent and may induce cardiotoxicity	
Carvone (Anti-MRSA)	(S)-Carvone	Caraway	Activity increased in combination
	(R)-Carvone	Spearmint	
Cetirizine	(S)-Cetirizine	Inactive	
	(R)-Cetirizine (levocetrizine)	Non-sedative anti-histamine, Potent and fewer side effect	
Citalopram	(S)-Citalopram (Escitalopram)	Potent selective serotonin reuptake inhibitor	
	(R)-Citalopram	20 times less potent than (s) enantiomer	
DOPA	(S)-Dopa (levodopa)	Parkinson's Disease	
	(R)-Dopa	Cause agranulocytosis	
Ethambutol	(S,S)-Ethambutol	Static in TB treatment	
	(R, R)-Ethambutol	Toxic may induce Blindness	
Ibuprofen	(S)-Ibuprofen (Dexibuprofen)	NSAIDs	
	(R)-Ibuprofen	Morning sickness	
Ketoprofen	(S)-Ketoprofen (Dexketoprofen)	Inhibition of cyclooxygenase activity	
	(R)-Ketoprofen	Less potent than S-form	
Ofloxacine	(S)-Ofloxacine (levofloxaxcine)	Active Isomer	
	(R)-Ofloxacine	Inactive isomer	
Omeprazole (PPI)	(S)-Omeprazole (Esomeprazole)	Increased bioavailability and lower the first pass metabolism and clearance	
	(R)-Omeprazole	Less active than (S) enantiomer	
Penicillamine	(S)-Penicillamine	Wilson's Disease	
	(R)-Penicillamine	Toxic may induce blindness	
Salbutamol	(S)-Salbutamol	Induce airway Hyper responsiveness, hence racemate is associated with some loss of bronchodilator potency	
	(R)-Salbutamol (levalbutamol)	*Produces significantly greater bronchodilatation than the equivalent dose of the racemate*	
Thalidomide	(S)-Thalidomide	Teratogen	
	(R)-Thalidomide	Sedative	

Suggested Readings

1. Burger AA. Guide to the Chemical Basis of Drug Design, NY, EUA, Wiley, 1983; p, 24-29.

2. Cayen MN (1991): Racemic mixtures and single stereoisomers: industrial concerns and issues in drug development. Chirality 3, p. 94-98.

3. Chiba M *et al.,* (2003). Prediction of hepatic clearance in humans from experimental animals and *in vitro* data. In drug metabolizing enzymes.

4. Cytochrome 450 and other enzymes in drug discovery and development (Fisher M.B., *et al.,* eds), pp. 453-481.

5. Drayer DE (1986). Pharmacodynamic and pharmacokinetic differences between drug enantiomers in human: an overview. *Clinical Pharmacology and Therapeutics.* **40(2):** 125-133.

6. Eichelbaum M (1995). Side effects and toxic reactions of chiral drugs: a clinical perspective. *Archives of Toxicology, Supplement.* **17:** 514-521.

7. Ekins S, Berbaum J, Harrison RK (2003). Generation and validation of rapid computational filters for CYP2D6 and CYP3A4. *Drug Metab. Dispos.* **31:** 1077-1080.

8. Ekins S, De Groot M, Jones JP (2001). Pharmacophore and three dimensional quantitative structure activity relationship methods for modeling Cytochrome P450 active sites. *Drug Metab. Dispos.* **29:** 936-944.

9. Erlenmeyer H, Leo M (1932). *Helv. Chim. Acta.* **15:** 1171.

10. Fontis Media and Marcel Dekker (2007). Demetri GB. Structural engineering of imatinib to decrease cardiac risk in cancer therapy. *Journal of Clinical Investigation.* **17(12):** 3650-3653.

11. Friedman HL (1951). Influence of Isosteric Replacements upon Biological Activity. Washington, EUA, National Academy of Science, n 206, p.295.

12. Guo A, Vangapandu S, Sindelar RW, Walker LA, Sindelar RD (2005). Biologically Active Quassinoids and Their Chemistry: Potential Leads for Drug Design. *Current Medicinal Chemistry.* **12:** 173-190.

13. Korolkovas A, Burckhalter J.H. Quimica Farmaceutica 1982, Rio de Janeiro, R.J. Editora Guanabara Dois, p.62.

14. Landoni MF, Soraci A (2001). Pharmacology of chiral compounds: 2-Arylpropionic acid derivatives. *Current Drug Metabolism.* **2(1):** 37-51.

15. Mehvar R, Brocks DR, Vakily M (2002). Impact of stereoselectivity on the pharmacokinetics and pharmacodynamics of antiarrhymic drugs. *Clinical Pharmacokinetics.* **41(8):** 533-558.

16. Park BK, Pirmohamed M, *et al.,* (1998). Role of drug disposition in drug hypersensitivity, a chemical molecular and clinical perspective. *Chem. Res. Toxicol.* **11(9):** 969-988.

17. Pollina E (1996). Design and synthesis of RGD mimetics as potent inhibitors of platelet aggregation. *J.Undergrad.Sci.* **3:** 119-126.

18. Reddy M. *et al.,* (2005). Physiologically based pharmacokinetic modeling: science and applications, John Wiley & Sons.

19. Stenlake JB (1979). Foundations of Molecular Pharmacology, Vol 2. The Chemical Basis of Drug Action, Londres, Inglaterra, Athlone Press, p, 213-290.

CHAPTER 15

COUNTERFEIT MEDICINES

Introduction

Various definitions exist for counterfeit medicines; the most accurate is that of the World Health Organization (WHO) which says: *"Counterfeit medicine is one which is deliberately and fraudulently mislabeled with respect to identity, composition and/or source. Counterfeit products may include products with the correct ingredients or with the wrong ingredients, without active ingredients, with insufficient active ingredients or with fake packaging"*. Similarly, according to FDA, *"Counterfeit medicine is fake medicine"*. It may be contaminated or contain the wrong or no active ingredient. They could have the right active ingredient but at the wrong dose. Counterfeit drugs are illegal and may be harmful to health. These definitions of counterfeits includes not only completely fake drugs, but also those that have been tampered with adulterated, diluted, repackaged or relabelled so as to misrepresent the dosage, origin or expiration date. This broad definition reflects the fact that adulterated or substandard drugs can be as dangerous as fake drugs and that all represent a fraudulent misrepresentation of the manufacturer's trademark.

In contrast to counterfeit medicines, substandard drugs are genuine products that are produced by legitimate or illicit manufacturers, which, due usually to poor manufacturing practice or improper storage conditions, do not meet agreed-upon standards for quality, purity, strength or packaging.

WHO defines Substandard Medicines as "genuine medicines produced by manufacturers authorized by the National Medicine Regulatory Authorities (NMRA), which do not meet quality specifications set for them by national standards". If substandard drugs are knowingly produced to make unlawful profit (produced cheaply and then sold as if full quality) they are considered to be counterfeit. Substandard drugs pose a serious problem as counterfeiting because substandard drugs can cause treatment failure and contribute to the emergence of drug resistant diseases.

There is another category of drugs which falls under the name of "Spurious Drugs". A drug shall be called as spurious if it is manufactured under a name which belongs to another drug, if it is an imitation of another drug or if it has been substituted wholly or partly by another drug or if it wrongly claims to be the product of another manufacturer. The term "Spurious Drug has been defined under Section 17-B of the Drugs and Cosmetics Act, 1940, as amended by the Drugs and Cosmetics (Amendment) Act, 1982. A stringent penalty for manufacture and sale of spurious drugs has also been prescribed under the Act. Spurious and counterfeit drugs and substandard drugs are not synonymous with each other and a clear line of demarcation is to be drawn between them (Table 15.1).

Prevalence of Counterfeit Drugs

The magnitude of the drug-counterfeiting problem is considerable and is difficult to determine as any true estimate of prevalence is difficult. The WHO estimates that up to 10% of the world's pharmaceutical trade, 25% in developing countries consists of fakes, whereas up to 25% of all drugs consumed in poor countries are thought to be counterfeit or substandard, according to the figures from the US Food and Drug Administration (FDA). The percentages are worse in certain areas: 38% in Southeast Asia, 48% in Africa; indeed a recent study of pharmaceuticals on sale in Nigeria's capital found that 80% were fake and 7% contained dangerous ingredients.

India, the world's largest manufacturer of generic drugs, has become a busy centre for counterfeit and substandard medicines. Experts says that the global fake-drug industry, worth about $90 billion, cause the deaths of almost 1 million people a year and is contributing to a rise in drug resistance. Estimates vary on the number of these drugs made in India. The Indian government says that 0.4% of the country's drugs are counterfeit and that substandard drugs account for about 8%. But independent estimates range from 12 to 25%. The number of people arrested for manufacturing and selling fake drugs rose from 12 in 2006 to 147 last year.

What are the Causes of Poor Quality of Drugs?

Poor drug quality has been linked to counterfeiting of medicines, chemical instability mainly in tropical climates and poor quality control during manufacture. Many factors contribute to the increased prevalence of substandard and counterfeit medications. Much of the counterfeit drug trade is probably linked to originate crime, corruption, the narcotics trade, the business interests of unscrupulous politicians and unregulated pharmaceutical companies. According to the WHO guidelines, factors that influence the prevalence of counterfeit drugs in any particular country include weak or absent drug regulatory authority, absence of a legal mandate for licensing of manufacture/import of drugs, lack of regulation by exporters and within free trade zones, proliferation of small pharmaceutical industries, complex transactions involving many intermediaries high demand for curative and preventive drugs and vaccines exceeding supply, high prices and inefficient cooperation among stakeholders. The WHO Essential Drug Program has failed in most countries because of personal financial interests at local, national and foreign levels or a black market. Studies indicate that a country's capacity to restrict dangerous drugs depends heavily on its wealth. It is quite surprising to know that almost a third of WHO member countries have poor means of controlling counterfeit medications. In these circumstances, the market for counterfeit and substandard drugs becomes a lucrative one. In addition, lack of good manufacturing practices (GMP) is common in local pharmaceutical industries in most developing countries because of many hurdles such as frequent power cuts and shortage of water. In addition to the existence of substandard drugs, assurance of the stability of pharmaceuticals marketed in developing countries (most of which have tropical climates) is a challenging issue as poor storage conditions, high temperature and high humidity conditions generally enhance chemical degradation and may alter the biopharmaceutical properties of the drugs as it has been shown for antibiotics such as tetracyclines. Finally, medicine sellers often exhibit lack of concern about expiration dates and storage conditions, especially in poor settings and in the absence of national control and this can increase the spread of substandard antimicrobials.

In contrast, in developed countries, other factors are involved in the spread of counterfeit medicines. For example, it is well known that underinsured or uninsured individuals and some states and local governments are turning to the internet and foreign pharmacies, particularly what they believe to be safe, reputable Canadian pharmacies, to find less costly medications. However, Internet pharmacies, even licensed ones in Canada, are increasingly buying from foreign sources themselves to meet American demand and thus import of counterfeit and substandard medications may be enhanced. Finally, certain antimicrobials such as artemisinin derivatives are not only confined to Asia and Africa but also to other countries of the industrialized world as they have a natural plant origin and tourists commonly buy them in the tropics as a standby treatment and they are also readily available on the Internet.

Consequences of Counterfeit Medicines

The use of low-quality drugs can result in adverse clinical outcomes such as lack of effect and treatment failure, risk of development of bacterial resistance, toxicity or side effects, all of which contribute to the burden of disease and consequently to excess mortality and morbidity. However, there are no reports (e.g., cohorts) that have studied these consequences of low-quality drugs in a systematic approach using adequate scientific methodology. According to some reports of WHO, tragedies caused by the counterfeit medicines include:

During the outbreak of meningitis epidemic in Nigeria in 1995, over 50,000 people were inoculated with fake vaccines, received as a gift from a country which thought they were safe, but unfortunately it resulted in 2,500 deaths.

The consumption of paracetamol cough syrup prepared with diethylene glycol (a toxic chemical used in antifreeze) led to 89 deaths in Haiti in 1995 and 30 infant deaths in India in 1998. Of the one million deaths that occur from malaria annually, as many as 200,000 would be avoidable if the medicines available were effective, of good quality and used correctly. A study conducted in South-East Asia in 2001 revealed that 38% of 104 antimalarial drugs on sale in pharmacies did not contain any active ingredients and had resulted in a number of preventable deaths. In 1999, at least 30 people died in Cambodia after taking counterfeit antimalarials prepared with sulphadoxine-pyrimethamine (an older, less effective antimalarial) which were sold as Artusenate.

Table 15.1 Difference between counterfeit, spurious and substandard medicines

S. No.	Counterfeit Drugs	Spurious Drugs	Substandard Drugs
1	The drug formulation may contains active drug, incorrect drug or without active drug	The drug formulation is without any active ingredient/salt	The drug formulation contains active drug but poor quality
2	It will resemble in packing, design, look with original brand.	It may or may not resemble in packing, design, look, etc. with original brand	It will resemble in packing, design, look with popular brand.
3	May not be injurious to health	May cause serious problems, even death of the patient	May cause serious problems due to low quality product
4	Sample will fail when tested in the laboratory	Sample may pass when tested in the laboratory	Sample may fail due to its poor quality standards
5	There is criminal intent behind producing and supplying these drugs	Criminal intent may or may not be there	There is no criminal intention behind supplying these drugs

Counterfeit Drugs in Developing Countries

Evidence suggests that a significant proportion of drugs consumed in the lower-income countries are of poor quality. Counterfeits are also significant in developing countries such as India, China, Brazil and Russia. Counterfeiting thrives in developing countries is because of high costs and limited resources, black market operations, lack of infrastructure and technical expertise to regulate and policy criminal activity, corruption and price controls. According to WHO 60% of counterfeit drugs are from low per capita nations, where it is estimated that more than 25% of drug supply is counterfeit. In low-resource countries, counterfeit medicines are commonly sold to treat life threatening and worlds most deadly infectious diseases such as malaria, tuberculosis, HIV/AIDS. A study conducted in 2004 found that 53% of the antimalarial drugs sold in South-East Asia are counterfeit medicines. This situation is worse in African countries, in Nigeria it is estimated that more than 85% of antimalarial chloroquine tablets are ineffective and in many other African countries more than 50% tablets are ineffective. Using of these drugs will increasing drug resistance in the patients and cause morbidity and mortality.

Counterfeit Drugs in Developed Countries

The European Union (EU) is predominantly threatened by a flood of counterfeit medicines, particularly those sold on the Internet. Estimation depicts that there is an increase in 15% of counterfeit sales in European countries and 20% of Europeans admitted in hospitals are purchasing prescription drugs without prescription and counterfeits have become serious public health problem over here. United States drug supply is among the most secure in the world and it is also affected to counterfeits by obtaining the drugs through unregulated channels and due to sophistication of counterfeit drug ring. WHO estimates that "5% to 7% of all drugs sold in United States have been tampered with mislabeled or otherwise fraudulent". United Kingdom was producing 500,000 counterfeit pills daily continuous to highlight the hazard of counterfeit pills in developed countries. To fight the prevalence of counterfeit drugs in developing countries the US Agency for International Development (USAID) joined with the US Pharmacopoeia Convention to promote the quality and safety of drugs used in USAID's priority health programs.

Evaluation of Counterfeit Drugs

In order to assess the quality of the drugs moving in the supply chain, it is enormously essential to estimate systematically the extent of the problem. To achieve this, informal drug samples are required to be drawn from different medical stores such as retailers, wholesalers, government hospitals where it is suspected that movement of spurious, counterfeit drugs may be more. For this, 15 informal samples should be collected from different drug stores i.e., 2 samples from wholesaler, 8 from the retailers (in the ratio of 1:1:1:1 (2 samples) from village, town, taluka and dist places respectively) and remaining 5 samples from the government hospitals. The ratio of samples collected from wholesalers to retailers is 1:4 and the plan is based on fact that ratio of that the wholesalers to retailers i.e., 5000:20000. Consumer association/Non-governmental organization along with circle drug inspector or assistant drug controller shall visit and collect the samples. Table 15.2 shows the different test adopted for different formulation to ensure the quality of the medication.

Table 15.2 Minimum quantity of samples required and tests
adopted for different formulations

S. No.	Formulation	Quantity of sample required	Tests adopted
1	Tablets/Capsules	30-40	Description, Identification, Assay, Disintegration
2	Dry powders/liquid injections (small volume parenterals 30ml)	6	Description, Identification, Assay and pH wherever possible
3	Liquid orals	100 ml	Description, Identification, Assay and pH wherever possible
4	Ointments/creams/gels	20 gm	Description, Identification, Assay and pH wherever possible
5	Ophthalmic and ENT liquid preparations/ointments/creams	4 samples	Description, Identification, Assay and pH wherever possible

Precautions to be taken during Sample Collection

- The quantity of sample taken must be from the same batch
- Samples collected shall have at least 6 months remain to expiry
- Minimum quantity of sample to be taken as mentioned in the table
- The sample should not be taken out of the original packaging
- The medicine labels and package leaflets should not be removed or damaged
- The sample collected should be kept under controlled conditions as per label requirements.

Legislative and Regulatory Authorities

The problem of spurious and counterfeit medicines was first addressed at international level in 1985 at the Conference of Experts on the Rational Use of Drugs in Nairobi, then in 1988 to protect health and safety of the patients World Health Assembly requested the Director-General of WHO to initiate programme for the prevention and detection of the export, import and smuggling of falsely labelled, counterfeited or substandard pharmaceutical preparations.

After more than 2 decades, in February 2006 WHO proposed the establishment international regulating body, International Medical Products Anti-Counterfeiting Taskforce (IMPACT), and it was endorsed by 160 participants on behalf of 57 national drug regulatory authorities, 7 international organizations, 12 international associations of patients, health professionals, pharmaceutical manufacturers and wholesalers. Then in the same year on 5 April 2006, the 12th International Conference of Drug Regulatory Authorities in Seoul, Republic of Korea, welcomed the establishment of IMPACT. At its core, IMPACT aims to build coordinated networks across and between countries in order to halt the production, trading and selling of fake medicines around the globe. IMPACT is a partnership comprised of all the major anti-counterfeiting players, including: international organizations, non-governmental organizations, enforcement agencies, pharmaceutical manufacturers associations and drug and regulatory authorities.

At national level Central Drug Standards Control Organization (CDSCO) is the Central Drug Authority to function against counterfeits. It will function to control over the import of drugs, to carry out inspections and rides over medical supply chain and quality control of medication. The Drug and Cosmetic Act 1940 and Rule 1945, which is a central piece of legislation regulates the manufacturing, packing, labeling, and sale of product or drug in India.

Methods for Analysis of Counterfeit Drugs

There has been a variety of innovative technologies from the pharmaceutical companies to reduce the counterfeiting and many believe that advances in these technologies will solve the problem of counterfeit in the drug supply chain.

These technologies include:

1. Radio-Frequency Identification (RFID)

2. Pharmacode/Bar code

3. Raman spectroscopy

1. **Radio-Frequency Identification (RFID):** Among these techniques RFID are the most promising track and trace technique that uses electronic devices to track and identify pharmaceutical products, by assigning individual serial numbers to the containers holding each product. RFID tags contain tiny radio transmitters which stores information electronically and read at short ranges a few meters *via* magnetic fields and then act as a passive transponder to emit microwaves or UHF radio waves i.e., electromagnetic radiation at high frequencies. Even though there are many barriers to widespread RFID like cost, complicated infrastructure required to track the drugs through the supply chain and unresolved questions regarding its possible effects on biological medicines it has benefits like better inventory management and reduction in theft and product loss throughout the supply chain.

2. **Pharmacode/(Bar code):** Pharmacode (also known as Pharmaceutical Binary Code) is another potential identification technology that would place a barcode on each drug package with a unique electronic product code that is used all over the world. Bar coding technology was traditionally chosen in pharmaceutical industry because of its three main features like:

   ➢ The kind of data required to appear on the bar code like numeric symbols, alpha-numeric or special characters.

   ➢ The amount of available space on which to print and the specific location of the bar code.

> Where the bar code needs to be placed near an edge, there is a considerable risk of misreads.

This technique is cheaper to installation than RFID but operating is expensive as it would require manual scanning.

3. **Raman Spectroscopy:** Raman spectroscopy is new non-invasive method for analysing the counterfeit drugs while they are still inside their packaging. This device could be used as a first line of defence against counterfeits and it is promise for its high chemical specificity and works by interacting the laser light with molecular vibrations, phonons other excipients results in shifting of energy which gives characteristic peak, which will helps in detecting the makeup of the compound. This method is conventional for the examination of many pharmaceutical products through their coating or capsules as well as through blister packs and white plastic bottles and so is used to detect counterfeit drugs.

In addition to track-and-trace technology, new authentication technologies could make it more difficult for counterfeiters to duplicate pharmaceuticals. These authentication technologies are:

- Overt – Visible and immediately apparent security features on the packaging or components, such as holograms, color-shifting ink or tamper-evident features.

- Covert – Visible but not immediately apparent security measures, often hidden features such as UV markers or micro batch codes.

- Forensic – Extremely covert security measures that require special equipment to detect.

These include imbedded chemical tags that can be tested for, and elemental analysis to verify composition.

How to Stop Counterfeiting?

The government and the regulatory authorities have a major role in servicing and coordination to fight against counterfeit drugs; most of the countries have enacted sufficiently tough laws to penalize counterfeit. In India government had set up an expert committee under the chairmanship of Dr. R. A. Mashelkar in February 2003 to recommend measures for strict the vigilance in the country and to tackle the problem of spurious drugs. In November 2003 the committee had recommended several changes in penal provisions of Drug and Cosmetic Act. The main recommendations made by the committee were:

- Severe vigilance must be maintained, with regular surprise checks.

- Enhancement of penalty and prison terms for sale and manufacturing of spurious drugs that cause serious harm or death, from life imprisonment to death sentence.

- Creation of competent national drug laboratories with high quality of testing facilities for checking the counterfeit drugs.

- There should be a penalty for those who are unable to produce documents in support of their purchase of drugs.

- Constitution of special courts for trial of offence under the Drugs & Cosmetics Act so that judicial proceedings can be expedited.

- There are no accessible testing services for fake drugs anywhere in the country so formation of a strong, well equipped Central Drugs Standards Control Organization, which could be given the status of central drug administration are recommended.

- There should be a provision for compounding of minor offences so that, these should be disposed of expeditiously, while prosecution is able to concentrate on serious cases in the appropriate courts.

Suggested Readings

1. Cockburn R, Newton PN, Agyarko EK, Akunyili D, White NJ (2005). The global threat of counterfeit drugs: why industry and governments must communicate the dangers. *PLoS Medicine*. **2(4):** e100.

2. Eliasson C, Matousek P (2006/2007). Non-invasive detection of counterfeit drugs using Spatially Offset Raman Spectroscopy (SORS). *Lasers for Science Facility Programme.*

3. Erhun W, Babalola O, Erhun M (2001). Drug regulation and control in Nigeria: The challenge of counterfeit drugs. *Journal of Health & Population in Developing Countries*. **4(2):** 23-34.

4. Gautam C, Utreja A, Singal G (2009). Spurious and counterfeit drugs: a growing industry in the developing world. *Postgraduate Medical Journal*. **85(1003):** 251-6.

5. Kelesidis T, Kelesidis I, Rafailidis PI, Falagas ME (2007). Counterfeit or substandard antimicrobial drugs: a review of the scientific evidence. *Journal of Antimicrobial Chemotherapy*. **60(2):** 214-36.

6. Mackey TK, Liang BA (2011). The global counterfeit drug trade: patient safety and public health risks. *Journal of Pharmaceutical Sciences*. **100(11):** 4571-9.

7. Newton PN, Amin AA, Bird C, Passmore P, Dukes G, Tomson G, *et al.,*(2011). The primacy of public health considerations in defining poor quality medicines. *PLoS Medicine*. **8(12):** e1001139.

8. Newton PN, Lee SJ, Goodman C, Fernández FM, Yeung S, Phanouvong S, *et al.,* (2009). Guidelines for field surveys of the quality of medicines: a proposal. *PLoS Medicine*. **6(3):** e52.

9. Outterson K, Smith R (2006). Counterfeit Drugs: The Good, the Bad, and the Ugly. *Alb LJ Sci & Tech*. **16:** 525.

10. Shakoor O, Taylor R, Behrens R (1997). Assessment of the incidence of substandard drugs in developing countries. *Tropical Medicine & International Health*. **2(9):** 839-45.

11. Shukla N, Sangal T (2009). Generic drug industry in India: the counterfeit spin. *Journal of Intellectual Property Rights*. **14:** 236-40.

CHAPTER 16

DRUGS AND SPORTS

Introduction

The issues related to drugs used in sports are varying, complex and are often interconnected. When people talk about drugs used in sports, they tend to be referring to elite athletes who use drug substances in order to enhance their performance. However, the use of drugs by sportspersons includes various other issues associated with it such as the sports ethics and the role of regulatory bodies. Doping is not a new phenomenon to sports community, looking at the history, since very beginning of sports i.e., 1904 Olympics, drugs are used in sports in order to enhance the performance. Sportspersons can face health hazards due to use of these drugs depending upon the type and way in which drugs are used. For example, harmful effects of steroid use. Other drugs may have undesired and adverse effects. In many regions, the sportspersons along with doctors/physicians are not well aware about the use/prohibit of drugs used in sports injury and for athletics. According to National Anti-Doping Agency (NADA) guidelines, there is a list of drugs or substances which are prohibited to be used in sports persons, but not all the athletes/coaches or physicians are aware about these drugs. Basically, there are three reasons why athletes and sportspeople may take drugs: as treatment medication for disease, to enhance performance or as recreational drugs. Sportspeople are as entitled to treatment of a medical condition as anyone else but both the sportsperson and the doctor must be aware of the prohibited substances in sports; Failure to which can lead to serious consequences.

An athlete could receive either a temporary or permanent ban from competing in that sport if he found guilty as per national anti-doping guidelines. Some drugs are permissible when not competing but not during competition. Some drugs are banned in some sports but not in others. Also there are some drugs which are not allowed at all times such as anabolic steroids.

Doping in Sports

Doping is the use of chemical substances or methods in order to alter the performance. It is unethical practice of sports and poses a risk to the health of sportsperson. The use of performance enhancing drugs or methods to gain a benefit over others is cheating. The term doping was originated from *dop*, which is an alcoholic drink used as a stimulant in ceremonial dances in 18th century. There are some other suggestions which indicate that the term doping is derived from the Dutch word *doop* for viscous opium juice, and has evolved to denote the use of performance enhancing drugs in sportspersons. According to the World Anti-Doping Code (developed by the World Anti-Doping Agency), doping should include the following statements in its definition;

- Presence of a prohibited substance or its metabolites or markers in the body of sportsperson/athlete.

- Refusing to submit to sample collection after being notified.

- Attempt to use the banned substance or method.

- Possession of any prohibited substance or method.

- Administering or attempting to administer a prohibited substance or method to an athlete.

- Failure to file athlete whereabouts information & missed tests.

- Tampering with any part of the doping control process.

- Trafficking and distribution of any prohibited substance or method.

Doping is the deceitful method of getting an advantage over other sportspersons in competition and also harmful to the health of the person. The use of performance enhancing drugs or methods is not a new phenomenon in sports and it dates to ancient times. However, the misuse of drugs in the sports seems to be increasingly more prevalent. The willing to win at any cost is thought to be the driving force for the athletes to use the banned drug substances. Enhancement of a performance by just a fraction of extra strength or fastness, make the athlete to win the gold medal and being a national hero. Some athletes will do almost anything to get an advantage in competition even after knowing the consequences of doping violations and the adverse effects associated with the use of steroids and other performance enhancing drugs. Furthermore, cheating of one athlete enforces another to cheat to succeed in competition. The use of performance-enhancing drugs is unfortunately on the upward trend.

Doping History: From Past to Present

Since antiquity, man has always tried to enhance his natural power; however, it is the craze of public for sports and records along with the progress in medicine research which made the drug abuse a social iniquity. Various miraculous medicinal products are often widely used during sporting competitions. Doping has been called the 'cancer of sport', and more importantly, young people are often persuaded to follow the senior professionals.

The drug abuse in sports is not a new problem amongst sportspersons; it is continuing form the ancient times. The use of performance enhancing drugs/doping methods has existed from very long time. The first recorded incident of doping violation was noted by Philostratus and Galerius in ancient Olympic Games held in the 3rd century BC. Furthermore, Ancient Greek Olympians who ate sheep's testicles in order to enhance their performance by increasing testosterone levels was noted in 8th century BC. In 1904 Olympics, Thomas hicks used brandy along with strychnine as a stimulant. He had also won the marathon, but later he died. Mixtures of brandy, cocaine, strychnine and caffeine were widely used by the sportspersons in order to increases their performance. In 1928, first rule against doping was built by the International Association of Athletics Federation (IAAF) by prohibiting the abuse of drugs in sports. In 1936 Olympics, German athlete was noted for the use of rudimentary testosterone preparations to increase the physical strength. Various armed forces (American, British, German, and Japanese) distributed amphetamines (as a substitute for cocaine) to their soldiers to stave off fatigue and injury, elevate mood and to improve the intensity of their fights. After that, use of amphetamines was passed over to the athletes in early 1950s. These drugs were used by Italian as well as Dutch cyclists to counteract the sensations of fatigue during exercise.

In 1960, during the Summer Olympics at Rome, a Danish cyclist was died during the 100 km team time trial race. Initially, it was thought that his death might be caused by high temperatures that day. His autopsy revealed the presence of amphetamines. Since then, there have been numerous doping suspicions and claims. In 1964, at the Olympic Games in Tokyo, some doping controls were set up in order to reduce the drug abuse in sports. However, doping in sport has not reduced but has expanded at a breathtaking rate in professional and elite athletes. In 1967, death of a British cyclist Tommy Simpson created pressure over various sports organizations to fight against doping in sports. As a result of this, the International Olympic Committee (IOC) sets up the Medical Commission against doping in sports. This Commission was built and worked in order to protect the health of athletes, to maintain the integrity for medical and sport ethics, and equality among all competitors. In 1968, first time the IOC made its doping controls and ordered the drug testing of competitors at the Winter Olympic Games, France and also at the Summer Olympic Games in Mexico City. Furthermore, the first full-scale testing of Olympic athletes has been done in 1972 at Summer Olympic in Munich, Germany. World's fastest man was divested of gold medal at the 1988 Olympic Games in Seoul, Korea for using Stanozolol (an anabolic steroid). The doping scandals were occurred almost at every sport competition, including Olympics, World Championships and even commonwealth games.

After all these scandals and events, IOC decided to arrange a World Conference on Doping for all the sports organizations and other parties involved in doping controls. The first World Conference on Doping was held on February 2-4, 1999 at Lausanne,

Switzerland. A document named *"Lausanne Declaration on Doping"* was produced in this conference which suggested the creation of an Independent International Agency against doping in sports. With agreement to terms of "Lausanne Declaration on Doping", the World Anti Doping Agency (WADA) was established on November 10, 1999, in Lausanne, Switzerland to promote, coordinate and monitor the fight against drug abuse in sports. WADA is an independent organization created through the collective initiative taken by IOC. WADA is responsible for the World Anti-Doping Code in order to harmonize the anti-doping rules and regulations in all sports and countries. The WADA code is adopted by more than 600 national as well as international sports organizations including IOC, International sports federations and NADOs.

The first person who tested in out-of-competition was a British sprinter named Dwain Chambers. He was found positive for the steroid tetrahydrogestrinone (THG) test conducted on August 1, 2003 and was suspended from all competitions for a period of two years and banned from the Olympics for life time. The Anabolic Steroid Control Act was passed by the U.S. Congress earlier in 2004. This bill included a list of anabolic steroids including various steroidal based drugs and their precursors which were banned for sales without a prescription. The list of these banned drugs was also adopted by famous baseball organization, Major League Baseball (MLB). In 2004, WADA took over the control of list of banned drugs/substances. Prior to 2004, athletes who tested positive for a level of caffeine greater than 12 micrograms per milliliter (about 8 cups of coffee) were banned from competition. WADA amended the list of banned substances in 2004 and also removed caffeine from the list of banned substances on the basis of research which showed that exceeding the amount of caffeine beyond allowed limit might cause the decrease in performance. Olympic gold medalist and track and field champion, Marion Jones retires from track and field in 2007 after admitting that she has used steroids prior to the 2000 Sydney Olympics. In December 2007, the IOC divested her of the three gold and two bronze medals won by her in 2000 Sydney Olympics.

Doping control (drug testing) and drug education of athletes is necessary in order to protect athletes from the harmful effects of drugs and also to maintain the quality and ethics in sports by providing an atmosphere for fair competition. The desire to win at all costs forces the athletes to adopt the illegal and unfair means so that they can take advantage over the other competitors. Due to better detection methods, the competitors are now trying to cheat by some different means such as by inducing natural physiological reactions, reactions and also to hide the evidence from the doping inspectors.

Role of WADA in Doping Control

In past years, the use of performance enhancing drugs by sportspersons has gained much attention. Various drugs such as anabolic steroids, stimulants, erythropoietin (EPO) and other ergogenic substances are being used by athletes to take the advantage in the competition. Several education and doping awareness programmes have been conducted by sports organizations. The World Anti Doping Agency (WADA) and the US counterpart, USADA are the most effective organizations to promote and coordinate the national and international anti-doping programmes. WADA has developed and implemented the World Anti-Doping Code and International Standards for harmonization and equality of anti-doping policies and regulations among different sport organizations and countries. This harmonization works to provide a solution to the previously raised problems associated with doping due to unorganized efforts. The adoption of code led to significant improvements in fight against doping.

The mission of WADA is to promote, coordinate and monitor the fight against drug abuse, i.e., doping, in sports. It has been established as Independent International Organization in 1999 after the Lausanne declaration produced in the first World Conference on Doping in sports. Its main focus is to promote the education about doping, research and development of anti-doping policies for all countries. WADA has achieved its key achievement in fight against doping by drafting and accepting World Anti Doping Code (2004) and continuous monitoring of doping regulations. World Anti Doping Code is the core document that consists of all the elements needed for harmonization of anti-doping rules, regulations and their implementation in various national and international sports organizations including International Olympic Committee (IOC), International Sports Federation, National Olympic Committee and other public authorities in different countries. It works on the basis of five International Standards (Testing Procedures, Laboratories, List of Prohibited Substances and Methods, Therapeutic Use Exemptions and for the confidentiality of personal information). The code has proven to be very effective tool to provide equality in anti-doping policies worldwide. International standards for the World Anti-doping Program are developed in conjunction with the signatories and member countries as approved by WADA. The main purpose of these international standards is to harmonize different technical and operational processes of anti-doping programs among different countries. World Anti-Doping Code and International standards are revised from time to time after consultation with signatories and member countries. The ultimate solution to prevent doping in sports can be achieved by implementing various education and awareness program amongst sportspersons and physicians to create a doping free environment in sports. WADA provides education to athletes about the ethical and technical guidelines through anti-doping programs. The main purpose of WADA is to protect the athlete's right for competing in doping free sports and to promote the equality among the competitors worldwide. By implementing various drug testing and anti-doping programs, the use of performance enhancing drugs by athletes and sportspersons has been reduced to some extent.

Doping Testing

Doping testing is necessary to perform, on routine basis, for all the sportspersons competing at national as well as international level. It is general practice to test all the athletes who are participating in competition as well as those who won medals in previous sports events and also there are provisions of random drug testing of sportspersons by their governing body for in competition and out-of-competition testing. Some drugs are allowed when out-of-competition but not allowed during competition. While, the drugs like anabolic steroids are banned for all times i.e., in-competition as well as out-of-competition. There are some drugs which are banned for use in some sports but allowed in others. Beta blockers are banned in shooting events because of its unfair advantage by suppressing the tremors. However, it would cause impair the athlete's performance. Drug substances like alcohol and caffeine are permissible only up to certain level.

Prohibited Substances

A wide variety of drugs have been used in sports for the performance enhancement. Prohibited list includes both drug substances and methods which are used for their potential to enhance performance in sports, poses a potential health risk to sportsperson and if its use dishonor the spirit of sport. Some substances or methods are included on the list because they have the potential to mask another prohibited substance or method. These drugs are used in combination with other drugs also in order to enhance the effect. Various examples include the use of digitalis for slowing down the heart rate, strychnine and caffeine for preventing the early fatigue, steroids for building muscle strength. Most commonly used drugs in doping are stimulants (amphetamines and other related compounds) and tranquillizers (meprobamate and barbiturates). Other drug substances used are analgesic agents such as morphine and its derivatives which may be used to reduce the pain due to injury or exertion so as to take an advantage over other competitors.

Anabolic steroids are the most commonly used substances for doping in sports which helps in building of muscle volume during training or exercise. Thus, these substances are known as muscle fertilizers. The 2014 Prohibited list of World Anti-Doping Code includes the following three categories of substances and methods:

- Substances and Methods Prohibited at All times
- Substances and Methods Prohibited In-competition
- Substances Prohibited in Particular Sports

There are five classes of prohibited substances (anabolic agents; peptide hormones, growth factors and related substances; beta-2 agonists; hormones and metabolic modulators; and diuretics and other masking agents) and three types of methods of doping (manipulation of blood and blood components; chemical and physical manipulation; and gene doping) which are banned at all times. Various substances and methods prohibited in-competition include stimulants, narcotic analgesics, cannabinoids, glucocoticosteroids. The most commonly used drug substances by athletes has been discussed below along with associated harmful effects on athlete's health.

Anabolic Steroids

Anabolic steroids are generally derived from male sex hormones. It is a generic term used for male sex hormones. Anabolic steroids (also known as anabolic androgenic steroids) are widely abused in sports to enhance body building and to improve the athletic performance. Along with their capacity to promote muscle growth and protein synthesis, these drugs also have many adverse effects including various neuropsychiatric disturbances, depression, mania, hypertension, cardiac arrhythmias, hepatic and renal dysfunction. Examples of the anabolic steroids as listed WADA list of prohibited substances 2014 are: androstenediol, androstenedione, danazol, methyltestosterone, nandrolone, stanozolol, DHEA, testosterone and related isomers as well as metabolites. In 1970s, athletes were using the synthetic steroids (e.g., nandrolone) and were easily detected by the conventional testing methods. However, the problem arose when use of endogenous steroids such as testosterone came into picture. Use of anabolic androgenic steroids led to disqualification of the Canadian sprinter from Olympics for life time. These steroids act by preventing protein breakdown in muscles and maintaining muscle mass. To increase muscle mass with use of steroids, the athletes must take high caloric diet (approx. 10000 calories/day) with rigorous exercise. Ergogenic effects of androgenic steroids are achieved at very high doses (50-90 times more than normal therapeutic dose). At this much high doses, there are increased chances of occurrence of more harmful or adverse effects of steroids. The common adverse effects associated with the use of anabolic-androgenic steroids include gynecomastia, hypertension, cardiac problems, hepatic and renal toxicity, aggressive behavior, depression and other neuropsychiatric disturbances. Some of the side effects, such as hepatotoxicity or nephrotoxicity, are reversible in nature and disappeared after the drug is stopped. However, chronic use of anabolic steroids leads to irreversible damages such as hepatitis, bleeding and tumors, etc. Acne and fluid retention are the most commonly associated complications with the use of steroids. There are also several other side effects that are gender specific. In males, the use of anabolic steroids might cause testicular atrophy, infertility, gynecomastia, increased risk of prostate cancer and baldness, while in case of females; it shows a different adverse effect profile like hirsutism, menstrual disturbances, male pattern baldness, clitoral hypertrophy. In males, chronic use of steroids causes negative feedback and inhibits the production of endogenous testosterone form testes and resulting in suppression of spermatogenesis. Anabolic-androgenic steroids may increase the risk of ischemic heart disease because it elevates LDL levels and reduces HDL levels. The use of anabolic-androgenic steroids increases stiffness of tendons which can lead to muscles breakdown and damage to joints. Further testing for anabolic-androgenic steroids poses a challenge to the authorities. Earlier, there was a lack of methods to detect and differentiate the exogenous testosterone from endogenous testosterone produced in the body. However, the International Olympic Committee and Anti-doping agencies have developed more accurate methods which can indirectly detect the exogenously derived steroids by measuring the urine testosterone: epitestosterone (T:E) ratio. There are strict legal implications and anti-doping rules for the use of steroids by athletes. Various education, training and counseling programs have also been initiated for increasing the awareness in order to stop the misuse of anabolic agents. Other banned substances include tibolone and anti-estrogens including the selective estrogen receptor modulators (SERMs) and aromatase inhibitors. If there are genuine reasons to prescribe such drugs, a TUE can be issued.

Peptide Hormones, Growth Factors and Related Substances

Peptide hormones and growth factors (FGF, VEGF) are being abused in sports to enhance the physical strength. Growth hormone and erythropoietin are now widely used by athletes in order to take an unfair competitive advantage. Various peptide substances and other related compounds prohibited for use in sports are:

- Erythropoietin (EPO)
- Chorionic Gonadotropin (hCG), Luteinizing Hormone and their related compounds
- Corticotropins (ACTH)
- Growth Hormone (GH) and its related factors
- Insulin-like Growth Factor (IGF-1)

Erythropoietin is one of the most well known substances used for doping purposes. In the past years, a large number of doping cases involving the use of erythropoietin has been detected. EPO is a peptide hormone which controls the synthesis of erythrocytes (RBCs) in body. It stimulates bone marrow to increase the production of red blood cells. The erythropoietin and its related substances are known as blood doping agents. Erythropoiesis-stimulating agents (ESAs) are used due to their capacity to increase the synthesis of RBCs and so that blood can transport more oxygen to the muscles. Doping experts, Paoli and Donati, have been reported that more than 500,000 individuals worldwide used EPO for doping purposes in 2004. The companies have achieved a sale of billions of dollars for EPO in 2004. Excessive use of EPO leads to increased hematocrit and hypertension. Adverse effects associated with misuse of EPO include the thickening of blood, reduced blood flow which further may lead to life-threatening thrombosis, stroke and in some cases it may cause the death due to occlusion of blood vessels. Chorionic Gonadotropin (CG), Luteinizing Hormone (LH) and their releasing factors are prohibited in males only. Use of gonadotropins can result in hypertrophy of the ovaries and hormone imbalance. Growth hormone helps in regulation of physical growth in adolescents. It also acts on the body to reduce fat deposits and helps in building of muscle mass. The growth factors such Fibroblast Growth Factors (FGFs), Hepatocyte Growth Factor (HGF), Vascular-Endothelial Growth Factor (VEGF) which affect muscle growth, protein synthesis, vascularization are also prohibited for their use in sports. Growth hormones are also used in combination with anabolic agents to increase the body-building which further doubles the associated risk. Excessive use of growth hormone and related compounds can lead to development of acromegaly, gigantism, metabolic and endocrine disorders. Corticotropin, also known as adrenocorticotropic hormone (ACTH), is produced by pituitary gland and acts on the adrenal cortex. Corticotropins regulate the synthesis and release of cortisol (body's natural steroid) which is responsible for producing euphoric effects and to create a sense of physical well-being. ACTH may produce a number of deleterious effects like body's immune system suppression, increased risk for infection.

Stimulants

Stimulants are also referred as psycho stimulants. Amphetamines and ephedrine are the typical examples of stimulants which have similar actions on body as that of adrenaline and noradrenaline which are naturally produced hormones in body. They increase the rate of metabolism and delay fatigue. The use of stimulants to enhance athletic performance is prevalent in Olympic sports. These stimulants are used to increase endurance and to reduce the fatigue during exercise. Ephedrine is commonly used for treatment of nasal congestion and other respiratory problems. Certain cold remedies contain ephedrine so those remedies are prohibited to be used in athletes. Potential harmful effects of these stimulants include psychiatric disturbances, headache, anxiety, insomnia, tremor, impaired decision making, confusion and restlessness. Amphetamines and ephedrine may also lead to the development of hypertension and tachycardia through stimulation of adrenergic receptors. Prolonged use of amphetamines can also cause dependence and precipitate withdrawal symptoms upon discontinuation of drug. Tolerance may also develop after chronic use of amphetamines. Despite the adverse effects and addictive nature of amphetamines, athletes still use these stimulants to gain a little performance advantage. Ephedrine is obtained form a Chinese plant named *Ephedra sinica*, also known as Ma-huang and also found in many dietary supplements. Phenylpropanolamine was commonly used by athletes for reducing body weight to take an unfair advantage in sports. Recently, Food Drug Administration (FDA) has banned this drug for marketing due to its serious adverse effects, e.g., Stroke. The potential health risks associated with use of these stimulants are headache, increased blood pressure, increased heart rate, weight loss, hallucination, convulsions, and heart attack.

Narcotics and Analgesics

Narcotics are used for alleviation of pain in serious injuries. The use of narcotics is prohibited in sports since 1967. Morphine, buprenorphine, diamorphine, fentanyl and its derivatives, methadone, pentazocine, pethidine are the typical examples of narcotics. Narcotics are primarily used by athletes' in-competition for increasing their pain threshold. The adverse effects of narcotics include loss of coordination, mood changes, inability to concentrate and other psychological problems. The major problem associated with the use of narcotics is the physical and psychological dependence because of its high addiction potential. Codeine is not included in WADA list of prohibited substances 2014. Only the stronger narcotics are banned for their use in athletes. However, it is recommended to avoid the use of codeine because screening of narcotics and codeine &

related compounds does not actually differentiate between two. In this case, non-steroidal anti-inflammatory drugs (NSAIDs) are the drugs of choice for relieving pain in sportspersons.

Beta-2 Agonists

Beta-2 adrenergic agonists are used for treatment of asthma due to its relaxing effect on bronchial muscles. Beta-2 agonists are used by athletes for doping for performance enhancement due to the dilation of bronchial muscles. Most of beta-2 agonists are banned by WADA. But in some cases, for an asthmatic patient, these can be used for medical reasons only after the approval of a therapeutic use exemption. As per the 2014 list of prohibited substances, all beta-2 agonists are banned except inhaled salbutamol (maximum limit 1600 mg over 24 hours) and inhaled formoterol (maximum limit 54 mg over 24 hours).

Diuretics

Diuretics are abused by athletes either for promoting weight loss by water elimination or to increase the excretion of other illicit substances i.e., for masking. For therapeutic purposes, these are used to treat high blood pressure and fluid accumulation (edema). These are banned in both in- and out-of-competition since 1988.

Other Banned Substances

World Anti-doping Agency and other International Sports Organizations have also banned many other substances in certain circumstances. Beta adrenergic blockers are banned in some sports events such as Automobile, Billiards, Golf, Shooting (also prohibited Out-of-Competition), Skiing/Snowboarding in ski jumping. Alcohol (ethanol) is prohibited (in-competition only) in particular sports like Air Sports, Archery, Automobile, Karate, Motorcycling, Power boating. The maximum allowed limit (for doping violation) of blood alcohol is equivalent to a concentration of 0.10 gm/L. In addition to banned substances, there are also banned doping methods such as blood doping, use of plasma expanders, gene doping.

Therapeutic Use Exemption (TUE)

Therapeutic Use Exemption (TUE) is an exemption that allows an athlete to use banned substance for therapeutic purposes only. The athlete can obtain a TUE for the use of prohibited substance or method for the treatment of a legitimate medical condition. In such cases, athletes should first check with their physician or sport's medical personnel to look if any alternatives are available. If there is no alternative, then athletes should apply for a TUE.

WADA has issued an International Standard for TUEs under the World Anti-Doping Code. According to this International Standard, all National and International Sporting

Organization must have a provision for the process of TUE requested by athletes with a legitimate medical condition such as asthma. TUE applications should be reviewed and managed by Therapeutic Use Exemption Committee (TUEC), comprised of a group of independent physicians. These TUECs would be responsible for the grant or rejection of such applications.

Doping Control in India

The National Anti-Doping Agency (NADA) is responsible for the doping control in India. It is funded by Ministry of Youth Affairs And Sports, Government of India. NADA works towards a vision of 'dope free' sport in India. The main functions of this organization are to promote, coordinate and monitor the various doping control program in sports in the country. India is one of the foundation members of World Ant-Doping Agency. The National Anti-Doping Agency (NADA) is a signatory member to Copenhagen Declaration on Anti-Doping and UNESCO International Convention against Doping, and under which it accepted the World Anti-Doping Code in March 2008. The anti-doping rules of NADA have been modified in compliance to the WADA code 2009. These rules came into force from January 2010 and applied to all athletes/sportspersons and concerned sports organizations across the country. There are three independent panels (Fig. 16.1) which look after the doping control and anti-doping violations in athletes. The primary functions of National Anti-Doping Agency are:

- Adopting and implementing Anti-doping rules and policies which conform to the World Anti-Doping Code.
- To work in coordination with other sports organizations and anti-doping organizations.
- Promoting anti-doping research & education.
- Sample collection and testing of sportspersons for doping, both in-competition and out-of-competition.
- Imposing sanctions/ban on athletes who violates the Anti-doping rules.

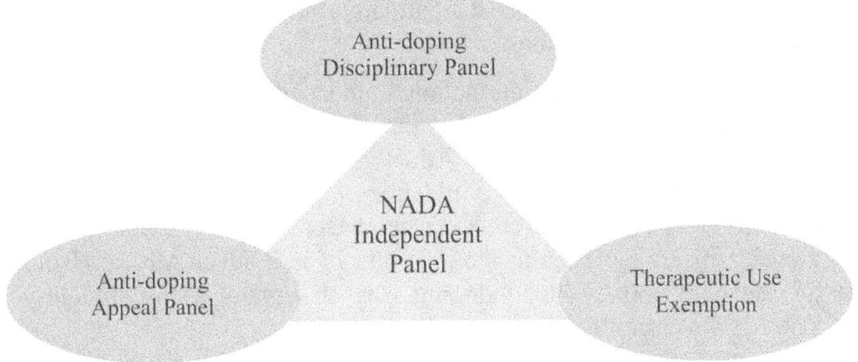

Fig. 16.1 Role of NADA in doping control.

Currently, there are 130 doping control officers (DCO) and chaperones for collection of dope samples of sportspersons across the country. The collected samples are tested in National Dope Testing Laboratory (NDTL) situated in New Delhi. NDTL is an autonomous body working under Ministry of Youth Affairs and Sports and is accredited by WADA for testing of blood as well as urine samples obtained from sportspersons. After doping sample testing, the laboratory reports the result to NADA and WADA.

NADA has also conducted various educational and awareness program about the anti-doping rules and regulation. The main focus of these programs is to increase the awareness and educate the athletes, coaches and other supporting staff about the updated list of prohibited substances or methods, adverse effects of doping in sports, responsibilities of athletes towards the ethics of sports and therapeutic use exemption process. In a telephonic questionnaire survey of awareness amongst medical doctors about doping in sports, it has been found that 63% of Doctors are not aware of WADA, only 68% of them knew partially (about anabolic steroids abuse in sports) of list of banned substances and not the complete classified groups of prohibited substances. Surprisingly, none of the doctors know about the TUE form and when to use it. Orthopedic surgeons had the maximum knowledge regarding doping matters and Gynecologists knew the least. Due to lack of knowledge or special educational programs about the awareness amongst physicians in many regions of India, the sports persons accidently use the drugs which are prohibited. Special educational programs should be conducted to promote awareness among medical doctors (Orthopedic Surgeons, Gynecologists) and Pharmacists about the effects of drugs and other substances, that are dangerous/illegal for athletes.

Athlete Biological Passport

The athlete biological passport (ABP) is a novel advancement in the fight against doping. Its fundamental principle is to monitor the selected biological variables (i.e., doping biomarkers) over time that indirectly reveals the effects of doping rather than to detect the doping substance or method itself. ABP is a turning point in the fight against doping. The ABP is an electronic record of an individual athlete's biological attributes, developed over time from multiple sample collections.

WADA, as the harmonized international independent anti-doping organization responsible for coordinating and monitoring the global fight against doping in sport, has taken the lead in the development of the Athlete Biological Passport concept. WADA's Athlete Biological Passport Operating Guidelines (ABP Guidelines) were approved by WADA's Executive Committee and took effect on December 1st, 2009. This first version contained a standardized approach to the profiling of individual Athlete Haematological variables for the detection of blood doping (the 'Haematological Module' or 'blood module'). The ABP is currently composed of two modules:

- *The Haematological Module*: Introduced in December 2009; aims to identify enhancement of oxygen transport, including use of erythropoiesis-stimulating agents (ESA) and any form of blood transfusion or manipulation. It considers a panel of biomarkers of blood doping that are measured in an athlete's blood sample.

- *The Steroidal Module:* Recently introduced on January 1st, 2014; aims to identify endogenous anabolic androgenic steroids when administered exogenously and other anabolic agents, such as selective androgen receptor modulators (SARMS). The Steroidal Module considers a panel of biomarkers of steroid doping measured in an athlete's urine sample.

The integration of ABP into the larger framework of a robust anti-doping program is the main objective of Anti-doping organizations in order: to identify and target athletes for specific analytical testing by intelligent and timely interpretation of passport data for both Haematological Module and Steroidal Module and; to pursue possible anti-doping rule violations (ADRVs) in accordance with World Anti-Doping Code (Code). WADA will continue to develop the ABP in consultation with stakeholders, by refining the present modules as well as adding new ones as they are finalized.

Suggested Readings

1. Anti-doping Rules and Regulations, National Anti-Doping Agency. Available online at: www.nada.nic.in

2. Dawson RT (2001). Drugs in sport - the role of the physician. *J Endocrinol.* **170(1):** 55-61.

3. Drugs in Sport. Available online at: http://www.ulster.ac.uk/scienceinsociety/ drugsin sport .html

4. The 2014 List of Prohibited substances, World Anti Doping Agency. Available online at http://www.wada-ama.org/Documents/World_Anti-Doping_Program/ WADP-Prohibited-list/2014/WADA-prohibited-list-2014-EN.pdf

5. Therapeutic Use Exemptions, WADA. Available online at: http://www.wada-ama.org/en/Science-Medicine/TUE/

CHAPTER 17

EXPIRED DRUGS

Introduction

Drugs have an important role in curbing the ailments and managing the health status of the patients but they have also an age beyond which their efficacy and safety becomes questionable. After attaining an age i.e., at the end of shelf life, drugs are called as expired drugs. The expiration dates on drugs are a critical part of information about the safety of the drug and ensure that drug will work as intended. According to the U.S. Food and Drug Administration (FDA), using expired medical products is risky and possibly harmful to our health. The requirement of the expiry date begins in the late 1970s, on the prescribed drugs. Sometimes following "EXP," the expiration date can be found printed on the label or stamped onto the bottle or carton. It is imperative to know and adhere to the expiration date on the medicine as expired medical products can be less effective or risky due to a change in chemical composition or decrease in potency with the course of time.

Improper storage such as exposure to the heat, light, humidity can contribute to the decreased effectiveness in medicines that have not reached their posted expiration date. Hence, it is important to store the medicines in the controlled conditions to ensure the proper shelf life of the medicines. The expired medicines should be disposed-off properly either by reading the label of the disposal instructions or should be disposed-off to the household trash.

It is important to know that once the expiration date has passed, there is no assurance that the expired medicines will be safe and effective, however it does not mean that a day after the expired date, drug will lose its potency.

Calculating the Expiry Date

For every new drug, a series of quality standards are established after conducting the clinical trials and before the regulatory permissions are sought. These are the manufacturing and testing specifications, which includes upper and lower limits for the amount of the Active Pharmaceutical Ingredient (API) in each dose unit (e.g., 300 mg per capsule). The final dosage form may be a mix of the API as well as fillers, binders and other ingredients to ensure the API is delivered to the body in a reliable and predictable manner. The date of manufacturing is expressed as month and year. Last day of the month mentioned in expiry date is considered as the deadline of consumption of the product.

To ensure the quality and safety, drug products are put through accelerated degradation testing, or "stress" testing, to estimate how fast a drug will deteriorate; in short, to ascertain the shelf life of the drug. There are ICH guidelines to ascertain the stability of drug products which divides the world into four distinguished climatic zones for this purpose of worldwide stability testing. Description of four climatic zones is shown in the figure shown below

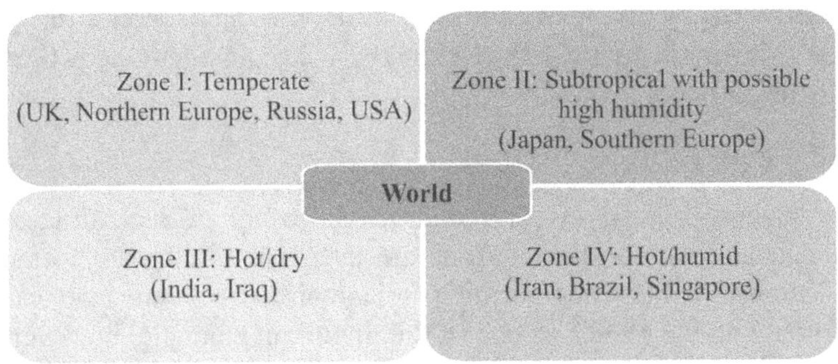

The shelf life should be determined by taking climatic zone(s) in which the products are to be marketed, into considerations. To ascertain the shelf life stability studies generally are carried out under different sets of temperature and relative humidity (RH) (Table 17.1).

Table 17.1 Storage conditions for stability studies of the drugs

Study	Storage conditions	Minimum time period covered by data at submission
Accelerated	40 °C ± 2 °C/75% RH ± 5% RH	6 months
Intermediate	30 °C ± 2 °C/65% RH ± 5%RH	6 months
Long term	25 °C ± 2 °C/60% RH ± 5% RH/ 30 °C ± 2 °C/65% RH ± 5% RH	12 months

The stress testing may include exposure to heat, light, oxidation, humidity, etc. After exposing over different time periods, API is quantified in the formulation to assess the efficacy of the drug. This process helps in understanding the stability of the drug as well as the degradation pathway of the drugs.

For liquid and injectable drugs, additional tests for bacterial purity and chemical stability are required. These quality checks are used to estimate that what will be the expiry date of the drug i.e., the date to which the manufacturer warrants the original product characteristics will be retained. Few other drug products are highly sensitive to moisture and hence, require dispensing in specialized containers with desiccants to trap moisture and enhance stability. Liquid antibiotics have very poor stability, so these drugs should be prepared when to be used. Few drugs ranging from vaccines to eye drops require refrigeration, which keeps the dosage form stable.

It is important to note that the expiry date of a drug is based on testing of previously unopened products that are maintained under the given conditions and stored in its original container or cover. Once the drug is exposed to light, heat and humidity, the stability of the drug could be compromised, but that doesn't mean that drug has become ineffective totally. Drug like Aspirin (acetylsalicylic acid) under the influence of humidity breaks down *via* hydrolysis to salicylic acid and acetic acid thereby giving a characteristic vinegar odour.

Safety of the Expired Drugs

The foremost concern related to expired drugs is safety of such drugs. There is no published data to suggest the harms from the use of expired drug formulations. The example of degraded tetracycline forming epianhydrotetracycline and causing kidney damage dating back to the 1960's, is one of the important example, however, that version of drug is not available anymore. In the lack of documented evidences, it is suggested that the degradation of the useful chemicals into the toxic compounds as rare phenomenon, if it occurs at all. However, there are very few case reports in which products of degradation are significantly more toxic than the original active pharmaceutical ingredient and human toxicity has been observed due to consumption of the expiry drug. Chloroquine can produce toxic reactions attributed to photochemical degradation. Phototoxicity has also been reported following administration chlordiazepoxide and nitrazepam. Antipenicilloyl antibodies were formed with the infusion of degraded Penicillin G.

Therefore, to maintain the safety of the drug, it should be made compulsory under the stability testing of the drugs that complete and proper information about the stability of drugs in the different time span and details should be given if expired products pose a safety risk over the period of time. A study conducted by the U.S. Food and Drug Administration covered over 100 drugs, prescription and over-the-counter showed that about 90% of them were safe and effective as long as 15 years past their expiration dates. It has been stated by the experts that most expired drugs are probably effective except few exceptions like nitroglycerin, insulin and some liquid antibiotics.

Regulatory Framework

In general, professions such as medicine and pharmacy are established as legal entities within a country that are enacted by the state lawmakers (legislature). Every country has different regulations on expired drugs. Manufacturing and sale of drugs are regulated by different governmental entities around the world. There may be different specific regulatory systems; but have a common goal of ensuring that drugs are safe and properly labelled. In the industrialized countries, these regulations have evolved to the point where they are rather extensive and, largely because the United States and European Union are the two largest markets in the world for drug manufacture and sale.

India

The medicines in India are regulated by the Drugs and Cosmetics Act 1940 and Rules 1945. The statue provides power to the central and state governments to ensure that only quality, safe and effective medicines are available for use. *The Drugs and Cosmetic Act 1940 and the Rules 1945, require the date of manufacture and the date of expiry of potency to be clearly and truly stated on the label or container of any specified imported drug or class of such drug, and prohibit the import of the said drug or class of drug after the expiry of a specified period from the date of manufacture.*

The regulation stipulates that, every medicine must have a date of expiry of its use. The date of expiry of potency is the date that is recorded on the container, label or wrapper as the date the product may be expected to retain potency not less than or not to acquire toxicity greater than required or permitted. The minimum potency required for a medicine is specified in the *pharmacopoeia* or other standard books. Rule 96 (*Manner of Labelling*) explains that the date of expiry is to be mentioned in terms of month and year which means medicine is recommended till the last day of the month. According to latest amendment, unsold medicines will be cleared out of pharmacies within 15 days of their date of expiry and drug inspectors will be empowered to cancel trade licences of erring pharmacies.

European Union

European Union has passed new legislation in 2005 for the compliance of the GMP in the drug preparations in accordance with ICH Q7 guidelines. The important regulations in the EU are amended as EU medicine legislation- Directive 2004/27/EC (2001/83/EC as amended) and have been transported into law in each of the member state and the United Kingdom. The manufacturer is responsible for demonstrating that the drug is safe for its intended use. Regulations are enforced at the national level, and each country in the EU has an authoritative body that is responsible for upholding compliance. The European medicine agency has given the guidance notes on the start of shelf-life of the finished product (CPMP/QWP/072/96/EMEA/CVMP/453/01) and the *Committees for Mutual Recognition and Decentralised Procedures* and *Quality Review of Documents product* information templates. According to the guidelines, the expiry date should be calculated from the date of release.

USA

In the US, drugs and cosmetics are regulated by Federal Food, Drug and Cosmetic Act. It is the role of the FDA to oversee the compliance with these regulations. The drugs require verifiable, mandatory compliance (such as FDA approval) before marketing. Under - *Current Good Manufacturing Practice for Finished Pharmaceuticals,* FDA has established requirements concerning the expiration date on a drug product as well as stability testing to assure the appropriateness of that date. Since each of the pharmaceutical products is unique, therefore, it is difficult to prepare single set of rules for all the products.

According to the CGMPs, the absence of an expiration date on any drug product packaged after September 29, 1979, except for those drugs specifically exempt by 211.137 (e), (f), and (g), is cause to initiate regulatory action against the product and/or the responsible firm.

OTC drug products meeting the exemption of 211.137 (g) may utilize accelerated testing programs to support the requirement that they are stable for at least three years. Information obtained from old stock, not previously the subject of stability studies, may also be utilized.

Any drug product intended for reconstitution and not bearing an expiration date for the unreconstituted product and another expiration date for the product after reconstitution is considered to be out of compliance with 211.137 (c). There must be separate stability studies to support each expiration date.

Table 17.2 Regulatory requirements on expired drugs in india, EU and USA

Contents	India	EU	USA
Authority	CDSCO	EMEA	FDA
Rules & Regulations	Drugs and Cosmetic Act	Article 11 of Directive 2001/83/EC	Food, drug and cosmetic act
Expiry date	Indicated as month, year	Indicated as month and year	Indicated as month and year

Expiry Dates for the Herbal Medicines

Herbal compounds are known to have a good effect on various diseases but usually their active compounds are unknown. For example, echinacea is effective for preventing or treating colds. However, its active ingredients have not been identified and isolated. Capsules of echinacea usually contain pieces of the root or rhizome. Since, the amount of active ingredient in each capsule cannot be verified, so is its stability over time. So, for herbal products without standardized active ingredients, any expiry date is going to be arbitrary – unrelated to product quality or safety. FDA does not require expiry dates to be placed on dietary supplements. In contrast to the FDA, Health Canada requires an expiry date to be assigned for herbal products. The EU regulations are strict and herbal products are treated as the drugs and expiry dates are to be assigned for the herbal products. India is the hub for the alternative therapies and herbal compounds are regulated under the Drugs and Cosmetic act, 1940.

Disposal of Expired Drugs

Use of expired drugs is hardy encouraged, but paradoxically there are several studies suggesting that drugs are equally safe and efficacious even after expiry date. There are certain grounds upon which we can say that we need to dispose off the expired drugs cautiously. Such reasons are mentioned as below:

1. *Social concern:* Improper disposal of expired drugs pose a risk of accidental exposure to children and intentional exposure in persons adopting drug abuse or self medication. In USA, out of improper medicine use reported to Poison Control Centers, almost 9% of the reports have described the use of drugs by the persons for whom drug was not prescribed, as a cause of occurrence of such reports. Alarmingly, involvement of 21% of the reports having accidental exposure was belonging to children 6 years and younger.

2. *Environmental concern:* Drug has a direct or indirect impact over the environment. Improper disposal of unused drugs contribute more towards the environmental hazards. Drugs consumed by humans or animals passes out either as metabolites or unchanged through excretory system and find their way into the sewage. Further, drugs disposed improperly also contaminate the environment. Even though water treatment plants are set in place to remove contaminants from water, but some drugs are not entirely removed by treatment process leaving their traces to recycle into human beings or animals. Cocaine, oral contraceptives, carbamazepine, and iodine contrast media are some of the examples. Cocaine has been detected in Po River in Italy. In Niagara River antidepressant drugs, carbamazepine and other antileptics, and lipid-regulating agents (statins) were detected.

   Seeing the gravity of this issue, a newer science called as "Ecopharmacovigilance" has emerged out which can be defined as science and activities concerning detection, assessment, understanding, and prevention of adverse effects or other problems related to the presence of pharmaceuticals in the environment, which affect human and other animal species.

3. *Economic impact:* Expired drugs signal wastage of resources in healthcare system where their beneficial potential could not be fully exploited. There are several

factors contributing towards the medicine leftover till their expiry date which are as following:

- Change in health status of the patient.
- Change in prescription of the patient.
- Over dispensing of the medicine due to large packaging.
- Non compliance of the patient.

Methods of Disposal of Expired Drugs

Though there cannot be any method of disposal of drugs universally applicable under all circumstances. Different regulatory agencies and scientific societies across the world have conflicting views on the methods and need of disposal of expired drugs. For consumers, federal guidelines issued by White House Office of National Drug Control Policy, recommends the steps of disposal process as depicted in figure below:

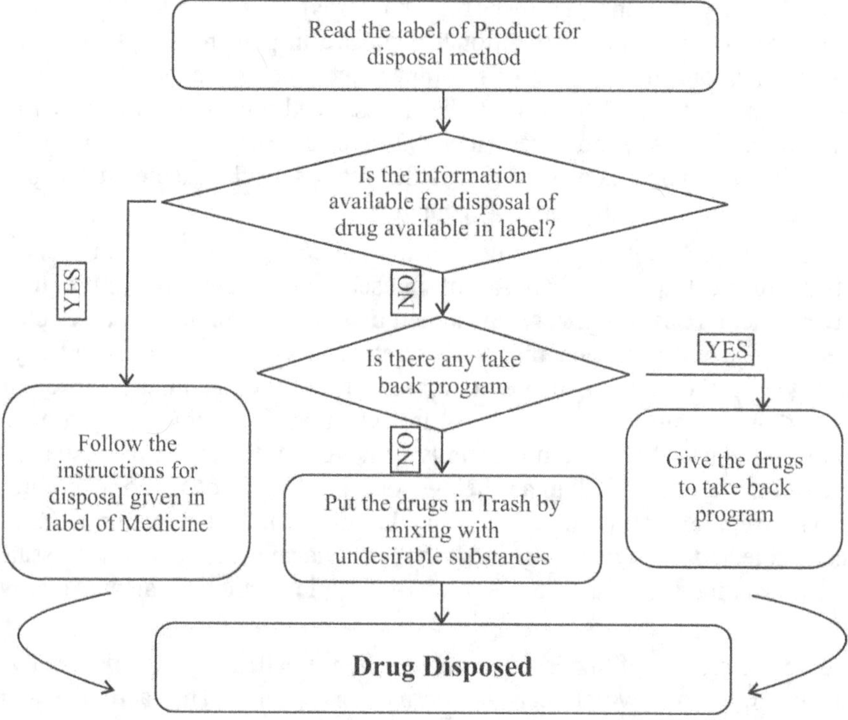

Foremost of the steps to be considered while disposing off the expired drug is to follow the instructions provided in label of the product. Instructions given in the label should never be overruled. For example, inhalers carry the information that they should be kept away from fire or incinerator and should not punctured, if this information is ignored and expired inhaler is thrown in a thrash to be incinerated, it may lead to an explosive incidence.

In case of lack of information on label, one should look for community take back programs for recycling of the drug. Drug Enforcement Administration (DEA) in collaboration with state and local law enforcement agencies, organizes National Prescription Drug Take Back Days throughout the United States of America to promote the culture of safe disposal.

In absence of both the above described options, the drugs may be disposed off through household trash but after making them not usable. To make them not usable, the drugs should be taken out of the packing and mixed with undesirable substances such as used coffee grounds or kitty litter. Such method may render the drugs non consumable and thus prevent accidental exposure to children and animals and intentional exposure in terms of drug abuse. Accidental exposure of some drugs like opioids has claimed many deaths in children.

Pharmacy, pharmaceutical companies, regulatory and health agencies also bear a responsibility for final disposal of the expired drugs or pharmaceutical wastes. If the community returns the drugs to the manufacturer or pharmacy then expert from manufacturing firm or pharmacy execute the process of disposal of drugs. Drug can be disposed off by using any of the following method

Landfill: This is the commonly practiced method of waste disposal since long back even for domestic wastes. This method seeks more stringent and scientific inclination while using it for drug disposal keeping in mind those drugs may serve as bane if not handled with care. Landfills range from conventional open uncontrolled dump to the novel engineered landfills of modern times. Types of landfills are depicted in the Fig. 17.1.

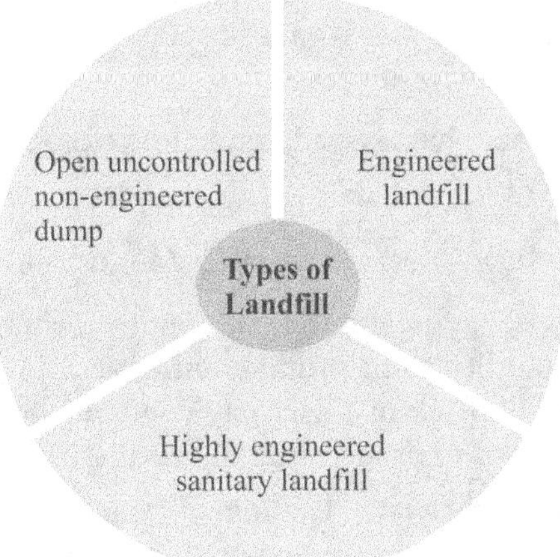

Fig. 17.1 Types of landfills.

Flushing in the Sewage

Disposing off the expired and unused drugs through flushing down in the sewerage has been a popular method because of its low cost and easiness to check the unintended use of the drugs. Liquid formulations are believed the most appropriate to be disposed through this method. But, environmental issues are raised by the environmental protection agencies throughout the world that discourage the practice of flushing the drug. Drug disposed through this method become a component of water resources and all drugs are not even removed from the water through water treatment plants, thus putting the population on risk of unintended exposure to the drug. Antineoplastic agents strictly should not be disposed through flushing as it may kill the aquatic flora.

Thermal Treatment

Drugs like antineoplastic agents or in the liquid formulations are subjected to medium and high temperature incinerations. Burning of drugs at low temperature in open is not recommended as it causes air pollution with toxic. At high temperature incineration is preferred which is done at a temperature ranging from 1400 to 2000 °C. But, under some emergency conditions, expired drugs are treated using a two-chamber incinerator at a minimum temperature of 850 °C, with a combustion retention time of at least two seconds in the second chamber.

Chemical Decomposition

If an appropriate incinerator is not available, then chemical decomposition can be used in accordance with the manufacturer's recommendations, followed by landfill. This method demands the chemical expertise for the process. Chemical inactivation is tedious and time consuming, and stocks of the chemicals used in treatment must be made available at all times. This method may be suitable only when small quantity of antineoplastic drugs is to be disposed off but for large quantities of antineoplastics, chemical decomposition is not practically recommended method of disposal.

World Health Organization has issued guidelines for Safe Disposal of Unwanted Pharmaceuticals in and after Emergencies.

Consequences of Improper Disposal or Non-Disposal

Improper disposal may pose a great threat to public health and environment if not disposed off properly. It may leak out in the environment to become part of chain. For example, drugs disposed in the sink or flush may contaminate the water resources. Some examples of possible hazards of improper drug disposal are summarized under.

1. Contamination of drinking water leading to unnecessary exposure of the drug to animals or human beings. Drug resistance of antimicrobial drugs may occur if the drugs at a very low concentration are being consumed by people through water resources.

2. Accidental exposures in children leading to their morbidity or mortality as several reports claim the deaths of children due to fentanyl transdermal patch consumption by the children. Transdermal patch contains the leftover drug even after the use of it.

3. Landfills where the drugs are disposed in trash may expose the animals or scavengers to the drug. Soil may also get contaminated with the drugs which again become a part of ecosystem.

4. Antibiotics, especially non-biodegradable, disinfectants and antineoplastic agents disposed into the sewage system may kill bacteria necessary for the treatment of sewage.

5. Antineoplastic agents flushed into watercourses may damage aquatic life or contaminate drinking water.

6. Burning drugs at low temperatures or in open containers results in air pollution with toxicants.

7. Improper disposal may allow expired drugs to be available for resale to the public.

Conclusive Remarks

Like, every other things drugs also have a life beyond which they are declared expired. Safety and efficacy past their expiry date has been a matter of conflicts. There's no single rule for expired drugs and supplements, owing to the variety of products, regulatory requirements, and other factors that can influence a safety and efficacy of the drug. There is no unanimous view over the safety or efficacy of expired drugs and also over the regulations pertaining to them. Further, the safe disposal of expired drugs put another challenge before us as improper disposal of drugs have impact on both environment and human beings apart from posing a threat of accidental exposure in animals and children. Therefore, there is a need of framing stringent regulations on use and disposal of expired drugs across the globe.

Suggested Readings

1. Bajaj S, Singla D, Sakhuja N (2012). Stability Testing of Pharmaceutical Products. *Journal of Applied Pharmaceutical Science.* **2(3):** 129-38.

2. Best practice guidance on the labelling and packaging of medicines. [Internet]2003 Jun[Cited on 2014 Jan 18] Available from http://www.mhra.gov.uk/home/groups/commsic/documents/publication/con007554.pdf

3. Bronstein AC, Spyker DA, Cantilena LR, *et al.,* (2009). 2008 Annual Report of the American Association of Poison Control Centers' National Poison Data System (NPDS): 26th Annual Report. *Clin Tox.* **47(10):** 911-1084.

4. Cohen, Laurie P (2000). Many Medicines Prove Potent for Years Past Their Expiration Dates. *Wall Street Journal.* **235(62):** pp.A1.

5. Government of India. Ministry of Health and Family Welfare. The Drugs and Cosmetic Act 1940 and the Rules 1945; Amended up to the 30 June, 2005. India.

6. ICH Guideline Q1A (R2). Stability Testing of New Drug Substances and Products, International Conference on Harmonization of Technical Requirements for Registration of Pharmaceuticals for Human Use. 2005.

7. Status of EMEA scientific guidelines and European pharmacopoeia monographs and chapters in the regulatory framework applicable to medicinal products [Internet] Availablefrom:http://www.ema.europa.eu/docs/en_GB/document_library/Scientific_ guideline/2009/10/WC500004008.pdf

8. United States of America. USFDA. Safe Disposal of Medicines. Disposal of Unused Medicines: What You Should Know; 2013.

CHAPTER 18

DRUG LAG

Introduction

A drug lag is any delay in drug availability in a particular region which could forestall the patients in that region from receiving certain treatment whereas the patients in another part of the world getting the benefit of the new treatment. There are two isoforms of drug lag exists, the first one is relative drug lag which is the delay in time between a drug being introduced in one country to another and the second is the absolute drug lag which is a measure of the quantity of drugs available in different countries. Drug development is an imperceptible process which involves various stages of scientific and objective evaluations. Preclinical trials are conducted to assess efficacy, toxicity and mechanism of action (MOA) of the drug followed by clinical trials involving human subjects in which the recommended administration dose and schedule is determined in order to establish the efficacy and safety evidences of the new agent as compared with the conventional one. A New Drug Application (NDA) is applied by the company after completion of trial in the regulatory unit for review. After the positive evaluation by the administrative authority, the approval is granted to the drug to be sold in that country. However, each country has its own laws and regulatory controls that govern pharmaceutical affairs for NDA in that region. The time needed for approval of an NDA depends on administrative authority of the country which ultimately leads to drug lag.

Historical Background

In 1972, Wardell for the first time mentioned the existence of a drug lag in his study in which he compared the time for introduction of new drugs in the United States (US) and the United Kingdom (UK). He reported a significant delay in the introduction of new drugs in the US and the lag was up to 7 years in five major therapeutic categories. It was finally concluded that the policies for approving new drugs were more relaxed in UK and more systematic program of post-marketing surveillance was there in UK when compared with US policies.

Predominantly, the drug lag in US was noticed after the thalidomide tragedy which hit the world in 1962. A sedative accustomed to prevent miscarriage, caused the birth of many thousands of malformed babies in Europe. In 1962, under the coercion of world picture shown against the drug, the congress finally passed an amendment according to which US FDA (Food & Drug administration) apart from dealing with the safety also would evaluate the efficacy of the drug. These added guidelines to FDA leads to significant drug lags. It was observed that mean drugs introduced were reduced to 16 per year in 10 years after the amendment get passed. It became difficult for manufacturing firms to introduce new drugs against the existing ones, so reducing competition within the trade also.

The drug lag issue get more augmented with the rise of the AIDS (Acquired Immuno Deficiency Syndrome) epidemic. It was estimated that only 46 new drugs approved by the US in 1985 and 1986 and found that 72 percent were available on average 5.5 years earlier in foreign markets which marked the slow pace of FDA with which it was approving drugs. Finally, the government responded positively and numerous of new reforms get introduced to combat the situation in US, specifically "fast track" approval of the AIDS drug AZT (Azidothymidine). The drug was found to be effective against the HIV (Human Immunodeficiency Virus) and found to save many lives. At last the drug got the approval within 2 years and made available for the patients. Different reforms enable patient's access to promising experimental medications. The drug lag issue get more worsened when the patients had to suffer or even die due to unavailability of the medications which were however available in other part of the globe. The issue came under the limelight when beta blockers, class of drug used for the management of cardiac arrhythmias were available in Europe in 1967 but not in US until 1976 as FDA concern with the long term effects of the drug.

Earlier there was a variation in drug lag among various European countries, but in 1995 European Medicines Agency (EMA) was established. Currently, the EMA presides common administrative body for all European member states which also prevent duplication of marketing authorization application review throughout EU (European Union) and also improved transparency for regulatory requirements and resulted in declining drug lag. Drug delay also rooted long in Japan where new drugs being granted Marketing Authorization Approval (MAA) several years after availability in Western countries. Further, the local clinical development (LCD) delays drug introduction in Japan. The drug lag also has a history in India. Earlier, India was less commercially appealing to the foreign companies due to its lack of Gross Domestic Product (GDP) and the submission lag was much longer. The submission lag rapidly decreased from 3885 days in the 1980s to 230 days in the 1990s demonstrating a positive relationship between rapid country GDP growth and a reduction in submission lag.

Determinants of Drug Lag

After the Thalidomide tragedy, the drug lag term was come forth for the first time but there are some other barriers which determines drug lag. The key determinants of drug lag in different countries which should be overcome in order to reduce drug lag in near future have been described here;

1. **Certificate of Pharmaceutical Product (CPP):** The only cause of bringing CPP into existence by the World Health Organization (WHO) was to ascertain the Good Manufacturing Practice (GMP) and quality status of the drug product. A drug only gets CPP when the authority grants approval to the drug in a country. The product complete information and regulatory status is embraced in the product's CPP. The time taken to issue a CPP varies between authorities but may take from 2 weeks up to 9 months. Furthermore, regulatory authorities sometimes require more than one CPP or that a CPP is issued with a marketed statement, which add further to drug lag, because despite a drug being approved, the company has to wait for product launch in the issuing market before it can request a CPP and thus submit for MAA review. The authorities should accept a single CPP from recognized, competent agencies as long as the GMP status of the manufacturing site is included.

2. **Lack of Harmonization:** It is apparent that a lack of harmonization among different countries can lead to duplication, more efforts and waste of resources which further leads to drug lag. The first harmonization which was established was the Association of South East Asian Nations (ASEAN) in 1967. The GMP harmonization will help to improve pharmaceutical trade between ASEAN member states by removing impeding barriers. The EU has seen a large reduction in drug lag, not just due to the establishment of the EMA but due to there being clear expectations of the agency and set approval timelines. The EMA has to commit to meet its 200 day approval timeline and it is upon this commitment which the agency is assessed. Both the EMA and ASEAN initiatives have been established for many years now and based upon the progress seen recently in the developing countries, it would be possible to suggest further harmonization for them as it is clear that harmonization is highly effective in reducing drug lag.

3. **Local Clinical Development (LCD) in Phase 3 clinical trial:** Phase 3 clinical trial which is conducted in India, China, Mexico and Vietnam comprises of LCD. Different ethnicities have different metabolisms which can sometimes mean variations in the actions of drugs on patients. Some countries have thus decided to implement LCD in order to protect their populations. To execute LCD is a burdensome and delay the introduction of new drugs in the market as an Investigational New Drug (IND) application has to be approved as a consequence of positive results followed by submission of a NDA in that country and a full

MAA review can then be undertaken. It has been observed that LCD when carried out in sequence with GCD (global clinical development) leads to delay in drug introduction so it is always suggested to carry both LCD and GCD in parallel. With the time LCD is losing its relevancy because of the introduction of GCD and only cause drug lag.

4. **Conventional guidelines:** The administrative units of some countries follow the same conventional guidelines for drug introduction which were made several decades ago. After 1962 amendment in US-FDA, a significant drug lag had been seen in US market but due to fast track and other priorities reform were introduced which help to overcome drug lag in US. In countries like India, the conservational guidelines are being followed which need strict reassessment and new priorities reforms should be introduced to lessen drug lag.

5. **GMP (Good Manufacturing Practice) & other approvals:** Most CPPs do not require separate GMP certificate as it is present in CPP's statement but authorities request for a separate GMP certificate which is an unnecessary duplication and waste of resources and delays in drug introduction. Further, pricing is also a very important aspect to be discussed. In actual, it is a certificate of agreement which decides the price of the drug in the market after MAA approval. The review and approval process for pricing is sometimes integrated into that of the MAA review, delaying the latter further.

6. **Additional testing:** In order to submit an MAA in the developing countries or the emerging markets, companies usually have to wait for an established regulatory authority such as the FDA or EMA to grant approval of that drug before applying approval in countries like in BRIC (Brazil, Russia, India, China) as additional testing is required that these countries have in order to comply with their local guidelines which finally leads to delay in drug introduction in these countries.

Analogy of Drug Lag

For the reason to understand the drug lag among the countries, 2 developed economies i.e., US and EU will be compared with the emerging one i.e., India, in terms of drug lag. US and EU are the developed market as most of the drugs are introduced there first nowadays. India has chosen as a representative emerging market due to the local presence of a large number of generic manufacturers and intellectual property rights. Drugs taken here for understanding the phenomenon of drug lag belongs to four major therapeutics categories i.e., Cardiovascular, Nervous system, anti-neoplastic and anti-microbial.

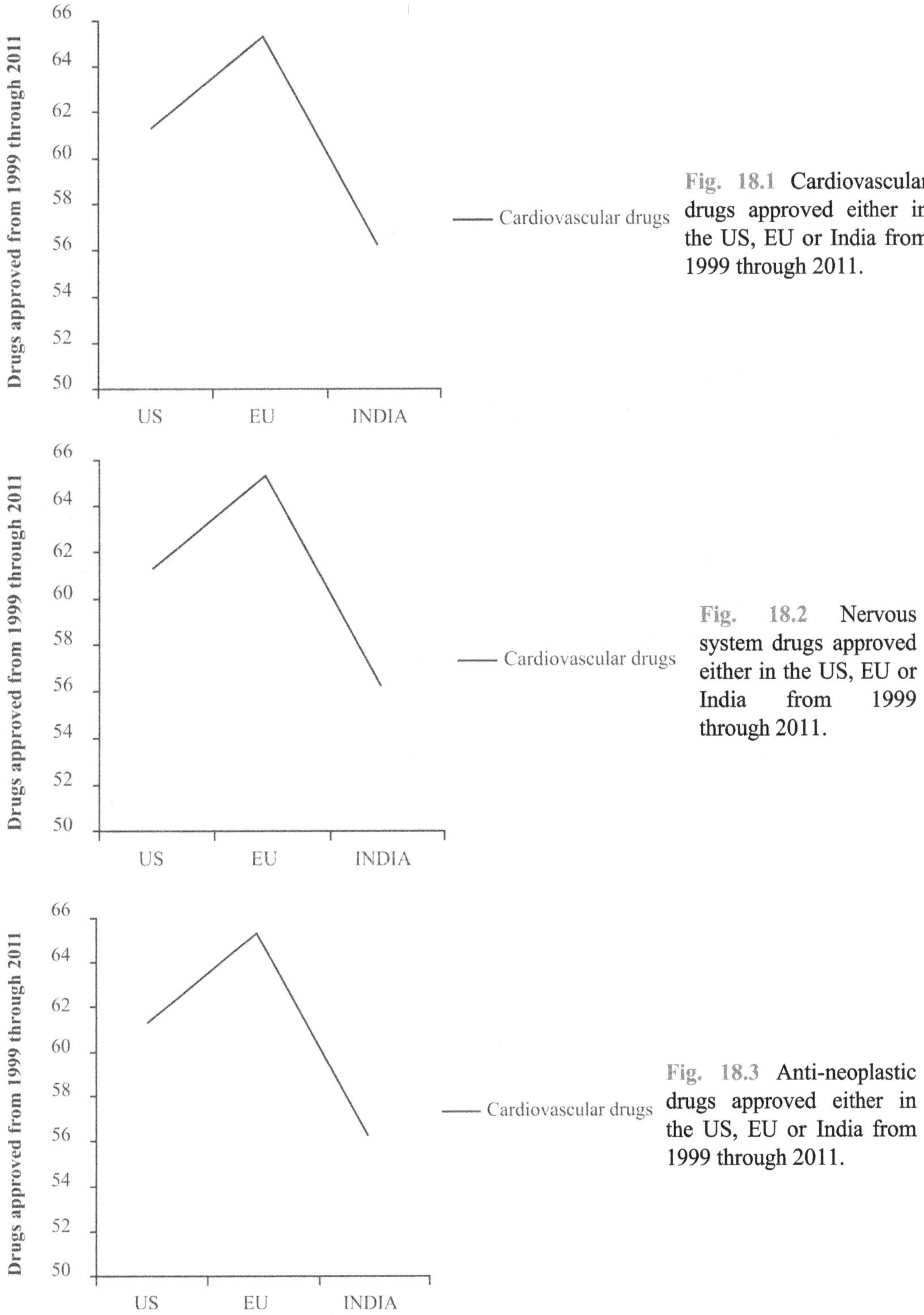

Fig. 18.1 Cardiovascular drugs approved either in the US, EU or India from 1999 through 2011.

Fig. 18.2 Nervous system drugs approved either in the US, EU or India from 1999 through 2011.

Fig. 18.3 Anti-neoplastic drugs approved either in the US, EU or India from 1999 through 2011.

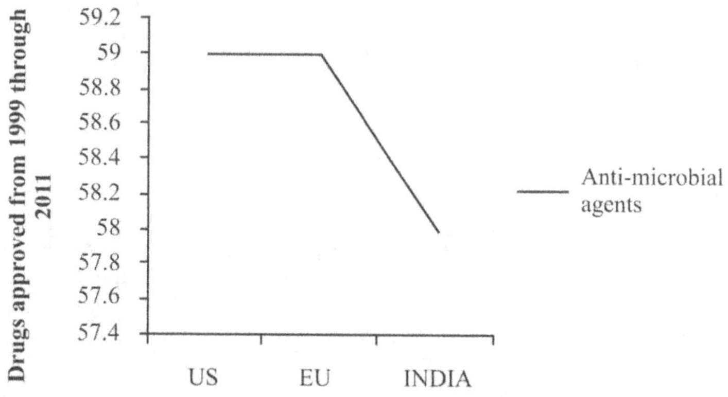

Fig. 18.4 Anti-microbial drugs approved either in the US, EU or India from 1999 through 2011.

Drugs approved in the four major therapeutic areas in three important regions of the world i.e., US, EU and India from 1999 through 2011 varies considerably. The absolute drug lags for the three regions US, EU and India have been shown in Figure 18.1-18.4; briefly, out of the 75 new cardiovascular drugs, 61 (81.33%) were approved in the US, 65 (86.66%) in the EU and 56 (74.66%) in India. About 70 new antimicrobial agents that were approved, 59 (84.28%) approved in the US, 59 (84.28%) in the EU and 58 (82.85%) in India. Of the 70 new antineoplastic agents, 64 (91.42%) were approved in the US, 54 (77.14%) in the EU and 44 (62.85%) in India. And of the 97 new nervous system drugs, 72 (74.22%) were approved in the US, 76 (78.35%) in the EU and 75 (77.31%) in India. India lags behind in comparison to the US and EU regions in terms of absolute drug lag in antineoplastic drugs and cardiovascular drugs but no significant difference was seen in case of antimicrobial agents and drugs for nervous system.

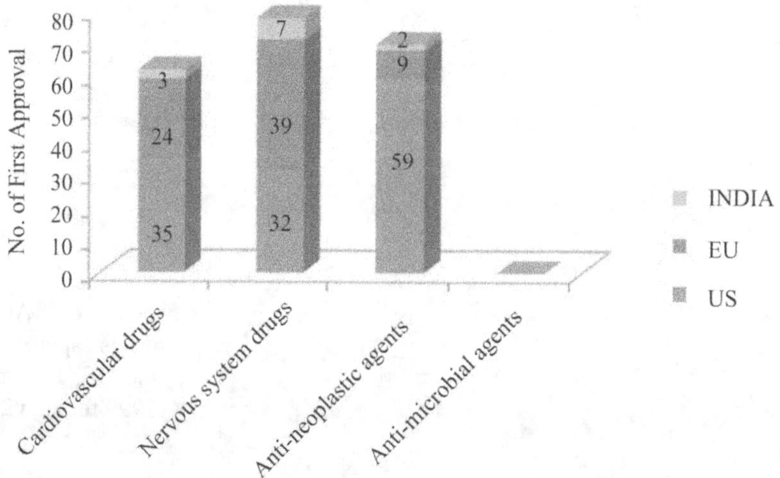

Fig. 18.5 First approval of drugs in US, EU and India (1999-2011).

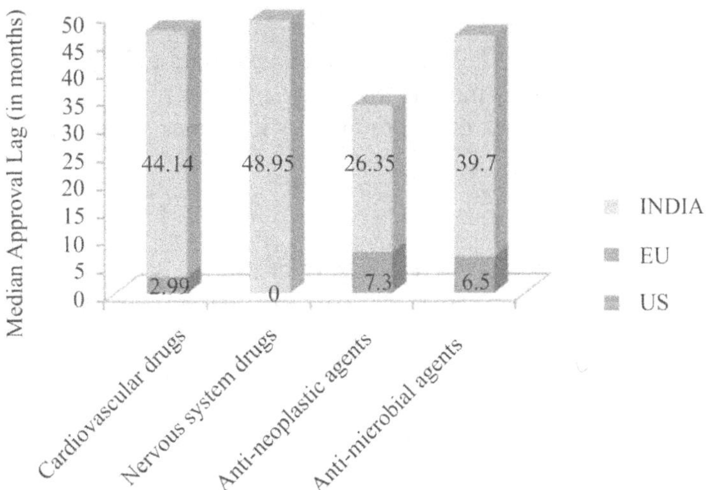

Fig. 18.6 Median approval lag in US, EU and India (1999-2011).

The relative drug lags for the US, EU and India has been shown in Fig. 18.5 and in Fig. 18.6. The US was the first to approve the majority of the new cardiovascular, nervous system, anti-neoplastic and anti-microbial drugs and the EU was slightly delayed. But, the substantial delay was observed for India in approval of new drugs in these categories. The median approval lag for India was 44.14, 48.95, 26.35 and 39.7 months respectively for cardiovascular, nervous system, anti-neoplastic and anti-microbial drugs than that for the US and even more than EU. US was first to approve majority of the new drugs in these categories, the relative drug lag for EU was not so high. Therefore, it may be assumed that the drug lag within the EU was merely a small delay in approval, which can be attributed to a delay within the start of development and may be a rather longer review period. But in comparison with the US and EU, a striking relative drug lag was observed for approval of new drugs in India. Delay in the start of development, delay in the progress of development and delay in review by the regulatory authority could be possible reasons behind these delays in approval of these drugs in India.

Pharmaceutical companies find risk to conduct registration trials in India simultaneously with US or any other developed market which can be one the cause of drug delay in India. Further, delay in commencement of drug development leads to delay in introduction of new drugs in India. As per World Trade Organization (WTO), from the year 2005, India granted product patent recognition to all new chemical entities (NCEs). But, before 2005, the relaxed patent law in India made foreign based companies to take risk if they would launch their patented drugs in Indian markets simultaneously with US or Europe. So, these foreign based companies do not take interest to take such a risk which further increased the delay of introduction of drugs in Indian market. The majority of huge international pharmaceutical firms have presence in India and that they might attempt to introduce their new product in India, at the same time with different markets. Now, due to product patent in India, the Indian pharmaceutical firms can't introduce patented medicine developed by the foreign international companies. With the introduction of product patents, Indian firms can shift the realm of focus from method development to developing new drug product so it further delay introduction of new drugs.

Conclusion

Developed regions which once had very lengthy drug lags, specifically the US and EU, have seen dramatic improvements over time due to the evolvement of their regulatory environments. As it is well known that drug development is being performed in the US and the EU concurrently, and the integrated data package may be used for NDAs in the US and the EU. Thus, there is a minimal time gap in new drug approvals between the US and the EU. And even the emerging markets like India in terms of its GDP has shown a significant reduction in the relative drug lag from 1960s and 2000s. Drug development is turning progressively globalized and to conduct the clinical trials in India is comparatively economical as compared to developed markets. However, there is a need to improve the regulatory processes in India to enhance the clinical trial and new drug approvals. The Indian regulatory authority has to take serious actions to minimize drug lag. Pharmaceutical companies should make an effort to enrol patients in international registration trials. More review staff should be hiring to fasten the approval process, and drug application requirements should be softened to make it easier for pharmaceutical companies to apply in India. By further reviewing the markets, it would be easier to target the areas where the specific regulatory barriers can be ameliorated.

Suggested Readings

1. Andersson F (1992). The drug lag issue: the debate seen from an international perspective. *International Journal of Health Services.* **22(1):** 53-72.

2. Hashimoto J, Ueda E, Narukawa M (2009). The current situation of oncology drug lag in Japan and strategic approaches for pharmaceutical companies. *Drug Information Journal.* **43(6):** 757-65.

3. Kataria BC, Mehta DS, Chhaiya SB (2012). Approval of antineoplastic agents in India: comparison with the US and EU regions. *International Journal of Basic & Clinical Pharmacology.* **1(1):** 13-21.

4. Kataria BC, Mehta DS, Chhaiya SB (2012). Drug lag for cardiovascular drug approvals in India compared with the US and EU approvals. *Indian heart journal.* **65(1):** 24-9.

5. Kataria BC, mehta DS, chhaiya SB. Approval of new nervous system drugs in India compared with the US and EU.

6. Kataria BC, Mehta DS, Mehta SJ (2012). Drug Lag for Antimicrobial Agents: Comparison of the US, EU and India Approvals. *National Journal of Medical Research.* **2(3):** 264-8.

7. Report of the working group on drugs and pharmaceuticals for the eleventh five-year plan (2007-2012), Planning commission of India. 2012.

8. Wardell W, Lasagna L, editors (1972). The "drug lag" and American therapeutics: An international comparison. Read before the Fifth International Congress of Pharmacology, San Francisco.

9. Wardell WM (1973). Introduction of new therapeutic drugs in the United States and Great Britain: an international comparison. *Clinical Pharmacology and Therapeutics.* **14(5):** 773.

10. Wardell WM (1974). Therapeutic implications of the drug lag. *Clinical Pharmacology and Therapeutics.* **15(1):** 73.

11. Wardell WM (1978). A Close Inspection of the Calm Look. *JAMA: The Journal of the American Medical Association.* **239(19):** 2004-11.

12. Wardell WM (1978). The drug lag revisited: comparison by therapeutic area of patterns of drugs marketed in the United States and Great Britain from 1972 through 1976. *Clinical Pharmacology and Therapeutics.* **24(5):** 499.

13. Wileman H, Mishra A (2010). Drug lag and key regulatory barriers in the emerging markets. *Perspectives in clinical research.* **1(2):** 51.

14. Yonemori K, Hirakawa A, Ando M, Hirata T, Yunokawa M, Shimizu C, *et al.,* (2011). The notorious "drug lag" for oncology drugs in Japan. *Investigational new drugs.* **29(4):** 706-12.

CHAPTER 19

DRUG POLICY-DIFFERENT STATES IN INDIA

Introduction

India is a vast country with a complex and diverse social, cultural, economic and political fabric. Health remains primarily a state subject. Although, health policy and drug policy are formulated and revised periodically by the Government of India (GoI), the major responsibility of their implementation lies with the state governments.

Within a few decades since independence India became self-sufficient in catering to the drug needs of its people and transformed itself from one of the highest priced nations to one with remarkably low drug prices. However, the contemporary challenges like economic liberalization and industrial policy reform (1991), globalization and decontrol measures and above all, the WTO agreement obligations, tend to make the matter of equitable access to essential medicines more elusive.

It has, therefore, become relevant that at all micro-levels, efforts are made to optimize people's access to medicines. Even within the confines of the national Pharmaceutical policy of India (2002), the state government with strong political commitment should strive for the same. Quite a good number of States in India namely Delhi, Himachal Pradesh, Madhya Pradesh, Karnataka, Orissa etc. have already formulated their drug policy.

Contemporary international drug policy seeks to control both the demand and supply of drugs through the criminalization of production, trafficking and use. Furthermore, adherence to the United Nations drug control conventions ensures that most nation states adopt a similar prohibition-oriented approach when formulating national drug control legislation. Recent research suggests that this can be problematic in some Asian countries where long standing cultural sanctions already existed for drug use; particularly those involving psychoactive plant products such as cannabis and opium.

With its focus on India, this chapter examines the impact of the punitive approach towards drugs in those societies and communities that have traditionally exerted socio-cultural controls over the use of mind-altering substances. The discussion highlights the unintentional but often harmful consequences of such drug control policies.

In framing, the discussion of this topic, it is important to note that the socio-cultural context of traditional drug use within many Asian countries means that experiencing an altered state of consciousness is only a part of the drug taking experience and not the ultimate goal of users. Indeed, norms controlling excessive and regular drug use have customarily governed socially and culturally accepted consumption of native mind-altering substances.

While such traditional use management strategies vary across Asian countries, it is possible to identify similarities that exist between these approaches to drug use and contemporary interventions that collectively fall within the so-called harm reduction paradigm. The defining feature of harm reduction program is their focus on the prevention of *harm* rather than the prevention of drug use itself. It can be argued, therefore, that as signatories to the 1961; UN Single Convention on Narcotic Drugs, many Asian countries have been required to move away from long standing approaches to control customary drug use. In many respects, there has been a subsequent shift from traditional drug use management to an emphasis one eradicating all drug use and trade. The implementation of law-enforcement-dominated policies has generated a tense relationship between contemporary legislation and culturally ingrained drug use patterns and associated management strategies.

This situation is compounded by changing patterns of drug use within India. This is the result of a number of interrelated factors; the rising popularity of new non-traditional forms of drug use introduced *via* tourism, urbanization and leakage from illicit drug production in the region. Indeed, evidence suggests that changes in policy may have contributed to increases in the use of harder forms of drugs and more harmful modes of consumption, notably drug injecting. Such a change in user behavior is particularly significant given the role played by injecting drug use in the transmission of HIV/AIDS and other blood borne infections. The management of this issue has become a cause for concern within the field of drug demand reduction and has serious implications for the development realities of many Asian countries.

Drug Policy of the State of Delhi

A comprehensive statement of the drug policy of the state of Delhi is necessary at this stage in order to provide a strong framework within which the different components would be implemented in the coming years. Such a policy statement would also clearly enunciate the social and economic goals, based on equity and care for the underprivileged, which are sought to be attained through this drugs policy.

The main elements of the policy are the following:

1. All the essential drugs needed for health care should be available at all times at all the health facilities of the state. These drugs should be safe, effective and of good quality.

2. The facilities and manpower needed for providing a good and continuing quality control and assurance system for the drugs being used will be strengthened.

3. The system for procurement, storage and distribution of drugs will be modified to ensure that drugs of good quality, obtained at competitive prices, are always available at the health units.

4. Rational use of drugs will be promoted. Rational use is the use of the most appropriate drug prescribed at the correct dose for the correct length of time. Medicines will be prescribed and ensuring as far as is possible that appropriate drugs only are prescribed.

5. Doctors at all public health facilities will be encouraged to prescribe drugs by their generic names. Procurement of drugs will also be by generic names.

6. There will be a strengthening of the health education programs of the government specially relating to drugs. This would promote rational use of drugs and enhance compliance. There would also be an acceleration of the continuing education programs for doctors and para-professional personnel in the field of drugs. This would include establishment of Drug Information Centre and development of links with non-governmental organization.

7. Research on all aspects of use of drugs will be an integral part of the drug policy in the state so that these results would be continuously utilized to modify the different components of the program for the benefit of the people. It is important, for example, to collect information as to what is happening at this time. A survey will be carried out by the best available professional consultancies available to understand the strengths and weaknesses of the present system. As each new mechanism will be introduced studies will be initiated to document the impact of such interventions.

It is important to emphasize that all these seven components of the drug policy for the state need to be implemented if the results are to be effective and make an impact:

1. Availability of safe and effective drugs

2. A good quality control and assurance system

3. Improved procurement, storage and distribution system

4. Rational prescribing of medicines

5. Prescribing by generic names

6. Strengthening of health education programs

7. Research on all aspects of drugs

It is the objective of the policy that a limited list of carefully selected drugs will always be available at all health centres and hospitals of the state. These medicines would be procured at reasonable prices, thus enabling the drug budget to be used for a much large number of persons than is now available. These drugs would be of good quality and there would be a good are being take, are of good quality, safe and effective. The prescribing of the drugs would be based on rational pharmacological and therapeutic knowledge and the patients would also be aware of the medicines they are getting and thereby actually take the medicines in the way they should be taken. Information about these essential medicines would also be available to the doctors and paraprofessional staff, wherever justified additional complementary medicine not on the essential list of drug would be provided through a mechanism established for this purpose. Each hospital, if it so desires could order drugs not on the common list of essential drugs but not more than 10% of the budget spent on drugs.

Drug Policy of the State of Jammu and Kashmir

Key Features of Drug Policy

Selection of Essential Drugs

1. The core concept of selection of essential medicines is that use of a limited number of carefully selected medicines based on Standard Treatment Protocols which lead to a getter supply of drugs, rational prescribing, reduction in costs and finally to better health outcomes.

2. Selection of Essential Drugs List has been proposed to be entrusted to an Expert Committee known as State Drug Committee which will comprise Clinicians, Microbiologists, qualified Pharmacists and independent experts besides senior functionaries of the departments like HODs. For Indian System Medicine, separate Committee has been proposed.

3. The EDL (Essential Drug List) would be revised after every two years so as to reflect therapeutic advances and changes in cost, resistance pattern and public health relevance.

4. There are some drugs which though not listed in the EDL are required for specific diseases/exceptional cases. Keeping this in view, a Complementary Drug List (CDL) would be drawn up and a provision of grants not exceeding 10% of the allocated budget for procurement of drugs shall be earmarked for purchase of drugs in the complementary drugs list.

5. The quantification of drugs would be done taking into consideration the parameters such as demand, lead time, transportation constraints and emergency needs as also the need to maintain buffer stock, keeping in view the state specific constraints of accessibility to remote areas.

6. Only drugs listed in the EDL shall be procured centrally.

7. There shall be appropriate inventory control system to prevent excessive stocking of individual items and also prevent stock outs.

8. Proper recall and disposal procedures shall be followed as per standard guidelines.

9. The Drug & Food Control Organization would be strengthened through a capacity building process by augmenting infrastructure, manpower and financial resources. The Drug Testing Laboratories would be strengthened by providing equipment, qualified analysts and other requirements as may be consistent with the work load. Approved private sector laboratories would also be involved in the process.

10. Efforts will be made to promote rational use of drugs in the state so that patients receive the medicines appropriate for their clinical needs in doses that meet the individual requirements for adequate period of time. In all the hospitals of the State, Drugs and Therapeutic Committees would be established.

11. The concept of essential drugs, rational drug use and generic prescribing shall be an integral part of basic and in-service training of health professionals. A Drug Information Centre would be established preferably in Government Medical Colleges to provide appropriate drug information.

12. Any advertisements and promotion of drugs will be required to provide complete drug information.

13. Pharmacovigilance centres would be established to monitor and document adverse drug reactions and events.

14. Operational research would be used to facilitate implementation, monitoring and evaluation of different aspects of drug policy. Monitoring and evaluation would take place at regular intervals and a complete external evaluation would be conducted after every five years. A mechanism for redressal of public grievances would also be developed and made effective.

15. Approved private sector laboratories under overall supervision of the State Government shall also be involved to ensure the quality of drugs in the state. Annual testing load and average testing time of existing Drug Testing Laboratories shall be fixed for proper accountability.

16. Sale, storage, use of drugs and record keeping specified under Schedule X of the Drugs and Cosmetics Act, 1940 shall be supervised and monitored effectively by the inspectorate working under Drug and Food Control Organization, J&K. Special checking squads under the leadership of Deputy Controllers will be constituted to undertake periodic inspections in this regard.

17. Schedule 'H' drugs shall be strictly dispensed on the prescription of Registered Medical Practitioners.

18. An Intelligence-cum-Legal Cell shall be established in the office Drug and Food Control Organization, J&K to facilitate busting of spurious drug rackets and their prompt prosecution. Efforts shall be made to provide incentives to informers giving information about spurious drugs. Efforts shall be made to rationalize number of drug licenses.

19. In order to prevent risks of misuse and marketing of drugs by quacks, wherever required, laws would be made and strengthened.

Drug Policy of the State of West Bengal

West Bengal has the oldest and probably the largest public health and government hospital-based health care delivery infrastructure and network. In the immediate pre-independence era (1940), the pharmaceutical industries of Bengal shared more than 80 per cent of the national drug production that has gradually been reduced to less than 8 per cent today (2004).

West Bengal remains one of the few states in India where the government subsidizes a major share of people's health care expenditure through the vast network of government health facilities. West Bengal is probably the pioneer state in India in promulgating the Central Medical Stores (CMS) concept and practicing the pooled procurement system for drug management in government hospitals. A carefully selected list of medicinal items, the so-called CMS catalogue list, much akin to the essential drug list (EDL) of World Health Organization (WHO) is given priority in such procurement. Around 70 percent of the population avail the government health care services and therefore enjoy the access to drugs that constitute an integral part of health care. The health department spends about 7 per cent of the total health budget, on drugs. Yet, people's access to essential medicines has remained far from satisfactory. There is a lot of scope for improvement in the drug management system in government hospitals in West Bengal.

Besides, the government also recognizes its obligation to address the legitimate need of people beyond the purview of government hospitals. The major responsibility of implementation of the National Drug Policy of India (NDP) lies with the state government. The State Drug Control Authority is entrusted with the regulatory mandates of the NDP. Harnessing and integrating the drug control activities in best interest of the people is a priority commitment of Government of West Bengal (GoWB). Yet many other matters relevant to the issue of ensuring people's access to essential medicines warrant appropriate attention. This assumes particular significance in view of the global economic and industrial reform process in general and the post-GATT pharmaceutical patenting regime in particular, along with their obvious impact in India. In order to set a balance between these newer challenges and people's health care and pharmaceutical care needs, the GoWB has decided to formulate its drug policy. This drug policy document will not merely mention the policy statement but also will outline the strategies and mechanisms towards implementation of the policy mandates and commitments.

Aims and Goals of the "State Drug Policy West Bengal"

1. To maximize equitable access to essential medicines by people
2. To promote rational use of medicines
3. To facilitate rational pharmaceutical management in government health facilities
4. To foster growth and sustainability of state level pharmaceutical industries (not sacrificing people's health goals and rights)
5. To ensure compliance of drug legislations/regulations and quality assurance

Drug Policy of the State of Madhya Pradesh

The M.P State Government made attempts from time to time to facilitate availability of drugs continuity of medicines at all Health Centres. For this the State Government made Store Purchase Rules, issued Guidelines as well as circulated guidelines received from the Government of India from time to time. In view of such rules, orders and instructions, medicines used to be purchased at State and District level by competent Authorities. But due to lack of availability and continuity of medicines, these arrangements could not fulfill the needs of common man. With a view, to remove such defects in purchase of medicines, the "Drug policy 2006" was enacted by the department. After implementation of "Drug Policy 2006" because of Centralized Drug Purchase Policy, the rates were minimized from 20 to 25 percentage of the cost of medicines. In the past, where district level officers used to purchase 100 to 125 types of medicines but after the Centralized System more than 350 types of medicines were made available. There was earlier no specified procedure for quality control of medicines at the district level. On the basis of the test report of the supplier used to be accepted as Quality Control Report and there was no specified procedure for testing the supplied drugs. Drug inspectors used to take samples at random and send it to the approved laboratories, the test reports were received too late, by the time the drugs were already consumed. In order to remove all these problems, Centralized Drug Policy 2006 was implemented in which there were 27 warehouses in 27 districts were arranged to keep medicines to meet the requirement of then total 48 districts. But, as there was no transportation facility, therefore, no interest was taken by the District Authorities to take the medicines from the warehouses (Drug stores) and so also to take the ownership of District Drug Store. As a result of this system, same type of medicines was purchased from two places.

As the Drug Policy 2006 was not started with full preparedness so the following problems cropped up during its implementation:

1. The Drug Cell was constituted but the adequate manpower was not made available.

2. The Drug Policy 2006 was started with 27 warehouses and 21 districts did not have the drug warehouses so there were problems of distribution.

3. As the Drug Stores were managed by private institutions so there was lack of effective management in Drug Stores.

4. There was problem of monitoring due to difficulties in running the software purchased and made available to the Drug Warehouses by Madhya Pradesh Laghu Udyog Nigam (MPLUN).

5. More time was consumed than required in finalization of rates of medicines/goods/instruments by MPLUN.

6. There were delays by MPLUN in diversions of the orders given by the Drug Cell.

After seeing the shortcomings of Drug Policy 2006 and problems faced in its implementation, it was decided to go for decentralization again. The meetings were held at various levels with district, division and state level officials and finally it was proposed to go for decentralized drug policy again so that district level procurement could be done as per their requirements, procured items could be inspected for its quality and payments released in time. Keeping this in mind the Drug Policy 2009 was proposed.

Objectives

1. To provide quality drugs and medicines at the right time to all patients in the health institutions in the state.

2. To ensure proper utilization of drugs/goods/equipments in all health institutions of the state.

3. For simplification of procurement procedure for advanced and modern equipments in the medical and health institutions.

Drug Policy of the State of Karnataka

The State has so far followed policy guidelines through the framework of successive five year plans developed by the Planning Commission, decisions of the Central Council of Health and Family welfare, Central health legislation and national health program developed by Central Government. Over a period of time, separate policies at the National level have been developed for Health (1983), which was revised in 2002, Education For Health Sciences (1989), Nutrition (1993), Drug Policy (1986 and 1994), Pharmaceutical Policy 2002, Medical Council of India (MCI) guidelines (1998, 1999 and 2000), Blood Banking have served the state well in developing its health system, and will continue to be used as guidelines for further growth.

A National Health Policy-2002 has been announced and provides a framework within which the Health Policy of the state would refashion the elements therein to meet the current needs of the state. The State Health Policy would be based on the specific needs of the state and recognize regional disparities.

Health, however, is constitutionally a state subject. Health needs, defined socio-epidemiologically, vary between states and even districts, requiring more specific planning. Health expenditure is met largely by the state budget, with 82% of public sector expenditure on health from State Government of Karnataka and 18% from Central Government. A comprehensive Karnataka State Policy for the Integrated Health Development and functioning of the health sector is, therefore, being articulated explicitly, for the first time. The Policy, with a string emphasis on process and implementation, will be an instrument for optimal, people oriented development of health services.

The State Health Policy would be based on the following premises-

- It will build on the existing institutional capacities of the public, voluntary and private health sectors.

- It will pay particular attention to filling up gaps and will move towards greater equity in health and health care, within a reasonable time frame.

- It will use a public health approach, focusing on determinants of health such as food and nutrition, safe-water, sanitation, housing and education.

- It will expand beyond a focus on curative care and further, strengthen the primary health care strategy.

- It will encourage the development of Indian and other systems of medicines.

- It views health as a reasonable expectation of every citizen and will work within a framework of social justice.

More importantly, it is intended to be guiding document that needs to evolve and be changed in response to changing Situations.

International Drug Control Policy

The global illegal drug trade represents a multi-dimensional challenge that has implications for U.S. national interests as well as the international community. Common illegal drugs trafficked internationally include cocaine, heroin, and methamphetamine. According to the US intelligence community, international drug trafficking can undermine political and regional stability and bolster the role and capabilities of organized crime in the drug trade. Key regions of concern include Latin America and Afghanistan, which are focal points in US efforts to combat the production and transit of cocaine and heroin, respectively. Drug use and addiction have the potential to negatively affect the social fabric of communities, hinder economic development, and place an additional burden on national public health infrastructures.

As an issue of international policy concern for more than a century, and as a subject of long standing U.S. and multilateral policy commitment, U.S. counterdrug efforts have expanded to include a broad array of tools to attack the international drug trade. Such approaches include combating the production of drugs at the source, combating the flow of drugs in transit, dismantling international illicit drug networks, and creating incentives for international cooperation on drug control.

Congress is involved in all aspects of US international drug control policy, regularly appropriating funds for counterdrug initiatives, conducting oversight activities on federal counterdrug programs, and legislating changes to agency authorities and other counter drug policies. For FY2012, the Administration has requested from Congress approximately $26.2 billion for all federal drug control programs, of which $2.1 billion is requested for international programs, including civilian and military U.S. foreign assistance. An additional $3.9 billion is requested for interdiction programs related to intercepting and disrupting foreign drug shipments route to the United States.

Through its appropriations and federal oversight responsibilities, the 112th Congress may choose to continue tackling several ongoing policy issues concerning U.S. international drug control policy, including

- The role of the Department of Defense in counterdrug foreign assistance.
- Challenges associated with sequencing alternative development and eradication programs.
- The effectiveness of U.S. efforts to promote international drug control cooperation.
- How to reduce drug trafficking-related violence and other harmful manifestations of the drug trade.

The 112th Congress may also choose to address authorizing legislation for the White House's Office of National Drug Control Policy (ONDCP), which, pursuant to Section 714 of P.L. 105-277, as amended, expired at the end of FY2010. ONDCP's primary purpose is to establish policies, priorities, and objectives for the overall U.S. drug control program, including domestic and international aspects.

Drug Policy for Pharmaceutical Companies

The basic objectives of government's policy relating to the drugs and pharmaceutical sector were enumerated in the Drug Policy of 1986. These basic objectives still remain largely valid. However, the drug and pharmaceutical industry in the country today faces new challenges on account of liberalization of the Indian economy, the globalization of the world economy and on account of new obligations undertaken by India under the WTO Agreements. These challenges require a change in emphasis in the current pharmaceutical policy and the need for new initiatives beyond those enumerated in the Drug Policy 1986, as modified in 1994, so that policy inputs are directed more towards promoting more internationally competitive. The need for radically improving the policy framework for knowledge-based industry has also been acknowledged by the Government. The Prime Minister's Advisory Council on Trade and Industry has made important recommendations regarding knowledge-based industry. The pharmaceutical industry has been identified as one of the most important knowledge-based industries in which India has a comparative advantage.

The main objectives of this policy are:

(a) Ensuring abundant availability at reasonable prices within the country of good quality essential pharmaceuticals of mass consumption.

(b) Strengthening the indigenous capability for cost effective quality production and exports of pharmaceuticals by reducing barriers to trade in the pharmaceutical sector.

(c) Strengthening the system of quality control over drug and pharmaceutical production and distribution to make quality an essential attribute of the Indian pharmaceutical industry and promoting rational use of pharmaceuticals.

(d) Encouraging R&D in the pharmaceutical sector in a manner compatible with the country's needs and with particular focus on diseases endemic or relevant to India by creating an environment conducive to channelizing a higher level of investment into R&D in pharmaceuticals in India.

(e) Creating an incentive framework for the pharmaceutical industry which promotes new investment into pharmaceutical industry and encourages the introduction of new technologies and new drugs.

In order to strengthen the pharmaceutical industry's research and development capabilities and to identify the support required by Indian pharmaceutical companies to undertake domestic R&D, a Committee was set up in 1999 by this Department by the name of Pharmaceutical Research and Development Committee (PRDC) under the Chairmanship of Director General of CSIR.

The recommendations of the PRDC in so far as they relate to the Pharmaceutical Policy have been taken into account while formulating the proposals on pricing aspects. The Pharmaceutical Research & Development committee has recommended in its report, submitted inter-alia, the setting up of a Drug Development Promotion Foundation (DDPF) and a Pharmaceutical Research & Development Support Fund (PRDSF). Necessary action in this regard has been initiated.

It has emerged that the domestic drugs and pharmaceuticals industry needs reorientation in order to meet the challenges and harness opportunities arising out of the liberalization of the economy and the impending advent of the product patent regime. It has been decided that the span of price control over drugs and pharmaceuticals would be reduced substantially. However, keeping in view the interest of the weaker sections of the society, it is proposed that the Government will retain the power to intervene comprehensively in cases where prices behave abnormally.

Ongoing Issues of Concern in the Area of Drug Demand Control in India

The authorities have clearly made efforts to alter provisions of the NDPS to take more account of the indigenous drug use culture within the country. That said, evidence suggests that Indian drug policy could be made far more effective and appropriate to national realities. This is crucial at a time when overall, "the drug situation is still in a benign stage in India, though moving in dangerous directions". While cultural norms in rural areas effectively restrict drug use to traditional forms and drug-related HIV is still relatively low within the national context of drug use, current trends suggest increasing levels of problematic non-traditional use and addiction. We suggest that in any assessment of contemporary Indian drug control policies, there are a number of key issues of concern:

- Most prevention efforts within India are, within the international framework laid down by the United Nations, currently based on experiences in predominantly Western countries. As such, they start from a position that considers all forms of drug use criminal and deviant. Thus, this leaves no scope for strengthening cultural mechanisms of use management or integrating them into contemporary legislation. For example, where institutional care appears unsustainable, practitioners could consider traditional forms of control such as the use of *dodapani* (a drink made from poppy pod) to wean users away from excessive opium or heroin consumption. Research suggests that cultural norms in India are far more efficient means of drug control, and have fewer negative side-effects than legislation inspired by global norms.

- Limited government funding means that the treatment of drug abuse is not widely available.

- Centres tend to provide services on a fee paying basis and the marginalized street level drug user consequently has limited options. In the city of Mumbai, for example, there are no treatment centres that cater to street level users with complications. Furthermore, the government hospital catering to the general population dislikes dealing with drug users because they are considered to be 'difficult' patients. Treatment for drug addiction is consequently not widely available and this sometimes results in use dying without receiving any care. There is a systematic reduction of government grants to drug treatment centres and the remuneration for the services of professionals is so minimal, that there are few takers. Under such conditions, there appears to be limited scope for an appropriate approach to care.

- Attempts at cost management by users in combination with the deteriorating quality of street drugs, have produced more risky forms of use; that is to say, injecting behavior. This has serious consequences for public health in some parts of India. A recent study found that the purity of heroin sold on the street varies from 3 percent to 12 percent. The Narcotics Drugs Control Board of India places the purity of street level heroin at 5 percent. In the northeastern part of the country, it seems that a shift to injecting drug use is also a result of time management issues. The behavior of a drug user in these areas of political instability is more dangerous than in other parts of the country.

- The approach of the Indian government is law enforcement led, with limited resources provided for treatment. This is unfortunate, since studies in other cultural settings show that efforts dominated by the law enforcement are not particularly effective. A high rate of drug incarceration as a strategy to control drug use has at best a marginal impact and does not lead to a significant undermining of the drug market. Indeed, experience from around the world reveals the cost effectiveness of appropriate treatment and harm reduction programs and interventions.

- By concentrating predominantly on the punitive aspects of UN legislation, the Indian authorities are currently failing to address adequately the issue of drug use within their own borders. Without an urgent change in approach, involving not only the refocusing of resources but also the recognition of traditional attitudes to the use and management of mind-altering substances, the nation may in the future face similar drug-related problems to those recently experienced in other countries in the region. Within the Islamic Republic of Iran, there is currently a high incidence of drug-related deaths and HIV/AIDS infection among injecting drug users while increasing problems surrounding the use of "amphetamine type stimulants" are to be found in Thailand. Specific national circumstances mean that no two countries experience identical patterns of problematic drug use. Yet the timely implementation of pragmatic and culturally appropriate policies within India would surely do much to prevent a repeat of such crises.

Suggested Readings

1. Annuradha KVIN (1999). The Narcotics Drugs and Psychotropic Substances Act, 1985. Drug Culture in India- A Street Ethnographic Study of Heroin Addiction in Bombay, Charles, *et al.*, Jaipur: Rawat Publishers p. 302-308.

2. Annuradha KVIN (2001). A flawed Act, Seminar. **504:** 50-54.

3. Bewley-Taylor D.R. (2001). The United States and International Drug Control: 1909-1997 Continuum, p. 176.

4. Charles M and Britto G (2002). Culture and the Drug Scene in India, Christian Geffary, Guilhem Fabre, Michel Schiray, Scientific Coordinators, Globalisation, Drugs and Criminalisation, Paris: UNESCO MOST and UNDP, 1: 4-30.

5. Charles M Nair, K.S and Britto Gabriel (1999). Drug Culture in India- A Street Ethnog   raphic Study of Heroin Addiction in Bombay; Jaipur: Rawat Publishers.

6. Charles M. (2004) Drug Trade Dynamics in India. Available from http://www.drugstat@free.fr.

7. Drug policy for pharmaceutical companies in India, 2002.

8. Drug policy of the national territory of Delhi, April 1994.

9. Drug policy of the state of J & K, January 2012.

10. MP Government Drug Policy, 2009.

11. Nissaramanesh B, *et al.,* (2005). The Rise of Harm Reduction in the Islamic Republic of Iran, Beckley Foundation Drug Policy Programme, Briefing Paper 8.

12. Proceedings of the Government of Karnataka, January 2004.

13. Roberts M, *et al.,* (2004). Thailand's War on Drugs, Beckley Foundation Drug Policy Programme, Briefing Paper 5.

14. State Drug Policy-West Bengal, November 2011.

15. Wyler LN (2011). International Drug Control Policy.

CHAPTER 20

NARCOTICS

In contemporary society, the drug has two connotations defining the positive and crucial role of drug in the medicines and another is self-destructing and socially deleterious effect of misuse. Human beings have used the drugs since thousands of years. Wine was used since the time of the early Egyptians; narcotics from 4000 B.C. The medicinal use of marijuana has been dated to 2737 B.C. in China. However, the active substances in these drugs were extracted only in the early 19th century A.D. There followed a time, when some of these newly discovered substances morphine, laudanum, cocaine were completely unregulated and prescribed freely by physicians for a wide variety of ailments. These were freely available and sold freely until the laws prohibiting the misuse of narcotics came into the force worldwide.

A narcotic, medically is any drug that produces sleep or stupor and relieves pain or alters psychological reaction associated with pain, induces lethargy due to its depressant effect on the central nervous system (CNS) or stimulates the CNS or produces the hallucination. Included in this medical definition are opium, opium derivatives (morphine, heroin, codeine) and synthetic opiates (methadone, demerol and oxycodone). In the United Nations treaty on narcotics, it embraces *Cannabis Sativa L* (marijuana), coca leaf and cocaine, sedatives and stimulants. The term "narcotic" is believed to have been coined by the Galen that refers to agents causing numbness and loss of feeling or paralysis. It is based on the Greek word ναρκωσις (narcosis), the term used by Hippocrates for the process of numbing or the numbed state. It is more of a legal term defining drugs regulated by government agency, though pharmacologically it is not of much use because of its varied usage. Narcotic drugs effect the central nervous system (CNS). Morphine is the standard or yardstick by which other narcotics are evaluated.

The Drugs and Cosmetics Act (DCA) 1940 and Rules (DCR) 1945 defined drug as an essential commodity and is required to be regulated in terms of its import, manufacture, sale and distribution. These legislations are applicable to the whole of India and to all categories of medicines whether imported or manufactured in India. The legislation is regulated by the Central Government (Ministry of Health & Family Welfare) in New Delhi, which is responsible for its overall supervision and enforced by State Government through its Food and Drug Administration to provide the non-adulterated, branded and non-spurious drugs. *There are 2 Schedules to the Act and 38 Schedules to the Rules framed under the Act.* It was in the year 1982, Schedules E, I and L were dropped, Schedules G and H were revised and Schedule X was introduced (Narcotics and psychotropic drugs). In 1988, Schedule M incorporating GMP (Good Manufacturing Practices) was amended and Schedule Y pertaining to clinical trials of newer drug formulations was incorporated.

According to the Narcotic Drugs and Psychotropic Substances Act, 1985, the term "Psychotropic Substances" are defined as any substance, natural or synthetic or any material or any salt or preparations of such substance or material included in the list of psychotropic substances specified in the Schedule to the Act.

Manufactured drugs: means (a) all coca derivatives, medicinal cannabis, opium derivatives and poppy straw concentrate; (b) any other narcotic substance or preparation which the central government may, having regard to the available information as to its nature, or to a decision, if any, under any International Convention, by notification in the Official Gazette declare to be manufactured drug; Central Government has declared certain narcotic drugs and preparations to be manufactured drugs.

Drug Control Strategy and Policy

The Narcotic Drugs and Psychotropic Substances Act, 1985 (NDPS Act) sets out the statutory framework for drug law enforcement in India. This Act consolidates the erstwhile principal Acts, viz. the Opium Act 1857, the Opium Act 1878 and the Dangerous Drugs Act, 1930. The NDPS Act also incorporates provisions designed to implement India's obligations under various International Conventions. Certain significant amendments were made in the Act in 1989 for controlling over chemicals and substances used in the manufacture of narcotic drugs and psychotropic substances. In order to give effect to the statutory provisions relating to these substances, an order, namely the NDPS (Regulation of Controlled Substances) Order, was promulgated by the Government of India in 1993 to control, regulate and monitor the manufacture, distribution, import, export, transportation etc. of any substance which the Government may declare to be a 'controlled substance' under the Act. The statutory regime in India consequently covers drug trafficking, drug related assets as well as substances which can be used, in the manufacture of narcotic drugs and psychotropic substances. Some further amendments were incorporated in the NDPS Act in 2001, mainly to introduce a graded punishment.

The Act empowers Central Government and the State Governments to make orders of detention with respect to any person (including a foreigner), if they are of opinion that it is necessary so to do with a view to prevent illicit traffic in narcotic drugs and psychotropic substances. The expression "illicit traffic" had been defined to include cultivation of any coca plant or gathering any portion of coca plants, cultivating the opium poppy or any cannabis plant, or engaging in the production, manufacture, possession, etc., of narcotic drugs or psychotropic substance.

In India, there is an alarming increase in the drug addicts because of the young nation. The most common drugs of abuse are ganja, hashish, opium and heroin. The abuse of pharmaceutical preparations like buprenorphine, codeine based cough syrups and painkillers like proxyvon has also assumed serious proportions.

According to the Narcotic Drugs and Psychotropic Substances Act, 1985, the addict is defined as a person addicted to any narcotic drug or psychotropic substance. Narcotic addiction is a combination of physical dependence (causing acute physical pains when drug is stopped), psychological habituation (emotional desire, craving or compulsion to obtain and experience the euphoria, daydreaming escape from reality) and body tolerance resulting from abuse or misuse of narcotic drugs. It has been shown that heroin can hook or make a user an addict with the first "fix" (injection). A heroin abuser can become a hopeless addict within a week. Addiction potency of morphine and other opiates are lesser than the heroine.

Drug abuse occurs if you take any drug for purposes other than for what it was intended or in any manner or in quantities other than directed. The abuse of drugs may lead to an addiction, now often referred to as drug dependence.

An addiction may be considered to be the compulsive and continued use of a drug, or the loss of control over its use, despite adverse consequences produced by the drug. Drug dependence has both psychological and physical characteristics. If unable to obtain the drug, the addicted person may experience symptoms of distress or withdrawal and a need to take the drug again. Recognizing the signs of addiction (to legal or illegal drugs) in someone else can be difficult. These signs vary from drug to drug and person to person. However, people who are addicted to one or more drugs often will exhibit changes in their behavior that may gradually affect personal relationships and work performance.

Criteria of Narcotics and Psychotropic Drugs Classification

Narcotics are defined as substances that bind at opioid receptors (cellular membrane proteins activated by substances like heroin or morphine). The classification is largely based on the action of these drugs on the central nervous system. These are therefore, categorized as stimulants, depressants, no effect and complex effect drugs. From a legal perspective, narcotic refers to opium, opium derivatives and their semi-synthetic substitutes.

Table 20.1 Classification of addictive drugs

Addictive drugs	Sub classification and Mode of intake	Short – term effects	Long – term effects
Narcotic Analgesics Pain killer or pain relieving drugs with opium like effects	• Natural sources – Opium (oral, inhalation); Morphine injection, Codeine oral (tablets and cough syrups) • Semi synthetic : Heroin (brown sugar) – injection, inhalation, chasing • Synthetic : Dihydrocodeinone,	Euphoria, thought process impairment, drowsiness, apathy, feelings of hunger and pain are not felt Overdose of heroin can cause convulsions, coma and death	Mood instability Reduced libido Constipation Respiratory impairments Physical deterioration
Stimulants Drugs which excite or speed up the central nervous system	• Amphetamines – oral • Cocaine – snorted	A heightened feeling of well-being, euphoria A sense of super-abundant energy Increased motor and speech activity Suppression of appetite Increased wakefulness	Chronic sleep problem Poor appetite Rapid and irregular heart beat Mood swings Amphetamine psychosis
Depressants Drugs which depress or slow down the functions of the central nervous system	• Barbiturates • Benzodiazepines	Relief from anxiety and tension Euphoria Lowering of inhibitions Poor motor coordination Impaired concentration and judgement Slurred speech and blurred vision Sedation, sleep with larger doses	Depression Chronic fatigue Respiratory impairments Impaired sexual function Decreased attention span Poor memory and judgement Chronic sleep problems

Table 20.1 *Contd...*

229

Addictive drugs	Sub classification and Mode of intake	Short – term effects	Long – term effects
Hallucinogens Hallucinogens are drugs which affect perception, emotions and mental processes	• LSD -Lysergic acid diethylamide (oral tablets) • PCP –Phencyclidine (snorted/smoked) • Mescaline (oral tablets) • Psilocybin (smoked)	Alterations of mood Distortion of the sense of direction, distance and time 'Pseudo' hallucinations Synesthesia – melding of two sensory modalities Feelings of depersonalization	Flash back or spontaneous recurrence of on LSD experience can occur Amotivational syndrome LSD precipitated psychosis
Cannabis	Ganja/Marijuana • Hashish/Charas • Hashish oil • Bhang Smoking	Mild euphoria Lowering of inhibitions Reddening of eyes Sense of smell, touch and taste are often enhanced Altered sense of time perception Impaired short-term memory Impairment of ability to perform complex motor tasks	Decreased cognitive ability Amotivational syndrome Psychosis Respiratory problems Sterility/impotence In women abusers, fetal damage can occur

Analgesics

Opium

Opium is the best-known analgesic. The word "opium" is derived from Greek word "Opion". The opium poppy (*Papaver somniferum L*) belonging to the family Papaveraceae, is an annual medicinal herb. The chemically related derivatives, such as the semi-synthetic alkaloids are termed as "Opiate" while "opioid" is used for both natural and synthetic drugs with morphine-like properties.

Opium is a drug distilled from the juice of the poppy flower. Natural alkaloids present in opium or poppy straw like morphine, codeine, thebaine, narcotine, papaverine are under the international control because of their potential for abuse. These opiates are used frequently as an analgesic, anti-tussive and anti-spasmodic in modern medicine. Morphine is the prototype of natural opiates and has strong analgesic potency which is used as a reference parameter for comparative purposes.

India is the only country authorized by the United Nations Single Convention on Narcotic Drugs (1961) to produce gum opium. The use of opium for medicinal purposes in India can be traced back as far back as 1000 A.D. where it finds mention in ancient texts such as "Dhanvantri Nighantu" as a remedy for variety of ailments. In Emperor Akbar, opium was cultivated extensively in the MP and Rajasthan regions. During the British East India Company Rule, collection of revenue from opium was made part of fiscal policy and various opium agencies such as the Bengal, Banaras, Bihar, Malwa agencies were formed over time.

After independence the Indian government checks and monitors its production and usage. Prior to 1950, the administration of the narcotics laws, namely, the Opium Act of 1857 & 1878 and the Dangerous Drugs Act 1930 are vested with the provincial government. The amalgamation of these agencies laid the foundation of the Opium Department in 1950, which is presently known as Central Bureau of Narcotics (CBN). The headquarters of the CBN was shifted from Shimla to Gwalior in 1960. All the three enactments mentioned above were repealed by the Narcotics Drugs & Psychotropic Substances Act, 1985 (NDPS Act, 1985).

Heroin

Heroin was developed as a "non-addicting" substitute for morphine in the 1870's. It was produced under the brand name "heroin" in 1898 by Bayer and Company, a German pharmaceutical firm. Though the word "hero", suggesting courage, daring and impressive power was the basis of the naming this drug, it is however, courage of illusory, self-destructive and socially damaging.

The heroin was obtained by acetylation of morphine and has narcotic and addictive qualities far exceeding those of morphine itself. This was one of the horrific tragedies of the medical world, as heroin was marketed as cure for morphine addiction and has instead addicted millions, before getting banned.

This diacetylmorphine drug or heroine produces an intense euphoria (an initial sweet surge of super-orgasmic intensity and then four or five hours of day-dreamy release). It causes tolerance to the body and the abuser is possessed by an over powering urge to take another "hit" (dose) because of the terrible pains. Due to its potency, heroin is "cut" (diluted or adulterated) with milk sugars, talcum or the powdered. It is usually mixed into a liquid solution and "mainlined" (injected into a vein), but it is also "snorted" (inhaled) and "dropped" (taken by mouth). How heroin exactly works was not known for years. What was known only was that, like opium and morphine, it depressed the central nervous system: the brain and spinal cord.

In our body, endogenous opioids include endorphins, enkephalins, and dynorphins act through the receptors and modulate the painful stimuli, regulate hunger and thirst, mood control, immune response and other processes. The reason that opiates such as heroin and morphine affect us so powerfully is that these exogenous substances bind to the same receptors as our endogenous opioids. There are three kinds of receptors widely distributed throughout the brain: mu, delta, and kappa receptors. These receptors, through second messengers, influence the opening of ion channels which in certain cases reduces the excitability of neurons. This reduced excitability is the likely source of the euphoric effect of opiates and appears to be mediated by the mu and delta receptors.

This euphoric effect also appears to involve another mechanism in which the GABA-inhibitory interneurons of the ventral tegmental area come into play. By attaching to their mu receptors, exogenous opioids reduce the amount of release of GABA. Normally, GABA reduces the amount of dopamine released in the nucleus accumbens. By inhibiting this inhibitor, the opiates ultimately increase the amount of dopamine produced and the amount of pleasure felt.

Chronic consumption of opiates inhibits the production of cAMP, but this inhibition is offset in the long run by other cAMP production mechanisms. When no opiates are available, this increased cAMP production capacity comes to the fore and results in neural hyperactivity and the sensation of craving the drug.

Morphine

It is the most potent pain killer and prescribed for the severe cases of chronic pain. It is found to be manufactured legally (white to brown powder or pill) and illegally (powder). It is antitussive and CNS depressant. It is still used as a yardstick for the analgesic activity of other narcotic drugs.

Codeine

Codeine is also known as morphine methylester or Methylmorphine. It is antitussive, CNS depressant and a powerful analgesic. It is a controlled substance and is prescribed for both pain relief as well as cough suppressant.

Synthetic Opoids

Hydrocodone: Dihydrocodeinone

Hydrocodone is a semi-synthetic opiate and is derived from thebaine. The therapeutic dose of 5 to 10 mg is pharmacologically equivalent to 60 mg of oral morphine. Hydrocodone is marketed as an advanced cough suppressant but can be obtained through prescription only.

Hydromorphone: Dihydromorphinone

Hydromorphone is derived from thebaine and is a semi-synthetic opiate. Its analgesic potency is from 2 to 8 times that of morphine. Hydromorphone is usually obtained by the abuser through fraudulent prescriptions or theft.

Oxycodone: Dihydrohydroxycodeinone

Oxycodone is similar to codeine and is a semi-synthetic opiate derived from thebaine. It is more potent and has a higher abuse and dependence potential. It is effective orally and is marketed in combination with aspirin or acetaminophen for the relief of pain. Addicts take these tablets orally and "mainline" the active drug after dissolving in water.

Stimulants

Stimulants are the class of drugs that are known to cause the stimulation of the CNS. These drugs increase alertness, reduce hunger and yield a feeling of self-confidence and well-being. They have approved medical uses, including: to curb appetite, to combat fatigue, sleepiness or mild depression. These drugs tend to be abused. Stimulation is followed by a let-down feeling or depressing, hangover, profound adverse effect on reasoning, judgment and reaction time. They can damage the body and mind, even kill in lethal overdose. Many stimulants are known, including: cocaine, amphetamine, methamphetamine, dextroamphetamine, benzphetamine, phenmetrazine, mephentermine and methylphenidate.

Stimulants are also known as pep pills, jolly beans, ups, uppers, eye-openers, wake-ups, wake-uppers and speed.

Amphetamines

Amphetamines and related drugs have a wide, important and essential use in medicine. They are used for treating a variety of mental disorders. Mood disturbances often improve with amphetamines; Slimming down the overweight. Amphetamine exerts a specific effect on the brain's appetite center. It also improves the obese person's mood and stirs them to activity. Treating narcolepsy, a disease characterized by an overwhelming compulsion to sleep. Amphetamine effectively counters narcolepsy, helps many patients to live normal lives; treating parkinsonism, a disease which results in rigidity of some muscles.

As stimulant, amphetamines stimulate the brain areas associated with vigilance, mood and heart action, sharpen alertness, curb hunger, banish sleep, dispel depression. Amphetamines, release "norepinephrine", and concentrate it in the brain's higher centers. This speeds up action of the heart and the metabolic process, through which the body converts food into the chemicals it needs.

Amphetamines, in their pure form, are a colourless liquid with a strong odour and a burning taste. These drugs also come as an odourless crystalline powder that are ingested orally or by injection. Amphetamines have been available since the 1930s. These drugs were used first as a nasal inhaler to treat cold and hay fever. But later found to stimulate the CNS.

The commonly abused amphetamines are: Benzendrine ("bennies"), Dexedrine ("dexies"), and Methedrine ("meth" or "speed"). These are available in the pure forms as well as in combination with tranquilizers and barbiturates as well.

When amphetamines are mainlined or injected, an ecstatic high occurs. This buoyant and lifting feeling subsides after a few hours, however, to reproduce the hyper-stimulation, the abuser gets a re-injection, this cycle can go on for days until the abuser is physically and mentally exhausted. Shaking, tension, itching and muscle pains are common among extreme drug abusers. Fatigue, malnutrition and emaciation, loss of self-control, impaired thinking and speech, quarrelsome, diarrhoea, paleness, dilation of eye pupils, hallucinations, visual and hearing are the main effects of the long term usage of the amphetamines.

Cocaine

Cocaine is the most powerful natural stimulant known to man. It works up a human's CNS. It causes physical and mental alertness when taken, including a feeling of surging body strength, followed by complete physical and mental exhaustion.

It is obtained from leaves of the coca plant found in Java, Taiwan and South America, mainly Peru, Bolivia, Chile, Colombia and Argentina. The active substance of the plant is alkaloid cocaine. In its pure form, cocaine is made up of shiny, white or colourless crystals. Hence, its common name is snow. The cocaine powder is odourless, but it has a bitter taste. It is also found in sterile solutions or tablets. It differs from other stimulants as it is completely banned and can be obtained only through illegal or criminal markets. Cocaine is sniffed, eaten or injected into a vain.

Cocaine is a quick-acting drug. Its effects are rapid from the time of intake. It is, indeed, "super-speed". It peps and speeds up the brain cells and mental power is sharpened, physical strength surges. Initially it causes euphoria or a sense of buoyant well-being, marked by a feeling of complete self-confidence, a feeling of being more than equal to any task or challenge, as well as pleasant hallucinations, visual and auditory. The peak "lift" lasts only briefly, however: only 15 to 30 minutes, although lesser effects linger up to 2 to 4 hours. The stimulation is followed often by a "crash" or collapse of the whole nervous system which is marked by: raw nerves, physical weakness, a feeling of gloom, all coming in a quick sudden, just as quickly as the "lift" had come. It may causes death from heart failure.

Heavy doses cause unclear speech, confused thinking, short temper, unease and tension, all signs of an impaired mind. When abused, it leads to social, intellectual and emotional breakdown, marked by mental instability, serious psychotic states and long-term personality disorders. Continued snorting or sniffing cocaine causes nasal ulcers and, in acute cases, perforates the dividing wall of the nose. Unhygienic "shooting" or "mainlining" cocaine leads to abscesses, sores and scars where the cocaine was injected.

Cocaine speeds up action of the heart, which gets overworked and results in: rapid breathing, soaring blood pressure, dilated pupils, stomach cramps, nausea, convulsions, vomiting, palpitations, sweating, severe headache, pallor and, sometimes, heart failure and death. It also numbs the tongue, causes the mouth to dry.

Sedatives

Sedatives are a big family of drugs which relax the nervous system. They calm the nerves, reduce tension and induce sleep. The best known are: the barbiturates, first produced in 1846 from barbituric acid. There are some 2,500 in the sedative family. Only about 30 are widely used medically. The sedatives are also known as: "goofballs", "sleeping pills", "downs", "downers", "sleepers" and "slumbers".

Signs and Symptoms of Abuse: Loss of appetite; Presence of needle Marks; Improper measurements of steps; Slurred Speech; Muscular incoordination; Drunk Appearance.

Barbiturates

Barbiturates are sedatives. They are among the most versatile depressant drugs. They are man-made. They depress the CNS. Used under medical supervision, barbiturates are impressively safe and effective. They are widely used and widely distributed legally, but more widely abused and misused illegally.

Barbiturates range from the short-acting, fast-starting pentobarbital sodium (Nembutal) and secobarbital sodium (Seconal) to the long-acting, slow-starting phenobarbital (Luminal), amobarbital (Amytal) and butabarbital (Butisol). The short-acting ones, known as "barbs" and "goofballs", are commonly abused. Barbiturates are taken as capsules and tablets orally.

In medically supervised doses, they mildly depress action of the nerves, skeletal muscles and heart muscles. They slow down the heart rate and breathing, lower the blood pressure, slow down the reflexes, distort the thinking, confuse and impair judgment. These drugs relieve pain by inducing sleep. In higher doses, the effects are like alcoholic drunkenness: confused mind, blurred vision, slurred speech, lurching walk, deep sleep. Large doses are potentially lethal. Barbiturates constitute a greater menace than other narcotics. The habitual abuser becomes a drug addict; when barbiturates are withdrawn, the user suffers considerable pain.

Barbiturate abusers react to barbiturate differently at different times: mildly at one time, acutely at other times. Confusion of the dosage taken usually leads to the overdose and death.

Hallucinogens

Hallucinogens cause hallucinations in their users. Hence their collective name: hallucinogens. These drugs are also called as psychedelics or psychotropics or psychotogens.

Hallucinogens can provoke in their users: Changes of sensation, distortions of perception, illusions, delusions and hallucinations. These drugs are known as mind-alterers, mind- benders. Hairs of the body stand, dilation of pupils and reddening of the eyes, hallucination, distortions of time and space, excessive giggling, psychotic behavior.

Mescaline or Peyote

Mescaline is a 3,4,5-trimethoxyphenethylamine. It is a colorless alkaline oil or oily crystalline material with a melting point of 35 °C-36 °C. Powdered form of mescaline can be obtained from "buttons" of the Mexican cactus peyote. It is soluble in water, alcohol, and chloroform but less soluble in ether. The sulfate or chloride salts form colorless crystals. As the mescaline salts are more soluble and more easily handled, these drugs have been used in the majority of psychological experiments. The active chemical of peyote, the alkaloid mescaline, was isolated in 1896 from the peyote cactus, *Lophophora williamsii.*

Mescaline is generally taken orally or can be mainlined. The average dose is 350 to 500 mg. The high or the effect of the mescaline appears after 1 or 2 hours and may last up to 5 to 12 hours. Because of its bitter taste, mescaline is often taken with tea, coffee, milk, orange juice, soda, or soft drink. The peyote button itself has a vile, fibrous taste.

The individual is usually in a state of extreme good humour and full of a feeling of intellectual and physical energy; a sense of fatigue rarely occurs. The user suffers sensation and perception impairment, loss of a sense of time, disorganization of thought and psychotic reactions. It is, therefore, a peril to the mind. Mescaline acts on the central nervous system.

Mescaline has severe cardiovascular effects there by speeding up the heartbeat and increasing the blood pressure. It also dilates the pupils, increases the blood sugar level, heightens the body temperature and causes heavy perspiration and nausea.

In high doses, mescaline lowers the blood glucose. In such cases, the user may suffer bloody diarrhea and fall into unconsciousness. Lethal doses produce convulsions, breath-arrests and heart failures. Death is due to respiratory failure. It can cause body tolerance and psychological dependence.

LSD

Dextro lysergic acid diethylamide tartarate-25 (LSD) is a man-made drug. It is among the most potent and most lethal of the narcotics drugs. It is described as "a brain eater".

An experimental study revealed that a single ounce can give 30,000 doses, thereby proving LSD as a very potent drug. It is 100 times more powerful than cocaine or peyote. A pin point of LSD is enough to blast a user's mind off to an uncertain journey. It affects the central nervous system primarily. It changes the user's mood and behaviour, perception and sensation. LSD is taken orally but can also be injected.

It is not a quick-action drug, except when injected into a vein and blood stream. When taken orally, in normal volunteers 1 or ½ µg per kg elevated the pulse rate from 84 to 90 per minute and stabilized the rate. It shows its effect within 20 minutes to one hour, however when injected, it activates in several minutes. Its effects last as long as 72 hours. LSD produced both sympathetic and parasympathetic activity. A speeding of heart and pulse beats, a rise in blood pressure and body temperature, cold and sweaty palms, shaking of limbs, a flushed face or paleness, widely dilated eye pupils, chills with goose pimples, nausea, convulsions, vomiting and loss of appetite. The effects disappear as the LSD action subsides. "Hallucinations," which LSD takers report, are among LSD's effects in this grouping. Sounds are "seen" or "felt," colours are "heard" or "tasted," objects "take life" and "pulsate", 3-D forms unfold in geometric or psychedelic patterns. It is a false sensory perception without the objective reality.

The abusive effect of LSD depends upon the dose of the drug and the emotional, intellectual and mental state of the abuser. It has the most unpredictable effects. The user may fear of losing mind, paranoia, mental imbalance, flashback (the victim may become insane or driven to suicide), heart failure, fatal convulsions, accidental death or injury.

Marijuana

Marijuana is a dry, shredded green and brown mix of flowers, stems, seeds, and leaves from the hemp plant (*Cannabis sativa*). The plant has more than 400 chemicals including 9-tetrahydrocannabinol (THC). Hashish, a more powerful derivative drug prepared from the resin of the hemp plant, contains 50% of the psychoactive THC. It is a concentrated form of marijuana and prepared by pressing it into cakes. It is a brown, sticky and crumbling substance.

Marijuana is the most popular illegal drug. Marijuana cigarettes are made from the leaves and tops of the plant. When smoked, THC is quickly absorbed from lungs into the bloodstream and rapidly distributed to most tissues and organs of the body. The metabolites are cleared from the body at a much slower rate than the other psychoactive drugs.

The effects of marijuana are almost immediate. The pulse quickens by as much as 50%, depending on the potency of the marijuana. Most users experience a mild euphoria and relaxation. There is variation in other effects but heightened sensory perception (e.g., brighter colors), laughter, altered perception of time, fevered eyes, blurred vision, slurred speech, and increased appetite has been reported with different users. After a while, the euphoria subsides, and the user may feel sleepy or depressed. Marijuana may produce anxiety, fear, distrust, or panic. High doses of marijuana may produce same behavioral effects as severe alcohol intoxication and many of the negative effects may linger for up to 6 hours after smoking marijuana.

Chronic marijuana smokers show evidence of decreased lung capacity and chronic bronchial irritation. It may impair body's immune system and lungs may be more susceptible to infections. Dried marijuana is occasionally contaminated by animal droppings containing *Salmonella* bacteria which can cause diarrhea, abdominal pain and fever.

Depending on the length of use and the potency of the marijuana used, the withdrawal symptoms are tremors, sweating, nausea, vomiting, diarrhea, irritability, and sleep disturbances. However, these withdrawal symptoms are usually mild compared with those of heavy opiate or alcohol use, and they rarely require medical attention. Although often misunderstood and misrepresented to the public, marijuana clearly is a drug of dependence. Regular use often results in the same type of drug dependence described for other substances. A person cannot smoke himself to death with marijuana but, can kill with enough purified or even just semi-purified THC, the psychoactive substance of marijuana.

Acute doses of marijuana can bring forth hallucinations; fragment the thoughts, personal unreality causing psychosis, aggressiveness and belligerency, delusions of grandeur and magical thinking, impairment of judgment and memory. Marijuana changes the social attitude of the user and they suffer in the hands of the drug abuse. Marijuana has no approved medical use. The appetite-enhancing, anti-convulsant or anti-depressant capabilities of this drug has been found to be inefficient without predictable effect, therefore, the drug was removed from the official drug lists of nearly all countries.

Research on Narcotic Drugs

Research on narcotic drugs in India, is very important element for narcotics control work as research can clarify the medicinal use of the narcotics and psychotropic drugs and the different issues on drug abuse problems and may lead to better solutions.

Conducting clinical trials with controlled drugs in particular for the treatment of breakthrough follows the standard procedure. Besides meeting, the ICH-GCP and Indian ICMR/CDSCO requirements, these clinical trials require additional narcotics compliances relating to storage, import-export quotas and movement of the investigational drug from the place of manufacturing to the place of consumption. This is closely monitored by Government of India (Central Bureau of Narcotics) and overseen by global regulatory watchdog (International Narcotics Control Board). The permissions sought at different levels are

Central level

1. Drugs Controller General of India (DCGI), New Delhi under the Ministry of Health is responsible for approvals for conducting clinical trials in India.
2. Central Bureau of Narcotics (CBN), Gwalior under the Ministry of Finance is responsible for approvals relating to manufacture and import of controlled drugs in India.
3. Central Excise Office - The Central Excise Office co-ordinates with CBN to oversee the activities of companies engaged in research or manufacture of controlled drugs located in their state including conducting a due diligence audit on behalf of CBN for the first application from a new company.
4. The Drug Enforcement Agencies (DEA), equivalent to CBN in India is responsible for issuance of the export license in response to the import certificate issued by CBN. At international levels, CBN provides reports to the INCB *via* NCB on annual quotas sanctioned for controlled drugs to India.

State level

State FDA office or Excise Agency oversees the manufacture and interstate movement of controlled drugs in their state.

In order to conduct a clinical trial in India using a narcotic drug, DCGI approval is sought for the study protocol which should compulsory follow Schedule Y. It is followed by application for the import certificate from CBN (valid for one year), to import the required quantity of investigational product for the number of Indian patients participating in the study. The protocol follows the Schedule Y and for manufacturing and management of the narcotics drugs follows schedule X.

Subsequently, an "export certificate" is required from CBN (valid for six months) to seek an "export certificate" from the DIA of the exporting country which must be approved within the category and quota permissible under the NDPS Laws (Narcotic Drugs and Psychotropic Substance) of the two countries. The validity of this NDPS license varies from State to State i.e., from one year to two years. This license has to be endorsed with the clinical trial investigational products and then transport permit have to be obtained from concerned zonal FDA office or state excise agency to move the medicine from depot to the hospitals. Again, the transport permit validity varies from State to State i.e., from fifteen days to two months.

After obtaining all these approvals and licenses, the investigational products can be shipped to the particular hospital and clinical trial on narcotic drugs can be initiated. The challenge in conducting narcotic clinical trial is mainly the time lines since there are several government agencies involved in controlling the narcotics and each of their license validity will be entirely different and overlapping, besides time-limiting factor. The filing requirements also vary from State to State and even intrastate too in India. However, the success of research on the controlled drugs lies in understanding the holistic picture of involvement of all regulatory agencies and making efficient project management plan to bring successfully the investigational products to the hospital that will surely bring down the drug abuse.

Conclusion

Drug abuse has become a severe socio-economic problem affecting the vulnerable age groups. The very essence of these wonderful analgesics have really marginalized due to the menace of the drug abuse. There should be reduction in the supply of narcotics and addicts should be rehabilitated with de-addiction measures.

Suggested Readings

1. A. Hoffer and H. Osmond (1967). The Hallucinogens. Academic press Inc. (London).

2. Bewley-Taylor D, Jelsma M (2012). Regime change: Re-visiting the 1961 Single Convention on Narcotic Drugs. *Int J Drug Policy*. **23(1):** 72-81. Epub 2011 Oct 12.

3. Holmes BB, Rady JJ, Fujimoto JM (1998). Heroin acts on delta opioid receptors in the brain of streptozocin-induced diabetic rats. *Proc. Soc. Exp. Biol. Med.* 1998 **218(4):** 334-40.

4. http://narcoticsindia.nic.in/NDPSACT.htm.

5. http://toxnet.nlm.nih.gov/cgi-bin/sis/search/a?dbs+hsdb:@term+@ DOCNO + 32 87 Inaba & Cohen, 2007.

6. Romesh Bhattacharji. India's experiences in licensing poppy cultivation for the production of essential medicines –Case study. 2007.

7. Synthetics & Other Opiates. Drug Free Workplace. 07 Sept. 2001 <http://www.drugfreeworkplace.com/drugsofabuse/synthetic.htm>

8. Takayanagi I, Koike K, Suzuki T (1990). Pharmacological properties of newly synthesized derivatives of (-)-6 beta-acetylthionormorphine and their interactions with opioid receptors. *Gen Pharmacol.* **21(5):** 605-11.

9. The Narcotic drugs and Psychotropic substances act, 1985.

CHAPTER 21

DRUG AND OFF-LABEL USE

Introduction

Whenever, a new drug is approved by the regulatory authorities, it is accompanied by an approved specific product label (package insert) as well. The drug label provides detailed information for safe and effective usage of drug along with the approved dose, dosage form, method of administration, indications for use and the target population. It also carries information for use in special populations, drug interactions, warnings, precautions and contraindications to use of the approved medicine. Broadly speaking, use of approved drugs in a manner not consistent with the information provided on its approved label is termed as off label/unlabelled/unapproved drug use. Thus, if the drug is used for an indication not specified in the product label, or at a dosage/in a dosage form or in a frequency or for a duration or *via* a route of administration or in a age group other than that mentioned on its approved label will constitute an off label use. In other words, off label drug use can belong to one or more of the following categories (Table 21.1). Though, such use may sometimes be clinically appropriate e.g., when there are no alternative therapeutic options and when potential benefits outweigh the risks or in informed patient with serious disease but on the other hand it is associated with number of ethical and safety issues. Sometimes it may do more harm than good, for example deaths were reported when propofol was used off label for sedation in the children in pediatric ICU. Another, often cited mishap is valvular heart disease in thousands of people after fenfluramine (anorectic drug, approved for short term use) was promoted for use in combination with phentermine for weight loss on long term basis. However, off label use is entirely separate from prescribing a medicine that has never been approved by the regulatory bodies for human use.

Table 21.1 Categories of off label drug use

Off label use categories	Description	Examples
Indication	Drug prescribed for an indication not mentioned in approved package insert	Sildenafil for pulmonary hypertension in children
Route of administration	Drug prescribed by a route not mentioned in product label	IV glucose solution *via* oral route for pain relief
Age	Drug used in age group which is not recommended in product label e.g., in children below certain age, adults > 80 years of age	Use of paracetamol in premature infants
Duration	Drug given for more or lesser duration of time than recommended	Frequently seen with antibiotics
Frequency	Drug is administered in lesser or more frequency than recommended	--
Dose/ Dosage form	Drug is used at a dose/in a dosage form not recommended on approved label	--

Extent of Off Label Drug Use

To figure out the nature and extent of off label prescribing practices of the physicians, a number of surveys and prospective studies have been conducted worldwide. It has been reported that off label drug use ranges between 7.5 to 40% for adults to as high as 90% among hospitalised pediatric patients. A nationwide representative survey (2006) of US office based physician practices in outpatient settings, found that 21% of total drug use (150 million drug encounters) was off- label. Out of this, more than 70% of off label drug use were not supported by scientific evidence of clinical efficacy. Further, it was found that for certain drugs, for example, gabapentin and oral dexamethasone, prescriptions were more frequent for the off label as compared to on-label uses (83% and 79% respectively). According to another study, off-label use without sound scientific evidence was common to the tune of 38% for anticonvulsants, 31% for allergy medications and 29% for the psychiatric medications, respectively. Table 21.2 gives a list of commonly encountered off label uses of certain drugs.

Table 21.2 Examples of off label drug uses

Drug	Off label uses by indication
Morphine	Pain in children
Propofol	Sedation in neonatal ICU
Sildenafil	Sexual dysfunction in females
Trazodone	Insomnia in elderly, refractory cases of insomnia

Table 21.2 *Contd...*

Drug	Off label uses by indication
Gabapentin	Restless leg syndrome, headache, bipolar disorder
Lignocaine (2-4%)	Topical anaesthetic agent in ophtahlmology
Alcohol injection	Painful blind eye
Omeprazole	Reflux related laryngitis
Ondansetron	Hyperemesis in pregnancy, in children
Mitomycin, 5 FU	Glaucoma
Glucose infusions through oral route	Pain relief in neonates and infants
Bevacizumab	Renal cell carcinoma, ovarian cancer
Rituximab	Idiopathic thrombocytopenic purpura
Cyclophosphamide	Ewing's sarcoma, osteosacoma
Dabigatran	Prophylaxis of thromboembolism after orthopedic surgeries
Propranolol, Atenolol	Chronic prophylaxis of migraine
Dexamethasone	Postoperative nausea
Azathioprine	Mouth ulcers, atopic dermatitis
Aspirin	Kawasaki disease
Erythromycin	Gastroparesis
Linezolid	Postinfective endocarditis
Atenolol	Hypertension in children
Nesiritide	Chronic stable heart failure for prevention of acute decompensation
Atypical antipsychotic agents	Substance abuse, obsessive- compulsive disorders, anxiety
Alendronate	Malignancy of hypercalcemia
Magnesium sulphate	Premature labour
Ciclopirox gel	Fungal dermatitis in babies

Thus, though the exact figures about such practice vary among studies, different regions and across different specialities, all of them unanimously point to the very existence of such off label use of drugs by the physicians in all parts of the world. In fact, as of today, off label use of drugs has become an integral part of the contemporary medicine. The off-label drug use is particularly more common for special patient populations e.g., pediatric age group, in diseases which occur less frequently (e.g., orphan diseases) and in palliative care settings. Studies conducted throughout Europe point out that at least one third of the hospitalized children and up to 90% of neonates in intensive care units receive such drug prescriptions. Another retrospective cohort study (2004) describes off-label medication use in hospitalized children, it was found that in 297,592 out of 355,409 patients at least one drug was used off-label. Moreover, it has been estimated that around 50-90% of drugs used in pediatric population today have never been actually studied in this population. The obvious reason for such a picture is the relative lack of conduct of clinical trials of new medicines in children, because until recently it was considered an unethical practice. As a result, many medicines currently being used in adults are insufficiently documented with regard to dosing, efficacy, and safety profile in the pediatric age group and thus, the results of clinical trials done in adults are often extrapolated for their use in children; which by definition fits into off label drug use.

Pros and Cons of Off Label Drug Use: Off-label drug use can't be simply classified as beneficial or harmful and as good or bad. It finds a prominent place in the medical practice as it has several advantages for the society.

1. It may offer patients earlier access to potentially valuable medicines and allow physicians to improve individual patient care based on emerging evidence.
2. It is critical to facilitating innovation in clinical settings. E.g., in oncology practice where off-label use of drugs might help the clinician to generate some proof of concept data which may then form the basis for future randomized controlled study.
3. It may be the only available option when all the approved therapies have failed for a particular disease condition or in an individual patient (i.e., in palliative settings).
4. Off-label use has the potential of establishing new uses for old drugs, as in the case of approval of thalidomide for multiple myeloma, after it was completely abandoned on account of its teratogenic effects.
5. In rare disease conditions (orphan diseases), such use may provide the only therapy available.
6. In practice areas like pediatrics, geriatrics and obstetrics when scientific and medical evidence justify off-label uses, physicians may promote patient's interests by prescribing medicines not well studied in these patient populations.
7. Off-label use may even become the standard of care for a particular health problem after well conducted research e.g., aspirin was widely used off-label long before its approval for use in rheumatic conditions, pain and cardiovascular conditions. Similarly, approval of botulinum toxin for the treatment of chronic migraine by FDA in 2010 was preceded by off label use.

On the other hand such a use is not without risks.

1. It can increase healthcare costs unnecessarily, when newer expensive drugs are selected over their approved cost-effective alternatives.
2. It may increase the likelihood of adverse drug events.

3. Off-label use offers the easiest way for the industry to subvert the cumbersome approval process and expand their product indications in the most cost-effective manner.

4. It may discourage evidence based practice by the physicians.

5. It shakes the consumer faith; in that there has been a full evaluation of the safety and efficacy of medications that are being prescribed to them.

6. Off-label use may affect innovation adversely, if the focus and resources are spent in widening the therapeutic uses of already approved drugs rather than developing targeted novel therapies.

7. It may encourage companies to conduct trials and seek regulatory approval for the easily approvable indications and not for the most profitable one because anyway after approval they will be able to sell their product for wider usage.

Perspectives of Stakeholders on Off Label Use: Different stakeholders (i.e., patients, physicians, industry, regulatory authorities and insurance agencies) of the health care have their own valid viewpoints. Industry obviously, would seek to promote off label drug use to expand their product markets. This in turn would ensure more profits for the industry as they evade the need of conducting costly and time consuming clinical trials; especially if their medicine is already in the market with widely accepted off label use. Physicians need freedom to exercise best of their clinical judgement for managing individual patients as well as the autonomy to innovate. Moreover, it appears to be justified when physicians do such off label use based on evidence from sources other than the product label (e.g., peer- reviewed literature in journals or based on opinion of experts like in oncology).

The consumer (patient) wants both, the safe and cost-effective evidence based medicine as well as the latest therapy which he/she presumes to be more superior to the current standard therapies. Many of the insurance/reimbursement companies, question the need to pay for unproven and costlier off label products, but some of the insurers for example Medicare and Medicaid do reimburse for the off label use. This issue of reimbursement is particularly important in reimbursing for cancer medications which are very costly. In US, the cost of off label drug use for 10 commonly prescribed anti-cancer agents was reported to be 4.5 billion $ in 2010. Regulatory authorities like US-FDA doesn't regulate off label drug use by the physicians.

Regulatory Stand on Off Label Prescribing: Despite large body of evidence in the literature regarding rampant off label use of drugs, there is no clear cut stand of regulatory authorities on such practice nor there are specific regulations governing such use or for evaluating their appropriateness. Most of the regulatory authorities in any part of the world (be it US, Japan, Europe, France), regulate only the market authorization of drugs. However, these agencies don't regulate the prescribing practice of the physicians. Thus, once a medicine is approved and is available in the market, the physicians are free to use such medicines outside the product label for other indications and patient groups in view of their professional judgement for the best interest of their patients. This is probably because, regulatory authorities recognise the fact that not all myriad patient needs encountered in real life clinical practice can be encompassed solely within the scope of approved drug label. Thus, off label drug use is not illegal practice on the part of clinicians but it can lead to malpractice liability if it doesn't conform to accepted standard of care like in any other area of medicine.

In India, Drug Controller General of India (DCGI) is regulatory body for approval of new medicines for use. It doesn't regulate off label use as the rest of the world. In 2004, a committee of Indian medical association was set up by the government of India to make specific guidelines governing the off label drug use. The committee strongly favoured the off label uses of drugs, when they were based on evidence, since it was of opinion that the approval of valid off label uses by the regulatory process is very slow. But, as of now, there is no concrete law on off label use of drugs in our country.

Regulations Governing Promotion of Off Label Uses: Regulations regarding promotion of pharmaceuticals by the industry have changed over time. In United States, after the 1938 Food, Drug and Cosmetic Act, the USFDA was empowered to regulate the promotional practices of the manufacturers for their approved medicines. It applied to any method of promotion whether through television, internet, advertisement in journals or distribution of materials to the physicians directly. This act indirectly restricted promotion of pharmaceuticals for off label uses because it prohibited manufacturers from introducing misbranded drugs in the market. Drug was labelled misbranded if its label included misleading information including any off label use also. But, subsequently, under the section 401 of the FDA Modernization Act of 1997, the manufacturers were allowed to distribute peer reviewed literature to the physicians on off label uses; subject to certain restrictions. Importantly, these restrictions included submitting the copy of materials to be distributed to healthcare professionals for FDA review at least 60 days prior to any such activity. The manufacturer, needed to commit that within six months of such promotion, it will submit supplemental NDA for relevant off label use of their product. Additionally, such information must be published in good quality peer reviewed journals and documents used for promotion should clearly mention that the said use is not FDA- approved.

Latest guidance issued by FDA in 2009 seems even more liberal on off label use of drugs. It allows distribution of information on unapproved uses of drugs without need to submit such materials for FDA review as well as submit a supplemental new drug application, as was needed before. This led to ever increasing promotion of off label uses by the manufactures. To deal with this scenario, FDA then introduced "Bad Ad" program in 2010 by which the consumers and physicians could report illicit drug promotional activities to FDA. This led to number of costly penalties for the pharmaceuticals for indulging in illegal off label promotional activities (Table 21.3).

Table 21.3 Penalties paid by pharmaceutical companies in recent years

Pharmaceutical company (year)	Off label drugs promoted	Settlement cost paid
Eli Lily (2009)	Olanzapine for dementia	1.4 billion US$
Novartis (2010)	Oxcarbazepine	422.5 million US$
Pfizer (2009)	Ziprasidone	301 million US$
Allergan (2010)	Onabotulinum A	600 million US$
Merck (2012)	Rofecoxib	950 million US$

Where Do We Go From Here?

Off label drug use is legal and is being widely practised worldwide. It has its own advantages and disadvantages. There is need to strike a balance between the innovation and physician autonomy on one hand with the evidence based health care on the other end. What is needed in such a situation is the more responsible prescribing by the physician, critically analysing the available information and robust pharmacovigilance systems in settings of off label use.

1. **Responsible Prescribing:** It would mean using the drug for some off label purpose only when it is appropriate. According to various recommendations for evaluating appropriateness of such use, it has been suggested that physician should answer few questions prior to using the drugs off label i.e., Is it supported by scientific evidence? Is it the only alternative available? (For e.g., all approved therapies have failed in patient for his disease condition), Do the possible benefits outweigh the risks? Has the patient/legal guardian been informed about it being off label use and whether consent has been obtained for the same?

2. **Evaluating Evidence Supporting Off Label use:** It is extremely important for the physicians to critically appraise the off label drug information available to them through journal articles or through internet etc. prior to using that evidence as a basis for the patient management. This includes searching for the strength of evidence, ensuring that the information is published in good quality peer-reviewed journal unlike in some industry sponsored supplement of publication and looking for any potential conflicts of interests as well. Equally important is to extensively review the scientific literature so as to form a balanced opinion for intended off label use and not solely base judgement on few selected studies favouring such use. Lastly, it is important to be sure that the evidence guiding the decision is actually answering both the safety and efficacy dimensions for intended use for the individual patient in question.

3. **Monitoring for the Safety of Off Label Use:** Since, the off label uses of the drugs are not studied in well designed large scale clinical trials, therefore monitoring the safety of such use through post marketing surveillance systems assumes utmost importance; given the fact that such use is not regulated at all. Various methods that can be applied to identify, analyse and monitor adverse drug events due to off label use of drugs include spontaneous ADR reports, observational epidemiologic studies including case-control and cohort studies and registries etc.

Suggested Readings

1. Dresser R, Frader J (2009). Off label prescribing: A call for heightened professional and government oversight. *J Law Med Ethics.* **37(3):** 476-396.

2. Gazarian M, Kelly M, McPhee JR, Grudins LV, Ward RL, Campbell T J (2006). Off label use of medicines: Consensus recommendations for evaluating appropriateness. *MJA.* **185(10):** 544-548.

3. Kinland E, Odlind V (2012). Off label drug use in Pediatric patients. *Nature Reviews.* **91(5):** 796-801.

4. Knopf H, Wolf IK, Sarganas G, Zhuang W, Rascher W, Neubert A (2013). Off label medicine use in children and adolescents: results of a population based study in Germany. *BMC Public Health* **13:** 631-50.

5. Mello MM, Studdert DM, Brennan TA (2009). Shifting Terrain in the regulation of off label promotion of pharmaceuticals. *N Engl J Med.* **360(15):** 1557-1564.

6. Stafford RS (2012). Off label use of drugs and medical devices: A review of policy implications. *Nature Reviews.* **91(5):** 920-25.

7. Ventola C Lee (2009). Off label drug information. *Pharmacology and Therapeutics.* **34(8):** 428-449.

8. Wittich CM, Burklc CM, Lanier LL (2012). Ten common questions and their answers about off label drug use. *Mayo Clin Proc.* **87(10):** 982-990.

SECTION – II

CHAPTER 22

DRUGS USED IN PREGNANCY

Introduction

Treatment options for pregnant women are limited and a highly complex individualized process. The ailment of mother has direct and indirect impact on the fetus development. The drugs used during pregnancy can also influence the internal milieu of the growing fetus. Optimization of the mother's health by using medicines or any alternate way can indirectly benefit the embryo or fetus by improving the uterine/placental environment in which, the embryo/fetus grows. On the other hand, the progression or continuation of mothers' disordered condition during pregnancy can have unfavourable consequence on the fetus as well as the mother. As for example, if a mother has a severe asthma attack or a prolonged seizure, the fetus may suffer an injury due to hypoxia. A mother having untreated hypertension is more likely to have a growth retarded infant or is having chance of preterm delivery with the associated risks of placental abruption and fetal hypoxia. Thus, the drug treatment in pregnancy is a situation of complex decisiveness. Drug treatment offers direct benefits to the mother and indirect benefits or potential risk to the embryo/fetus.

The Tragedy of Thalidomide Prescription in Pregnancy

Thalidomide tragedy in early 1960s is a landmark in the drug history. This is the greatest of all drug disasters. Thalidomide had been introduced, and welcomed, as a safe and effective hypnotic and anti-emetic. It rapidly became popular for the treatment of nausea and vomiting in early pregnancy. Tragically, the drug proved to be a potent human teratogen that caused major birth defects in an estimated 10,000 children in the countries in which it was widely used in pregnant women. It is an example of a drug that may profoundly affect the limbs development after only brief exposure. This exposure, however, must be at a critical time in the development of the limbs. The thalidomide induced phocomelia developed during the fourth, through the seventh weeks of gestation because it is during this time that the arms and legs develop. The thalidomide disaster led to the establishment of the drug regulatory mechanisms, of today.

Pathophysiological basis of Drugs Affecting Fetus

Different modalities have been described for the mechanism of action of drugs, leading to potential risks during pregnancy. These include;

- *Directly teratogenic:* They can act directly on the fetus causing damage or abnormal development leading to birth defects or death.

- *Placental function alteration:* They can also, alter the function of the placenta usually by constricting blood vessels and reducing the blood supply of oxygen and nutrients to the fetus, from the mother and thus, resulting in a baby that is underweight and underdeveloped.

- *Changing myometrial activity:* Moreover, they can cause the muscles of the uterus to contract forcefully; indirectly, injuring the fetus by reducing the blood supply or triggering pre-term labor and delivery.

- Altered biochemical & functional dynamics.

Developmental Period In Relation to Effect of Drug

Fetus stage of development is very susceptible to the drug's affect. As, there is inadequate information regarding the effects of drugs in the period of conception and implantation, it is a broad suggestion to all the women wishing to conceive to withdraw all unnecessary medications 3-6 months before conception. The drugs having a long $t_{1/2}$ are going to affect the fetus even if consumed days/months before conception. Drugs taken early in pregnancy (15-21 days after fertilization) during the period of blastogenesis mainly act in an all or nothing fashion i.e., causing termination of the conceptus or not affecting it at all. The next stage between 3rd week and 8th week after fertilization is the time of organogenesis and, embryo is highly vulnerable to congenital malformations by the drugs. Drugs reaching the fetus during this stage may cause a abortion, an obvious birth defect, or a subtle defect, that is perceived later in life. At 9th week the embryo is referred to as a fetus. This phase is primarily attributed to maturation and growth of the fetus. Drugs exposure during this period may alter the growth and function of normally formed organs and tissues. So, in summary;

- < 3 weeks: "all or none" effect
- 3rd to 8th week: True teratogenicity, covert embryopathy
- 9th week to term: Altered growth, biochemical & physiological functions

Key Physiological Changes in Pregnancy and Effect on Pharmacokinetics

Pregnancy is a physiologic process having unique changes in the body that affect the pharmacokinetics of medications, used by pregnant women. Hemodynamic changes during pregnancy include 30-50% increase in blood volume, increase in cardiac output and increase in heart rate by 10-20% and 25% decrease in systemic vascular resistance. Glomerular filtration rate (GFR) increases in similar proportion. This leads to decrease in plasma concentration of the drugs especially, those excreted by kidney. The overall increase in plasma volume contributes to lower circulating concentration of some drugs in a pregnant woman and possibly to sub-therapeutic drug levels. The volume of distribution of fat soluble drugs increases due to increase in body fat during pregnancy. Plasma albumin concentration has apparent decrease during pregnancy and consequently the excretion of unbound drugs is increased by kidney and liver. This is somewhat counterbalanced by the increase in volume of distribution of highly protein bound acidic drugs e.g., anticonvulsants. The increase in alpha-1 acid glycoprotein level leads to increase in protein binding of basic drugs. Progesterone causes decrease in transit time in the gastrointestinal tract, which is more apparent particularly in the third trimester, thus delaying the onset of effect of the drug. In respiratory system, there is increased minute ventilation and greater tendency to pulmonary edema. Increased pro-coagulants (factor VIII, vWF, fibrinogen), decreased protein S leads to increased tendency for coagulation. Insulin resistance, dyslipidemia may be precipitated, sometimes leading to gestational diabetes.

The use of other common medications during pregnancy, such as antacids, iron and vitamins causes binding of some drugs in the gastrointestinal tract. Intramuscular absorption of drug is generally more rapid due to increased blood flow; which enhances systemic drug absorption and the rate of onset of action. High levels of estrogen and progesterone affect hepatic enzyme activity, leading to drug accumulation or decrease elimination of some drugs.

Placental Transfer of Drugs

Placenta acts as a functional barrier and transporter between fetal blood and maternal blood. This performs diverse functions like nutrition, respiration, metabolism, excretion and endocrine activity to maintain fetal and maternal well-being. The teratogenic or pharmacological effects of a drug on the fetus are produced, only after it crosses from maternal circulation to fetal circulation through the placenta by diffusion. The drugs disposition in the fetus and its transfer through placenta are dependent on the physiochemical properties of the drug, such as protein binding, pH difference, lipid solubility and molecular weight of the drug. Only free unbound drug crosses the placenta. As, there is a pH difference exists between fetal (pH 7.2) and maternal (pH 7.4) plasma leading to slightly more acidic nature of fetal plasma. This facilitates the drugs of weak bases to cross the placenta more aptly. Lipid solubility and lower molecular weight

(< 500 g/mol) are the complimentary factors for the passage of drugs through placenta. The increase in molecular weight between 500-1000 g/mol leads to lower permeability of the drugs, while some drugs with a high molecular weight (> 1000 g/mol) cannot cross the placental membrane. However, in the third trimester drug permeability is augmented due to increased maternal and placental blood flow, decreased thickness and increased surface area of the placenta.

Use of Medication during Pregnancy

A variety of chronic diseases and pregnancy linked complications necessitate drug treatment of pregnant women in about 8% subjects worldwide. Many times, medications are consumed by women without the knowledge of being pregnant. A drug other than a vitamin or mineral supplement was prescribed in about 64% of pregnancies, and almost half of pregnant women were on medications without having a safety evidence for use during pregnancy. Dietary herbal supplement are consumed by approximately 13% of pregnant women. Use of drugs, either as prescription or nonprescription (over-the-counter) is seen in more than 90% of pregnant women. Sometimes, even social drugs such as tobacco or alcohol or illicit drugs are found to be taken during pregnancy. Certain drugs might be harmful to the unborn child which is a typical problem in medical treatment of pregnancy. Among, all birth defects about 2-3% are the consequences of drugs usage.

However, treatment of medical ailments in pregnant women and fetus by using the drugs is an essentiality. Vitamins and minerals are the basic requirement of pregnancy. Some common symptoms associated with pregnancy, such as aches and pains, nausea and vomiting, and edema needs drug treatment. Situations having temporal association but not related to pregnancy such as upper respiratory infections, urinary tract infections and gastrointestinal upsets also need to be treated. Pre-existing chronic conditions such as epilepsy, hypertension or psychiatric disorders compels the subject to continue the prescribed medications. Disorders, those are related to pregnancy such as pregnancy induced hypertension, preterm labor with immature lung in the fetus and induction of labor are the requisites for medications.

Teratogenicity

'Teratogen' word was derived from "terato" meaning monster and "gen" to give rise to, so teratogens 'give rise to monsters' (not really). A particular birth defect may have multifactorial etiologies like genetics, environmental agents, medications, physical conditions as well as these are caused by different mechanisms, whereas chemical or drug exposures resulted into a specific pathogenic process with varied outcomes depending upon factors such as embryonic age, duration and dose of exposure and genetic susceptibility. Maternal pharmacokinetics including drug administration, distribution, metabolism, and excretion, may also play as determinants of teratogenicity. Still the mechanistic explanations of the birth defects caused by drug exposures are not fully apprehended. It has been identified that at least six major teratogenic mechanisms are associated with medication use: folate antagonism, neural crest cell disruption, endocrine disruption, oxidative stress, vascular disruption and specific receptor- or enzyme-mediated teratogenesis. Many medications classified as class X are associated with at least one of these mechanisms.

Folate Metabolism Alteration: Elevated plasma homocysteine levels due to disturbances of folate metabolism may not itself cause neural tube defects, but is a biomarker of alteration in the methylation cycle which may result in neural tube defects. Intracellular accumulation of homocysteine results into increased levels of *S*-adenosylhomocysteine, which acts as a competitive inhibitor of many methyltransferases. This leads to perturbations in gene expression, protein function and the lipid and neurotransmitter metabolisms. On the other hand, the decreased remethylation of homocysteine to methionine leads to decreased levels of *S*-adenosylmethionine, which is the most important methyl-group donor in the methylation cycle. This inadequate gene and amino acid methylation results in deranged neural development. Disturbed folate metabolism is thought to have significant causal association with orofacial clefts, limb reduction defects, anal atresia and urinary tract anomalies. There are evidence that folic acid supplementation, alone or in multivitamins have protective effect on the occurrence of these birth defects to some extent, although the evidence is not as strong and consistent as for neural tube defects. Therefore, it is attributed that medication that act as folate antagonists may cause various birth defects through similar mechanisms.

Neural Crest Cell Disruption: Induction, migration, proliferation and differentiation of neural crest cells are programmatically designed process. A variety of molecular signals and receptors are implicated in neural crest cell development. Fibroblast growth factors, integrins, cadherins, endothelins and their receptors and Pax3 are necessary for the fine tuning of the complex developmental process of neural crest cells. It has been observed that drugs that interfere with these pathways, such as bosentan, which is indicated for the treatment of pulmonary hypertension and to reduce new digital ulcers associated with systemic sclerosis, may induce neural crest-related malformations. There are *in vivo* and *in vitro* experiments suggesting that alteration in the levels of folate and/or homocysteine cause abnormalities of cardiac neural crest cell migration. Vitamin A (retinoic acid) homeostasis is necessary for normal development, which is reflected by the neural crest-related malformations seem to be associated with abnormal levels of retinoids. Retinoids used in the treatment of dermatologic conditions, such as tretinoin, isotretinoin and etretinate may also be involved in disturbances of retinoid homeostasis.

Endocrine Disruption and Sex Hormones: The actions of drugs including diethylstilbestrol (DES), oral contraceptives and hormones used in fertility treatment, and other endocrine disrupting chemicals (EDCs), such as bisphenol A and phthalates *in utero* have been of concern because of their possible impact on the developing reproductive systems, especially since treatment of pregnant women with the synthetic estrogen DES led to an increased risk of vaginal adenocarcinoma in their daughters. This can also be explained by the facts that the capability of the placenta to reduce the transfer of estradiol, plasma binding and metabolism of this endogenous hormone to less active estrogens may be important defence mechanisms for the fetus to reduce the actions of estradiol, which are apparently not operational for the synthetic estrogen DES. This affect is not limited to drugs of endocrine systems only. The enteric coatings for oral medications, such as mesalamine and omeprazole, may be a source of EDC exposure, which contain phthalates. This may affect human male reproductive development due to their anti-androgenic properties. But in epidemiologic studies, omeprazole and mesalamine have not been associated with an increased risk of major birth defects.

Male development is more amenable to endocrine disruption than female development because of its hormone dependence. Suppressed testosterone production may result in hypospadias, excess estrogen exposure also suppresses the production of insulin-like factor-3 by fetal Leydig cells. This peptide is responsible for the growth of the gubernaculum, which regulates testicular descent. This signifies the role of estrogen exposure in the induction of hypospadias. On the contrary, epidemiologic studies could not confirm this, since prenatal estrogen exposure, including pharmaceutical estrogens, does not seem to be related to hypospadias and cryptorchidism.

The other proposed mechanisms by which EDCs could affect development of male reproductive systems, include perturbation of the androgen signalling pathway (e.g., suppression of androgen receptor expression), resistance to anti-Mullerian hormone (AMH) and inhibition of enzymes involved in the inactivation of sex steroids. Polycyclic aromatic hydrocarbons and their metabolites have also shown to inhibit the signalling pathways, but their pharmacological mechanism of action has not been completely understood.

Oxidative stress: Wide spectrum of birth defects, including skeletal malformations, limb defects, neural tube defects, cleft lip/palate and cardiovascular defects are correlated to the presence of oxidative stress. Several drugs like thalidomide, phenytoin, valproic acid, class III antiarrhythmic drugs, iron supplements and various chemotherapeutic drugs are known to induce oxidative stress, which is suspected to be their main teratogenic mechanism. Proteratogens including phenytoin are bioactivated by embryonic prostaglandin-H synthases (PHSs) and lipoxygenases (LPOs), which are highly expressed during embryonic and fetal period. This is necessary for the formation of reactive oxygen species (ROS) and subsequent macromolecule damage in the developing embryo.

Vascular Disruption: Blood supply from maternal to fetal circulation is determined by maternal circulation, uterine-placental unit, the placental-fetal unit or the fetus itself. The vascular disturbances in the above units include hyperperfusion, hypoperfusion, hypoxia and obstruction. Exposure to vasoconstrictive substances in pregnancy, could decrease placental or fetal blood flow or affect the development of blood vessels, thereby changing the structure and/or anatomy of the vasculature. Epidemiologic studies have shown that vasoactive therapeutic drugs like misoprostol, aspirin, ergotamine and pseudoephedrine have associations with the vascular disruption defects. The structural anomalies caused by such vascular disruption are determined by the gestation period, the site and severity of tissue damage and the secondary adhesion of necrotic tissue with adjacent organs or the amnion.

Specific Receptor or Enzyme-mediated Teratogenesis: Many medications act through specific receptor or enzyme to produce their effect. Some notable ones are angiotensin-converting enzyme and angiotensin II receptors, hydroxymethylglutaryl-coenzyme A reductase, histone deacetylase, cyclooxygenase-1, N-methyl-D-aspartate receptors, 5-Hydroxytryptamine receptors and transporters, γ-Aminobutyric acid receptors, carbonic anhydrase.

1. **Angiotensin-converting enzyme and angiotensin II receptors:** The two types of angiotensin system modifier drugs commonly used as antihypertensive medications include the angiotensin-converting enzyme (ACE) inhibitors and the AT II receptor antagonists. These may disrupt the fetal rennin-angiotensin system and thereby impair fetal development. The decrease in fetal renal vascular tone may contribute to a human malformation syndrome that is typical for exposure to ACE inhibitors during the second and third trimesters of pregnancy, characterized by renal tubular dysgenesis and oligohydramnios, their sequelae, including limb contractures and pulmonary hypoplasia, and hypocalvaria. The two angiotensin II receptor subtypes, AT_1 and AT_2, are expressed in early development. However, the developmental effects of ACE inhibitors during the first trimester are controversial. A recent study has shown an increased risk of cardiovascular and central nervous system malformations associated with ACE inhibitors. The effects of the less often studied AT II receptor inhibitors are considered to be similar to those of ACE inhibitors.

2. **Hydroxymethylglutaryl-coenzyme A reductase:** Cholesterol is as an essential product of the mevalonate pathway. In embryonic tissues, cholesterol has immense role in the normal growth patterns, synthesis of steroid hormones, signaling domains in plasma membranes and activation of Hedgehog morphogens. Hedgehog proteins are key regulators of embryonic growth, patterning and morphogenesis of many structures. So, down-regulation of the synthesis of these proteins may lead to birth defects. Inhibition of hydroxymethylglutaryl-coenzyme A (HMG-CoA) reductase, the rate-limiting enzyme in the mevalonate pathway by the use of statins may lead to a wide range of disorders. In epidemiologic studies, this has not been proven among pregnant women subjects using lower dose and frequency of statin, however, a recent study could not confirm this hypothesized pattern.

3. **Histone deacetylase:** Histone Deacetylase Inhibitors (HDACIs) are a new class of prospective anticancer agents and have been shown to inhibit migration, invasion, and angiogenesis, and induce differentiation, cell-cycle arrest, and apoptosis in many cancer cell lines. These compounds have shown antitumor activity in animal models

and in patients. Histone deacetylase (HDAC) has essential role in embryonic development, and this has been shown by the HDAC1 knockout mice. However, effects of HDAC inhibition in the pathogenesis of human birth defects are not established. Drugs that inhibit HDACs include vorinostat, valproic acid, trichostatin-A and salicylates. On the other hand, boric acid, an inactive ingredient used in pharmaceutical preparations and as an antibacterial product in non-prescription products, has shown induction of hyperacetylation in somites.

4. **Cyclooxygenase-1:** Cyclooxygenase (COX)-1 has important role in cardiac, midline and diaphragm development. Inhibition of COX-1 by non-selective Non-steroidal anti-inflammatory drugs (NSAIDs) may be involved in the induction of above organ defects. It is also known that, COX-2 is not expressed during embryogenesis in rats, which suggests that COX-2 has least role in NSAID-induced teratogenicity noted in this species. So, these defects were associated with exposure to drugs with a relatively high COX-1/COX-2 ratio in rats and rabbits. Acetylsalicylic acid irreversibly inhibits COX by acetylation, and seems to be associated with a higher incidence of malformations than other NSAIDs in animal studies. It was known that first trimester exposure to NSAIDs did not have significant association with birth defects in humans, but in recent epidemiologic studies an increased risk of orofacial clefts and cardiovascular defects, especially cardiac septal defects have come into picture.

Table 22.1 Examples of some identified teratogenicity

Drug	Trimester	Effect
ACE inhibitors	All, especially 2nd & 3rd	Renal damage
Aminopterin	First	Multiple gross anomalies
Amphetamines	All	Suspected abnormal developmental patterns, decreased school performance
Androgens	2nd & 3rd	Masculinization of female fetus
Antidepressants (Tricyclic)	Third	Neonatal withdrawal symptoms (with clomipramine, desipramine, and imipramine)
Barbiturates	All	Chronic use can lead to neonatal dependence.
Busulfan	All	Various congenital malformations; low birth weight
Carbamazepine	1st	Neural tube defects
Chlorpropamide	All	Prolonged symptomatic neonatal hypoglycemia
Clomipramine	3rd	Neonatal lethargy, hypotonia, cyanosis, hypothermia
Cocaine	All	Spontaneous abortion, abruptio placentae, and premature labor; neonatal cerebral infarction, abnormal growth & development
Cyclophosphamide	First	Various congenital malformations

Table 22.1 *Contd...*

Drug	Trimester	Effect
Cytarabine	1st, 2nd	Various congenital malformations
Diazepam	All	Chronic use may lead to neonatal dependence
Diethylstilbestrol	All	Vaginal adenosis, clear cell vaginal adenocarcinoma
Ethanol	All	Risk of fetal alcohol syndrome and alcohol-related neurodevelopmental defects
Etretinate	All	High risk of multiple congenital malformations
Heroin	All	Chronic use leads to neonatal dependence
Iodide	All	Congenital goiter, hypothyroidism
Isotretinoin	All	High risk of CNS, face, ear, and other malformations
Lithium	First	Ebstein's anomaly
Methadone	All	Chronic use leads to neonatal dependence
Methotrexate	First	Multiple congenital malformations
Methylthiouracil	All	Hypothyroidism
Metronidazole	First	May be mutagenic (from animal studies)
Misoprostol	First	Möbius sequence
Mycophenolate mofetil	First	Malformations of the face, limbs, and other organs
Organic solvents	First	Multiple malformations
Penicillamine	First	Cutis laxa, other congenital malformations
Phencyclidine	All	Abnormal neurologic examination, poor suck reflex and feeding
Phenytoin	All	Fetal hydantoin syndrome
Propylthiouracil	All	Congenital goiter
Smoking	All	IUGR; prematurity; sudden infant death syndrome
Streptomycin	All	Eighth nerve toxicity
Tamoxifen	All	Spontaneous abortion or fetal damage
Tetracycline	All	Discoloration and defects of teeth and altered bone growth
Thalidomide	First	Phocomelia and many internal malformations
Trimethadione	All	Multiple congenital anomalies
Valproic acid	All	Neural tube defects, cardiac and limb malformations
Warfarin	First	Hypoplastic nasal bridge, chondrodysplasia
	Second	CNS malformations
	Third	Risk of bleeding. Discontinue use 1 month before delivery.

Systems of Drug Categories in Pregnancy

Several countries have made the categorization of medications on basis of risk and benefit of their use during pregnancy. Some examples include:

- In 1979, the United States Food and Drug Administration (FDA): A, B, C, D, X category system

- Australian Drug Evaluation Committee (ADEC): A, B1, B2, B3, C, D, X category system
- Germany: G1-11 category system

FDA's First-Generation Regulations for Pregnancy and Lactation Labeling

In 1962, thousands of babies were born in Western Europe with severe limb deformities due to thalidomide disaster in Europe. Thalidomide was marketed as a sleeping pill and was used widely by women of reproductive age. A FDA medical officer, Dr. Frances Kelsey, helped prevent the approval and marketing of thalidomide in the United States. This hazardous consequence becomes an eye-opener for health care providers. Specific requirements for pregnancy, labor and delivery, and nursing mothers were first published by FDA in 1979 (21 CFR 201.57). The 1979 regulations established the 5 pregnancy categories (Table 22.2).

Table 22.2 FDA pregnancy categories

Category	Definition	Examples
A	Adequate and well-controlled (AWC) studies in pregnant women have failed to demonstrate a risk to the fetus in the first trimester of pregnancy (and there is no evidence of a risk in later trimesters).	Thyroid hormones, Folic acid, Prenatal vitamins
B	Animal reproduction studies have failed to demonstrate a risk to the fetus and there are no AWC studies in pregnant women, *or* animal studies demonstrate a risk and AWC studies in pregnant women have not been done during the first trimester (and there is no evidence of risk in later trimesters).	Acetaminophen, Amoxicillin, Loperamide
C	Animal reproduction studies have shown an adverse effect on the fetus, there are no AWC studies in humans, *and* the benefits from the use of the drug in pregnant women may be acceptable despite its potential risks. *Or* animal studies have not been conducted and there are no AWC studies in humans.	Diclofenac, Rifampicin
D	There is positive evidence of human fetal risk based on adverse reaction data from investigational or marketing experience or studies in humans, *but* the potential benefits from the use of the drug in pregnant women may be acceptable despite its potential risks (e.g., if the drug is needed in a life-threatening situation or serious disease for which safer drugs cannot be used or are ineffective).	Paroxetine, Phenytoin, Tetracycline

Table 22.2 *Contd...*

Category	Definition	Examples
X	Studies in animals or humans have demonstrated fetal abnormalities *or* there is positive evidence of fetal risk based on adverse reaction reports from investigational or marketing experience, or both, *and* the risk of the use of the drug in a pregnant woman clearly outweighs any possible benefit (e.g., safer drugs or other forms of therapy are available).	Thalidomide, Finasteride, Isotretinoin, Retinoic acid, Warfarin, Misoprostol, Live vaccines, Iodides, Androgens, Diethylstilbestrol, Antimetabolites

Each category was defined by the presence or absence of data, the source of the data (animal and/or human) and the results of the studies (positive findings or negative). Some categories (D and X) also included consideration of the drug's benefits to the mother as well as the potential risks to the fetus. Based on the category, the regulation described where the information should appear on the label and provided required language and structured sentences to include in the various label sections. The regulation also allowed omission of certain subsections, if there were no data available or if the drug was not systemically absorbed. The *primary goal* of these labeling regulations was to inform counseling between a physician and a patient planning a pregnancy, to provide evidence based, risk/benefit guidance prospectively, before an embryofetal exposure occurred.

Shortcomings

FDA realized that the 1979 labeling regulations for pregnancy and nursing mothers had inconsistencies in practice. Several limitations noted were;

1. The risk/benefit considerations that define categories C, D, and X are not always appreciated by prescribers.
2. Clinicians incorrectly assume that categories imply that drugs in a particular category carry a similar degree of risk for developmental abnormalities in humans.
3. The categories do not distinguish between supporting data from animals and humans.
4. Hard to remember
5. May be misleading
   - Up to 60% of category X drugs have no human data
   - No information on degree of risk
   - A drug may end up in category X, simply if it has no utility in pregnancy
   - Rarely updated

FDA's Second-Generation Pregnancy and Lactation Labeling Regulations: Understanding the Proposed Rule

With development and implementation of the Physician Labeling Rule (PLR), FDA transformed the prescription drug label into a better communication tool in which information is better organized, clearly presented, and more easily located. The Proposed Rule for Pregnancy and Lactation Labeling is the final piece of PLR, creating a detailed and defined framework in which to present and what is not known about the use of drugs during pregnancy and breastfeeding.

Three major informational parts are required for any drugs to be used in the pregnant and lactating subjects under the proposed regulations. These include;

- Summary of the risks involved
- Clinical considerations
- Data

Summary of Proposed Pregnancy Labeling Regulation

Elements	Content
Pregnancy registry statement	If available, contact information for pregnancy registry
Background risk statement	"All pregnancies have a background risk of birth defect, loss, or other adverse outcome regardless of drug exposure. The fetal risk summary below describes (*name of drug(s)*) potential to increase the risk of developmental abnormalities above the background risk."
Fetal risk summary	Based on all available data, this section characterizes the likelihood that the drug increases the risk of developmental abnormalities in humans and other relevant risks. More than 1 risk conclusion may be needed. **For drugs that are systemically absorbed**: • When there are human data, a statement describes the likelihood of increased risk based on this data (framework for statement provided in proposed rule). This statement is followed by a brief description of the findings. • A standard statement describes the likelihood of increased risk based on animal data (not predicted to increase risk, low likelihood, moderate likelihood, high likelihood, or insufficient data). **For drugs that are not systemically absorbed**: • "(*Name of drug*) is not absorbed systemically from (*part of body*) and cannot be detected in the blood. Maternal use is not expected to result in fetal exposure to drug."

Table Contd...

Elements	Content
Clinical considerations	This section provides information on the following topics: • **Inadvertent exposure** (known or predicted risk to the fetus from inadvertent exposure to drug before pregnancy is known) • **Prescribing decisions** for pregnant women: • Describe any known risk to the pregnant woman and fetus from the disease or condition the drug is intended to treat • Information about dosing adjustments during pregnancy • Maternal adverse reactions unique to pregnancy or increased in pregnancy • Effects of dose, timing, and duration of exposure to drug during pregnancy • Potential neonatal complications and needed interventions • **Drug effects during labor and delivery**
Data	Human and animal data are presented separately, with human data presented first. • Describes study type, exposure information (dose, duration, timing), and any identified fetal developmental abnormality or other adverse effects • For human data, includes positive and negative experiences, number of subjects, and duration of study • For animal data, includes species studied and describes doses in terms of human dose equivalents (provide basis for calculation)

Pregnancy Registries

This is the most practical means to collect information on safety and experience during pregnancy.

A Pregnancy Registry means,

- A pregnancy drug exposure follow-up study
- A prospective epidemiologic study that actively collects information on medical product exposure & associated infant outcomes when exposure occurred during pregnancy

Rationality and necessity of Pregnancy Registries:

- Lack of data on birth defects in developing countries
- Large scale deployment of medicines: Malaria, HIV, Leishmaniasis
- High prevalence of other diseases (TB, Malnutrition, parasitic diseases, HIV): exposure to other teratogenic treatments
- Concerns about safety in pregnancy could undermine public confidence in life-saving therapies

Flow chart of steps of pregnancy registries:

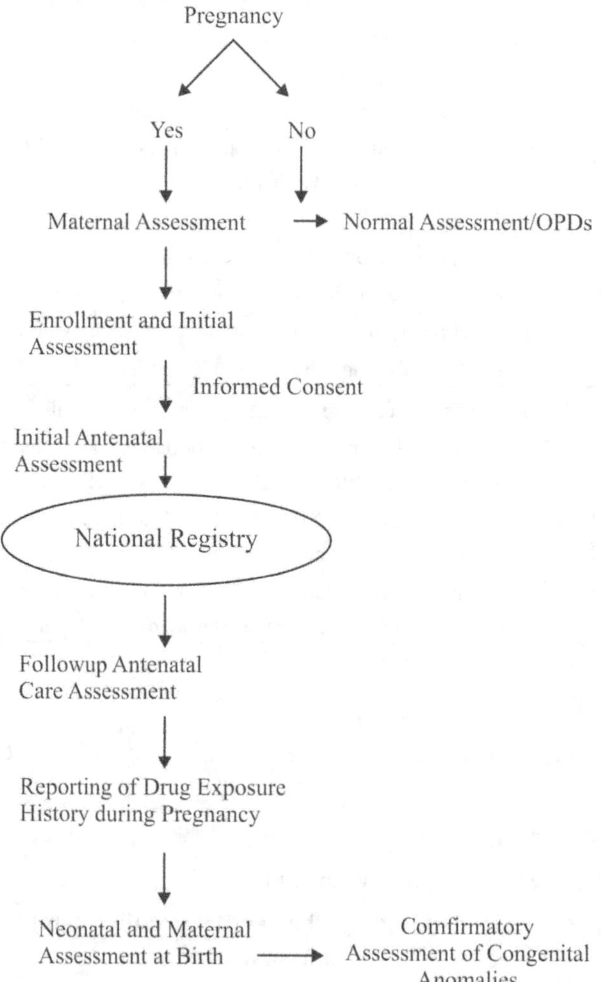

Points to Remember: Safer Mode of Prescribing in Pregnancy

- Do not start any medication unless clearly indicated.
- Do not discontinue medicines that successfully maintain the maternal condition unless there are clear indications to do so.
- Ask about and document non-prescription medications.
- Have a pregnancy medication reference available.
- Use older medicines with longer record of use.

- Check blood levels and consider increased and/or more frequent dosing,
  - Increased volume of distribution, hepatic and renal clearance.
  - Increased production of binding proteins-free drug levels are better.
- Educate and negotiate the patient,
  - Pregnant women more likely to stop needed medications.
- Report adverse outcomes.
- Remember that few drugs are absolutely contraindicated.
- Since the thalidomide disaster, medicine has been practiced as if every drug were a potential human teratogen when, in fact, fewer than 30 such drugs have been identified.
- *Mother risk program*: women need counseling about fetal exposure to drugs, chemicals, and radiation and teratogenic risk.
- Clinicians to provide such counsel must have information up-to-date and evidence-based.
- Risk of a neonatal abnormality in the absence of any known teratogenic exposure is about 3%.

Principles of Diagnostic Imaging

- Little evidence that radiation exposures < 5 rads have significant fetal effects
- NIH consensus statement says that MRI be reserved for 2nd and 3rd trimester if possible, but can be performed in pregnancy

Fetal Therapeutics: An Emerging Area

Maternal administration of

- *Corticosteroids:* To stimulate fetal lung maturation when preterm birth is expected.
- *Phenobarbital:* Near term, can induce fetal hepatic enzymes responsible for the glucuronidation of bilirubin.
- *Phenobarbital:* Means of decreasing the risk of intracranial bleeding in preterm infants. However, large randomized studies failed to confirm this effect.
- Antiarrhythmic drugs for fetal cardiac arrhythmias. Although their efficacy has not yet been established.
- Zidovudine decreases by two thirds transmission of HIV from the mother to the fetus, and use of combinations of three antiretroviral agents can eliminate fetal infection almost entirely.

Conclusion

Research into medication safety during human pregnancy involves ethical considerations. Pregnant and lactating women are usually excluded from clinical trials and results from animal studies need not apply to human population. Hence, choice of medications to be used in pregnant and lactating subjects is a risk covering situation. Most clinicians have a rather restricted approach to the use of drugs during pregnancy. There is fear of causing fetal harm, even death through medication use in pregnancy, which resulted in many confront to clinical research about the safety of drugs in pregnancy. Therefore, major safety aspects of medications in pregnancy are actually obtained through case reports, epidemiological studies and animal studies. However, all of which have limitations, and thus determining risks of a drug use during pregnancy is difficult.

Pregnancy exposure registries, which prospectively monitor the outcomes of pregnancies exposed to certain drugs, can provide some information about major risks associated with use of these medications during pregnancy. However, although the FDA produced guidelines in 2002 for the conduct of these registries and actively promotes their use, pregnancy registries monitor only a small proportion of medications that could be used during pregnancy.

Obstetricians vary in their knowledge about the risks and safety of medications when used during pregnancy, the level of training they receive about the teratogenic potential of medications, the resources, they utilize to obtain information about the effects of medications on the fetus, and their participation in monitoring activities that can generate new information about these effects. There is need for generating accurate and current information about the effects of medications when used during pregnancy. This information should be readily available to health care providers in an updated form. Obstetrician–gynecologists would benefit from improved residency training about the risks and benefits of medication use during pregnancy. Increased awareness of and participation in pregnancy registries that monitor the effects of medication use during pregnancy could provide some of this needed information.

Suggested Readings

1. Andrade SE, Gurwitz JH, Davis RL, Chan KA, Finkelstein JA, Fortman K, McPhillips H, Raebel MA, Roblin D, Smith DH, Yood MU, Morse AN, Platt R (2004). Prescription drug use in pregnancy. *Am J Obstet Gynecol.* **191(2):** 398-407.

2. Bánhidy F, Lowry RB, Czeizel AE (2005). Risk and benefit of drug use during pregnancy. *Int J Med Sci.* **2(3):** 100-6.

3. Bozzo P, Einarson TR, Koren G, Einarson A (2011). Nausea and vomiting of pregnancy (NVP) and depression: cause or effect? *Clin Invest Med.* **34(4):** E245.

4. Carson G, Cox LV, Crane J, Croteau P, Graves L, Kluka S, Koren G, Martel MJ, Midmer D, Nulman I, Poole N, Senikas V, Wood R, Society of Obstetricians and Gynaecologists of Canada (2010). Alcohol use and pregnancy consensus clinical guidelines. *J Obstet Gynaecol Can.* **32(8 Suppl 3)**: S1-31.

5. Djokanovic N, Klieger-Grossmann C, Pupco A, Koren G (2011). Safety of infliximab use during pregnancy. *Reprod Toxicol.* **32(1)**: 93-7.

6. Feibus KB (2008). FDA's proposed rule for pregnancy and lactation labeling: improving maternal child health through well-informed medicine use. *J Med Toxicol.* **4(4)**: 284-8.

7. Katzung Bg, Masters SB, Trevor AJ (2009). Basic and Clinical Pharmacology. 11th Ed. McGraw-Hill.

8. Koren G, Nickel S (2010). Sources of bias in signals of pharmaceutical safety in pregnancy. *Clin Invest Med.* **33(6)**: E349-55.

9. Koren G, Nulman I (2010). Drugs in pregnancy: associations, causation, and misperceptions. *Arch Pediatr Adolesc Med.* **164(5)**: 494-5.

10. Koren G, Pastuszak A, Ito S (1998). Drugs in pregnancy. *N Engl J Med.* **338(16)**: 1128-1137.

11. Koren G, Sarkar M, Einarson A (2010). Safety of using montelukast during pregnancy. *Can Fam Physician.* **56(9)**: 881-2.

12. Koren G (2011). Fetal risks of maternal pharmacotherapy: identifying signals. *Handb Exp Pharmacol.* **205**: 285-94.

13. Koren G (2011). SSRIs in late pregnancy: the risk of neonatal respiratory distress and seizures. *Acta Psychiatr Scand.* **123(4)**: 318.

14. Kraemer K (1997). Placental transfer of drugs. *Neonatal Netw.* **16(2)**: 65-7.

15. Law R, Bozzo P, Koren G, Einarson A (2010). FDA pregnancy risk categories and the CPS: do they help or are they a hindrance? *Can Fam Physician.* **56(3)**: 239-41.

16. Matok I, Levy A, Wiznitzer A, Uziel E, Koren G, Gorodischer R (2012). The Safety of Fetal Exposure to Proton-Pump Inhibitors During Pregnancy. *Dig Dis Sci.* **57(3)**: 699-705.

17. Matok I, Pupco A, Koren G (2011). Drug exposure in pregnancy and heart defects. *J Cardiovasc Pharmacol.* **58(1)**: 20-4.

18. Morgan MA, Cragan JD, Goldenberg RL, Rasmussen SA, Schulkin J (2010). Obstetrician-gynaecologist knowledge of and access to information about the risks of medication use during pregnancy. *J Matern Fetal Neonatal Med.* **23(10)**: 1143-1150.

19. Pupco A, Bozzo P, Koren G (2011). Selective serotonin reuptake inhibitors and risk for major congenital anomalies. *Obstet Gynecol.* **118(4):** 959-60.

20. Sachdeva P, Patel BG, Patel BK (2009). Drug use in pregnancy; a point to ponder! *Indian J Pharm Sci.* **71(1):** 1-7.

21. Van Gelder MM, van Rooij IA, Miller RK, Zielhuis GA, de Jong-van den Berg LT, Roeleveld N. Teratogenic mechanisms of medical drugs. Hum Reprod Update 2010; **16(4):** 378-394.

CHAPTER 23

DRUGS USES IN PEDIATRICS

Introduction

Developments in pediatric clinical pharmacology and pharmacokinetics have markedly improved the rational use of drugs in children. Children are a major part of world population, accounting approximately 29% of world population. Growth of nation is measured through multiple indicators and among them infant mortality rate (IMR) is a crucial one. According to World Fact Book of Central Intelligence Agency, 2010 report infant mortality rate ranges from 1.78 per 1000 live births in that year in Monaco to 178.13 in Angola country. Out of 224 countries surveyed, 57 countries have the rate above 45 with India having IMR rate 49.13. Similarly, mortality in children under 5 years old in 2008 was estimated at 65 per 1000 live births in world.

Clinical management of disease in pediatric patients has seen remarkable progress in the recent past. Important principles of pediatric pharmacotherapy are discussed in this chapter. Pediatric patients, are generally defined as those younger than 18 years, however to be specific, premature means newborn born before 37 weeks of gestational age; neonates means those between 1 day and 1 month of age; infants means 1 month to 1 year age; children means 1 to 11 years age; and adolescents means 12 to 16 years age. The authors have tried to represent with notable examples of subjective differences in pediatrics with reference to pharmacokinetics of drugs, efficacy and toxicity, and multitude factors modifying pediatric pharmacotherapy.

Pros and Cons of 'off-label' Drug use in Pediatrics

Evidence based prescription i.e., clinical trial generated evidence for rational use of medications in pediatric age group constitutes less than 15% of all drugs, currently marketed and less than half of those specifically intended for children. Many medicines are prescribed to the pediatric population on an unlicensed or 'off-label' basis which is most prevalent in complex diseases such as cancer, cardiovascular or renal diseases. In patients admitted into hospital especially in intensive care, 36%-67% of children receive off-label prescriptions. Similarly, among the outpatient prescription off-label use of drugs is seen in 11%-37% of the cases. This wide off-label use can be ascribed to of lack of reliable data in the pediatric population. This is because of inadequate clinical trials in the pediatric population leading to limited availability of pharmacokinetics, pharmaco-dynamics, efficacy, and safety data; inaccurate dosing in pediatric subjects due to the lack of pharmacokinetics or dose-finding studies; unexpected and delayed expressing ADRs in pediatrics; pediatric maturation, growth and development being susceptible to drug-induced alterations.

The use of off-label drugs poses the child to a high risk of adverse reactions. The extemporaneous prescription for pediatrics has significant errors. These errors are dependent upon the age of the subject, the therapeutic area, and the adaptation of simple method to find out pediatric dose from setting and in most cases it is due to the need to adapt. In a very simplistic manner, an adult dose according to the difference in weight and body surface of a child. Quoting the joint, WHO-UNICEF report of 2006: "Children are not small adults when taking a drug". The pharmacokinetics of a drug i.e., absorption, distribution, metabolism and elimination of a drug vary widely between adults and children and is also associated with a continuous change at par with the stage of development. The risks of off-label use of drugs may therefore be due to overdose (increase in adverse reactions), ineffectiveness of the drug (for dosing) and use of a formulation which is not appropriate

According to US surveillance study in 2001, there were 244,000 outpatient visits of children under 15 years of age due to ADRs. The study of NEISS-CADES (National Electronic Surveillance System-Cooperative Adverse Event Surveillance project) incorporated active surveillance of 63 US hospitals and opined, that the incidence of ADRs was equal to 2 out of 1000 people among the under 15 years of age group. Further analysis has shown that younger children are at greatest risk. Half of registered ADRs were seen in the age group less than 4 years. Children under 5 years of age were having 4 times higher risk of ADRs than the children who attend schools (5.8/1000 compared to 1.1/1000). ADRs leading to disasters have been well known. Like, thalidomide associated phocomelia, chloramphenicol induced gray baby syndrome and sulphonamide therapy associated kernicterus. Seal limb deformity is a well defined and evidence based teratogenic effect of thalidomide. Thalidomide also can cause multiple congenital fetal abnormalities including limb deformities, polyneuritis, nerve damage, and mental retardation. This thalidomide disaster brought into regulatory actions related to drug safety in the current medical practice. Chloramphenicol induced gray baby syndrome was first identified in two neonates who died after higher doses of chloramphenicol (100-300 mg/kg/day); and immediately before their death the serum concentrations of chloramphenicol were 75 and 100 mcg/mL. Clinical presentation of patients with gray baby syndrome comprises of abdominal distension, vomiting, diarrhea, a characteristic gray color, respiratory distress, hypotension, and progressive shock. Similarly phenytoin, a widely used antiepileptic has shown to cause teratogenicity like hypoplastic phalanges, cleft lip palate, microcephaly. Isotretinoin is used to treat severe acne vulgaris, a common ailment in girls. This drug is also a potent teratogen leading to craniofacial, heart and CNS defects. Kernicterus was a major problem in neonates receiving sulphonamides treatment. Displacement of bilirubin from protein-binding sites in the blood by sulphonamides can cause hyperbilirubinemia, which results in accumulation of bilirubin in the brain and induces encephalopathy in infants.

Dose calculation in pediatric subject is another potential area for medical error. Often the dose is calculated based on age of the child based on certain crude formulas. Sometimes instead of age child's bodyweight or body surface area is taken into consideration and as a ratio basis the dose is calculated from the adult dose. In applying above functions, the wide difference between the pediatric subject and the adults on the parameters like bioavailability, pharmacokinetics, pharmacodynamics, efficacy, and adverse-effect information are often kept overruled. It is to be noted that differences in age, organ function, and disease state in pediatric subject, than the adult; can have significant impact on the above parameters. So, dosage regimens cannot be simply extrapolated on basis of age, body weight or surface area of a pediatric patient; assuming them as small adults. Though, during the past few years pediatric pharmacokinetics and pharmacodynamics have been the subject of research in many clinical trials, more studies and analysis are the need of the time to obtain the correlation between pediatric pharmacokinetics with the outcomes of efficacy, adverse effects, or quality of life.

A Look into Clinical Studies in Pediatrics

The major force withholding the pharmaceutical industry to develop drugs and derive guidelines on optimal dose calculation for children, apart from a few therapeutic areas, is the marginal profits and are unlikely way to cover the costs of a clinical trial. Because of, the continuous metabolic changes and the maturation of the organ systems, there is need of studies to be carried out in different age groups (newborns, infants, children, adolescents).

The FDA's Pediatric Drug Development page is a great place to find information on pediatric studies. FDA just posted the most recent metrics for studies performed between September 27, 2007 and September 30, 2010 related to the Best Pharmaceuticals for Children Act (BPCA) and the Pediatric Research Equity Act (PREA). During that period, 305 studies including 111,986 patients were completed. Most studies enrolled many fewer patients, typically under 300, except one Rotarix vaccine study enrolled 36,755 patients (more than 30% of the 111,986 patients referenced above). Among these, highest numbers of studies were performed on efficacy and safety accounting about 202 studies. The Food and Drug Administration Amendments Act of 2007 (FDAAA), emphasized the need for transparency in evaluating products in pediatric patients. It required that all pediatric findings be described in the product labeling (package insert), even if the results were negative or inconclusive. As of 21 December 2010, 394 labeling changes had been made based on the pediatric studies performed in response to pediatric legislative initiatives. Under FDAAA, manufacturers are granted of additional 6 months of market exclusivity for pediatric use on submission of pediatric study reports. Applicants are eligible for pediatric usage exclusivity only if the pediatric study reports are submitted to FDA at least nine months prior to the expiration of the product's existing marketing exclusivity.

European Medicines Agency (EMEA) has made laws enforceable from 2007, as well as providing guidelines in order to conduct studies in pediatrics and has established some incentives for pharmaceutical companies, including the extension of one year for the duration of the patent for those products used for experimentation on children. It was reported that researchers found 41% of studies in pediatrics had the potential for bias. This assessment was conducted using the Cochrane Collaboration tool. This tool is used to assess internal validity and the risk of bias directly in studies.

Finally, the need for additional pharmacological or therapeutic research brings up the issue of ethical justification for conducting research. Investigators proposing studies and institutional review committees approving human studies must assess the risk-benefit ratio of each study to be fair to children who are not in a position to accept or reject the opportunity to participate in the research project.

Pharmacokinetics in Pediatrics

Last two decades have seen quite progress in pharmacokinetics research in pediatric patients. Factors those have contributed to this progress are: (a) availability of sensitive and specific analytic methods to measure drugs and their metabolites in small volumes of biologic fluids and (b) increasing application of clinical pharmacokinetics in optimization of drug therapy. Pharmacokinetics of many drugs differs in pediatrics than adults and also varies among different pediatric age groups (premature infants, full-term infants, and older children) due to gradual maturation in enzyme system and receptors. Prescription of many drugs for infants and children are not available in suitable dosage forms. For example, extemporaneous liquid dosage forms (amiodarone, captopril, omeprazole, and spironolactone) are prepared for infants and children who cannot swallow tablets or capsules. Injectable dosage forms of some drugs (aminophylline, methylprednisolone, morphine, and Phenobarbital) are diluted to accurately measure small doses for infants. Dilution or reformulation of dosage forms thus raises questions about the bioavailability, stability, and compatibility of these drugs. Because of low volume of drugs to be administered and limited access to intravenous sites, modified methods must be used for delivery of intravenous drugs to infants and children. Administration of oral drugs to young patients is a difficult task for nurses and parents. Similarly, ensuring compliance and accurate administration of pharmacotherapy in pediatric patients poses a special challenge.

Absorption

Age-Related Trends

Young Infants: Reduced peristalsis with prolonged gastric emptying time.

Neonates: Greater intragastric pH (> 4) relative to infants.

Older Infants: Enhanced lower GI motility.

Pharmacokinetic Implication

Slower rate of drug absorption (e.g., increased T_{max}) without compensatory compromise in the extent of bioavailability.

Clinical Implication

Potential delay in onset of drug action following oral administration. A variety of methods are used to administer drugs to children, the most common of which involve extravascular routes. A therapeutic agent administered by means of any extravascular route must overcome chemical, physical, mechanical, and biologic barriers in order to be absorbed. Developmental changes in absorptive surfaces such as the gastrointestinal tract, skin, and pulmonary tree can influence the rate and extent of the bioavailability of a drug.

A. Gastrointestinal tract

The oral route is the principal means for drug administration to children and therefore the drug absorption part of this review will focus on drug absorption from the gastrointestinal tract. The most important factors that influence drug absorption from the gastrointestinal tract are related to the physiology of the stomach, intestine and biliary tract. The developmental differences in the physiological composition and function of these organs can alter the rate and/or extent of drug absorption.

1. Changes in intraluminal pH can directly impact both drug stability and degree of ionization, thus influencing the relative amount of drug available for absorption. These changes in gastric pH (developmentally or caused by the use of proton pump inhibitors) might result in clinically important changes in the absorption of weak organic acids such as phenobarbital and phenytoin, necessitating adjustment of the amount of antiepileptic drug administered to the individual patient. During the neonatal period, intragastric pH is relatively elevated (greater than 4) consequent to reductions in both basal acid output and the total volume of gastric secretions. Thus, oral administration of acid-labile compounds such as penicillin G, ampicillin and nafcillin produces greater bioavailability in neonates than in older infants and children.

2. Additionally, the ability to solubilize and subsequently absorb lipophilic drugs can be influenced by age-dependent changes in biliary function. Immature conjugation and/or transport of bile salts into the intestinal lumen results in low intraduodenal levels despite blood levels that exceed those of adults.

3. Gastric emptying time is prolonged throughout infancy and childhood consequent to reduced motility that may retard drug passage into the intestine, where the majority of absorption takes place. As a consequence, the rate of absorption of drugs with limited water solubility such as phenytoin and carbamazepine can be significantly altered resulting from these changes in gastrointestinal motility. Similarly, intestinal motor activity matures throughout early infancy, with consequent increases in the frequency, amplitude, and duration of propagating contractions. Unfortunately, few studies have systematically evaluated the effect of these developmental changes on drug absorption in infants and children. The few bioavailability studies that have examined the absorption of drugs (e.g., phenobarbital, sulphonamides, and digoxin) and nutrient macromolecules (e.g., arabinose and xylose) suggest that the processes of both passive and active transport are fully mature in infants by approximately four months of age. Generally, the rate at which most drugs are absorbed is slower in neonates and young infants than in older children; thus, the time required to achieve maximal plasma levels is prolonged in the very young.

4. Although, it is generally assumed that intestinal surface area is reduced in early life, the average intestinal length as a percentage of adult values exceeds other anthropometric measurements throughout development. Villous formation begins at eight weeks of gestation and matures by week 20, rendering it unlikely that reductions in the surface area of the small intestine contribute to reduced absorption. Furthermore, age-associated changes in splanchnic blood flow during the first two to three weeks of life may influence absorption rates by altering the concentration gradient across the intestinal mucosa.

5. Despite their incomplete characterization, developmental differences in the activity of intestinal drug metabolizing enzymes and efflux transporters have the potential to markedly alter drug bioavailability. The duodenal-jejunal biopsy has shown that epoxide hydrolase and glutathione peroxidase activities demonstrate little age dependence, whereas the intestinal activity of cytochrome P-450 1A1 (CYP1A1) appears to increase with age. However, there is decrease in activity of glutathione-S-transferase activity in distal duodenal biopsy from infancy through early adolescence, as reflected by reduced apparent oral clearance of busulfan, a substrate for this enzyme. Little is known about the development and expression of the efflux transporter P-glycoprotein. Changes in the intestinal microflora during infancy are suggested by the finding that the urinary excretion of metabolites such as digoxin reduction products produced by bacterial (enzyme) degradation is age dependent.

B.   **Other extra vascular sites**

1.   **Percutaneous:** Enhanced percutaneous absorption during infancy may be accounted for, in part, by the presence of a thinner stratum corneum in the preterm neonate and by the greater extent of cutaneous perfusion and hydration of the epidermis (relative to adults) throughout childhood. The ratio of total body surface area to body mass in infants and young children far exceeds that in adults. Thus, the relative systemic exposure of infants and children to topically applied drugs (e.g., corticosteroids, antihistamines, and antiseptics) may exceed that in adults, with consequent toxic effects in some instances. The increased exposure can produce toxic effects after topical use of hexachlorophene soaps and powders, salicylic acid ointment, and rubbing alcohol. Interestingly, a study has shown that a therapeutic serum concentration of theophylline can be achieved for control of apnea in premature infants less than 30 weeks' gestation after topical application of gel containing a standard dose of theophylline. A transdermal patch formulation of methylphenidate has been approved for use in children 6 to 12 years of age for treatment of attention deficit hyperactivity disorder (ADHD). The patch can be applied once daily and can remain on during normal activities such as bathing, swimming, and exercising.

2.   **Intramuscular:** Reduced skeletal-muscle blood flow and inefficient muscular contractions (responsible for drug dispersion) may reduce the rate of intramuscular absorption of drugs in neonates. However, the influence of these factors on bioavailability may be off-set by the relatively higher density of skeletal-muscle capillaries in infants than in older children. Accordingly, evidence supports the concept that intramuscular absorption of specific agents (e.g., amikacin and cephalothin) is more efficient in neonates and infants than in older children. Phenobarbital has been reported to be absorbed rapidly, whereas diazepam absorption may be delayed. Thus, intramuscular dosing is used rarely in neonates except in emergencies or when an intravenous site is inaccessible.

3.   **Rectal:** The bioavailability of extensively metabolized compounds administered rectally may be enhanced in neonates and very young infants, most likely owing to the developmental immaturity of hepatic metabolism rather than to enhanced mucosal translocation. However, infants have a greater number of high-amplitude pulsatile contractions in the rectum than do adults, which can enhance the expulsion of solid forms of drugs, effectively decreasing the absorption of drugs such as erythromycin and acetaminophen.

4.   **Inhalation:** Intrapulmonary administration of drugs (inhalation) is increasingly being used in infants and children. Although the principal goal of this route of administration is to achieve a predominantly local effect, systemic exposure does occur, as evidenced by the suppression of cortisol that

occurs in association with inhaled corticosteroid therapy. Developmental changes in the architecture of the lung and its ventilatory capacity (e.g., minute ventilation, vital capacity, and the respiratory rate) most likely alter the patterns of drug deposition and consequent systemic absorption after the intrapulmonary administration of a drug. Unfortunately, current investigations have focused on the effects that either the device or the formulation has on the delivery and deposition of inhaled drugs rather than on the rate and extent of their pulmonary absorption.

Distribution

Age-Related Trends

Young infants have decreased fat, decreased muscle mass, increased extracellular and total body water spaces.

Pharmacokinetic Implication

Increased apparent volume of distribution for drugs distributed to body water spaces.

Clinical Implication

Requirement of higher weight-normalized (i.e., mg/kg) drug doses to achieve therapeutic plasma drug concentrations.

Drug distribution is influenced by a variety of drug-specific physiochemical factors (pKa, molecular weight, partition coefficient) and physiologic factors specific to the patient including the role of drug transporters, blood/tissue protein binding, blood, and tissue pH and perfusion. However, age-related changes in drug distribution are primarily related to developmental changes in body composition and the quantity of plasma proteins capable of drug binding. Age-dependent changes in body composition alter the physiological ''spaces'' into which a drug may distributed.

1. **Extracellular fluid:** Several factors lead to lower plasma concentrations for hydrophilic drugs as neonates and young infants have comparatively larger extracellular space and total body water, coupled with adipose stores that have a higher water/lipid ratio than in adults. As a percentage of total body weight, total body water comprises of 94% in fetuses, 85% in premature infants, 78% in full-term infants, and 60% in adults. Extracellular fluid volume also is markedly different in premature infants compared with older children and adults. The extracellular fluid volume (as percentage of body weight) varies widely in different age groups as 50% in premature infants, 35% in 4 to 6 months old infants, 25% in children less than 1 year old, and 19% in adults. This has been reflected from observed gentamicin distribution volumes of 0.48 L/kg in neonates and 0.20 L/kg in adults. It has also been observed that the distribution volume of tobramycin is largest in premature infants and has a downward trend with increases in gestational age and birth weight of the infant.

2. **Plasma protein and drug binding:** The extent of drug binding to proteins in the plasma may influence the volume of distribution of drugs. The freely circulating unbound part of drug gets passage from the vascular space into other body fluids and, thereby drugs tissue distribution occurs. The portion of drug which is in bound form in plasma is mainly associated with plasma proteins. The significant contribution among plasma proteins is from albumin and globulins such as alpha-1-acid-glycoprotein. Several factors influence these proteins concentrations in the body e.g., age, nutrition, and disease. In case of highly protein bound drugs, alteration in the composition and amount of the circulating plasma proteins can have significant effect, as the free part of drug may get manifold concentration. The presence of fetal albumin (which has reduced binding affinity for weak acids) and an increase in endogenous substances (e.g., bilirubin and free fatty acids) capable of displacing a drug from albumin binding sites during the neonatal period may also contribute to the higher free fractions of highly protein-bound drugs in neonates. A reduction in the quantity of total plasma proteins in the neonate and young infant increases the free fraction of drug, thereby influencing the availability of the active moiety.

3. **Adipose tissue distribution:** The influence of age on the apparent volume of distribution is not as readily apparent for lipophilic drugs that are primarily distributed in tissue. However, for drugs having gradual redistribution from adipose tissue to systemic circulation, the quantity of adipose tissue could have significant effect. In case of neonates, there is substantially low amount of body fat than in adults, which may affect drug therapy. As for example, highly lipid-soluble drugs like diazepam are distributed less widely in infants (apparent volume of distribution ranged from 1.4 to 1.8 L/kg) than in adults (apparent volume of distribution ranged from 2.2 to 2.6 L/kg).

4. **Drugs through breast milk:** There is chance for certain drugs to be channelized from the breast milk of lactating mother to the child. So, indirectly the child gets exposed to the drugs, which are taken by the mother. The American Academy of Pediatrics have enlisted number of drugs which may pose problems for the infants, if taken during lactation such as bromocriptine, ergotamine, lithium, anticancer medications (e.g., cyclophosphamide, cyclosporine, doxorubicin, methotrexate) and all drugs of abuse [e.g., amphetamine, cocaine, heroin, marijuana, and phencyclidine (PCP)]. The risk of passage through breast milk has also been seen in case of nuclear medicines and radio-contrast dye. It has been observed that some drugs upon prolonged period use by the mother, may also possess adverse effects among the nursing infant, such as acebutolol, aspirin, atenolol, clemastine, phenobarbital, primidone, sulfasalazine, and 5-aminosalicylic acid have. So, it is recommended that mother should avoid using any drug during pregnancy and while breast-feeding, unless the benefits of using medication outweigh the risks associated with.

5. **Drug transporters:** ATP binding proteins such as P-glycoprotein can influence drug distribution because these transporters can markedly influence the extent to which drugs cross membranes in the body and whether drugs can penetrate or are secreted from the target sites. Thus, drug resistance to antibiotics or epilepsy may be dependent on these drug transporters and their effect on drug distribution. A single study of the expression of P-glycoprotein in the central nervous system in tissue obtained post mortem from neonates born at 23 to 42 weeks of gestational age suggests a pattern of localization similar to that in adults late in gestation and at term. However, the level of expression of P-glycoprotein appeared to be lower than that in adults.

6. Other factors associated with development and/or disease such as variability in regional blood flow, organ perfusion, permeability of cell membranes, changes in acid-base balance and cardiac output can also influence drug binding and/or distribution.

Drug Metabolism

Age-Related Trends

Young Infants: Immature isoforms of cytochrome P-450 and phase II enzymes with discordant patterns of developmental expression.

Children 1-6 yr: Apparent increased activity for selected drug metabolizing enzymes (DME) over adult normal values.

Adolescents: Attainment of adult activity after puberty.

Pharmacokinetic Implication

Young Infants: Decreased plasma drug clearance early in life with an increase in apparent elimination half life.

Children 1-6 yr: Increased plasma drug clearance (i.e., reduced elimination half life) for specific pharmacologic substrates of DMEs.

Clinical Implication

Young Infants: Increased drug dosing intervals and/or reduced maintenance doses.

Children 1-6 yr: For selected drugs, need to increase dose and/or shorten dose interval in comparison to usual adult dose.

Expression of several Phase I and Phase II drug metabolizing enzymes involved in drug biotransformation are considerably modified during fetal development. According to Dotta and Chukhlantseva (2012) drug metabolizing enzyme system undergoes three main categories of developmental stages, as follows;

(a) Enzymes expression in peak during whole or part of fetal period, but being silenced or expressed at low levels within 1-2 years after birth, for examples:

CYP3A7, Flavin-containing monooxygenase-1 (FMO1), sulphotransferase-1A3/4 (SULT1A3/4), SULT1E1, and maybe alcohol dehydrogenase-1A (ADH1A).

(b) Enzyme expression steady during whole fetal period, and postnatal, there is increase in their expression, for examples: CYP2A6, 3A5, 2C9, 2C19, 2D6, 2E1, and SULT1A1.

(c) Enzyme expression initiated in the third trimester, and substantial increase in their expression occurs within the first 1-2 years after birth, for examples: ADH1C, ADH1B, CYP1A1, 1A2, 2A 6, 2A7, 2B6, 2B7, 2C8, 2C9, 2F1, 3A4, FMO3, SULT2A1, glucuronosyltransferases (UGT), and N-acetyltransferase.

Drug metabolism is substantially slower in infants than in older children and adults. Distinct patterns of isoform-specific developmental changes in the biotransformation of drugs are apparent for many Phase I (primarily oxidation) and Phase II (conjugation) drug-metabolizing enzymes. (Table 23.1) Selected examples are summarized below.

Table 23.1 Major pathways of drug elimination

Pathway	Incidence (%)
Renal excretion (unchanged drug)	25
Cytochrome P450 metabolism	
CYP3A4	30
CYP2D6	20
CYP2C9/CYP2C19	10
UDP glucuronosyltransferase (UGT)	10
Other	5

A.   Phase I metabolism

Distinct patterns of isoform-specific developmental expression of cytochrome P450 isozymes (CYPs) have been observed postnatally. Within hours after birth, CYP2E1 activity surges, and CYP2D6 becomes detectable soon thereafter. CYP3A4 and CYP2C (CYP2C9 and CYP2C19) appear during the first week of life, whereas CYP1A2 is the last hepatic CYP to appear, at one to three months of life. Metabolism of drugs such as theophylline, phenobarbital, and phenytoin by oxidation also is impaired in newborn infants. However, the rate of metabolism is more rapid with phenobarbital and phenytoin, than with theophylline, perhaps because of the involvement of different cytochrome P450 isozymes. Thus, a child with asthma often requires markedly higher doses on a weight basis of theophylline compared with an adult. Because of, decreased metabolism, doses of drugs such as theophylline, phenobarbital, phenytoin, and diazepam should be decreased in premature infants.

CYP3A4: The slope of decreasing or increasing activity, respectively, can vary substantially for each enzyme. Also, in the level of activity large variations are noted. As such, the CYP3A4 activity in the first 2 to 3 years of life can even exceed adult levels. Midazolam undergoes biotransformation through CYP3A4/5 and its plasma clearance after intravenous administration is about five times more (1.2 to 9 ml/min/kg), over the first three months of life. Similarly, another drug i.e., carbamazepine, which is primarily degraded by CYP3A4, has greater plasma clearance in children relative to adults. This is the reason for higher mg/kg doses administration of the drug in children to produce therapeutic plasma concentration.

CYP2D6: Psychotropic medications like nortriptyline can develop suboptimal, therapeutic, or potentially toxic concentrations, depending on the individual's rate of drug metabolism. The CYP2D6 gene locus is highly polymorphic with more than 75 allelic variants identified. Consequently, poor (PM), intermediate (IM), extensive (EM) and ultrarapid (UM) metabolizer phenotypes are observed. Inheritance of two recessive loss-of-function alleles result in the "poor-metabolizer phenotype", which is found in about 5-10% of Caucasians and about 1-2% of Asian subjects. At the other end of the spectrum, in 1-2% in Caucasians the presence of CYP2D6 gene duplication/multiplication events is most often associated with enhanced clearance of CYP2D6 substrates and sometimes, leads to toxicity due to increased formation of pharmacologically active metabolites. Finally, although the CYP2D6 activity does not appear to change significantly after infants reached a postmenstrual age of 42 weeks, the activity might still change due to inhibitors of CYP2D6. Inhibitors that are well recognized are the selective serotonin reuptake inhibitors (SSRIs). Paroxetine and fluoxetine are potent inhibitors of CYP2D6 whereas, fluvoxamine and venlafaxine are not. For a clinical standpoint, it is advisable to use low doses when prescribing CYP2D6 substrates in patients taking CYP2D6 inhibitors.

CYP2C9: Total clearance of phenytoin by CYP2C9 and, to a lesser extent, by CYP2C19 surpasses adult values by 2 weeks of age. Phenytoin apparent half life is prolonged (~75 hour) in preterm infants but decreases to ~20 hr in term infants less than one week postnatal age and to ~8 hr after two weeks of age. Saturable phenytoin metabolism does not appear until approximately 10 days of postnatal age, demonstrating the developmental acquisition of CYP2C9 activity. The clearance of unbound S-warfarin, a substrate of CYP2C9, was substantially greater in prepubertal children than among pubertal children and adults even after adjustment for total body weight.

CYP1A2: Theophylline clearance is not fully developed for 4 to 5 months. Two additional observations about theophylline metabolism by CYP1A2 in pediatric patients should be noted. First, in premature infants receiving theophylline for treatment of apnea, a significant amount of its active metabolite caffeine may be present, unlike the case in older children and adults. Second, theophylline clearance in children 1 to 9 years of age exceeds, the values in infants as well as adults. Clearance of caffeine, metabolized by demethylation (mediated by CYP1A2), declines to adult values when girls reach Tanner stage II (early puberty) and boys reach Tanner stages IV and V (late puberty), this represents sex difference in the ontogeny of CYP1A2.

CYP3A7: CYP3A7, the predominant CYP isoform expressed in fetal liver, may protect the fetus by detoxifying dehydroepiandrosterone sulfate and potentially teratogenic derivatives of retinoic acid. The expression of CYP3A7 peaks shortly after birth and then declines rapidly to level that are undetectable in most adults.

B.   Phase II metabolism

The ontogeny of conjugation reactions (i.e., those involving phase II enzymes) is less well established than the ontogeny of reactions involving phase I enzymes.

Glucuronidation (glucuronyltransferases): According to available data, the sulphation pathway is well developed but the glucuronidation pathway is undeveloped in infants. Although acetaminophen metabolism by glucuronidation is impaired in infants compared with adults, it is partly compensated for by the sulfation pathway. The cause of the tragic chloramphenicol- induced gray baby syndrome in newborn infants is decreased metabolism of chloramphenicol by glucuronyltransferases to the inactive glucuronide metabolite. This metabolic pathway appears to be age related and may take several months to 1 year to develop fully, as evidenced by the increase in clearance with age up to 1 year. Interestingly, higher serum concentrations of morphine are required to achieve efficacy in premature infants than in adults, in part because infants are not able to metabolize morphine adequately to its 6-glucuronide metabolite (20 times more active than morphine). This is balanced to some degree by the fact that the clearance of morphine quadruples between 27 and 40 weeks of postconceptional age.

Methylation (Thiopurine methyltransferase): The knowledge of pharmaco-genetics and pharmacogenomics now is being applied to patient care in some instances. 6-Mercaptopurine (6-MP), a drug commonly used in pediatric leukemias, undergoes catabolism that is facilitated by thiopurine methyltransferase (TPMT). The inherited deficiency (an autosomal recessive trait), which occurs in 6% to 11% of patients, is primarily explained by three polymorphisms in the TPMT gene (*2, *3A, and *3C). Children homozygous for one of the variant alleles require 6-MP dose reduction of approximately 90%, and heterozygotic children need a dose reduction of approximately 50% to achieve survival rates observed in patients receiving full doses in the absence of TPMT deficiency. Thus, TPMT screening is recommended to identify patients with genotypes associated with TPMT deficiency that may benefit from dose reductions to prevent toxicity.

Elimination of Drugs

Maturation of renal function is a dynamic process that begins during fetal organogenesis and is complete by early childhood. The developmental increase in the glomerular filtration rate relies on the existence of normal nephrogenesis, a process that begins at 9 weeks of gestation and is complete by 36 weeks of gestation, followed by postnatal changes in renal and intrarenal blood flow. The glomerular filtration rate is approximately 2 to 4 ml per minute per 1.73 m^2 in term neonates, but it may be as low as 0.6 to 0.8 ml per minute per 1.73 m^2 in preterm neonates. The glomerular filtration rate rises rapidly during the first two weeks of life and then increases steadily until adult values are reached at 8 to 12 months of age.

Similarly, tubular secretion is immature at birth and reaches adult capacity during the first year of life. Collectively, developmental changes in renal function can dramatically alter the plasma clearance of compounds with extensive renal elimination and thus, constitute a major determinant of the age appropriate selection of a dose regimen. Pharmacokinetic studies of drugs such as ceftazidime and famotidine, which are excreted primarily by the glomeruli, have shown correlations between plasma drug clearance and normal maturational changes in renal function. For example, tobramycin is eliminated predominantly by glomerular filtration, necessitating dosing intervals of 36 to 48 hours in preterm newborns and of 24 hours in term newborns. Failure to account for the ontogeny of renal function and to adjust aminoglycoside dosing regimens accordingly can result in the exposure of infants to potentially toxic serum levels of these drugs. Because of, immature renal elimination, chloramphenicol succinate can accumulate in premature infants. Although, chloramphenicol succinate is inactive, this accumulation may be the reason for an increased bioavailability of chloramphenicol in premature infants compared with older children. Furthermore, concomitant administration of medications such as betamethasone and indomethacin may alter the normal pattern of renal maturation in neonates.

Thus, for drugs with extensive renal elimination, both maturational and treatment associated changes in kidney function must be considered and used to individualize treatment regimens in an age-appropriate fashion.

Pharmacodynamics of Drugs in Pediatrics

Pathophysiologic and pharmacodynamic differences between children and adults are numerous. Clinical presentation of chronic asthma differs as children present almost exclusively with a reversible extrinsic type of asthma, whereas adults have nonspecific, non atopic bronchial irritability. This explains the value of adjunctive hypo sensitization therapy in the management of pediatric patients with extrinsic asthma. Although, it is generally accepted that development can alter the action of and response to a drug, little information exists about the effect of human ontogeny on interactions between drugs and receptors and the consequence of these interactions (i.e., the pharmacodynamics). For example, the apparent developmental differences in the pharmacodynamics of famotidine in neonates are directly associated with the reduced plasma clearance of the drug owing to the developmentally dependent reductions in the glomerular filtration rate. However, data on certain other drugs appear to support the existence of true age-dependent differences either in the interaction between a drug and its specific receptor (e.g., warfarin and cyclosporine) or in the relation between the plasma level and the pharmacologic effect of a given drug (e.g., sedation associated with midazolam).

Drug receptor binding affinity is variable in children and adults. For example, digoxin necessitates higher maintenance dose administration in infants than in adults, because of, lower binding affinity of Na^+-K^+ ATPase receptors in the myocardium for digoxin and increased entrapment of digoxin by neonatal erythrocytes compared with adult erythrocytes. Owing to rapid growth during adolescence, insulin requirement increases substantially than old age patients. Recent evidence of the age-dependent expression of intestinal motilin receptors and the modulation of antral contractions appears to have implications with respect to the prokinetic effects of erythromycin in preterm infants. Clearly, any assessment of pharmacodynamics in children must take into consideration the influence of ontogeny on the efficacy or safety of a given drug with respect to age-dependent differences.

Adverse Effects of Drug Specific to Pediatric Use

Apparent pharmacogenetic determinants of the action of a drug may contribute to the age-dependent differences in the response to treatment of children with certain well-defined diseases (e.g., asthma and leukemia) and to the likelihood of severe adverse events (e.g., the hepatotoxicity of valproic acid is increased in young infants). Promethazine now is contraindicated for use in children younger than 2 years because of the risk of severe respiratory depression. Chloramphenicol toxicity is increased in newborns because of immature metabolism and enhanced bioavailability. Similarly, propylene glycol, which is added to many injectable drugs, including phenytoin, phenobarbital, digoxin, diazepam, vitamin D, and hydralazine, to increase their stability, can cause hyperosmolality in infants. Benzyl alcohol was a popular preservative used in intravascular flush solutions until a syndrome of metabolic acidosis, seizures, neurologic deterioration, gasping respirations, hepatic and renal abnormalities, cardiovascular collapse, and death was described in premature infants. A decline in both mortality and the incidence of major intraventricular hemorrhage was documented after use of solutions containing benzyl alcohol was stopped in low-birth-weight infants. Tetracyclines are contraindicated for use in pregnant women, nursing mothers, and children younger than 8 years because these drugs can cause dental staining and defects in enamelization of deciduous and permanent teeth, as well as a decrease in bone growth. However, the Centers for Disease Control and Prevention has recommended the use of doxycycline for initial prophylaxis following suspected bioterrorism related exposure to *Bacillus anthracis* (anthrax); the potential benefits outweigh potential risks among infants and children. Similarly, quinolones cause growth retardation in children.

Some drugs may be less toxic in pediatric patients than in adults. Aminoglycosides appear to be less toxic in infants than in adults. In adults, aminoglycoside toxicity is related to both peripheral compartment accumulation and the individual patient's inherent sensitivity to these tissue concentrations. Although, neonatal peripheral tissue compartments for gentamicin have been reported to closely resemble those of adults with similar renal function, gentamicin rarely is nephrotoxic in infants. This dissimilarity in the incidence of nephrotoxicity implies that newborn infants have less inherent tissue sensitivity for toxicity, than do adults. This finding emphasizes the need for identifying specific indications for the effective and safe use of drugs in pediatric patients.

Pre-marketing trials are able to provide information about the benefits of drugs, but do not manage to establish a safety profile. Therefore, spontaneous reporting of suspected ADRs becomes an important means to promote reasonable warning signs: from the description of a few cases, significant regulatory actions may derive in order to protect pediatric age groups. The reports are verified and compared with data from reports presented in international networks like national ADR monitoring centers or international centers like WHO UMC (Uppsala Monitoring Centers). In order to complete, the safety profile of a drug it is necessary to carry out post-marketing epidemiological studies aimed at a long-term recovery of all the events that occur during monitoring. The primary objective of a good pharmacovigilance activity is the definition of the risk/benefit ratio. For a more precise and consistent verification of this report there are continuous investments in key inputs, and there is the contribution of a careful and continuous scientific evaluation of what are called "weak signals". Greater the transparency and simplification of procedures in the pharmacovigilance field, the greater the hope of positive benefits in terms of public health and improved safety.

Dosage Regimen for Pediatrics

Dosing regimens commonly used for pediatrics are based on age dependent differences in drug disposition. Many drugs have quite differences in the dose and the dosing interval used in children and those used in adults. The most reliable pediatric dose information is usually that provided by the manufacturer in the package insert. However, such information is not available for the majority of products. Recently, the FDA has moved toward more explicit expectations that manufacturers test their new products in infants and children. Still, most drugs in the common formularies, e.g., National Formulary and Physicians' Desk Reference, are not specifically approved for children.

Most drugs approved for use in children have recommended pediatric doses, generally stated as milligrams per kilogram or per pound body weight. In the absence of explicit pediatric dose recommendations, an approximation can be made by any of several methods based on age, weight, or surface area. These rules are not precise and should not be used if the manufacturer provides a pediatric dose. The pediatric dose should never exceed the adult dose.

Children

Age (Young's rule):

Dose = Adult dose × [Age in years/(Age + 12)]

Weight (somewhat more precise is Clark's rule):

Dose = Adult dose × (weight in Kg/70)

or

Dose = Adult dose × (weight in lb/150)

Calculations of dosage based on age or weight are conservative and tend to underestimate the required dose. Doses based on surface area are more likely to be adequate (Table 23.2).

Dose = Adult dose × (Surface area in m^2/1.76)

Table 23.2 Approximate weight and body surface area

Age	Weight (Kg)	Surface area (m^2)
Newborn	3	0.2
3 months	6	0.3
1 year	10	0.45
5.5 year	20	0.8
9 years	30	1
12 years	40	1.3
14 years	50	1.5
Adult	60	1.7
Adult	70	1.76

Infants

In the absence of complete pharmacokinetic data or established dosing guidelines, a method to approximate the initial dose for an infant on the basis of the established dose for adults has been proposed that uses descriptors of body size, such as ideal body weight adjusted for height, body-surface area, and the apparent volume of distribution. This method is illustrated by the following equations,

Infant dose if volume of distribution is < 0.3 liter per kilogram = infant's body surface area (in square meters ÷ 1.73 m^2) × the adult dose and

Infant dose if volume of distribution (determined from the literature) is ≥ 0.3 liter per kilogram = infant's body weight (in kilograms $\div$ 70 kg) $\times$ the adult dose.

Neonates

1. In neonates, age is primarily considered variable. It is calculated as gestational age (GA, weeks) is the weeks of pregnancy at birth, postnatal age (PNA, days) are the days since birth, postmenstrual age (PMA, weeks) are the weeks of pregnancy + the postnatal weeks since birth.

2. Besides age size is most relevant variable. While body weight (/kg) is used most commonly in the clinical setting, it is recognized that there is a non-linear relationship between weight and metabolism.

3. Body surface area ($/m^2$) was subsequently proposed

4. An allometric power model ($kg^{0.75}$) might be an even more appropriate scaling because of the observation of a linear relationship between the logarithm of basal metabolic rate and weight with of slope of 0.75. This allometric $kg^{0.75}$ power model may be used to scale metabolic drug clearance. This has recently been documented for propofol clearance.

Therapeutic Drug Monitoring (TDM)

Therapeutic Drug Monitoring (TDM) focuses on achieving and maintaining a drug concentration within a therapeutic range. Even within the therapeutic range, however, some patients do not achieve the expected pharmacologic effect, and others experience toxic adverse effects. In general, TDM samples should be drawn at "steady state" serum concentrations. TDM is indicated for drugs having narrow therapeutic range, wide interindividual variability, pharmacogenetic variation, no significant clinical indicator to measure efficacy, both sub and supra therapeutic range will have devastating results.

In pediatric subjects, the drugs require TDM are theophylline, aminoglycosides, immunosupressants (cyclosporine, tacrolimus, sirolimus, mycophenolate mofetil), antiepileptics (Carbamazepine, Valproic acid, Phenobarbitone, Phenytoin), anticancer drugs (6 mercaptopurine, irinotecan, 5-fluorouracil) and for digoxin when the desired therapeutic effects are not observed after administration of a standard dose.

It is not needed for drugs having wide therapeutic range like penicillins, benzodiazepines, vitamins and antiulcer drugs. Not all drugs can be monitored by plasma concentrations. For example, diazepam metabolites manifest a large proportion of the desired pharmacologic effect but cannot be monitored effectively by measuring the parent drug. Similar problems are encountered with drugs that are comprised of a mixture of enantiomers, one of which is significantly more active. For many other drugs (e.g., antidepressants, certain sedatives), there is no direct correlation between serum concentrations and effect.

Drug Interactions

Drug interactions can occur at every pharmacokinetic stage. Prior or concomitant administration of another drug leads to modification of the magnitude or duration of action of one drug (index drug). Only limited data are available regarding the influence of immature enzyme systems on drug interactions in infants and young children, due partly to obvious ethical and practical issues. Also, it rarely is feasible to distinguish drug interactions from other coexisting factors, such as disease processes and environmental factors (e.g., diet). Some of these drug interactions are described below.

1. Drug interactions in the gastrointestinal tract may decrease the oral bioavailability of the index drug. Absorption of many drugs such as cephalosporins and fluoroquinolones can be impaired significantly by concomitant oral administration of calcium, magnesium, iron, or aluminum compounds.

2. The hepatic enzyme system is the key field of drug interaction due to induction and inhibition effects of large number of drugs. Commonly prescribed medications in children, such as erythromycin, ciprofloxacin, cimetidine, and omeprazole, have inhibitory effects on hepatic enzymatic systems, reducing the metabolism of drugs such as theophylline, codeine, beta blockers, antidepressants, corticosteroids, warfarin, and metronidazole. In such cases, toxicity may occur. In contrast, rifampin, phenobarbital, carbamazepine, and phenytoin are potent enzymatic inducers that increase the metabolism of other drugs metabolized by the liver, decreasing their plasma concentration and effect. In this case, the dose of the index drug may need to be increased.

3. Renal elimination may be decreased by concomitant administration of medications, especially for drugs that are actively excreted by the tubule. For example, salicylates can inhibit tubular secretion of methotrexate, leading to toxicity.

Role of Developmental Pharmacologist

The increasing knowledge concerning pharmacotherapy in relation to translational science (use of microarrays, DNA-chips, and biomarkers) results in situation where the integration of this new knowledge into daily pharmacotherapy is getting more and more complicated. Based on patient-specific information there is a continuous search for an optimal balance between the safety and efficacy of the pharmacological treatment. In addition, developmental pharmacologists have a seat in committees dedicated to the optimal use of medication in many health care institutions because of their specific expertise. Many times they chair these pivotal committees being the expert in pharmacotherapy. In addition they often are also chairing committees determining which drugs should be on the National Essential Medicines List and Drug Formulary and which ones not. There is clearly a need to initiate clinics in Developmental Pharmacology where patients treated with several medications (polypharmacy), patients with (severe) adverse medication events, and patients who will need pharmacogenetic consultation can be seen and supported. There are several major areas of research that ultimately will improve the patient care and the educational activities in the field of developmental pharmacology and the major ones are pharmacogenetics, population pharmacokinetics, and therapeutic drug monitoring.

Suggested Readings

1. Allegaert K, de Hoon J, Naulaers G, Van De Velde M (2008). Neonatal clinical pharmacology: recent observations of relevance for anaesthesiologists. *Acta Anaesthesiol Belg.* **59(4)**: 283-8.

2. Available at: http://www.emaxhealth.com/3275/researcher-details-biases-pediatric-studies-good

3. Available at: http://www.fda.gov/downloads/Drugs/DevelopmentApprovalProcess/DevelopmentResources/UCM049870.pdf

4. Available at: http://www.fda.gov/downloads/ScienceResearch/SpecialTopics/PediatricTherapeuticsResearch/UCM163159.pdf

5. Available at: http://www.fda.gov/Drugs/DevelopmentApprovalProcess/DevelopmentResources/ucm190622.htm

6. Available at: http://www.who.int/whosis/whostat/EN_WHS10_ Full.pdf

7. Available at: https://www.cia.gov/library/publications/the-world-factbook/rankorder/2091rank.html

8. Dotta A, Chukhlantseva N (2012). Ontogeny and drug metabolism in newborns. *J Matern Fetal Neonatal Med.* **25** Suppl 4: 83-4.

9. Kearns GL, Abdel-Rahman SM, Alander SW, Blowey DL, Leeder JS, Kauffman RE (2003). Developmental pharmacology--drug disposition, action, and therapy in infants and children. *N Engl J Med* **349(12)**: 1157-67.

10. Nahata MC and Taketomo C (2008). Pediatrics. Pharmacotherapy A Pathophysiologic Approach: DiPiro JT, Talbert RL, Yee GC, Matzke GR, Wells BG, Posey LM. 7th ed. New York. McGraw Hill, pp. 47-56.

11. Napoleone E (2010). Children and ADRs (Adverse Drug Reactions). *Ital J Pediatr* **36:** 4.

12. Tabor E (2009). FDA requirements for clinical studies in pediatric patients. *Regulatory Focus* **14:** 16-21.

13. Van den Anker JN (2010). Developmental pharmacology. *Dev Disabil Res Rev* **16(3):** 233-8.

CHAPTER 24

DRUGS USES IN GERIATRICS

Introduction

Demographic structure of the world is rapidly changing with the fastest growing age group of 60 and older. WHO has projected that this group of population will expand by three times from 600 million to 2 billion between the years 2000 to 2050. Further, predictions suggest that the number of the very elderly (85+) will show the greatest growth. This demographic change referred to as "grey tsunami" has significant impact on the health, social, and economic sectors of all countries. Health care system is now burdened with the enlarging proportion of elderly population. Mortality rate among this group is mainly from two components: one from the 'traditional' communicable disease but, also from hastily increased rates of, chronic, non-communicable diseases.

Health care management in geriatrics integrates treatment of diseases, individual health care and psychological care with additional services for housing, home care, nutrition, activities of daily living, socialization programs, as well as financial and legal planning. Treatment of diseases in this population needs to be individualized and to be focused on unique needs of the elderly person. Ageing is a process of gradual and significant morphological and functional changes due to which aged body is different physiologically from the younger adult body with decline of various organ systems. The reduction in physiological reserve in organ systems makes the elderly susceptible to some peculiar diseases and complications get precipitated from mild problems. Functioning of all body systems got affected, which leads to altered pharmaceuticals, pharmacokinetic, and pharmacodynamic phases of the pharmacotherapy. In the pharmaceutic phase age-associated sensory and cognitive losses and decreased manual dexterity must be considered. Accounting the above facts, pharmacotherapy in geriatrics becomes one of the most complex areas in medicine.

In a broad way, the altered pharmacological response of drugs in older people can be ascribed to changing and differing physiology and psychology due to ageing process. Changes in physiology with ageing may alter the drug handling by the human body including absorption, distribution, biotransformation, and excretion of drugs. Absorption of drugs is restricted by dryness of the mouth caused by diminished salivary glands and delayed gastric emptying of solids and liquids in the gastrointestinal tract. Similarly, distribution of drugs is influenced by decline in body fat and muscle mass. Diminution in hepatic function leads to slow biotransformation of drugs, resulting in an altered first-pass effect of orally administered drugs. Altered first-pass effect may precipitate into drug toxicity due to overt plasma and tissue concentration of some drugs. Regarding drug elimination, it is to be noted that decreased renal function in older subjects is in par with young infant and in both of these groups there is increase in the half-life elimination for drugs that are eliminated primarily unchanged in the urine.

Age-related physiologic changes also influence the pharmacodynamic phase of drug therapy, including alteration in homeostatic mechanisms, changes in receptor site response, and variation in the permeability of the blood-brain barrier. These individuals may have more pronounced cognitive side effects from certain drugs. All of these alter a drug's mechanism of action.

Identification of specific drug-related problems is one of the major hurdles in elderly treatment. There is increased chance of aggravation of trivial symptoms and increased incidence of adverse drug reactions and interactions. The major factors contributing to these are polytherapy, non-compliance with drug regimen, and substance misuse, abuse and addiction. Adverse drug reactions are particularly cumbersome in case of elderly, leading to 20 to 25% of hospital admissions in individuals over the age of 65 years. Polypharmacy is often a predictive factor. The use of multiple medications concurrently, is a concern of elderly health care providers and it has been projected that approximately 15% of population comprises of elderly ones, take 25% to 31% of all prescription medications. Another important area is the potential for improper administration and use of potentially inappropriate medications, and the possibility of errors that could result in dangerous drug interactions.

Psychological variation such as substantial memory loss or other types of cognitive impairment are unlikely to be adequately monitored. This incapacitates elderly to adhere to their own scheduled pharmacological administration, and account to 25% to 50% of skipping doses and noncompliance to treatment.

These changes often influence drug kinetics, the effectiveness and the side effect profile of many drugs necessitating change in the dosage regiments, dosage form, and route of administration. Thus, many similarities in this manner in which the young and the elderly respond to medications can be anticipated.

Special Drug Considerations in the Elderly

Factors Influencing Drug Responses in Elderly

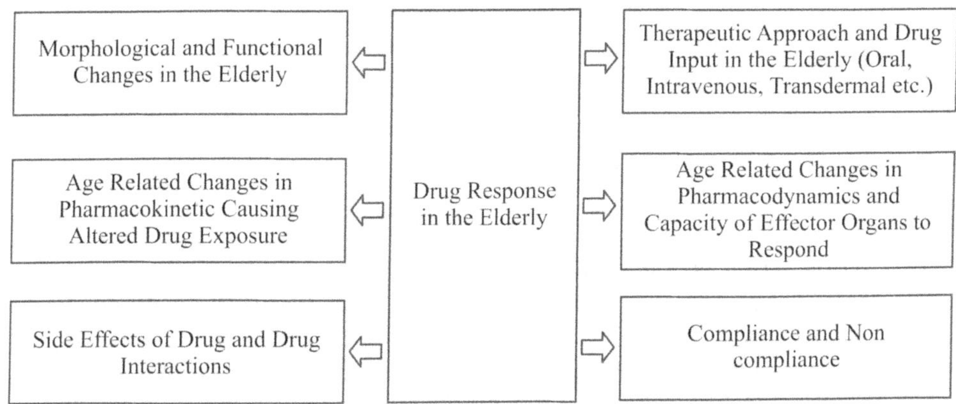

Drug responses are influenced by all the steps involved i.e., drug prescription, drug administration and pharmacotherapy, pharmacokinetics, pharmacodynamics and the effector organ systems. Some though may not all changes in these steps due to the effect of older age leads to alteration in drug responses in the elderly as compared to young adult.

A.   **Morphological and functional changes in the elderly**

Ageing is a process which starts from the day of birth. The rapidity and manifestations of ageing depend on a variety of individual factors, including heredity, lifestyle, dietary pattern, exercise, presence of chronic disease, and social and occupational stress. Irrespective of all of the above, some generalized physiological changes happens automatically in all individuals, including decline in rate of cell division, deterioration of specialized non-dividing cells, loss of elasticity and increased rigidity in connective tissue, and loss of reserve functional capacity.

Altered functioning of all body organ systems pertaining to ageing affects the pharmacotherapy in all aspects, such as drug intake, pharmacokinetic, and pharmacodynamic. Elderly may experience aggravated and paradoxical drug response and adverse drug effects than young adult individuals because of the decreased functional reserve in a variety of body systems (e.g., cardio-reno-vascular, cerebral). There is lack of a safety margin with which the individual can cope with drug effects. The pharmacodynamic effects are altered owing to age-related changes in the structure, number, or sensitivity of drug receptors, enzyme systems and effector organelles in the elderly. Certain characteristics are to be looked after while considering the treatment of an elderly patient, such as biological age, comorbidities, etc. Presence of these specific features, makes pharmacotherapy in geriatrics one of the most complex areas in medicine.

Characteristic morphological and functional changes of the elderly

Biological age
Co-morbidities
Changed symptomatology of disease
Changed course of disease
Complications of disease
Loss of adaptability
Reactivity to drugs
Social and environmental stress in elderly

Older individual often have five to ten disease diagnoses, each of which has one or more proved beneficial therapies. This will increase exposure of the subject to bundles of prescription, as well as nonprescription medications and accelerates the potential for drug interactions. Evidence based medicines are in favor of developing dramatically effective medications for several disease, but the fact is that most of them are being tested in healthy young adults. The exposure in the elderly population is very limited; still these are used as the treatment options in elderly ailments. Therefore, drug-drug and drug-disease state interactions are much more frequently observed in this age group.

Regarding drug interactions the role of psychotherapeutic agents is of utmost importance. Elderly subjects have a declined cognitive status, and these medications additively or synergistically depress the sensorium, are especially troublesome in the elderly. This type of drug interaction contributes to poor self esteem in the elderly patient and results in improper and exaggerated diagnosis of mental dysfunction in elderly including senile dementia.

It is worthwhile to consider extra precaution for dosing and monitoring of the effects of medications in the elderly. The above mentioned morphological and functional factors are relatively newly discovered and have not previously been given wide attention. Therefore, dosing in the elderly is not as exact as in the young adult. In case of pediatrics specific dosages formulations and general formulae for dose calculations have been extensively worked out; however, only for a very few drugs has an exact dosage been identified for the elderly. Most of the time dose calculation in the elderly is based upon creatinine clearance status; however, because of the multitude of factors affecting drug therapy in the elderly, this type of solitary attitude/equations may not serve the whole purpose, rather it will make the treatment unnecessarily complex.

All of these morphological and functional alterations leading to specific differences in pharmacotherapy of the elderly points to the fact, that geriatric care should be complex and systematic. It should adhere to the following key points, such as (a) continuous for long term and permanent; (b) combined with psychotherapy, social intervention, etc.; (c) professional skilled care with active approach.

B.   **Therapeutic approach in the elderly**

Geriatric care should be professional and combination of general and lay care. It is to be actively provided even if individual elderly person does not request it. Therapy must be holistic with a combinational approach of pharmacotherapy, therapeutic diet and other methods.

Therapeutic approach in an elderly individual

> Pharmacotherapy
> Therapeutic diet
> Radiotherapy
> Rehabilitation
> Psychotherapy
> Ergotherapy
> Balneotherapy
> Social rehabilitation
> Other methods Sensitive approach tolerance, etc.

Pharmacotherapy in geriatrics is influenced by several factors as mentioned above including polypharmacy for number of coexisting diseases, preference for symptomatic therapy over causal therapy, high risk of adverse effects of drugs, and specific changes in pharmacokinetics and pharmacodynamics. Polypharmacy or multipresciption (polytherapy) aimed at coexisting polymorbidity of the patient leads to higher incidence of side effects with often atypical presentation.

C.   **Age related changes in pharmacokinetics**

Absorption

Starting from the oral cavity to enteron, the entire gastrointestinal (GI) tract i.e., drug absorption site is more or less physiologically altered with ageing. The reducing activity of salivary glands leads to dryness of oral cavity, stomach pH may increase, blood flow may decrease, and gastric motility may be delayed. The significance of these changes for drug absorption is controversial. For most of the drugs, it has been shown that, despite above changes and prolonged transit time in the GI tract, drug absorption remains adequate.

Distribution

Ageing significantly decreases body mass. Though, both muscle and adipose mass reduces, the proportionate reduction in muscle that makes up lean body tissue is more, which shifts the body mass to increased fat stores. Body water content decreases by 10% to 15% by 80 years of age. Reduction in serum albumin (by approximately 20%) results in an increase in free drug concentration of drugs. This is of importance in case of highly protein bound drugs such as warfarin and phenytoin.

Plasma protein binding is an important aspect in drug metabolism. There are two important drug-binding plasma proteins: albumin and α1-acid glycoprotein. Albumin binds to acid compounds or drugs such as warfarin, whereas α1-acid glycoprotein has affinity for lipophilic and alkaline drugs such as propranolol. Several factors influence serum proteins level such as, chronic disease, nutritional deficits, immobility, and age-related liver changes. The significance of decreased serum proteins is realized when highly protein-bound drugs compete for decreased protein-binding sites. The result can be greater levels of free or unbound circulating drug and, therefore, potential toxicity.

Body mass alteration may lead to significant variation in total amount of drugs in elderly patients. A water-soluble drug has low volume of distribution (Vd) in elderly patients. It is taken up more readily by lean tissue or muscle and attains higher serum concentrations in patients with less body water or lean tissue. Conversely, a lipid soluble drug has high Vd. This type of drug is retained in body fat, resulting in a higher Vd. This increase in Vd can lead to increased half lives and drug accumulation in elderly patients. For example, diazepam has a half life (t1/2) of approximately 20 hours in a young adult, but the $t_{1/2}$ can exceed 70 hours in the older adult. In addition, some drugs, such as tricyclic antidepressants (TCAs) and long acting benzodiazepines, pass more readily through the blood brain barrier, causing more pronounced central nervous system (CNS) effects. Elderly patients who are treated for depression and anxiety may experience fatigue and confusion from drug therapy because antidepressant and antianxiety agents more readily cross their blood brain barrier.

Changes in drug distribution

Central compartment volume	— or ↓
Peripheral compartment volume	
Lipophilic drugs	↑↑
Hydrophilic drugs	↓↓
Plasma protein binding	
Binding to albumin	↓
Binding to α1-acid glycoprotein	— or ↑

Biotransformation and Elimination

Hepatic metabolism

Drug biotransformations occur in quantitatively important amounts in the liver, gastrointestinal tract, kidneys, lung, and skin. However, nearly all organs have some metabolic activity. Liver has primary role in drug biotransformation. As the body ages, the size and weight of the liver generally decrease, splanchnic blood flow diminishes, and activity of microsomal drug-metabolizing enzymes decreases. With the shrinking of liver, fewer hepatic cells are present to break down drugs. As hepatic function declines, drugs may be metabolized more slowly, resulting in an altered first-pass effect of orally administered drugs. First-pass effect refers to the amount of a drug that is removed from the bloodstream during the first circulation through the liver after intestinal absorption. Altered first-pass effect leads to increased plasma and tissue concentration of some drugs and can result in drug toxicity. Impaired liver function also results in elevated levels of active metabolites of drugs.

In vivo drug biotransformations are commonly separated into Phase I and Phase II biotransformations. Phase I biotransformations are catalyzed by membrane-bound enzymes found in the endoplasmic reticulum and Phase II biotransformations occur predominantly in the cytosol, with the exception of the UDP-glucuronosyl-transferases that are membrane bound to the endoplasmic reticulum membranes. Phase I biotransformations are primarily catalyzed by enzymes of the cytochrome P450 monoxygenase system (CYP450), with the important members of this enzyme family for drug biotransformations being CYP3A, CYP2D6, CYP2C, CYP1A2, and CYP2E1.

Phase I biotransformations catalyzed by CYP3A have most consistently been shown to be decreased in ageing, with the decrease on the order of 10-40%. The drugs studied that are prototype CYP3A substrates and exemplify this are midazolam and triazolam. The result of this decrease in drug biotransformation is decreased metabolic clearance and increased exposure to drug of the individual at a given dose. The clinical consequence of this is that older patients treated with a given dose of triazolam experience increased sedation and impaired task performance. Quantitatively significant CYP3A activity in the gastrointestinal wall, which catalyzes biotransformation of drugs prior to and during absorption, has been demonstrated. However, it is unknown if this is altered in ageing as well. There is some suggestions that Phase I biotransformations catalyzed by CYP2C are decreased with age, with modest decreases in clearance of warfarin (CYP2C9) and phenytoin (CYP2C19) reported in older individuals. However, this is much less well established. Similarly, Phase I biotransformation by CYP1A2 may be somewhat decreased in older individuals, and decreased theophylline and caffeine clearances have been reported. However, this too is not well established.

Phase II biotransformations are little changed with ageing, based on studies of glucuronidation, sulfation, and acetylation. Prototype substrates studied for glucuronidation have been lorazepam and oxazepam; for sulfation, acetaminophen; and for acetylation, isoniazid and procainamide.

Genetic polymorphisms for the Phase I enzymes (CYP2D6 and CYP2C19) and the Phase II enzymes (N-acetyltransferase and the methyltransferases thiopurine methyltransferase, catechol O-methyl transferase, and thiol methyltransferase) may significantly alter exposure to relevant drug substrates. Evaluation of the frequency of polymorphic variants with increasing age has consistently shown that the same frequencies occur in older individuals as in younger individuals.

Changes in the drug biotransformation and elimination

Biotransformation and elimination pathways	Status in the elderly	Drugs elimination affected
Renal elimination		
Renal elimination	↓↓	All aminoglycosides, vancomycin, digoxin, procainamide, lithium, sotalol, atenolol, dofetilide, cimetidine
Hepatic elimination		
Phase I metabolic pathway		
CYP3A	↓	Alprazolam, midazolam, triazolam, verapamil, diltiazem, dihydropyridine calcium channel blockers, lidocaine
CYP2C9 and CYP2C19	— or ↓	Diazepam, phenytoin, celecoxib
CYP1A2	— or ↓	Theophylline
CYP2D6	— or ↓	Tricyclic antidepressants, beta blockers like metoprolol, propafenone, timolol, antipsychotics like haloperidol, risperidone
CYP2E1	— or ↓	Acetaminophen, chlorzoxazone, ethanol
Multiple Phase I metabolic pathways		Imipramine, desipramine, trazodone, hexobarbital, flurazepam
Phase II reactions		
Glucuronidation	—	
Sulfation	—	
Acetylation	—	

Renal elimination

The most consistent and predictable age-related change in drug pharmacokinetics is that of renal clearance of drugs. These changes may necessitate adjustment in administration schedule and dosage strength. Most drugs are eliminated from the body by the kidneys after they are metabolized. Excretion rate of drugs depend on renal blood flow, glomerular filtration rate, active renal tubular secretory processes and urea and creatinine clearance. All these functions are diminished during the ageing process. After 40 years of age, renal blood flow declines and the glomerular filtration rate (GFR) drops approximately 1% a year and accelerates with advancing age. In many of the elderly these renal changes may be further complicated by other medical problems such as infections, nephrosclerosis, congestive heart failure, diabetic neuropathy, and dehydration. Many of the drugs commonly used in the treatment of geriatric patients (e.g., certain cardiac drugs, diuretics, and antipsychotic drugs) can further diminish renal function.

Although, there is considerable variability in this decline, an approximation of the decline in glomerular filtration rate has been usefully characterized by the Cockroft–

Gault equation and this is considered as a guide to drug dosing. For men, creatinine clearance can be estimated from this equation as follows:

CLCR (mL/min) = (140 − age) (weight in kg)/72 (serum creatinine in mg/dL)

For women, this estimate should be reduced by 15%

In general, when a drug is being eliminated exclusively by the kidneys, one may also take the following approach to determine the adjusted daily dose of a drug:

Adjusted daily dose = Dose for normal renal function × (Patient's creatinine clearance/Normal creatinine clearance)

Drugs that are eliminated primarily by glomerular filtration, including aminoglycoside antibiotics, lithium, and digoxin, have an elimination clearance that decreases with age in parallel with the decline in measured or calculated creatinine clearance. The renal clearance of drugs undergoing active renal tubular secretion also decreases with ageing. For example, the decrease in renal tubular secretion of cimetidine has been shown to parallel the decrease in creatinine clearance in older patients. On the other hand, the renal clearance/creatinine clearance ratio of both procainamide and N-acetylprocainamide decreases in the elderly, indicating that with ageing the renal tubular secretion of these drugs declines more rapidly than creatinine clearance does.

Changes in pharmacokinetic parameters are results of physiological changes of the organism in the process of ageing, pathological changes in the body and external influences.

Factors influencing pharmacokinetic parameters in elderly

Pharmacokinetic parameters	Physiological changes in ageing	Pathological changes	External factors
Absorption	Increased pH of gastric fluid, smaller resorption surface, slower bowel motility	Achlorhydria, constipation, diarrhoea, gastrectomy, malabsorption syndrome, pancreatitis	Antacids (enteral), anticholinergics, cholestyramine, drug interactions
Distribution	Decreased cardiac output, decreased volume of circulating fluid, higher proportion of fat tissue, lower plasmatic albumin	Cardiac insuficiency, dehydratation, edemas, ascites, hepatopathy, malnutrition, kidney insufficiency	Drug interactions
Biotransformation	Liver involution, decreased enzyme activity, decreased liver perfusion	Hepatopathy, fever, malnutrition, thyroid disease	Dietary habits, drug interactions, smoking
Elimination	Decreased kidney perfusion, decreased glomerular filtration, decreased tubular secretion	Hypovolemia, kidney insuficiency	Drug interactions

D.   Age related changes in pharmacodynamics

Modification of all major organ systems due to ageing affects the pharmacokinetic disposition of the drug. Similarly, there is change in the impact of drugs on the body i.e., change in pharmacodynamic aspect of drug. Few studies are available regarding age-related pharmacodynamic changes in elderly adults. Drug–receptor interactions are found more in number and in an exaggerated manner in the elderly population. This has been ascribed to increased sensitivity of the receptor to the drug or decreased capacity to respond to drug-induced signaling of receptors. In addition, there is alteration in the quantity and affinity of receptors. The CNS effects of drugs are commonly found to be exaggerated in the elderly patient. Particularly egregious are the agents with anti-cholinergic affects, such as the psychotropic drugs, tricyclic antidepressants, antispasmodics and antihistamines. The anti-cholinergic effect induced by these agents can lead to excessive dry mouth, blurred vision, constipation, and even an exacerbation of benign prostatic hyperplasia. Caution should be used if these agents are prescribed at all. Other factors attributed to ageing leading to alteration in drugs response include changes in receptor site response, alteration in homeostatic mechanisms and variation in the permeability of the blood-brain barrier. Cognitive side effects are more prominent in association with above conditions.

Similarly, the sedative effects of agents may be intensified in elderly patients. The benzodiazepines and potent analgesic agents are examples of drugs for which older patients are particularly susceptible to this adverse effect. Overprescribing, or typical prescribing without considering the potential for exaggerated effect, can lead to over sedation and a greater risk of falls and fractures.

The cardiovascular system can be affected by changes due to ageing. Orthostatic hypotension is more common in the elderly because of a loss of the baroreceptor reflex and changes in cerebral blood flow. Moreover, drugs that lower blood pressure or decrease cardiac output put the elderly patient at risk for a syncopal episode.

Changes in pharmacodynamic parameters

Changed sensitivity of target tissues
Reduced number of receptors
Altered drug–receptor signal transduction
Increased penetration through blood-brain barrier
Altered homeostasis of elderly body

E.   Side effects of drugs

Elderly subjects are at high risk of drug induced adverse effects. Most of the side effects can be due to polytherapy and comorbidities. Other factors contributing to increased adverse reactions and drug interactions seen in the elderly can be explicated by ageing related changes such as reduced liver function and resultant decrease in drug metabolism, declined renal glomerular filtration rate and resultant decrease in renal elimination, changed drug-receptor signaling response and increased permeability of the blood-brain barrier. Geriatric physicians should be aware of these changes and their potential harm which will aid in minimizing drug induced adverse effects in elderly subjects. Adverse drug reactions are particularly problematic in elderly patients leading to 20 to 25% of hospital admissions in individuals over the age of 65 years.

The correlation between polytherapy and incidence of adverse drug effects has been investigated in several studies over the past three decades, and has demonstrated that the likelihood of adverse drug effect increases with the number of drugs prescribed. There is a disproportionate increase in both total and severe adverse drug reactions when more than five drugs are coadministered. Adverse drug effects also are more likely in older patients when certain drugs, such as tricyclic antidepressants, theophylline, warfarin or digoxin are among the drugs prescribed. However, the absolute number of drugs the patient concurrently receives is probably the best predictor of an adverse drug event. CNS side effects like confusion are the common conditions seen in elderly subjects and the drugs associated with this are psychotropic drugs, anticholinergics, oral antidiabetics, digoxin, corticosteroids, etc.

Measures for prevention of side effects

Limiting polytherapy
Better assessment before prescribing
Dose calculation
Increasing compliance
Therapeutic drug monitoring (TDM)
Monitoring and interpreting side effects
Improving communication – feedback
Real availability of safe and effective drugs
Easy access for treatment facility

Drug interactions

Factors increasing risk of drug interactions
Polytherapy (Allopathy and alternative system medicines)
Long-term pharmacotherapy
Incorrect dosage
Inappropriate combination of drugs
Narrow therapeutic window
Self prescription!!!

Contd...

<table>
<tr><td>

Dangerous interactions
Hypoglycemia
Increased disposition for bleeding
Induction of arrhythmias
Convulsions
Hypertonic crisis

Risky drug groups
Antidiabetics (sulfonylurea, metformin)
Oral anticoagulants (warfarin)
Digoxin
Antiepileptics
Psychotropic and Tricyclic antidepressants

</td></tr>
</table>

F.   Compliance and Non-compliance

Compliance to treatment is a big hurdle in older age, because of an incapability of an older to understand and correctly follow the instructions of a physician.

Statistics has shown that almost 60% of patients do not adhere to the order of medication intake as it was prescribed. This is specifically true about people living alone. With this regard the value of social compliance is also important. It has been seen that among the subjects on concomitant administration of 5 drugs, total compliance is only 33-44%; on combination of 10 drugs, compliance is only 10-20%. The noncompliance can be of various forms: abuse of medication (50%), additional self-prescription (20%), incorrect dosing (10%) and incorrect timing of administration.

Factors with negative influence on compliance

Factors	Examples
Cognition deficit	Dementia, confusion
Lack of communication	Physician-patient, nurse-patient, caregiver-patient, etc.
Improper form of drug	Parenteral route for daily intake
Inability to apply medication	Tremor, hand deformity
Polytherapy/multiple drug prescribing	Multimedication
Sensory impairment	Vision, hearing
Social factors	Maladjustment, fear of expose about disease

Medications to halt ageing

So, many clinical studies and experimental studies have been performed to stop the ageing. But, all are with inadequate evidences. However, for many years there have been discussions about medications influence on the process of ageing, so called *geriatrics*, which are divided to genuine and non-genuine. *Non-genuine geriatrics* has beneficial effects on common symptoms in older age. These include vitamins, trace elements, enzymes, stimulants and others. Whereas, *genuine geriatrics* are substances which interfere ageing process itself, and tried to slow down the ageing. Mechanisms of ageing are inadequate and a definitive statement about substance considered as genuine geriatrics cannot be provided. The substances tried in this group include a whole group of adaptogens, mostly of herbal origin e.g., ginseng; It is used as tonic, stimulant, protective, metabolic and antisclerotic medication.

Basic Rules and Complexity of Therapy of Elderly

Though the geriatric medicine seems to be complex, it should not dither us from adapting this in routine practice. It is to be noted that unawareness of these fundamentals with inadequate compliance of elderly patient can lead to iatrogenic trauma, which is mostly a result of multiprescription, inappropriate dosing, adverse drug reactions and drug interactions.

The Commonest Problems in Rational Pharmacotherapy of the Elderly

Inaccurate diagnosis
Polytherapy
Incorrect drug (drug group) indication
Inaccurate dosing
High risk of adverse drug effects and drug interactions
Non-compliance of the patient

In recent years the focus on medical care for the aged has changed from passive care to active cure. The ageing population wants a cure for the ageing process – something that will halt the changes.

Prescribing Guidelines for the Elderly

1. When prescribing new medications review the following issues
    a. Is medication necessary?
       (i.e., is there a nonphamacologic treatment?)
    b. Determine therapeutic endpoints
    c. Assess: risks '*vs*' benefits
    d. Can one medication treat more than one condition?
    e. Administration time matches existing medicines?
2. Identify all drugs by generic name and drug class
3. All drugs prescribed should have clinical indications.
4. Know the side effect profile of drugs you prescribe
5. Understand ageing pharmacokinetics and how to decrease ADE's

Contd...

6. Stop all drugs without known benefit

7. Stop all drugs without clinical indication

8. Always attempt to substitute less toxic drug

9. Avoid negative prescribing cascade

   (i.e., treating one ADE with another drug)

10. Brown Bag inventory (Annual or biannually)

    a. Request assistant go thru OTC's, Creams and "left over" medications and record for you (Because 25 % of prescription drugs not recorded).

    b. Most effective is coincides with annual major check- ups.

    c. Reception staff to automatically remind patient when they schedule appointments to bring in all medications for a "Brown Bag inventory".

    d. Offer to throw away outdated and unused meads.

Principles of Drug Prescribing in Hospitalized Elderly Patients

Admission:

(a) Review all medications (include relevant OTC, herbal, vitamins, etc.), diet habit of patient prior to hospitalization

(b) Assess previous compliance

Avoid unnecessary polypharmacy by:

(a) Using drugs that treat more than one condition (e.g., beta-blockers for both hypertension and angina pectoris) when practical.

(b) Discontinue drugs unnecessary in hospital (e.g.. simultaneous use of proton pump inhibitors, H_2 blockers and antacids for acidity problems).

Safe prescribing habits:

When initiating a new medication:

(a) Choose agents whose pharmacokinetic properties in elderly patients are known.

(b) Begin with a short-acting agent but by discharge convert to an agent that is given once or twice daily in order to enhance patient compliance and reduce caregiver burden at home.

(c) In multiple medications, consider drug interactions and treat with alternatives.

(d) When the maintenance dose of a medication is not established, "start low and go slow", to allow time to titrate the dose against the desired clinical effect.

(e) Consider reduced renal and hepatic function status and use the corrected dose (e.g., digoxin).

Adverse drug events (ADEs):

Anytime a patient develops new or unexplained medical problem consider ADE as a cause: e.g., delirium, hypotension, arrhythmias, renal failure, electrolyte disorders, constipation.

Contd...

> At time of discharge:
>
> (a) Review medications that were taken by patient prior to admission and evaluate which should be renewed on discharge.
>
> (b) Review all discharge medications with the patient and family, and provide written instructions.

Geriatric Medicine and Clinical Pharmacology

The multidisciplinary health care team is championed by geriatric medicine as the optimal means of providing care for the complex older patient with multiple concurrent illnesses. The clinical pharmacologist has a key role on this team, working closely with the primary geriatric medicine clinician, the clinical pharmacist, and other members of the team to individualize and modify complex drug therapy regimens as the clinical status of the older patient evolves over time.

During the past 30 years, clinical pharmacologists have conducted the research that has defined the pharmacokinetics of ageing. This work, particularly in the area of drugs that undergo renal clearance, has contributed importantly to patient safety and well being. Looking to the future, the research opportunities to define drug pharmacodynamics and altered drug risk/benefit relationships in older patients are abundant. Similarly, teaching rational use of drugs for older patients and placing this into a geriatric medicine perspective is an important role for the clinical pharmacologist. The number of physicians trained as geriatric clinical pharmacologists is inadequate to meet either the research or educational needs, and attracting physicians and training them to do geriatric clinical pharmacology is a continuing challenge.

Clinical pharmacology has an important role to foster the linkage of the principles of geriatric medicine and disease-based therapeutics. In geriatric medicine advances in understanding the interplay of multiple concurrent illnesses and how this may result in a common path to patient disability and death has allowed definition of the frailty syndrome. In addition, the concept of competing morbidity, such that in the older patient successful treatment of one illness may result not in restoration of health, rather in the more obvious clinical presentation of another concurrent illness, has advanced clinical decision making and end of life care. The clinical pharmacologist has an important role in teaching the changing balance of risk and benefit for specific drug therapy intervention in the context of the individual older patient and their specific concurrent illnesses. The research opportunities in this area for the clinical pharmacologist are both challenging and exciting.

Conclusion

Finally, clinicians must check at the patient holistically, not focus solely on drug therapy; should include quality of life. Improvement in nutrition, use of alternative therapies when possible, and promotion of general health and fitness may result in reduced medication requirements in geriatric patients.

Suggested Readings

1. Carroll D (2006). Principles of Pharmacotherapy in Elderly Patients. In Pharmacotherapeutics for advanced practice: a practical approach. Wolters Kluwer 2nd edition, Page 55-65.

2. Drug therapy considerations in older adults. Available at: http://www.pharmacy.ca.gov/publications/health_notes_drug_therapy.pdf.

3. Fried LP, Tangen CM, Walston J *et al.,* (2001). Frailty in older adults: Evidence for a phenytype. *J Gerontol A Biol Sci Med Sci* **56:** M146-M156.

4. Jambhekar SS and Breen PJ (2009). Basic Pharmacokinetics. Pharmaceutical press. Chicago.

5. Katzung Bg, Masters SB, Trevor AJ (2009). Basic and Clinical Pharmacology. 11th Ed. McGraw-Hill.

6. King SA. Pharmacotherapy In Geriatrics: Cause For Concern. Available at: http://www.dcmsonline.org/jax-medicine/1998journals/august98/geriatrics.htm.

7. Klotz U (2009). Pharmacokinetics and drug metabolism in the elderly. *Drug Metab Rev* **41:** 67-76.

8. Starner CI, Gray SL, Guay DRP, Hajjar ER, Handler SM and Hanlon JT (2008). Geriatrics. In Pharmacotherapy A Pathophysiologic Approach: DiPiro JT, Talbert RL, Yee GC, Matzke GR, Wells BG, Posey LM. 7th ed. New York. McGraw Hill, pp. 2349-67.

CHAPTER 25

DRUG AND HEPATIC DYSFUNCTION

Introduction

Liver is of utmost importance in drug biotransformation and excretion of drugs. Every drug introduced in the body is metabolized by liver leading to formation of inactive metabolites or activation of inactive drugs. Apart from metabolism, liver also is a route of excretion of drugs through biliary secretion.

The liver is exposed to every drug introduced in the body and more than 1000 drugs, toxins and herbs are known to cause hepatotoxicity. Drug induced hepatotoxicity is underestimated and underreported. About 20-40% of fulminant hepatic failure is caused due to drugs. Bromfenac, Pemoline and Troglitazone are examples of drugs withdrawn due to hepatotoxicity.

Drugs need to be used cautiously in pediatric age group, in elderly patients, patients on polypharmacy, infections with hepatic involvement, where hepatotoxic drugs need to be given for a longer time, in conditions with underlying liver disease, post operative after liver resection, in conditions with hepatic malignancies etc. Adults are generally more susceptible to hepatotoxicity than are children and women are more commonly affected than men. Hispanics and blacks are more susceptible to drug induced liver injury. Apart from race, pediatric age and sex, there is also some genetic predisposition for hepatotoxicity. Host factors like obesity, malnutrition, coexisting diabetes mellitus, renal failure and AIDS enhances the susceptibility to hepatic damage.

Drugs Causing Hepatotoxicity

Common classes of drugs include-

(i)   *Antibiotics:* Ampicillin, amoxicillin-clavulanic acid, oxacillin, cephalosporins, tetracycline, sulfonamides, erythromycin, trimethoprim-sulfamethoxazole

(ii) *Anti tubercular drugs:* Isoniazid, rifampicin

(iii) *Antiretroviral drugs:* Zidovudine, ribavirin, nevirapine, efavirenz

(iv) *Lipid lowering agents:* Statins, clofibrate, nicotinic acid, ezetimibe

(v) *Oral hypoglycemics:* Rosiglitazone, troglitazone

(vi) *Antiepileptics:* Phenytoin, carbamazepine, valproic acid, chlorpromazine

(vii) *NSAIDs:* Diclofenac, indomethacin, tolmetin, sulindac, ibuprofen, ketoprofen, mefenamic acid, celecoxib

(viii) *Anti-tumour drugs:* 6-Mercaptopurine, azathioprine, L-asparaginase, mithramycin, vincristine, cyclophosphamide, carmustine

(ix) *Antihypertensive agents:* Methyldopa, hydralazine, lisinopril, labetalol

Mechanisms of Hepatotoxicity

There are various mechanisms of hepatic injury reported in the literatures. It is widely recognized that drug-induced liver injury (DILI) is mediated by two chief mechanisms: *intrinsic and idiosyncratic hepatotoxicity.* Intrinsic hepatotoxins cause hepatocellular damage in a predictable dose-dependent manner directly by the drug or indirectly by its metabolite and it is reproducible. The latent period of intrinsic hepatotoxicity is short and usually consistent. The majority of drugs lead to idiosyncratic liver injury and can be classified into metabolic and immunological categories.

- *Interference with bilirubin transport and conjugation:* Interference with bilirubin transport leads to hyperbilirubinemia. Example: Rifampicin.

- *Cytotoxic injury:* Direct hepatic parenchymal injury by drug or its metabolite. Example: Paracetamol, INH.

- *Cholestasis:* Impaired biliary secretion. Example: Steroid induced Jaundice.

- *Mixed cytotoxic/cholestatic injury:* Few drugs have both mixed pattern of injury E.g.: Para aminosalicylic acid.

- *Fatty liver (steatosis):* Tetracycline is known to cause fatty liver, more commonly in females.

- *Chronic active hepatitis, cirrhosis and sub-acute necrosis:* The clinical features are mild and subclinical. Example: α-methyldopa, nitrofurantoin and isoniazid.

- *Liver tumors:* Oral contraceptive pills are known to cause hepatic adenomas.

Clinical Features

The onset of clinical features may vary from 5-90 days after exposure of drug. The manifestations of drug-induced hepatotoxicity are highly variable, ranging from asymptomatic elevation of liver enzymes to fulminant hepatic failure. It is important to distinguish between hepatic injuries from hepatic dysfunction. As hepatic injury, may present as asymptomatic transaminitis, where as clinical features appear when hepatic dysfunction sets in.

The injury may suggest a hepatocellular injury, with elevation of aminotransferase levels as the predominant symptom, or a cholestatic injury, with elevated alkaline phosphatase levels (with or without hyperbilirubinemia) being the main feature. Clinical differentiation between the two mechanisms of action cannot be made. The biochemical manifestations reflect the histological pattern of injury.

1. *Asymptomatic elevations in aminotransferases:* Asymptomatic elevations in aminotransferases may be encountered with some drugs, continuation of drugs does not lead to progressive elevation of liver enzymes. E.g., Phenytoin, methyl dopa, tacrine, quinidine.

2. *Elevated aminotransferase levels with acute hepatocellular injury:* In drug-induced acute hepatocellular injury the ALT levels are increased to more than twice the upper limit of the reference range and alkaline phosphatase levels remain within the reference range or are minimally elevated. Whereas elevation of aspartate aminotransferase (AST) greater than ALT, especially if more than 2 times greater, suggests alcoholic hepatitis. For example, acetaminophen, NSAIDs, ACE inhibitors, nicotinic acid, INH, sulfonamides, erythromycin, and antifungal agents such as griseofulvin and fluconazole.

3. *Elevated aminotransferase and bilirubin levels:* Elevation of bilirubin levels suggests worse prognosis. Increasing hepatocellular injury with subfulminant or fulminant necrosis leads to elevation in bilirubin levels. Subfulminant hepatic failure most commonly results from acetaminophen, halothane, methoxyflurane, enflurane, trovafloxacin, troglitazone, ketoconazole, dihydralazine, tacrine, mushroom poisoning, ferrous sulfate poisoning, phosphorus poisoning, and cocaine toxicity.

4. *Elevated alkaline phosphatase (acute cholestatic injury) levels:* Acute intrahepatic cholestasis is divisible into 2 broad categories (a) cholestasis without hepatocellular injury (bland jaundice or pure cholestasis) and (b) cholestasis with variable hepatocytc injury. In bland cholestasis the ALP level is barely elevated (not more than twice) with normal cholesterol levels, whereas in cholestasis with inflammation ALP is elevated more than thrice with elevated cholesterol levels.

Histological Classification of Hepatic Injury

The following morphological patterns have been seen in Drug Induced Hepatic Injury. Acute hepatitis, with or without cholestasis, is the most common histological pattern of drug-induced liver injury. Drug-induced chronic hepatitis is rare, but fibrosis and cirrhosis can occur with drugs such as methotrexate, while autoimmune hepatitis-like disease can result with drugs such as minocycline.

- Acute hepatitis and cholestatic hepatitis
- Acute liver failure (Necrosis with marked inflammation/Necrosis with little or no inflammation)

- o Microvesicular steatosis with little or no inflammation (Microvesicular/ Macrovesicular)
- o Chronic hepatitis (Autoimmune hepatitis marker-negative/Drug-induced autoimmune hepatitis)
- o Cholestasis
- o Granulomatous hepatitis
- o Steatosis/steatohepatitis
- o Vascular abnormalities.

Hepatic necrosis is associated with 8-200 fold increase in AST and ALT with minimal increase in ALP. Usually acute toxic steatosis is microvesicular and chronic steatosis is macrovesicular. In microvesicular steatosis the transaminases are 5-15 times elevated. Cholestatic injury is further classified as cholestasis with or without significant inflammation. In bland cholestasis the ALP level is barely elevated (not more than twice) with normal cholesterol levels, whereas in cholestasis with inflammation ALP is elevated more than thrice with elevated cholesterol levels.

Mixed injury (hepatocellular + cholestatic) is characteristic of drug induced hepatic injury.

Example of Drugs causing Hepatotoxicity with Pattern of Involvement

Histological pattern	Drugs
Hepatocellular	Phenytoin, Dapsone, Sulfonamides and Para-aminosalicylic acid
Microvesicular steatosis	Tertracycline, Valproate and Aspirin

Cholestasis
  - Bland cholestasis
  - Cholestasis with Inflammation
	
	Anabolic steroids/Oral contraceptive pills
	Erythromycin, Chlorpromazine

Granulomatous	Allupurinol, Carbamazepine, Methydopa, Quinidine.

Monitoring and Drug Modifications

ATT induced hepatic injury occurs most commonly in the initial two month after initiation of treatment, major proportion being affected in the initial 15 days. Two weekly monitoring is recommended to identify patients who develop early drug induced hepatotoxicity.

The severity of liver dysfunction is classified according to the WHO Toxicity Classification standards: Mild (ALT/AST ≤ 3 times ULN, or TBil ≤ 2 times ULN), Moderate (3 times ULN $<$ ALT/AST ≤ 5 times ULN, or 2 times ULN $<$ TBil ≤ 5 times ULN) and Severe (ALT/AST/TBil > 5 times ULN).

In case of hepatotoxicity, all drugs are stopped and liver function tests are monitored twice weekly. Once the LFT is normal drugs are serially introduced in low dose and gradual increase in dose, ethambutol is introduced first followed by isoniazid, rifampicin and pyrazinamide.

Differential Diagnosis

Drug induced hepatotoxicity may sometimes mimic infection induced hepatic injury and needs to be differentiated from acute viral hepatitis, autoimmune hepatitis, shock liver, cholecystitis, cholangitis, Budd-Chiari syndrome, alcoholic liver disease, cholestatic liver disease, pregnancy-related conditions of liver, malignancy, Wilson disease, hemochromatosis and coagulation disorders.

Management

Awareness of drugs causing hepatotoxicity and avoiding its use is of utmost importance. Prevention also includes increased vigilance during preclinical drug development and clinical trials. Early recognition and withdrawal of the offending drug is essential in minimizing liver injury. In majority of situations there is no specific treatment available and stopping the drug is usually the only option. Good supportive care is what is required after the offending drug has been stopped. Maintaining calorie intake, adequate fluids and electrolyte balance is essential. Symptomatic treatment for pruritis, fever, and rash is administered. For management of pain in patients with liver disease lower doses of acetaminophen (2-3 grams/day) or tramadol 25 mg thrice daily may be used. For neuropathic pain gabapentin/pregabalin may be used. NSAIDs should be avoided in patients with preexisting liver disease.

Prompt use of N-acetylcysteine after acetaminophen overdose and intravenous carnitine for valproate-induced mitochondrial injury are exceptions. In drug induced fulminant hepatic failure emergency liver transplantation is increasingly opted for the outcome of acute liver failure is determined by etiology, the degree of hepatic encephalopathy present upon admission, and complications such as infections.

Suggested Readings

1. Andrade and Tulkens (2011). Hepatic safety of antibiotics used in primary care. *J Antimicrob Chemother* **66(7):** 1431-46.

2. Batt AM and Ferrari L (1995). Manifestations of chemically induced liver damage. *Clin Chem.* **41:** 1882-1887.

3. Devarbhavi H, Singh R, Patil M, Sheth K, Adarsh CK, Balaraju G (2013). Outcome and determinants of mortality in 269 patients with combination anti-tuberculosis drug-induced liver injury. *J Gastroenterol Hepatol* **28(1):** 161-167.

4. Farrell GC (1997). Drug-induced hepatic injury. *J Gastroenterol Hepatol* **12(9-10):** S242-50.

5. Lee WM (2003). Drug-induced hepatotoxicity. *N Engl J Med* **349(5):** 474-485.

6. Navarro VJ, Senior JR(2006). Drug Related Hepatotoxicity. *N Engl J Med* **354:** 731-9.

7. Pugh *et al.,* (2009). Drug-induced hepatotoxicity or drug-induced liver injury. *Clin Liver Dis* **13:** 277-94

8. R Ramachandran, S Kakar (2009). Histological Patterns in drug-induced liver diseases. *J Clin Pathol* **62:** 481-492.

9. Singanayagam A, Sridhar S, Dhariwal J, Abdel-Aziz D, Munro K, Connell DW *et al.,* (2012). A comparison between two strategies for monitoring hepatic function during antituberculous therapy. *Am J Respir Crit Care Med* **185(6):** 653-659.

10. Tostmann A, Boeree MJ, Aarnoutse RE, de Lange WC, van der Ven AJ and Dekhuijzen R (2008). Antituberculosis drug-induced hepatotoxicity: concise up-to-date review. *J Gastroenterol Hepatol* **23:** 192-202.

CHAPTER 26

DRUG AND RENAL DYSFUNCTION

Introduction

This chapter is dedicated to the description of principles of using different drugs in patients with compromised renal functions. The chapter begins with a brief description of general concepts about altered renal functions which are relevant for understanding of concepts discussed later in the chapter. It is expected that the reader is able to use the principles in clinical practice after reading the chapter.

Definition of renal failure: In simple terms renal failure is a state of renal functions where kidneys are not able to maintain the urinary output adequate to remove toxins from the body.

Types of renal failure: Two types of renal failure have been defined in medicine: Acute and chronic renal failure.

Acute Renal Failure (ARF): It develops suddenly within a matter of hours to days leading to accumulation of urea and other toxins in the body. ARF has been classified into pre-renal, renal and post-renal ARF depending on the insults. The description of causes of ARF is beyond the scope of this chapter. Management of this condition involves use of drugs directed at the primary etiology and supportive functions. Dialysis may be used for supporting renal functions. New criteria have been proposed for evaluation of ARF. The terminology has been recently modified to Acute Kidney Injury (AKI) and a new classification system RIFLE has been extensively validated for use in acute renal injury. ARF is characterized by rapid changes in renal functions followed by there may be complete functional recovery (potentially reversible) or renal functions stabilize at sub-normal levels. This state is called a state of chronic renal failure.

Chronic Renal Failure (CRF): It has been defined as kidney damage for three or more months, as defined by structural or functional abnormalities of the kidney, with or without decreased GFR manifested by pathologic abnormalities or markers of kidney damage, including abnormalities in the composition of the blood or urine or abnormalities in imaging tests and GFR < 60ml/min/1.73 m^2 for 3 months of more with or without kidney damage. Renal functions are relatively stable and change over a period of days to months. End-stage renal disease is characterized by a stage of compromised renal functions presenting clinically as uremic syndrome. This syndrome is potentially life-threatening if toxins are not removed from the body by renal replacement therapy. Excellent medical reviews are available on causes of CRF. Drug therapy is primarily supportive and is directed at co-morbidities of CRF.

Monitoring and stages of renal failure: Renal functions have been described in terms of GFR. Estimation of GFR involves use of molecules which are cleared from circulation by kidneys. Inulin, para-aminohippuric acid, creatinine and urea are some of these. Inulin clearance provides the best estimates of GFR but, the practical issues associated with use and monitoring of inulin preclude its use in routine clinical practice. Creatinine is the most practical candidate for estimation of GFR in clinical practice. More details about use of molecules for estimation of GFR can be found in physiology text-books. Stages of renal failure have been described conventionally on the basis of GFR. Table 26.1, describes the stages of CRF on the basis of GFR. Although, a lot of criticism is seen in medical literature for using GFR as a marker of severity of renal disease for GFR alone not being predictive of mortality and presence of other co-morbidities which can modify the outcomes of disease. As of now, GFR is considered the best marker of overall renal functions.

Table 26.1 Stages of CFR on basis of GFR

Stage	GFR, mL/min per 1.73 m^2
0	> 90
1	90
2	60-89
3	30-59
4	15-29
5	< 15

Compensatory Changes in CRF

The kidneys in CRF patients undergo compensatory changes which make for loss of function of some nephrons. The changes include compensatory hypertrophy of remaining nephrons and hyperfiltration which can lead to their sclerosis and progressive renal functional compromise. Worsening of systemic inflammation is also seen in these patients with increase in levels of inflammatory markers.

Pharmacokinetic Considerations in Patients with Renal Failure

A number of changes are seen in patients with renal failure which affect absorption, distribution, metabolism and elimination of drugs. All these changes may require dose modification of drugs. Changes in intra-gastric pH modify the absorption of many drugs. All gastrointestinal hormones including gastrin levels are increased due to decreased breakdown leading to decrease in pH, motility and blood flow. Increased incidence of mucosal ischemia also poses challenges to drug absorption from gastric mucosa and is said to be responsible for GI bleeding in these patients. Renal impairment may change the apparent distribution volumes of a number of drugs by changing fluid balance, circulating proteins, levels of endogenous molecules and toxins, altered vascular permeability and drug protein binding. These changes are relevant only in case of drugs which show high-degree of plasma-protein binding like valproate and warfarin or have very low volumes of distribution like vancomycin. Changes in total body water and third space collections also modify the concentration of drugs in central compartment.

Drug Elimination in Patients with Renal Failure

Kidneys play an important role in elimination of drugs or their metabolites from the body. Glomerular filtration, secretion, and metabolism of drugs by kidneys play a major role in elimination of drugs from the body. A number of significant changes take place in metabolism and excretion of drugs in patients with chronic renal failure which will be discussed in detail in the following sections. These are the changes which mandate dose modifications for various agents in patients with compromised renal functions. Additionally, effect of uremia on hepatic enzymes also leads to modification of hepatic elimination of drugs and endogenous metabolites (hepato-renal syndrome). This also requires dose and drug modification in these patients.

Drug Transporters in Patients with Chronic Renal Failure

Chronic renal failure is known to affect elimination of drugs by changes in filtration of drugs. The disease process can also affect the expression of a number of transporters involved in drug elimination process. Tubular transporters belong to two major groups of families: ATP-binding cassette and solute carriers. They are involved in either secretion or reabsorption of drugs from tubules into urine. Few studies have tried to explore the changes induced in levels of these transporters in CRF. Reductions in expression of CYP1A, organic anion transporter 1-2-3, K1/K2, P1-4C1, P-gp were seen in animals models of CRF. This could lead to intra-renal accumulation of drugs and reduced clearance of drugs eliminated by this route. Changes induced in hepatic microsomal enzymes also lead to decreased metabolism of a number of drugs and ultimately necessitating drug dose modification.

Phase I and phase II metabolic reactions are all slowed in patients of CRF. Although kidneys do not contribute significantly towards metabolism of drugs, the slowing of reactions may have important implications for some of them in patients with compromised renal functions. This change may lead to increased incidence of adverse drug reactions in these patients unless dose modification is done.

Drug Therapy Related Issues in Patients with CRF

A number of issues related to drug therapy are seen in patients with compromised renal functions. Besides altered pharmacodynamics of drug by a number of mechanisms, altered pharmacokinetics of drug remain the most important modifiable factors for preventing drug related problems. Pharmacodynamic issues include increased incidence of nausea and vomiting decreasing the compliance and impaired drug absorption from GIT, altered responsiveness to CNS active agents, dyselectrolytemia leading to altered responses to a number of drugs like digoxin. Pharmacokinetic issues remain the most easily modifiable drug related factors which can improve the outcomes of pharmacotherapy.

Assumptions for Dose Modifications in CRF

Estimation of appropriate dose regimen in patients with compromised renal functions is done on the basis of estimated remaining renal functions and prediction of total body clearance. Several approaches to estimate the remaining renal functions are available. These approaches are based on similar assumptions. Pharmacodynamic alterations in the body of uremic patient are not considered in various schemes of dose modifications. The first and foremost assumption is that creatinine clearance accurately predicts the renal functions. Serum creatinine levels may be the most practical biomarker for renal functions, but it is not the best marker as discussed previously. Also, at very low GFR, calculations based of serum creatinine levels do not correctly predict the renal functions. Another assumption is that all drugs follow a pharmacokinetic profile which is independent of dose. Since, a number of pharmacodynamic alterations do take place in CRF patients, this assumption may not hold true for all the drugs. Other processes involved in drug elimination process are not altered and continue to function as in normal person. For all the drugs, it is assumed that the absorption and distribution processes are not modified and it is only the elimination process as predicted by creatinine clearance which is affected by CRF. It is assumed that the renal functions remain stable over the duration of dosing and the formulas for dose calculations do not work in rapidly changing renal functions. The last assumption is that the target concentration remains the same in these patients. As discussed previously, these assumptions do not hold true in many ways. Contemporary science does not have any substitutes for these assumptions and this introduces limitations in the dose calculation process.

Dosage Adjustment According to Renal Functions

To minimize dosing errors in patients with CRF and reduce the number of adverse drug events, dose modification is one of the strategies followed clinically along with aggressive monitoring and providing therapies aimed at improving renal functions.

Estimation of serum creatinine concentrations is the single most important parameter which can affect the dose calculations significantly. Creatinine clearance is estimated from the serum concentrations using either Cockcroft-Gault or Modification of Diet in Renal Disease study (MDRD) equation.

$$\text{Creatinine Clearance (males)} = \frac{(140 - \text{age}) \times \text{weight}}{72 \times \text{serum creatinine}}$$

Where age is in years, weight in kilograms and serum creatinine is in milligrams per deciliter. If μmol per liter is used, then calculation are done using the formula 88.4 μmol/L = 1 mg/dL. For calculation of creatinine clearance in females, the formula is multiplied by 0.85. If patient is obese, the Ideal Body Weight (IBW) is used in calculations.

$$\text{IBW} = 50 \text{ kg} + (2.3 \text{ kg} \times \text{number of inches over 5 feet})$$

This equation assumes creatinine clearance to be equivalent to GFR.

The other equation that can be used in clinical situations is MDRD4 equation. This equation also predicts estimated GFR from serum creatinine and is given for males by:

$$\text{eGFR} = 186 \times (\text{Serum creatinine})^{-1.154} \times (\text{Age})^{-0.203}$$

For females the eGFR is calculated by

$$\text{eGFR} = 186 \times (\text{Serum creatinine})^{-1.154} \times (\text{Age})^{-0.203} \times 0.742$$

This equation gives eGFR in ml/minute/1.73m^2 and uses age in years and serum creatinine in milligrams/deciliter.

Other method of determining creatinine clearance is direct measurement of serum and urinary creatinine levels and putting the values in formula

$$Cl_{cr} \text{ (ml/min)} = C_u \times 100/C_p \times 1440$$

Where, Cl_{cr} is creatinine clearance, C_u is concentration of creatinine in 24 hour urine sample, C_p is creatinine concentration in serum at midpoint of urinary sampling interval. Factor of 100 is used when C_{cr} is provided in μg/L and 1440 is to convert 24 hours into minutes.

Once we have the estimated GFR, new dose can be calculated assuming that drug clearance is equal to creatinine clearance, dosing interval is not modified and average target concentration remains the same by using the formula

$$C_{avg} = D/Cl \times t$$

Where t is the dosing interval.

$$D_N/Cl_N \times t = D_O/Cl_O \times t$$

Where, D_N is the new dose, Cl_N is the new drug clearance, D_O is the old dose and Cl_O is the previously known clearance and t is the dosing interval used for calculating the average drug concentration.

Critical Analysis of Various Methods for Calculating Estimated GFR

The assumptions mentioned previously may not hold well in all the clinical situations. This leads to introduction of error in estimation of GFR. The use of age in years introduces some error because the age of 2 individuals may differ by 364 days but still in years it will be same. There could be errors in calculating weight of individual because of balance used, with or without clothes or rounding off. The equation may give erroneous results when used in patients with severe muscle loss. Cl_{cr} is not predictive of GFR in states of severely compromised renal functions. In such situations, this formula overestimates GFR.

MDRD equation considers four variables to estimate GFR. It does not consider weight but includes race. Inclusion of race limits the predictability of this equation to certain races only which were included in clinical studies for generating data for developing this equation while excluding others.

Commonly used drugs requiring dose modification in patients with renal failure*

Antihypertensive agents	Dosage adjustment (percentage of usual dosage) based on GFR (mL per minute per 1.73 m^2)		
Drug	**Usual dosage**	**> 50**	**10 to 50**	**< 10**
Enalapril	5 to 10 mg every 12 hours	100%	75 – 100 %	50%
Fosinopril	10 mg daily	100%	100%	75 to 100%
Lisinopril	5 to 10 mg daily	100%	50 to 75%	25 to 50%
Ramipril	5 to 10 mg daily	100%	50 to 75%	25 to 50%
Acebutolol	400 to 600 mg	100%	50%	30 to 50%
Atenolol	5 to 100 mg	100%	50%	25%
Bisoprolol	10 mg	100%	75%	50%
Nadolol	40 to 80 mg	100%	50%	25%
Amiloride	5 mg	100%	50%	Avoid
Spironolactone	50 to 100 mg	Every 6 to 12 hours	Every 12 to 24 hours	Avoid
Thiazides	25 to 50 mg	100%	100%	Avoid
Fluconazole	200 to 400 mg	100%	50%	50%
Itraconazole	100 – 200 mg	100%	100%	50%
Ertapenem	1 gm	100%	100%	50%
Meropenem	1 – 2 gm	100%	50%	50%
Clarithromycin	250 – 500 mg	100%	50 - 100%	50%
Ciprofloxacin	500 – 750 mg orally	100%	50 – 75%	50%

Contd...

Antihypertensive agents	Dosage adjustment (percentage of usual dosage) based on GFR (mL per minute per 1.73 m^2)			
Drug	**Usual dosage**	**> 50**	**10 to 50**	**< 10**
Norfloxacin		100%	50%	Avoid
Sulfamethoxazole	1 gm every 8 to 12 hours	Every 12 hours	Every 18 hours	Every 24 hours
Trimethoprim	100 mg every 12 hours	every 12 hours	Every 12 hours (GFR > 30); every 18 hours (GFR 10 to 30)	Every 24 hours

Summary and Conclusion

State of compromised renal functions warrants modification of pharmacotherapy. Besides avoiding drugs, with known nephrotoxic potential, alteration in dose or dosing intervals can be done to avoid adverse drug reactions in the individuals. Dose modifications are based on estimation of remaining renal functions using creatinine clearance as biomarker for GFR. Nomograms and mathematical equations are available for the same. Cockgroft-Gault equation and MDRD equations can be used for estimating creatinine clearance. MDRD equation gives better results in patients with GFR < 60 ml/min. Both these equations have certain assumptions suffer from some limitations which warrant intensive clinical monitoring of the patient for adverse effects.

Suggested Readings

1. Diebel L, Kozol R, Wilson RF, Mahajan S, Abu-Hamdan D, Thomas D (1993). Gastric intramucosal acidosis in patients with chronic kidney failure. *Surgery*. **113:** 520-6.

2. Dzhavad-Zade MD, Karaev ME (2004). Gastrointestinal hormones in the blood serum of patients with chronic renal failure. *Urologiia*. 56-8.

3. Johnson CA, Levey AS, Coresh J, Levin A, Lau J, Eknoyan G (2004). Clinical practice guidelines for chronic kidney disease in adults: Part I. Definition, disease stages, evaluation, treatment, and risk factors. *Am Fam Physician*. **70:** 869-76.

4. Myrna Y. Munar, Harleen Singh (2007). Drug Dosing Adjustments in Patients with Chronic Kidney Disease. *Am Fam Physician*. **75(10):**1487-1496.

5. Naud J, Michaud J, Beauchemin S, Hebert MJ, Roger M, Lefrancois S, *et al.,* (2011). Effects of chronic renal failure on kidney drug transporters and cytochrome P450 in rats. *Drug Metab Dispos*. **39:** 1363-1369.

6. Srisawat N, Hoste EE, Kellum JA (2010). Modern classification of acute kidney injury. *Blood Purif*. **29:** 300-7.

7. Ventkateswaran PS, Jeffers A, Hocken AG (1972). Gastric acid secretion in chronic renal failure. *Br Med J*. **4(5381):** 22-3.

CHAPTER 27

DRUG AND MALNUTRITION

Problem Status of Malnutrition

Malnutrition is a complex condition in which many deficiencies occur simultaneously. Protein energy malnutrition (PEM) is considered to be a global problem, especially for vulnerable children, infants, and institutional elderly who can be afflicted with PEM that accounts for high child mortality and morbidity. There were 925 million malnourished people in the world in 2010, an increase of 80 million since 1990. The largest number of undernourished people (million) in 2005-2007, according to the Food and Agriculture Organization of the United Nations is about 237.7 million in India. The incidence of PEM in industrialized societies is not rare, although it is usually secondary to renal, hepatic, or neoplastic diseases or surgery.

The prevalence of nutritional indicators in the form of underweight, stunting, and wasting in children under 5 years of age is one of the ways of assessment of nutritional status of the population. The available data indicate that the a huge disparity persist in the 21st Century with about 40% prevalence of moderate underweight in Bangladesh and Yemen to 2.2% in Brazil and 1.3% in the USA. So, prevalence of nutritional indicators is lowest in Western countries such as the United States and highest in much less developed countries such as Bangladesh and Yemen.

Malnourished children suffer from impaired immunity, which increases the likelihood of infection, disease, and death. Disease, in turn, can cause poor nutrient absorption, altered metabolism, and lack of appetite, leading to inadequate nutritional intake. In fully 56 % of all child deaths, undernutrition is a contributing factor; 83 % of these deaths are associated with mild or moderate rather than severe malnutrition. Malnutrition plays a role in the deaths of about 16,000 young children every day, virtually all of them in the developing world. That is a yearly toll of almost 6 million, about the same as the population of Denmark, Jordan, or Laos. Eliminating malnutrition would remove one-third of the global burden of disease and increase child survival.

What causes Malnutrition?

It includes many different clinical syndromes with protean manifestations. PEM is the state reached when the body's need for protein and energy fuels is not satisfied by the diet. Protein deficiency seldom occurs without a concomitant deficit of other nutrients; however, this may be one of the most important nutritional determinants of drug metabolism, pharmacokinetics, and effects. The immediate causes of malnutrition are inadequate dietary intake and disease. Underlying causes include inadequacies in access to food; in health services and a sanitary environment; and in people's caring practices for their children, eating behaviors, and personal hygiene. PEM can result of a disease state. In the latter case, diseases such as anorexia nervosa, cancer, and AIDS often lead to low food intake, inadequate nutrient absorption/utilization, or increased requirement of, or exaggerated loss of, nutrients. Approximately, 50% of cancer patients will become malnourished during the course of their disease, and this can lead to impaired tolerance to chemotherapy and impaired immune function. PEM also occurs in up to 65% of elderly hospitalized patients. The malnourished often have several concomitant diseases; including cancer, gastrointestinal diseases, acquired immunodeficiency syndrome (AIDS) are also associated with PEM. Therefore, drugs are as widely used as in the well-nourished. The pathophysiological profile in malnutrition can alter pharmacokinetic processes, drug responses and toxicity. This review summarizes the available knowledge on nutrient-drug interactions in malnourished subjects.

Micronutrient Deficiency

Micronutrients are essential daily dietary requirements which needed in very minute quantity and deficiencies of these key vitamins and minerals, like iron, vitamin A, zinc, and iodine; are associated with onset of disease and even severity. Worldwide, 2 billion people suffer from deleterious effects of micronutrient deficiencies; 37% suffer from anemia, 35% are at risk for iodine deficiency, and 20% are at risk for zinc deficiency. Zinc deficiency, adversely affects physical and reproductive growth, and neurodevelopment. Studies say that in pre-school age children, Vitamin A deficiency affects 25% and 18 % of women. Vitamin A deficiency weakens immunity and leads to infection, a range of eye problems including blindness, and an increased risk of childhood disease and death (child mortality by an average of 23%). In the developing countries, nearly, 50% of all young children don't receive enough iron in their diets, endangering their mental and physical development. Iodine deficiency disorders can result in irreversible mental retardation, goiter, reproductive failure, and increased child mortality whereas, Iron deficiency affects pregnancy, impairs cognitive development, and reduces work productivity. Severe iron-deficiency anemia increases the probability of disability and death among women of childbearing age.

Overnutrition

Worldwide, overweight and obesity increased alarmingly and known as the "nutrition transition," which found to be due to primarily increased intake of fats and processed carbohydrates and reduced physical activity. Overweight and obesity are measures of excess weight relative to height for children and adults (measured by body mass index (BMI), or weight/ height^2). Individuals experiencing intrauterine growth retardation or stunting in the first two years of life face a higher risk of obesity and/or non communicable diseases (NCDs) in adulthood: diabetes, hypertension, stroke, cardiovascular disease, and some forms of cancer. However, NCDs, often precipitated by poor nutrition, presently account for 60 % of global deaths and 46 % of the global burden of disease; the overall impact of diseases and injuries at the individual and societal level. By 2020, NCDs and obesity are predicted to cause 73 % of all deaths and 60 % of all disease. Among school-age children, 155 million are overweight and 40 million are obese whereas, about 1.1 billion adults are overweight and 300 million obese.

Maternal Nutrition

As we all know, in pregnancy physiology of body completely behaves differently (*see details in Chapter 22*) and hence maternal nutritional status is very important. As per the evidence, malnourished mothers suffer higher rates of morbidity and mortality, and are more likely to experience poor pregnancy outcomes, such as low birth weight, birth defects, hemorrhage, eclampsia, and other high-risk deliveries. Although, a mother's energy and nutrient needs increase during pregnancy and lactation hence require proper nutrition.

Assessment of Nutrition Status

A comprehensive nutrition assessment is the first step in formulating a patient-specific nutrition care plan. Nutrition assessment has four major goals:

(a) identification of the presence of factors associated with an increased risk of developing malnutrition, including disorders resulting from macro- or micronutrient deficiencies (under-nutrition), obesity (overnutrition), or impaired metabolism;

(b) determination of risk of malnutrition-associated complications;

(c) establishment of estimated nutrition needs; and

(d) establishment of baseline parameters against which to measure nutrition therapy outcomes.

A comprehensive nutrition assessment should include a nutrition- focused medical, surgical and dietary history, a nutrition focused physical examination including anthropometrics and laboratory measurements. Nutrition assessment provides a basis for determining the patient's nutrition requirements and the optimal type and timing of nutrition intervention.

Anthropometric Measurements

Anthropometric measurements, gross measurements of body cell mass, are used to evaluate LBM and fat stores. The most common measurements are weight, stature (height or length, depending on age), head circumference (for children younger than 3 years of age), and measurements of limb size, such as skin fold thickness, mid-arm muscle circumference, wrist circumference, and waist circumference. Bioelectrical impedance analysis (BIA) is also an anthropometric assessment tool. These parameters are used to compare an individual with normative standards for a population and as repeated measurements in an individual to monitor response to a nutrition care plan. In adults, nutrition-related changes in anthropometric measurements occur slowly; several weeks or more are usually required before detectable changes are noted. In infants and young children, however, changes may occur more quickly. Acute changes in anthropometric measurements, specifically weight and skin fold thickness, usually reflect changes in hydration status, which must be considered when interpreting these parameters, particularly in hospitalized patients.

Below are some Indicators of Malnutrition

1. Child growth indicators: How are they defined?

   - *Underweight:* weight for age < –2 standard deviations (SD) of the WHO Child Growth Standards median

   - *Stunting:* height for age < –2 SD of the WHO Child Growth Standards median

   - *Wasting:* weight for height < –2 SD of the WHO Child Growth Standards median

   - *Overweight:* weight for height > +2 SD of the WHO Child Growth Standards median

2. Low birth weight has been defined by WHO as weight at birth of < 2500 grams (5.5 pounds).

3. Body mass index (BMI) (kg/m2) or (lb/in2) Interpretation for adults

(a)	< 16	Severe malnutrition
(b)	16-16.9	Moderate malnutrition
(c)	17-18.5	Mild malnutrition
(d)	19-25	Healthy (19-34 years of age)
(e)	21-27	Healthy (older than 35 years of age)
(f)	25-30	Overweight (19-34 years of age)
(g)	27.5-29.9	Overweight (older than 35 years of age)
(h)	30-40	Moderate obesity
(i)	> 40	Severe or morbid obesity

4. Anemia in children under 5 years of age and pregnant women as a haemoglobin concentration < 110 g/l at sea level.

5. Vitamin A: A plasma or serum retinol concentration < 0.70 µmol/l indicates subclinical vitamin A deficiency in children and adults, and < 0.35 µmol/l indicates severe vitamin A deficiency.

6. Iodine: Median urinary iodine concentration:

   (a)   < 20 µg/l: Severe deficiency

   (b)   20-49 µg/l: Moderate

   (c)   50-99 µg/l: Mild deficiency

   (d)   100-199 µg/l: Optimal

   (e)   200-299 µg/l: Risk of iodine-induced hyper-thyroidism

   (f)   ≥ 300 µg/l: Risk of adverse health consequences

7. Visceral Proteins Used for Assessment of Lean Body Mass: Serum visceral proteins are of greatest value in assessing uncomplicated semi starvation and recovery.

   (a) *Albumin:* It is assumed that a low serum protein concentration in states of under-nutrition reflects the hepatic protein synthetic mass, and therefore indirectly reflects the functional protein mass of other organs such as heart, lung, kidney, and intestines. Albumin remains one of the most widely used biochemical markers of malnutrition and has long been used in population studies. It is, however, a relatively insensitive index of early protein malnutrition because there is a large amount normally found in the body (4 to 5g/kg of body weight), it is highly distributed in the extravascular compartment (60%), and it has a long half-life (18 to 20 days). However, chronic protein deficiency in the setting of adequate nonprotein calorie intake leads to marked hypoalbuminemia because of a net ALB loss. Serum ALB concentrations of 2.5g/dL or less can be expected to exacerbate ascites and peripheral, pulmonary, and GI mucosal edema as a result of decreased colloid oncotic pressure.

   (b) *Transferrin:* TFN is a glycoprotein that binds and transports ferric iron to the liver and reticuloendothelial system for storage. As a surrogate marker of nutrition status, TFN will decrease in response to protein depletion before serum ALB concentrations decrease because it has a shorter biologic half-life (8 days), and there is less of it in the body (less than 100 mg/kg of body weight). Serum TFN concentrations may be determined by direct measurement or can be estimated indirectly from measurement of total iron-binding capacity, where TFN = (total iron-binding capacity × 0.8) − 43. In iron deficiency, hepatic TFN synthesis is increased, resulting in increased serum TFN concentrations unrelated to protein status.

(c) *Prealbumin:* It is the transport protein for thyroxin and a carrier for retinol-binding protein. The body's content of prealbumin is low (10 mg/kg of body weight), and it has a very short biologic half-life (2 to 3 days). Prealbumin may be reduced in as few as 3 days after calorie and protein intake is significantly decreased, or when hyper catabolism or severe metabolic stress (trauma or burns) is present. Because of its short half-life, it is most useful in monitoring the short-term, acute effects of nutrition support or deficits. As with ALB and TFN, serum prealbumin concentrations are depressed in those with liver disease as a consequence of decreased hepatic synthesis. Increased serum prealbumin concentrations have been noted in patients with kidney disease as a result of impaired excretion.

Clinical Presentation of Under-Nutrition

Malnutrition is manifested with protean manifestations affecting every organ systems of the human body. The clinical features also depend upon the age, previous body weight, associated disease conditions and severity of deficiency of nutrition and duration of such deficiencies. In adults under-nutrition or prolong starvation mainly presents as marasmus. Two classic types of under-nutrition presentation in pediatric age group are marasmus and kwashiorkor. Marasmus is characterized by loss of weight, disappearance of subcutaneous fats leading to loss of skin turgor and muscle atrophy, all these leading to gauntness. Plasma albumin may deplete from its normalcy.

Kwashiorkor, in the other hand manifests aggressively with inadequate growth, loss of muscular tissue, fluid retention, oedema and hepatomegally. Hair discoloration to crazy pavement dermatological patches along with psychological alterations and impaired immune status make the subject proan to multitude of bacterial and viral infections. Even in some cases these two conditions present simultaneously leading to marasmic-kwashiorkor.

Overnutrition/Obesity on Drug Disposition

Obesity is defined as BMI > 95th percentile for age and sex of individuals, results in altered body composition i.e. increased proportion and absolute amount of adipose tissue as well as an increase in lean body mass, blood volume, cardiac output, and organ size, furthermore, effect physiology of body. In pediatric population, obesity can result in an expansion of blood volume, resulting in increased stroke volume and cardiac output. Generally speaking, malabsorption of drugs is more likely to occur with the primary malabsorptive procedures such as jejunoileal bypass and pancreato-biliary diversion. The lipophilicity of a drug determines the extent to which obesity influences the volume of distribution and ultimately whether dosing should be based on actual or adjusted body weight. Highly lipophilic drugs, such as lidocaine, thiopental, phenytoin, verapamil, and most benzodiazepines, have an increased volume of distribution in severely obese patients. Absorption of drugs evaluated to date appears to be unchanged owing to obesity; however, the data are very limited. Severely obese patients who have undergone bariatric surgery for weight loss are more likely to experience altered drug absorption that may affect the clinical responses to therapy. Modest increases in volume of distribution have also been reported for aminoglycosides, heparin, ibuprofen, methylxanthines, prednisolone, and vancomycin, suggesting that an adjusted body weight rather than actual body weight (ABW) be used to avoid toxicity. However, the most accurate approach to adjust for the excess body mass is unknown and appears to be different depending on the characteristics of individual compounds. Therapeutic drug monitoring is recommended when applicable to optimize therapy. Although the protein binding of acidic drugs is unchanged, the free fraction of basic drugs may be decreased. Similarly, changes in hepatic drug clearance are variable. Phase 1 reactions and phase I acetylation appear to be unaffected by obesity, but the phase II glucuronidation and sulfonation pathways are enhanced. Obesity may also affect systemic clearance of highly extracted drugs such as aminoglycosides and unmetabolized procainamide. Both glomerular filtration and tubular secretion also appear to be increased. Renal clearance of drug that, mediated by both glomerular filtration and active secretion, such as digoxin and cimetidine, is relatively unchanged in obesity.

Early dosing recommendations suggested that initial dosing must be based on ideal body weight (IBW) as it was thought that the drug distributed only into lean body mass. Schwartz and colleagues determined that, when the volume of distribution is corrected for total body weight, it is significantly smaller when compared with normal weight subjects. For example, the distribution of aminoglycosides into excess body weight is estimated to be about 40% of that distributed into ideal body tissue. Initial dosing of aminoglycosides in obese patients may be determined by adding 40% of the excess weight to the patient's IBW, with subsequent dosage adjustments based on serum drug levels and clinical status. A similar controversy exists for optimizing theophylline dosing in obese patients and whether actual or IBW should be used to calculate the initial theophylline loading dose. The differences in theophylline volume of distribution based on IBW and ABW increases as the degree of obesity increases. The recommendation is that theophylline dosing in patients with mild to moderate obesity, be based on ABW but that IBW be used when initiating therapy in severely or morbidly obese patients. Hepatic drug metabolism may also be altered in patients with nonalcoholic steatohepatitis (NASH), including enhanced glucuronidation and sulfonation, causing a faster drug excretion compared with normal-weight subjects. There is alteration in CYP2E1 expression and activities in obese patients (increased) with nonalcoholic fatty liver disease, including NASH resulting in alteration in metabolism of compound like, fatty acids, ketones, and ethanol. The metabolic pathways of fatty acids and other xenobiotics may lead to the release of free radicals, which can cause lipid peroxidation and liver injury, including mitochondrial damage. In patients with hepatic inflammation or fatty liver, these oxidative stress changes may have role and may also be more susceptible to the toxic effects of drugs resulting to impaired metabolism.

Alteration in Pharmacokinetics in Undernutrition

PEM has been shown to alter drug metabolism and dynamics in children and in animal models. In children, PEM reduced the clearance of isoniazid, and acetanilide. Animal models of PEM have shown reductions in the clearance of doxorubicin and acetaminophen, and altered oxidative drug metabolism, conjugation, and protein binding. PEM induced alterations in drug metabolism and dynamics appear to be multifactorial processes and a complete understanding of the effect of nutritional status on drug pharmacokinetics would be highly desirable for effective clinical treatment.

There are very few data of diet and nutritional status in human which shows important environmental variables determining the pharmacotoxicological properties of chemicals. Clinical risk of toxicity appears to be higher in malnourished children. Rehabilitation studies suggest that a number of these pharmacological abnormalities can be reversed. Recently, intense effort has been initially directed at studying drug kinetics in grade III malnutrition, namely kwashiorkor and marasmus. Studies on drugs and nutrients indicate, delayed or decreased absorption, reduced protein binding of several drugs, fluctuations in volume of distribution, altered hepatic oxidative drug biotransformations and conjugations, reduced elimination of conjugates and reduced elimination of renally excreted drugs. The estimated steady-state levels of a few drugs suggest accumulation. Bioavailability problems are seen in some drugs due to divergent effects of pharmacokinetic processes during malnutrition. Therapeutic inadequacies and toxicities need careful evaluation in malnourished children.

Single dose pharmacokinetics studies were preferred in severely malnourished children. During the study, a number of abnormalities were seen in drug metabolism during the acute phase of malnutrition. For practical purposes, it is important to consider steady-state levels and data in mild and moderate forms of growth-retarded children; drug-induced nutritional deficiencies can occur more easily in these populations. There must be monitoring of drug plasma concentrations in malnourished children as per published reports, particularly for those drugs which have dose dependent kinetics and narrow margins of safety.

As malnutrition is associated with multifactorial diseases, so use of drugs to combat those ailments is common among them. Again the drugs are handled by the body by the four cardinal processes of absorption, distribution, metabolism and excretion. These processes are dependent on the status of organ system of body, which are affected to a greater extent during malnutrition. The interrelationship between food, nutritional status and drug is a complex process and it needs good understanding of the specific fields of interaction which are of practical relevance and clinical significance. Proper management i.e. rational drug use in these cases requires knowledge of sound pharmacokinetic and pharmacodynamic principles relevant in this scenario of malnutrition and the factors modifying the fate of drugs in body. Nutrient drug interaction and nutritional pharmacotoxicological interactions are basically caused by physical, chemical, physiological and pathophysiological interaction between drugs, nutrients and human body. Therefore, the nutritional status has significant effect o the drug pharmacokinetics and pharmacodynamics.

Organ System Alteration Influences Drug Handling

We will discuss the effect of malnutrition on the organ systems and their significant effect on drug kinetics in body.

A.   **Gastrointestinal system**

The mucosal epithelium of GI tract is having rapid turnover of cells. In the nutrient deficient condition mucosa suffers much due to impaired cell proliferation, migration and maturation leading to loss of crypt of villus, loss of surface area. This results in reduced mucous and enzyme production, altered intestinal flora, scretory antibodies are reduced. Functional representation of these causes impaired absorption, altered peristalsis and delayed gastric emptying, increased or decreased intestinal transit time, pancreatic and billiary insufficiency, reduced enterohepatic circulation, maldigestion, vitamin and mineral deficiency and bacterial over-growth and infestation.

B.   **Hepatic changes**

Liver has major role in body metabolism of endogenous to exogenous products. Dietary deficiency leads to alteration in the structural and functional status of liver, though permanent changes do not occur due to malnutrition. Kwashiorkor causes fat infiltration of hepatocytes leading to fatty liver. There is decreased protein synthesis in liver leading to alteration in plasma protein levels. All these leads to derangement in biotransformation process of drugs, reduced hepatic and billiary excretion, reduced enterohepatic circulation, decreased first pass metabolism of drugs.

C.   **Body composition and metabolic changes**

Malnutrition results in loss of body water, initially extracellular and later intracellular also. Depletion of glycogen stores both from liver and muscles, reduced blood glucose and poor insulin response causes impaired glucose tolerance. Loss of body deposit of fats and accumulation of triglycerides in liver (Fatty liver) leads to elevated serum free fatty acids. Reduction in protein synthesis and reduced muscle proteins leads to decrease in lean body mass and basal metabolic rate. Hypoalbuminemia with increased alpha-1 acid glycoproteins leads altered plasma protein binding of drugs. Body electrolytes i.e. sodium, potassium, magnesium are reduced due to loss of body tissues and also due to associated malabsorption and diarrhea. All these leads to alteration in protein binding, receptor and drug interaction, reduced volume of distribution and tissue uptake and alteration in drug retention and excretion.

D.   **Renal function**

Reduction in renal blood flow and glomerular filtration results in perturbed renal clearance of drugs.

E.   **Cardiovascular changes**

Reduction in plasma volume, decreased cardiac function leads to low blood pressure, decreased cardiac output and prolonged circulation time. All these leads to decline in organ blood flow and decreased tissue perfusion. So drugs cannot reach the site of action and leads to reduced efficacy.

F.   **Endocrine function**

In malnutrition hormonal alteration also occurs due to the stress factor and deranged protein status. In pediatric malnutrition the marasmic children are more adaptive than kwashiorkor subjects. The marasmic children have high rise in cortisol levels and they live at own expenses of muscle and adipose mass. The kwashiorkor children being unadaptive, there occurs oedema, fatty liver with high rise in growth hormone levels. Thyroid hormone is also depleted. All these leads to altered intermediary metabolism of drugs, deranged protein binding, drug receptor interaction, distribution and biotransformation of drugs.

G.   **Immune status**

Impaired immune function leads to more proan for infections, which requires more use of drugs. Altered drug kinetic status complicates this situation.

Pharmacokinetic Changes

A.   **Drug absorption**

Under malnutrition, the extent of absorption of most of the drugs was not significantly affected except few drugs like apirin, metronidazole, phenytoin, tobramycin, caffeine, paracetamol, penicillin, phenobarbitone, quinine, sulphadiazine and sulphame-thoxazole, were found to be significantly increased, which is probably due to the effects of decreased clearance or a prolonged half-life. Ideally, in pharmacokinetic studies, rate is measured as Ka (h^{-1}) and extent of absorption, F (%), as $AUC_{oral} \times Dose_{i.v}/ AUC_{i.v} \times Dose_{oral}$. In the case of, oral penicillin administered to fasted PEM children, F was decreased in underweight children by 36% compared with 55% in controls, increased in marasmus by 66% compared with 55% in controls and in kwashiorkor by 83% compared with 55% in controls. Contrasting results were also documented for quinine. The extent of absorption of oral quinine was increased, whereas the extent of intramuscular absorption was not significantly affected. For chloroquine, the peak plasma concentration and extent of absorption are lower in kwashiorkor than in healthy children, which might be of clinical significance.

Rate of absorption (Ka) was significantly increased for sulphadiazine and significantly decreased for sulphamethoxazole, tetracycline, rifampicin and anticonvulsants in children with PEM. In children with different categories of PEM, the Ka of chloramphenicol was significantly decreased in children with marasmic-kwashiorkor only, whereas it was significantly increased for oral penicillin in children suffering from kwashiorkor only. Absorption of nutrients given as medicaments, such as vitamin A, B_{12}, iron and fat and peptides are declined in PEM. Thus nutrient deficiency in the gastrointestinal tract may influence several steps in the bioavailability pathway and it is not possible to predict these by general rules. It is also necessary to quantify absorption in malnutrition with specific references to other pharmacokinetic parameters.

B.   Protein binding and distribution

The interaction of drugs and protein molecules profoundly influences the distribution of a drug in body compartments and its biological activity which is produced by the free form of the drug. The variability in drug-protein binding leads to alteration in other pharmacokinetic parameters such as volume of distribution, half life and elimination of drugs. Clearance always depends directly upon the free form of the drug. Several nutrients such as fatty acids, tryptophan, bilirubin, hormones like thyroxine also play a role in modifying protein binding of several drugs. Malnutrition, which causes reduction in plasma albumin and increases acid glycoprotein, and deranged the above nutrients leads to significant changes in protein binding of drugs. The practical significance of this deranged drug-protein binding is not so well studied in malnutrition subjects. In the presence of low protein binding, drugs with low extraction ratio have increased hepatic clearance. But this fact does not hold good in malnutrition, where the hepatic and renal function are also deranged.

The protein binding of several drugs was significantly reduced in kwashiorkor including cloramphenicol, cloxacillin, digoxin, ethionamide, flucoxacillin, para-aminosalicylic acid, penicillin, phenobarbitone, salicylate, streptomycin, sulphamethoxazole, thiopentone. The drugs which have increased protein bindings in kwashiorkor include chloroquine, dicoumarol, ethambutol, gentamicin, isoniazid, rifampicin, phenytoin, quinine. However, for quinine protein binding expressed as a % of bound drugs, was not significantly different in both the control group (94%) and the PEM children (93%).

Drug is distributed in the body by compartmental system. After equilibrium is reached, drug distribution can be assessed by apparent volume of distribution. The drugs which have small volume of distribution, the increase in free fraction of drug owing to reduced protein binding will significantly alter its pharmacokinetics and pharmacodynamics. For drugs, with larger volume of distribution, such changes are not significant. The volume of distribution though decreased in kwashiorkor but not significant, for acetanilide, amikacin, chloramphenicol, isoniazid, metronidazole. In marasmus condition, chloramphenicol and penicillin have shown insignificant increase in volume of distribution. There were contrasting results for 4 drugs (gentamicin, quinine, streptomycin and theophylline). In the case of gentamicin, children with kwashiorkor documented decreased Vd. In contrast, in children who were underweight, marasmic or experiencing marasmic-kwashiorkor had an increased Vd of gentamicin. In the case of theophylline, erratic Vd was found. In the case of, streptomycin, children with kwashiorkor exhibited an increased Vd, whereas children with marasmus or underweight had a decreased Vd.

Based upon these, drawing of any clinical conclusions regarding changes in protein binding and volume of distribution will not be satisfactory, because there is alteration in multiple facets of drug handling like the plasma protein status and also hepatic and renal functions. However, for highly protein bound drugs, having narrow margin of therapeutic index and requiring biotransformation and renal clearances, toxicities are expected in extreme cases of malnutrition.

C.   Biotransformation of drugs

Metabolism is a cardinal factor influencing drug clearance and followed by drug concentration and effects. This process is carried out by group of enzymes in the endoplasmic reticulum of several organ systems of the body including liver, intestinal mucosa, skin, lungs, kidney, and placenta. Nutrients have shown significant influence on the biotransformation of drugs by affecting enzyme systems to several associated steps.

Role of nutrients in biotransformation

- *Macronutrients:* The macronutrients like carbohydrate, protein and fat affects overall cell functions, protein synthesis and phosphatidylcholine synthesis.

- *Vitamins:* Vitamins have also wide effects like vitamin E as coenzymes, riboflavin for flavoprotein synthesis, nicotinic acid as coenzyme in oxidation and reduction reactions, folic acid in one carbon transfer reactions, ascorbic acid as coenzyme in hydroxylation reactions and in absorption of iron.

- *Trace elements:* These have important role like selenium and zinc in haem synthesis, magnesium in electron transfer, potassium in membrane structure and calcium in bone turnover. Enzymes require elements as prosthetic group like cobalt, copper, iron, molybdenum, selenium, zinc. Elements having regulatory role and role in hormone action are calcium, chromium, iodine, magnesium, manganese, sodium and potassium.

- *Endogenous cofactors:* Cofactors like glucose, aminoacids, glutathione, glycine, S-adenosylmethionine are involved in conjugation reactions of drug metabolism.

Most metabolic biotransformation occur at some point between absorption of the drug into the general circulation and its renal elimination. A few transformations occur in the intestinal lumen or intestinal wall. In general, all of these reactions can be assigned to one of two major categories called phase 1 and phase 2 reactions. Phase 1 reactions, in which enzymes carry out oxidation, reduction, or hydrolytic reactions, and leading to polarization of the drug product by introduction of functional groups. In phase 2 reactions enzymes form a conjugate of the substrate. Phase 2 enzymes facilitate the elimination of drugs and the inactivation of electrophilic and potentially toxic metabolites produced by oxidation. While many phase 1 reactions result in the biological inactivation of the drug, phase 2 reactions produce a metabolite with improved water solubility and increased molecular weight, which serves to facilitate the elimination of the drug from the tissue.

- *Phase 1 reactions:* In severe malnutrition, when dietary protein intake is considerably reduced, enzymes responsible for oxidative metabolism are impaired resulting in higher steady-state concentrations of drugs such as theophylline, acetanilide and phenobarbitone.

- *Phase 2 reactions:* Conjugation reactions require enzymes like glucuronosyl transferase for glucuronidation, glutathione transferase for glutathione conjugation, sulfotransferase for sulfation, N-acetyl transferase for acetylation, transmethylase for methylation, glycine transferase for glycine conjugation. Drastic reduction in dietary proteins will lead to depletion in these enzymes leading to decreased clearance of drugs such as isoniazid, sulphadiazine, chloramphenicol and paracetamol.

D.   Clearance and half-life

Clearance of drugs is mainly through two important organs of body i.e. liver and kidney, though other organs have also role for specific drugs.

1. *Hepatic clearance:* Among drugs that are primarily metabolised in the liver, the total clearance is significantly decreased with a correspondingly increased half-life has been seen for acetanilide, caffeine, chloramphenicol, isoniazid, and metronidazole. All of these have been related to kwashiorkor condition. The total clearance of quinine was significantly decreased in poorly categorised malnourished children and kwashiorkor, but significantly increased in children with all categories of PEM except kwashiorkor. Similarly, the total clearance of chloramphenicol was either significantly decreased in kwashiorkor or unaffected in marasmus and marasmic kwashiorkor.

2. *Renal clearance:* The effects of PEM on total clearance of drugs that are primarily eliminated by the kidneys are also studied. Cefoxitin and penicillin have significant decrease in clearances, though their half-life was not affected

significantly. However, for aminoglycosides like gentamicin, amikacin and streptomycin, there was no influence of PEM on the total clearance. Streptomycin has an increased plasma half-life in children with kwashiorkor, but no change in children who were underweight or had marasmus only. This was probably a result of the presence of oedema in kwashiorkor, which enhances the volume of distribution of streptomycin.

Plasma half-life of chloramphenicol, paracetamol, phenobarbitone, sulphadiazine and sulphamethoxazole were significantly increased due to protein energy malnutrition, whereas that of aspirin, chloroquine, isoniazid, phenytoin, gentamicin and tobramycin is not significantly affected.

Solutions

1. Growth Monitoring and Promotion and Behavior Change Communication: The control on malnutrition is well, when accompanied by successful behavior change communication, growth monitoring and attending promotion programs. These points have the potential to bring about a 3-% point reduction in stunting per year (when observed over five years).

2. Food or Cash Provisions by governments and non-government organizations though different programs

3. Micronutrient Interventions: National programs to reduce micronutrient malnutrition have used two primary strategies: supplementation and food fortification, with some additional attention to dietary diversification and genetic modification of food crops to boost micronutrient content, as with Golden Rice fortified with vitamin A, Iodized salt is the most common fortified food.

4. Addressing the Nutrition Transition: Solutions to overweight and obesity often focus on promoting physical activity; on changing eating habits to less processed foods lower in fat, sugar, and salt; and on food policy.

5. Nutrition Interventions in the Presence of HIV and Malaria: The infants must be under investigation if, mother suffering from any HIV. Appropriate infant feeding practices can limit mother-to-child transmission of HIV, occurring in an estimated 30 % of infants born to HIV-positive mothers. WHO/UN recommendations advocate for replacement feeding by HIV-infected mothers when replacement milk is acceptable, feasible, affordable, sustainable, and safe; otherwise, breastfeeding is recommended during the first months of life.

Despite the noted benefits of micronutrient supplementation, there is evidence that iron supplementation can exacerbate malaria among young children. Revised WHO guidelines now recommend that in place of universal supplementation, iron and folic acid supplementation in malaria-endemic areas target only those who are anemic and at risk of iron deficiency.

Parenteral Nutrition

Lack of oral nutrient intake during parenteral nutrition (PN) leads to mucosal atrophy of the bowel along with a reduction in gastric, biliary, pancreatic, and intestinal secretions. Bacterial overgrowth can result in a progressive decline in intestinal function owing to impaired motility and depressed enzyme activity. This may alter the rate and extent of absorption of specific nutrients as well as various drugs. Decreases in nutrient absorption include fat, iron, peptides, and vitamins A and B12 as well as drugs such as chloramphenicol, chloroquine, tetracycline, and rifampin. PN has been observed to decrease hepatic drug and xenobiotic metabolism in animals and humans. Drug metabolism may be altered due to jejunal and ileal mucosal hypoplasia and hypofunction as parenterally administered nutrients bypass the intestine. Patients receiving a postoperative 2,000 kcal PN regimen providing all nonprotein calories as dextrose showed a 34% reduction of mean antipyrine clearance after 7 days of total parenteral nutrition compared with unfed controls. This effect was seen also in patients receiving a 1,600 kcal dextrose-based regimen Moreover, patients receiving a 2,000 kcal PN regimen in which 500 kcal were provided as lipid, mean antipyrine clearance was not significantly different from that of the unfed control group. This study suggested that hepatic CYP1A activity might be affected by different total parenteral nutrition regimens.

Conclusion

Protein energy malnutrition is a public health problem affecting a great number of children throughout the world. PEM significantly decreased total clearance and increased the half-life of many drugs primarily metabolised in the liver, which may indicate a need for modifications of the doses of these drugs in the acute phase management of PEM. Despite the global burden of PEM and treatment of the affected children with numerous medicines, there have been so few studies that have looked at the effect of PEM on the pharmacokinetics of drugs in children. The World Health Organisation (WHO), in collaboration with UNICEF, Save the Children, Médicins Sans Frontières and the International Paediatric Association, has launched a major campaign entitled "Make Medicines Child Size". This welcome initiative will result in increased research in relation to medicines for children in developing countries.

Suggested Readings

1. Abernathy DR, Greenblatt DJ (1986). Drug disposition in obese humans: An update. *Clin Pharmacokinet* **11**: 199-213.

2. Blouin RA, Kolpek JH, Mann HJ (1987). Influences of obesity on drug disposition. *Clin Pharm* **6**:706-14.

3. Burgess P, Hall RI, Bateman DN, Johnston ID (1987). The effect of total parenteral nutrition on hepatic drug oxidation. *J Parenter Enteral Nutr* **11**: 540-3.

4. Chessman KH, Kumpf VJ (2008). Assessment of nutrition status and nutrition requirements. In Pharmacotherapy A Pathophysiologic Approach: DiPiro JT, Talbert RL, Yee GC, Matzke GR, Wells BG, Posey LM. 7th ed. New York. McGraw Hill, pp. 2349-67.

5. Denke M, Wilson J (1998). Protein and energy malnutrition. In Harrison's Principles of Internal Medicine: Fauci A, Braunwald E, Isselbacher K, Wilson J, Martin J, Kasper D, Hauser S, Longo D (editors). 14th ed. New York. McGraw Hill, pp. 452-4.

6. El Mouzan MI, Foster PJ, Al Herbish AS, Al Salloum AA, Al Omar AA, Qurachi MM (2010). Prevalence of malnutrition in Saudi children: a community-based study. *Ann Saudi Med.* **30(5):** 381-5.

7. Emery MG, Fisher JM, Chien JY, *et al.,* (2003). CYP2E1 activity before and after weight loss in morbidly obese subjects with nonalcoholic fatty liver disease. *Hepatology.* **38:** 428-35.

8. Greene JB (1988). Clinical approach to weight loss in the patient with HIV infection. *Gastroenterol Clin North Am.* **17(3):** 573-86.

9. Gura KM, Chan LN (2008). Drug Therapy and Role of Nutrition. Chapter 18. Available at: http://anhi.org/learning/pdfs/bcdecker/Drug_Therapy_Role_of_Nutrition.pdf.

10. http://www.fao.org/economic/ess/food-security-statistics/en/

11. http://www.prb.org/pdf07/Nutrition2007.pdf

12. http://www.prb.org/pdf07/Nutrition2007.pdf.

13. http://www.prb.org/Publications/Datasheets/2007/2007WorldPopulationDataSheet.aspx

14. http://www.prb.org/Publications/Datasheets/2007/2007WorldPopulationDataSheet.aspx

15. Krishnaswamy K (1989). Drug metabolism and pharmacokinetics in malnourished children. *Clin Pharmacokinet.* **17 (Suppl 1):** 68-88.

16. Lieber CS (2004). CYP2E1: From ASH to NASH. *Hepatol Res* **28:** 1-11.

17. NLIS Country Profile Indicators Interpretation Guide. WHO. Available at: http://whqlibdoc.who.int/publications/2010/9789241599955_eng.pdf

18. Oshikoya KA, Sammons HM, Choonara I (2010). A systematic review of pharmacokinetics studies in children with protein-energy malnutrition. *Eur J Clin Pharmacol.* **66(10):** 1025-35.

19. Reilly JJ, Weir J, McColl JH, Gibson BE (1999). Prevalence of protein-energy malnutrition at diagnosis in children with acute lymphoblastic leukemia. *J Pediatr Gastroenterol Nutr.* **29(2):**194-7.

20. Schwartz SN, Pazin GJ, Lyon JA, Ho M (1978). A controlled investigation of the pharmacokinetics of gentamicin and tobramycin in obese patients. *J Infect Dis* **138:** 499-505.

21. Strauss SG, Lynn AM, Bratton SL, Nespeca MK (1999). Ventilatory response to CO_2 in children with obstructive sleep apnea from adenotonsillar hypertrophy. *Anesth Analg* **89:** 328-32.

22. Sullivan DH, Sun S, Walls RC (1999). Protein-energy undernutrition among elderly hospitalized patients: a prospective study. *JAMA.* **281(21):** 2013-9.

23. Traub SL, Johnson CE (1980). Comparison of methods of estimating creatinine clearance in children. *Am J Hosp Pharm* **37:** 195-201.

24. Visram N, Friesen EG, Jamali F (1987). Theophylline loading dose in obese patients. *Clin Pharm* **6:** 188-189.

25. Williams ML, Mager DE, Parenteau H, Gudi G, Tracy TS, Mulheran M, Wainer IW (2004). Effects of protein calorie malnutrition on the pharmacokinetics of ketamine in rats. *Drug Metab Dispos.* **32(8):** 786-93.

CHAPTER 28

CLINICAL IMPLICATION OF FIXED DOSE COMBINATIONS (FDC)

Introduction

In recent time, drug therapy is widely changed to improve the patient compliance and the disease treatment. Designing of Fixed Dose Combinations (FDC's) is one of the important from the public health prospective. There was guideline developed by the international organization (WHO) and by regulator (US-FDA/ICMR/CDSCO). Now days, FDC's are commonly used in the clinical practice and particularly found to be useful in the management of HIV, malaria and tuberculosis. FDC's is usually described drug combination of two or more active drugs present in a dosage form. Whereas, US-FDA broaden the term by defining it as combination product or a product composed of any combination of a drug and a device or a biological product and a device or a drug and a biological product or a drug, device, and a biological product.

Advantage, Disadvantage and Pharmacoecomonic Consideration of FDC

The most important consideration is that there should be real clinical benefits in the form of increased efficacy with reduced incidence of adverse effects, but such claims should be supported by evidence. Patient's compliance, low inventory, less manufacturing cost and multiple targeting in microbial therapy is the other advantages of FDC's.

The control and regulation of the FDC's are well in the developed countries whereas in the developing and under developing countries regulation are in bad condition and has been an alarming increase in irrational FDC's. The implementation of product patent regime in developing countries restricts many companies for manufacturing the drugs under the regulation and hence, manufacturing industries find various alternatives to sustain themselves in the market place and combination products for newer indications was an attractive alternative. WHO described 18 fixed dose combinations in their 14th list of essential medicine, but despite of there are several irrational combinations are available and widely prescribed by physician in developing and under developed countries. Study from developing country showed 80% of the FDC's prescribed are not from the recommended WHO list. These are actually leads to financial burden, resistant strains of bacteria and increase the adverse effects.

Role of Regulatory Organization and other Issue in Developed and Developing Countries

The regulatory requirements for approval of FDC is usually vary from country to country. So, important aspect for regulator is to evaluate the pharmacokinetic profile of the drugs in combination and pharmacological effects or risks and benefits ratio. Irrational FDC's may be minimized by preparing guideline which should provide guidance to the industry and control the developing new FDC's. Pharmaceuticals industry is rapidly growing in developing nation and same time excess numbers of FDC's are also available in the market for diseases like, cold, tuberculosis, malaria, HIV etc. More than one-third of all the new drug products introduced in the market are fixed dose combination (FDC's) preparations. Availability of the FDC's varies in developed and developing countries such as 10% of the new products are FDC's in Japan, whereas in European countries, it is approximately 56%, whereas epidemiological data of developing countries are not available.

There are several rational FDC's designed to increase the efficacy (β-lactam + β-lactamase inhibitors), duration (β-lactam + tubular secretion inhibitors) or to reduce the side effect of the drug (levodopa + l-amino acid decarboxylase inhibitors) etc. but few irrational FDC's like NSAID's and NSAID's, NSAID's and muscle relaxant etc. Experts have expressed serious concerns over the marketing of increasing number of irrational FDC's by pharmaceutical companies which unnecessarily increase financial burden, adverse effects, and decrease quality of life of patients. The practice of polypharmacy is the advantageous but, it may be widely misused and hence, highly debatable issue. The World Health Organization (WHO) issued a list of 325 essential drugs with 18 FDC's, but available FDC's are quite a large number compared to the WHO list. Particularly in developing countries market; FDC's are available for various disease conditions and most of FDC's preparations are vitamins, cough suppressants, anti-diarrheal, iron preparations, antacids, analgesics etc. Presently most of regulatory bodies treated FDC's as a new drug, since these combining two or more drugs, should be pass through the efficacy, and bioavailability study including the toxicity profile.

Clinical Pharmacologist View *Vs* Clinician Consideration (Rationale and irrational drug combination)

The rationale behind the FDC's combination is to increase the efficacy or reduce the side effect of the individual drugs but, should not be combined together just because they can be taken together.

The FDC's are rational if it has a well defined, and documented therapeutic indication and if specific mechanism exists to justify the combination for example cotrimoxazole, pyrimethamine + sulfadoxine, levodopa + carbidopa etc. So, in absence of such mechanisms a FDC's is irrational because titration of doses for individual drugs is not possible. There may be dumping of dose which lead to difficulty in identification of cause of side effects moreover pharmacokinetics of drugs may change after the combination and not match. So, it has been assumed that FDC's without well defined, well documented and specific mechanisms are harmful and undesirable to use in the clinical practice. But, theoretical disadvantage of FDC's is often inconsequential and further there is a convenience, compliance and less cost in combination compared to single ingredient product.

Presently, prescribing FDC's has become the integral part in medical practice. The major excuse is better patient compliance and some of infectious diseases being resistant to treatment with an individual drug. With the escalating cost of drugs and poor drug compliance due to adverse effects, which further magnifies the problem, both for the prescriber as well as the patient.

The selection of optimal dose and optimal combination has remained largely a matter of trial and error. There are number of irrational combinations which are not approved in any developed country but are being marketed in the developing countries. It is always important to check rationality by keeping various factors like dose titration issue, safety concern; satisfaction of pharmacokinetic measurements besides this all the benefits should be evident. So, an absolute requirement is the clinical need for FDCs. The ingredients should all be necessary and should contribute towards the therapeutic goal. The ingredients should be compatible with each other which should not disturb the bio-availability of the resultant compound.

Conclusions

Presently better future approach and corrective measure are required because pharmaceutical industry is rapidly growing in the world market. So, marketing scientifically sound drug combination would add value to this business. At the same time academia has the opportunity of contributing by conceptualizing and documenting the value for FDC's. FDC's screening is already a practice in many developed and developing countries to evaluate its efficacy, safety and rationality.

Presently, there is no existing guideline for fixed dose combination in most of the developing countries. Most of the regulatory bodies usually monitor of drug withdrawn in country. Pharmacovigilance committee keeps vigilance on the drug use in the market and their rational combinations. Their main aim is to make available of safer and economic substitutes of the drug or its combination and with better benefit/risk ratio. Regulators must examine formulations time to time, including the combinations alleged at different forums at national and international level of being irrational or harmful or in effective in the context of present existing published literature. The development of FDC's is becoming increasingly important from the public health prospective and some of the combinations are well accepted by international organization in the management of HIV, malaria and tuberculosis. FDC's are the advantages in many contexts but its limitation become many irrational combinations. So, in near future a strong regulation, better guidelines and better operational pharmacovigilance system are required to regulate FDC's formulations.

Suggested Readings

1. Chakraborti A. Fixed dose combinations in therapy, www.expresspharmaonline.com

2. Dreedhar D, Subramanian G, Udupa N (2006). Combination drugs: Are they rationale? *Current Science.* **91(4):** 406.

3. Gabriels GA, McIlleron H, Smith PJ, Folb PI, Fourie PB (2007). Modification to improve efficiency of sampling schedules for BA/BE testing of FDC anti-tuberculosis drugs. *Int J Tuberc Lung Dis.* **11(2):**181-8.

4. Herrick TM, Million RP (2007). Tapping the potential of fixed-dose combinations. *Nat Rev Drug Discov.* **6(7):** 513-514.

5. http://whqlibdoc.who.int/hq/2005/a87017_eng.pdf

6. http://www.cdsco.nic.in/html/Drugsbanned.html

7. Jonker DM, Visser SA, Vander Graaf PH, Voskuyl RA, Danhof M (2005). Towards a mechanism based analysis of pharmacodynamic drug-drug interactions. *Pharmacol Ther.* **106:** 1-18.

8. Kastury N, Singh S, Ansari KU (1999). An audit of prescription for rational use of fixed dose drug combinations. *Indian J Pharmacol.* **31:** 367-369.

9. Office of Combination Products, Food and Drug Administration, USA: www.fda.gov/oc/combination/21 CFR Part 3.2(e).

10. Oyugi JH, Byakika-Tusiime J, Ragland K, Laeyendecker O, Mugerwa R, Kityo C *et al.,*(2007). Treatment interruptions predict resistance in HIV-positive individuals purchasing fixed-dose combination antiretroviral therapy in Kampala, Uganda. *AIDS.* **21(8):** 965-71.

11. Pensi T (2007). Fixed dose combination of lamivudine, stavudine and nevirapine in the treatment of pediatric HIV infection: a preliminary report. *Indian Pediatr.* **44(7):** 519-21.

12. Rao RB, Goldfrank LR (1998). Fixed-dose combination therapy: panacea or poison? *Intensive Care Med.* **24(4):** 283-285.

13. Satoskar RS (1986). The expanding role of pharmacologist in the changing Indian scene. *J Postgrad Med.* **32:** 111-3.

14. Shenfield G (2005). Prescribers and drug withdrawals. *Aus Prescr.* **28:** 54-55.

15. Stanton T, Reid JL (2002). Fixed dose combination therapy in the treatment of hypertension. *J Hum Hypertens.* **16(2):** 75-78.

CHAPTER 29

DRUG-DRUG INTERACTIONS

Introduction

Drug-drug interactions are an important cause of adverse drug reactions and are of wide concern especially in patients with chronic diseases such as diabetes, cancer and cardiovascular diseases, where most of the time multiple drug therapy is mandatory. The problem of drug interactions was first recognized over 100 years ago, when an adrenal extract administration produced arrhythmias in a dog anesthetized with chloroform. Today, with the development of new, complex and high potency therapeutic agents and widespread use of multiple drug therapy, the probability for drug interactions is also increased. Although, drug regulatory authorities keep strict watch on new drug development and approval process to ensure its safety profile, the interaction potential of a drug is not always predictable or evident. It is well illustrated by the example of calcium channel blocker, mibefradil. It is voluntarily withdrawn all over the world within a month of its launch due to its serious drug interaction potential.

In epilepsy, diabetes, cardiovascular diseases, cancer and other chronic disease states, it becomes mandatory to administer several drugs simultaneously whenever the patient suffer from another illness. In addition to this, patient may also self-administer over the counter (OTC) drugs and alternative and complementary medicines, which further increases the probability and risk of drug interactions.

The vast medical literature containing wide number of medical reports of disastrous drug interactions raised the awareness among physicians, pharmacists, nurses, scientists and regulatory authorities. However, in order to predict the possible consequences of the drug interactions, physician and pharmacist must be aware of all the medicines that the patient is already taking along with over the counter (OTC) drugs and alternative and complementary medicines with their interaction potential. The knowledge about pharmacokinetic and pharmacodynamic of drug will allow him to handle the worst situations arising from drug interactions.

Definition

Drug Interactions

An interaction is said to occur when the effects of one drug are altered by the presence of another agent, food, drink or an environmental chemical agent. The combined or net effect of such interaction may be:

- Synergism or additive effect of one or more drugs
- Antagonism of effect of one or more drugs
- Alteration of effect of one or more drugs
- Production of idiosyncratic effects

The net effect of such interaction may be beneficial or harmful. The clinically relevant drug interaction may lead to significant change in condition of patient or underlying disease. This chapter reviews on epidemiology, pharmacoeconomics, types, factors, mechanisms and strategies to avoid or prevent the drug interactions.

Pharmacoepidemiology

It is difficult to give an exact and accurate incidence of drug interactions, because different published reports have variably used the definitions of clinically significant and non-significant interactions. Between 1970s and 1980s, various studies reported the incidence rate between 2.2% and 70.3% for ambulatory, hospitalized, or nursing home patients. On the basis of review of nine epidemiological studies, the incidence of drug-drug interactions is ranged from 0% to 2.8% in hospital admissions. In one landmark, often-cited study by Grymonpre and colleagues that was published in 1988, drug interactions were found to be the main cause for roughly 2.8% of all admissions among persons older than 50 years who were taking medications. Other studies have examined and quantified the risk of drug interactions for specific treatments. For example, a study on 104 patients who were treated with warfarin, significant increases were found in length of hospital stay (a mean increase of 3.14 days) and in prothrombin-time results (a mean increase of 24%) among those who received an interacting drug (55%), compared with those who did not. In Boston Collaborative Drug Surveillance Program (BLDSP 1972) reported around 3600 adverse drug reactions (4.3%) in 83000 drug exposures, out of these, 234 (6.5%) adverse drug reactions were only due to drug-drug interactions. In a retrospective study, Goldberg et al. (1996) reported that the incidence of potential drug interactions is increases as the number of total medications increased, ranging from 13% for two drugs to 82% for seven or more medications. In a prospective study, Herr et al. (1992) examined medications being used by all patients at admission to the emergency department and medications added by emergency department physicians. It has been reported that upon admission 30.3% of patients were at risk of a potential drug interactions, which is increased to 47.4% after being treated in the emergency department. Similarly in the Harvard Medical Practice Study, Leape et al. (1992) reported that around

20% of adverse events were drug related in acute hospital admitted patients, out of which 8% were attributed to drug interactions. There are few community-based studies that reported the incidence of drug interactions. Rupp et al., (1992) reported the 4.1% incidence of drug interaction in their US Community Pharmacy Study, while Swedish study reported the incidence about 1.9%.

Although, the overall incidence of potentially significant adverse drug interaction is less than 1%, it is still a major problem in terms of quality of life, health care cost to the patient and society. Drug interactions are also a major cause of adverse drug reactions and may lead to an increased risk of hospitalization and morbidity and mortality.

Susceptible Patients and Population

Certain population and patients such as the elderly, extensive metabolizer, those with hepatic or renal failure and those are on multiple drug therapy are at increased risk of interactions. Of these, multiple drug therapy or polypharmacy is most common. Goldberg et al. (1996) reported that the incidence of drug interaction increased as the number of total medications increased, ranging from 13% for two drugs to 82% for seven or more medications.

Due to disease, ageing physiology, the incidence of drug interaction is increases in elderly and seriously ill population. Patients with chronic disease states or with hepatic or renal failure, patient undergoing complicated surgical procedure and those with more than one prescribing physician are on high risk of drug interactions. For example, the potential interactions are as high as 75% in the HIV population with an actual incidence of clinically significant interactions is 25%. This increased risk of interactions is mainly due to their multiple drug therapy and impaired body homeostasis. In addition, to such population, drug interaction may occur only in some individuals but not in others. The consequences of drug metabolism based interactions may differ greatly because of differences in the rates of drug metabolism and in susceptibility to hepatic drug metabolizing enzyme induction which could lead to extensive, or slow or ultra-extensive metabolism.

Pharmacoeconomics

Accepting the statistic from Grymonpre and colleagues, that drug-drug interactions cause roughly 2.8% of all hospitalizations, Hamilton and colleagues stated, "Using a cost-of-illness model, this could represent 245, 280 hospital admissions/year, costing the health care system $1.3 billion". In a nursing home setting, 70% of the potential drug interactions involved in some loss of action of one or more drugs. Drug-drug interactions are actually quite commonplace and are responsible for considerable patient morbidity and mortality. Growing and sobering evidences implicates that drug interactions as a major factor for hospital admissions, treatment failures, avoidable complications and subsequent healthcare costs to patient and society. In US drug interaction are responsible for 3-10% of hospital admissions of older patients, which cost an estimated $20 million annually. The medical literature also suggests that up to 2.8% of hospitalizations are of due to adverse drug interactions. Drug interactions compromises human health and incur costs. Conjoint administration of two or more drugs may produce a response greater that that was anticipated, a decrease in effectiveness of one or both drugs or an unanticipated drug toxicity. One case report involving an interaction of fluoxetine and selegiline required a 15 day hospitalization, emergency room visits, ambulance services, magnetic resonance imaging, electrocardiogram, laboratory tests, and consultations. The resultant total medical expenditures for treatment of this single case of interaction-induced illness were $17,213. Although the overall incidence rates of drug interactions is quite low (less that 1%), the quality of life and cost to the patient and society are equally or more important. Therefore, the impact of adverse drug interactions remains a matter of wide concern.

Factors Affecting Drug Interactions

There are various drug and patient related factors (Table 29.1) responsible for occurrence of clinically important drug interactions. They are very important as they markedly influence the incidence of drug interactions. Certain classes of drugs have high risk of clinically significant interactions (Table 29.2) such as drugs with narrow therapeutic index, steep dose response curve and saturated hepatic metabolism.

Table 29.1 Drug and patient related factors affecting drug interactions

Drug-related factors	Patient-related factors
Drug with narrow therapeutic window	Age/Sex
Drug with low bioavailability	Race
Drug with steep dose response curve	Genetic polymorphisms
Drug with saturated hepatic metabolism	Body weight
Drug with high potency	Tobacco use, smoking and alcohol use
Drug with problematic pharmacokinetics	Dietary pattern
Drug concentration in blood and tissue	Concomitant disease
Physiochemical characteristics of drug formulation	Impaired function of target organs (liver, kidney)
Dose, dosing schedule and duration of drug therapy	Multiple drug therapy
Route of administration	
Rate and extent of drug metabolism	
Extent of protein binding	
Volume of distribution of affected drug	
Drug stereochemistry	

Table 29.2 Examples of drugs with high risk of interaction

Drug with concentration dependent toxicity	Digoxin, aminophylline, carbamazepine, phenytoin, primidone, clindamycin, cyclosporin, clonidine, lithium, aminoglycosides, cytotoxic agents, warfarin
Drugs with steep dose-response curve	Vancomycin, verapamil, sulphonylureas, levodopa
Drug with saturable hepatic metabolism	Phenytoin, theophylline
Others	Immunosuppressive agents (cyclosporin, tacrolimus, glucocorticoids), oral contraceptives, anti-epileptics, anti-arrhythmic drugs

Classification of Drug Interactions

1. **Pharmacokinetic Drug Interactions:** Interactions results due to alterations in absorption, distribution, metabolism and elimination characteristics of drug.
2. **Pharmacodynamic Drug Interactions:** Interactions results due to the influence of combined treatment at the site of biological action and gives altered pharmacologic actions at a standard plasma concentration.

On the basis of, net effect that produced by combination of two drugs, drug interactions may be classified as

1. **Additive or Synergistic Drug Interactions:** Interactions in which the net effect of concomitantly administered drugs is equal to or greater than the sum of their individual effects.
2. **Antagonistic Drug Interactions:** Interactions in which the net effect of concomitantly administered drugs is less than the sum of their individual effects. There may be pharmacological antagonism, physiologic antagonism, biochemical antagonism or chemical antagonism.

Mechanisms of Drug Interactions

The most common underlying mechanisms involved in drug interactions (Table 29.3) can be divided as,

Table 29.3 Potential mechanisms of drug interactions affecting pharmacokinetics of drugs

Affected Process	**Mechanisms**
Absorption	Changes in gastric pH
	Adsorption and chelation
	Changes in gastrointestinal flora
	Changes in gastric emptying and intestinal motility
	Changes in intestinal blood flow
	Alterations in active and passive transport
	Changes in presystemic clearance
	Changes in condition of GIT
Distribution	Protein binding and displacement

Table 29.3 *Contd...*

Affected Process	Mechanisms
Metabolism	Inhibition of phase I and II drug metabolizing enzymes
	Induction of phase I and II drug metabolizing enzymes
	Genetic polymorphisms of phase I and II drug metabolizing enzymes
Excretion	Alterations in urinary pH
	Alterations in active transport systems
	Alterations in renal blood flow

A. Drug Interactions that have Pharmacokinetic Basis

B. Drug Interactions that have Pharmacodynamic Basis

One drug interaction may often involve more than one mechanism. Pharmacokinetic drug interactions: These type of drug interactions may occurs due to alterations in absorption, distribution, metabolism and excretion pattern of one drug by another drug and may results in change in drug concentration at the site of biological activity which may lead to decreased efficacy or toxicity.

A. Drug Interactions that have Pharmacokinetic Basis

1. **Drug Interactions affecting Absorption:** As the oral route is the most common route for drug administration, drug interactions influencing absorption are most likely occurs within gastrointestinal tract (GIT). In GIT, absorption of a given drug occurs through mucus membrane and it is determined by various factors such as pKa value and lipid solubility of drug, physiochemical properties of the formulation, gastric pH, gastric emptying and intestinal motility, gastrointestinal flora, chelation and adsorption, changes in active and passive transport, alterations in presystemic clearance, changes in hepatic cytochrome P450 isozymes activity, changes in intestinal P-glycoprotein activity.

   (i)   *Changes in Gastric pH:* It is well understood that drug in non-ionized form is more lipid soluble, therefore it most rapidly absorbable across the mucus membranes. However, extent of non-ionized form of drug is depends on the pH of its surrounding environment, the pKa value of drug, physiochemical properties of formulation. Also, it is well known fact that the basic drugs are better absorbed in acidic medium and acidic drugs are better absorbed in basic medium because non-ionized form of drug exists in greater extent. Thus interaction may occur when one drug produces basic environment may decrease the absorption of compounds needing acidic environment. For example, change in pH due to antacid administration may decrease the bioavailability of ketoconazole, as it requires acidic pH for optimal absorption.

(ii) *Adsorption and Chelation:* Certain drugs can interact within GIT by forming an insoluble and non-absorbable chelates and complexes. A good example of this interaction is provided by tetracycline, which forms insoluble complex with iron, calcium, aluminum, magnesium leads to reduced serum tetracycline concentrations.

(iii) *Changes in Gastrointestinal Flora:* In the large bowel of gastrointestinal tract, bacterial flora predominates; therefore drugs that are well absorbed from the large bowel are more likely to be affected by alterations in intestinal flora. In about 10% of individuals, digoxin is extensively metabolized by intestinal bacteria. Therefore, broad-spectrum antibiotics (such as erythromycin and tetracyclines) induced inhibition of bacterial flora may double the plasma concentration of digoxin with subsequent toxicity at therapeutic dose.

(iv) *Changes in Gastric Emptying and Intestinal Motility:* A drug that changes the rate of gastric emptying can change the rate of absorption of other concurrently administered drug. Anticholinergic drugs induced delay in gastric emptying markedly (approximately 50%) reduces the bioavailability of levodopa.

(v) *Alterations in Intestinal Blood Flow:* Theoretically, a drug that alters the intestinal blood flow, may affect the absorption of lipophilic compounds.

(vi) *Alterations in Active and Passive Transport:* It has been identified that various intestinal transporters are located on the brush border and basolateral membrane of the enterocyte. Recently, competitive inhibitory potential of quinolone antibiotics for these transporters has been documented as an additional mechanism for drug interactions.

(vii) *Changes in Presystemic Clearance:* Cytochrome P4503A4 and 5 are gastrointestinal drug metabolizing isozymes that highly expressed in the intestine and responsible for drug activation by phase I oxidative metabolism. P-glycoprotein, a multidrug resistance gene product, expressed in a variety of tissues including at the luminal surface of the intestinal epithelium and they extrudes an unchanged drug from the enterocyte into the lumen. Although, both CYP 3A4/5 and P-glycoprotein are substrate specific, they also have significant number of common substrates. Therefore, both are key players in drug-drug interactions.

Cytochrome P450 isozymes are major drug metabolizing enzymes and present in higher concentrations in hepatocytes. They are mainly responsible for phase I oxidative metabolism. More than 90% of drug oxidations are attributes to six main isozymes viz. CYP1A2, CYP2C9, CYP2C19, CYP2D6, CYP2E1, and CYP3A4. Therefore, they are most important determinant of the systemic bioavailability of orally administered drugs.

As, the P-glycoproteins block absorption of drug in the gut, they are considered as the part of the "first-pass effect". They are also acts as "gate keepers" for later cytochrome P450 actions. The inhibition and induction of intestinal CYP 450 isozymes and P-glycoprotein results in direct changes in drug absorption. If one drug is a substrate of both P-glycoprotein   and CYP3A4, and second drug is an inhibitor of both P-glycoprotein and CYP3A4 (e.g. ketoconazole, erythromycin), then the first drug will be absorbed in increased amounts. Because, CYP3A4 is inhibited, high levels of unmetabolized drug will enter the blood. The effect of P-glycoprotein blockade is to "open the gates" so that the later actions of CYP3A4 will be increased and therefore first drug will be absorbed in large amounts.

A potential suicide inhibition of CYP3A4/5 by grapefruit juice is another important example of drug interactions that results in a minimum threefold increase in rate of absorption with subsequent toxicity of the concomitantly administered drug. This type of drug interaction can also results in decreased therapeutic efficacy of prodrugs that requires CYP3A for its conversion to active metabolites.

(viii)   *Toxic Effects on the Gastrointestinal Tract:* The rate of absorption also depends on the condition of gastrointestinal tract. If one drug affects or damage the stomach or small intestine, then absorption of some another drugs may be reduced. For example, the absorption of phenytoin and verapamil can be reduced (approximately 20-35%) in patients taking cytotoxic drugs (e.g., methotrexate, carmustine, vinblastine) for the treatment of malignant disease. These types of drug interactions mostly reduce therapeutic effect of drug.

2. Drug Interactions affecting Drug Distribution

Protein binding and Displacement: The main and most important underlying mechanism for such interactions is changes in extent of protein binding and drug displacement from the site of protein binding. Generally, the drug displacement interaction is described as a decrease in the plasma protein binding of one drug caused by the presence of another one, which competes for the same binding sites of protein, leads to an increased free or unbound concentration of the displaced drug. This type of interactions are much more likely to occur with agents having high tendency (approximately more than 80%) to bound with plasma proteins, with high hepatic extraction ratio, with narrow therapeutic index and with small volume of distribution.

It is well understood that acidic drugs (i.e. penicillin, sulphonamides, doxycycline and clindamycin) are strongly bound to albumin and basic drugs (i.e. erythromycin) strongly bound to alpha-1-acid glycoprotein. Although, albumin can bound both acidic as well as basic drugs as it contains both acidic and basic groups, it only weakly bound to basic drugs. Therefore, the interaction between basic drugs and albumin are not clinically significant.

Drug displacement interactions may have beneficial or harmful effects. Phenylbutazone may competitively displace the salicylates from the proteins, resulting in strong analgesic and anti-inflammatory effect. In most of the cases, the increased effectiveness of the displaced drug is not very significant. Some time they may have serious consequences such as interaction of anticoagulants and antidiabetic drugs. Excessive amount of anticoagulants can produce increased bleeding tendency, and increased antidiabetic agents may lower blood sugar by undesirable levels which may leads to emergency.

3. **Drug Interactions affecting Drug Metabolism:** Generally, the process of metabolism converts the active lipophilic compounds to inactive and ionized metabolites for renal elimination. The liver is the prime site of drug metabolism. Most of the time, the drug is metabolized in liver through nonsynthetic (phase I) and synthetic or conjugative (phase II) metabolic reactions. Phase I reactions mainly include oxidation, reduction and hydrolysis and occur in the membrane of hepatocyte endoplasmic reticula. Phase II reactions mainly involve conjugation of the compound with such as glucuronic acid, sulphate, or glycine and occur in cytosol of the hepatocyte. Co-administration of dietary substances, especially fruit juices, along with certain drugs, leads to serious pharmacokinetic as well as pharmacodynamic interactions. Fruit juices (e.g., grapefruit juice) thought to inhibit biochemical processes in the intestine and also intestinal CYP3A-mediated metabolism.

(i) *Phase I (Non-synthetic) Drug Metabolism:* Phase I metabolic reactions mainly involve a superfamily of mixed function monooxygenase system, most commonly called as cytochrome P450 isozymes. Till date in humans at least 14 families, 22 subfamilies and 36 CYP enzymes have been identified. Of these, the three main families i.e., CYP1, 2 and 3 account for 70% of the total hepatic P450 content. Of the many isozymes, CYP1A2, CYP2C8/9, CYP2C19, CYP2D6, CYP2E1 and CYP3A4/5 are responsible for about 95% of all therapeutic drug oxidation. Drug interactions related these enzymes are results from enzyme inhibition, suppression and induction by their inhibitors and inducers (Table 29.4) and due to genetic polymorphisms. There are various factors that affect the activities of CYP enzymes (Table 29.5).

Table 29.4 Some drug substrates, inducers, and inhibitors of the
major cytochrome P450 isoforms

P-450 isoform	Substrates	Inducers	Inhibitors
CYP1A2	Flutamide, clomipramine, clozapine, tacrine, imipramine, olanzapine, warfarin, zileuton, ropinirole	Charcoal-broiled meat, omeprazole, cigarette smoke	Fluoxamine, isoniazid, furafylline, mexiletine, cimetidine, ciprofloxacin,
CYP2A6	Halothane	Phenytoin	Tranylcypromine

Table 29.4 *Contd...*

P-450 isoform	Substrates	Inducers	Inhibitors
CYP2C9	Celecoxib, diclofenac dronabinol, ibuprofen, flurbiprofen, losartan, fluvastatin, glimepiride, diazepam, diclofenac, indomethacin,	Barbituratees, dexamethasone, aminoglutethimide, barbiturates, carbamazepine, griseofulvin, nafcillin, phenytoin, primidone, rifampin	Sulphaphenazole, amiodarone, cimetidine, clopidogrel, co-trimoxazole, disulfiram, efavirenz, fluconazole, fluvastatin
CYP2C19	Clomipramine, carisoprodol, citalopram, mephenytoin, phenytoin, rabeprazole, R-warfarin	Rifampicin	Tranylcypromine, efavirenz, felbamate, fluconazole, fluoxetine, fluvoxamine
CYP2D6	Clomipramine, amitriptyline, carvedilol, codeine, desipramine, dexfenfluramine, dextromethorphan, efavirenz, encainide, flecainide, fluvoxamine, haloperidol	CYP 2D6 appears relatively resistant to enzyme induction.	Amiodarone, chloroquine, cimetidine, diphenhydramine, haloperidol, mibefradil, paroxetine, perphenazine, propafenone, propoxyphene,
CYP2E1	Enflurane, halothane	Isoniazid	Disulfiram
CYP3A4	Acetaminophen, alfentanil, alprazolam, amlodipine, amiodarone, atorvastatin, bepridil, bromocriptine, buspirone, carbamazepine, cisapride, citalopram, clarithromycin, cyclophosphamide, prednisolone, quetiapine,	Aminoglutethimide Barbiturates carbamazepine dexamethasone efavirenz glutethimide griseofulvin nevirapine phenytoin primidone	Clarithromycin, danazol, delavirdine, erythromycin, fluvoxamine, grapefruit juice, indinavir, isoniazid, itraconazole, ketoconazole, metronidazole
CYP4A1	Testosterone	Clofibrate	

Table 29.5 Various factors and affected CYP enzymes

Factors	CYP enzymes
Nutrition and metabolism	1A2, 3A
Smoking	1A2
Other environmental carcinogens and pollutants	1A2, 3A
Disease	1A2, 2BC, 2C, 2D6, 3A
Medications	1A2, 2BC, 2C, 2D6, 3A

Source: Kashuba, 2001.

(a) *Mechanism of Enzyme Inhibition:* There are several mechanisms of enzyme inhibition and one drug can interact by multiple mechanisms such as reversible, irreversible or mechanism-based inhibition (or suicide inhibition). Of these, reversible inhibition is most common and occurs, when interacting drug forms weak bond with CYP isozyme without permanent inactivation. This inhibition may be both competitive and noncompetitive in nature and its magnitude is mainly determined by affinity of substrate and inhibitor for the CYP isozyme, concentration of inhibitor at the binding site of enzyme. For example, ketoconazole and ritonavir are reversible inhibitor of CYP3A isozyme. In some cases, inhibitor binds to a CYP isozyme and undergoes oxidation to a nitroalkane species, which then forms a reversible complex with the reduced heme in the CYP isozyme (e.g., interaction between the macrolide antibiotics with CYP3A).

In irreversible or suicide inhibition, CYP-mediated formation of a reactive metabolite occurs, which then covalently and irreversibly binds to catalytic site of CYP isozyme and inactivates it permanently. The degree of this type of inactivation is depends on total concentration of CYP isozyme, inhibitor to which CYP isozyme is exposed and rate of new isozyme biosynthesis.

(b) *Mechanism of Suppression:* Number of mechanisms and factors were described for suppression of drug metabolizing activity of various isozymes. Majority of investigations reported the changes in drug metabolism pattern during viral, bacterial infections, surgery and bone marrow transplantation. In addition, various experimental studies demonstrated that IL-1, IL-6 and TNF-alpha suppresses (approximately by 80%) the activity of CYP isozymes be decreasing the mRNA synthesis. There are few clinical reports that documented the reduced activity of drug metabolizing enzymes during the administration of therapeutic interferon and interleukins.

(c) *Mechanism of Induction:* In comparison to inhibition of CYP450 enzyme, its induction is not a major and immediate concern because induction occurs gradually with subsequent decrease in therapeutic outcome. However, inhibition of CYP enzymes occurs rapidly that leads to profound toxicity with serious consequences. Generally, an increase in activity CYP 450 enzymes occurs due to its increased synthesis through receptor-mediated transcriptional activation or mRNA stabilization.

Cigarette smoke, charcoal broiled food items indoles containing foods (cauliflower, cabbage, Brussels sprouts) and certain drugs (such omeprazole) induce the CYP1 family through mRNA stabilization. In addition to these, azole nucleus containing antifungal drugs causes induction of CYP2 family through transcriptional CYP2C gene activation and mRNA stabilization. Recently, various studies reported the involvement of pregnane-X receptor

(PXR) and cAMP-dependent phosphorylation process in induction of CYP enzyme activity.

(d) **Genetic Polymorphisms:** Genetic polymorphisms occur due to by chance processes or may have been induced by various external agents such as viruses or radiations. These polymorphisms are responsible to produce distinct subgroups of individuals within the population that have different ability to metabolize the same drug. They may be fast, slow or ultra extensive metabolizers. Most commonly and clinically important polymorphisms were reported for CYP2D6, CYP2C9 and CYP2C19, CYP3A4, CYP3A5, and CYP3A7 isozymes. Variability in the inter-individual responses to drugs is often caused by genetic polymorphisms in CYP2D6, also termed the debrisoquin/sparteine genetic polymorphism in reference to the drugs that are its substrates that lead to its discovery. For CYP enzymes, subject to genetic polymorphism, most subjects will be extensive metabolizers (EM, the normal condition), some will be ultra-extensive metabolizers (UEM, or high metabolism), some will have reduced metabolism, and others will have no metabolism (PM, no enzyme or poor metabolizers). The expression of particular gene for corresponding CYP enzyme and transporter determines its extent of activity and ultimately the rate of metabolism. Ethnic variability may exist (Table 29.6).

Table 29.6 Examples of CYP alleles and their significance

CYP Enzyme	Population	Percentage (%)
2C19*2 or *3	Asians	13%-20% reduced activity or no active 2C19
2D6*2xN	Ethiopians/Saudis	30% ultra extensive activity
2D6*10	Asians	Up to 80% reduced activity
2D6*17	African-Americans	5% reduced activity

(ii) **Phase II (Synthetic) Drug Metabolism:** Various isozymes (such as UDP-glucuronyl-transferases, sulfotransferases, acetyl transferases, glutathione-S-transferases and methyltransferases) involved in conjugation reactions. As phase II metabolism process having wide number of conjugative enzymes, their inhibition or induction is not much clinically important. In phase II drug metabolizing enzymes, only UDP-glucuronyl-transferase is most important, as it is most common enzyme involved in conjugative reactions. It is reported that many drugs competitively inhibits the UDP-glucoronyl-transferases, but actual significance of such inhibitions is not explored. Also, there is no sufficient data related to mechanism of induction of phase II drug metabolizing enzymes. In recent time, it is reported that UDP-glucoronyl-transferases and glutathione-S-transferases can be induced, but clinical significance of such induction is still unexplored. However, it has been reported that co-administration of zidovudine and rifampicin results the rapid and increased clearance of zidovudine suggesting the role phase II drug metabolizing enzymes in drug interactions.

Genetic polymorphisms: Like phase I drug metabolizing enzymes, genetic polymorphisms were also reported for phase II drug metabolizing enzymes such as glutathione S-transferase (GST) M1, T1 and P1, sulfotransferase 1A1 (SULT1A1), catechol-O-methyltransferase (COMT).

4. **Drug Interactions affecting Excretion:** Drug interactions can occurs when interacting drug affects the urinary pH, active transport systems and renal blood flow thereby alters the excretory pattern of the affected drug. Drug interactions affecting excretion are usually occurs at the stage of glomerular filtration, tubular secretion and tubular reabsorption.

   (i) *Alterations in Urinary pH:* In renal tubules, non-ionized form of drug is unable to diffuse into the renal tubule cells and will therefore be lost in the urine. Therefore, any drug that produces alkaline urine enhances the excretion of weakly acidic drugs and agents that produces acidic urine enhances the excretion of weakly basic drugs. For example, sodium bicarbonate administration gives rise to alkaline urinary pH, thereby increases excretion and shorten the duration of action of phenobarbitone. This beneficial drug interaction is implicated in the management of phenobarbitone poisoning. In another case, to manage amphetamine poisoning, urinary acidification is usually recommended to enhance amphetamine excretion.

   (ii) *Alterations in Active Transport Systems:* In kidney, proximal tubular active system plays very important role in tubular secretion. This is the most common site where most of the renal drug interactions occur. Many organic anionic and cationic drugs and metabolites selectively compete for these transport sites for tubular secretion. A well-known and beneficial drug interaction between probenecid and penicillin to increase serum concentration and therapeutic benefit of penicillin. Recently, it is reported that P-glycoprotein plays an important role in transporting a large variety of drugs into the lumen. Number of experimental studies demonstrated that plasma concentration of certain drugs could be increased by inhibition of renal P-glycoprotein. As quinolones (e.g., macrolides, erythromycin, azithromycin) and azole moiety containing antifungal agents can bind and inhibit the P-glycoprotein, they may cause clinically significant drug interactions.

   (iii) *Alterations in Renal Blood Flow:* As renal blood supply is controlled by renal vasodilatory prostaglandins (e.g., PGE_2, PGI_2), inhibition of their synthesis by certain drugs may reduced the renal secretion of other co-administered drugs. Patient on lithium therapy should be closely monitored if NSAIDs (e.g., diclofenac) are prescribed for him. Because, NSAIDs inhibits the synthesis of vasodilatory prostaglandins and therefore the renal excretion of lithium is significantly reduces with subsequent rise in serum levels.

B. Drug Interactions that have Pharmacodynamic Basis

Generally these types of interactions are additive, synergistic or antagonistic in nature that is pharmacodynamic interactions results in increasing or decreasing the therapeutic effect of drugs.

1. **Additive/Synergistic Drug Interactions:** An interaction in which two concurrently administered drugs acting by the same mechanism produces the net effect equal to that expected by simple addition. For example, the concomitant administration of aspirin and paracetamol will produce additive analgesia, as they both are acts by the same mechanisms. Other examples are shown in Table 29.7.

Table 29.7 Examples of additive or synergistic drug interactions

Interacting drug	Pharmacological effect
NSAID and warfarin	Increased risk of bleeding
ACE inhibitors and potassium sparing diuretics	Increased risk of hyperkalemia
Verapamil and β-adrenergic antagonists	Bradycardia and asystole
Neuromuscular blockers and aminoglycosides	Increased neuromuscular blockade
Alcohol and benzodiazepines	Increased sedation
Thioridazine and halofantrine	Increased risk of QT interval prolongation
Clozapine and co-trimoxazole	Increased risk of bone marrow suppression

Source: Lee and Stockley, 2001

2. **Summative Drug Interactions:** When two drugs gives rise to the same overt response independent of their mechanism of action, and their combined effect is equal to the algebraic sum of their individual effects, then drug interaction is having summation effect.

   For example, the concomitant administration of aspirin and codeine will produce analgesia and the combined effect is called summation, as they both are acts by the different mechanisms.

3. **Synergistic Drug Interactions:** When the concurrent administration of two drugs produce the combined effect greater than their algebraic sum of their individual effects, then drug interaction is having synergistic effect. In this case, two drugs act at different sites and one drug (called as synergist) increases, the effect of the second drug by changing the absorption, distribution, metabolism and excretion pattern. In synergism, the activity of affected drug may be increased or duration of action may be prolonged.

   For example, combined administration of procaine and adrenaline increases the duration of action of procaine.

4. **Antagonistic Drug Interactions:** Interactions in which the combine effect is of two co-administered drug is less than the sum of the effects of the drugs acting separately, is called as antagonistic drug interactions. Antagonism may be of different types:

   (i) *Pharmacologic Antagonism:* When antagonist interferes with the formation of agonist-receptor complex then it is known as pharmacologic antagonism. An antagonist, diphenhydramine reduces the effect of an agonist like histamine by preventing it from combining with its receptor.

   (ii) *Physiologic or Functional Antagonism:* When two agonist acting on different target sites counterbalance each other by producing opposite effects on the same physiological function, then it is called as physiologic antagonism. For example, the effect of histamine on blood pressure can be counterbalance by norepinephrine.

   (iii) *Biochemical Antagonism:* It is just opposite of synergism i.e. one drug indirectly decreases the amount of a second drug that would otherwise be available to its site of action in the absence of antagonist. Phenobarbital induces the hepatic microsomal drug metabolizing enzymes responsible for the biotransformation of other drugs.

   (iv) *Chemical Antagonism:* When biological activity of one agent is diminished or abolished by a chemical reaction with other agent then it is called as chemical antagonism. For example, neutralization of excess gastric acid by any of the antacid and antagonism of anticoagulant effect of heparin by toludine blue or protamine.

5. **Interactions due to Disturbances in Fluid and Electrolyte Imbalance:** The effects of certain drugs especially those acts on myocardium, neuromuscular transmission and kidney, may be alter by changes in body electrolytes composition, because their pharmacological effect is determined by the electrolyte composition. Most clinically important and highly concerned drug interaction is the potentiation of effect of digoxin and other cardiac glycosides by diuretics and other drugs which decrease plasma potassium concentration. Serious hyperkalemia due to combined administration of angiotensin converting enzyme (ACE) inhibitors (e.g., ramipril, enalapril) and potassium supplement because ACE inhibitors also have potassium sparing effect.

Strategies for Avoiding and/or Preventing Drug Interactions

The potential for drug interactions is growing day by day due to continued development of many number of new, high potency drugs. As multiple drug therapies are usually being used in the treatment of various chronic diseases such as diabetes, epilepsy, cancer and cardiovascular diseases, therefore probability of drug interactions is also increasing.

Other than drug interactions, drugs may interact with various foods, drink, nutrients, alternative medicines etc. Also, drug interactions may occur due to physical, pathological condition of patients.

It is therefore an urgent and important need of time to avoid and or prevent the drug interactions for appropriate and effective use of drugs for well being of humans. Although, it is not solely depends on one person, we can able to attain the said goal by team efforts of physicians, pharmacists, nurses, patients, and society. For better management of drug interactions, Hansten and Horn recommended a five-class categorization system of analysis and management of drug interactions (Table 29.8).

Table 29.8 Classification scheme for management of drug interactions

Class 1	Avoid administration of the drug combination. The risk of adverse patient outcome precludes the concomitant administration of the drugs.
Class 2	Combination should be avoided unless it is determined that the benefit of co-administration of the drug overweighs the risk to the patient. The use of an alternative to one of the interacting drug is recommended when appropriate. Patient should be closely monitored if the drugs are co-administered.
Class 3	Several potential management options are available: use of an alternative agent, change in drug regimen (dose, interval), or route of administration to minimize the interaction, or monitor patient if drugs are co-administered.
Class 4	Potential for harm is low and no specific action is required other than to be aware of the possibility of drug interaction.
Class 5	Available evidence suggests no interaction.

Source: Hansten and Horn, 1999.

However, following strategies may be useful to avoid and or prevent the drug interactions

1. Avoid completely the use of drugs that are likely to be involved in drug interactions in a given condition.

2. Don't add a drug with known drug interaction potential if it is not clearly indicated in a given condition.

3. If possible, delay the initiation of other drug with known interaction potential

   For example, antimicrobial drugs are usually administered for limited period, therefore it is possible to start other therapy followed by antimicrobial therapy to avoid drug interaction.

4. Take concomitant disease condition into consideration before prescribing other therapy

For example, renal or hepatic failure and other chronic disease states may alter the pharmacokinetic and pharmacodynamic of prescribed therapy, therefore physician must be well aware with concomitant disease condition so that by modification of drug regimen he can significantly reduced the risk of drug interactions.

5. Choose a drug with the least interaction potential. After choosing an adequate drug for a given indication with consideration of other concomitant patient factors, agent with a least interaction potential should be selected. For example, levofloxacin or gatifloxacin are better options in comparison to ciprofloxacin as formers have less interaction potential for drug metabolizing enzymes.

6. If possible, avoid drugs with serious adverse effects to reduce the potential and serious consequences of unpredictable drug interactions.

7. Avoid concurrent use of drugs having same adverse effect profiles to minimize the potential risk of unpredictable drug interactions. For example, incidence of neutropenia is increased with concurrent administration of zidovudine, ganciclovir, trimethoprim-sulphamethoxazole.

8. Use the drugs at smallest effective doses and lowest effective concentration. As most of the time drug associated adverse effects are dose- and concentration-dependent. Therefore, drugs involved in interactions should be used at smallest effective doses and lowest effective concentration to reduce the significance of potential drug interactions.

9. Use dose staggering method or strategy. In drug interactions affecting absorption, chelation or changes in gastric pH may reduce the absorption of affected drug. In such cases, dose staggering is the most useful method to minimize absorption related drug interaction. By keeping a gap of 1-2 hours between administrations of two medications, it is possible to minimize absorption related drug interactions. For example, decreased bioavailability of ketoconazole and itraconazole due to concomitant administration of antacids.

10. Monitor and follow up the patient regularly for early detection and reducing the drug interactions.

11. Educate and counsel the patient about purpose of his therapy, drug administration technique, dosing schedule, sign and symptoms of drug toxicity and expected time for improvement of his disease condition.

Conclusions

With increasing availability of new classes of highly potent drugs, number of complex chronic disease states, increasing tendency to use multiple drug therapy, the incidences for clinically significant drug interactions is also increasing and it is rather alarming. Drug interactions are also a matter of wide concern as it is leading cause of drug related adverse drug reactions. It is still a considerable problem in terms of the global number of patients at risk and the potential for morbidity and mortality. They are also responsible decreased drug efficacy or increased drug activity with subsequent toxicity.

Therefore, it is an urgent need to develop various strategies to avoid or prevent the drug interactions for appropriate use of drug to enhance its therapeutic outcome. This aim can be fulfilled by team efforts of physicians, pharmacists, nurses, patients and society in this direction.

Suggested Readings

1. Ameer B., and R.A. Weintraub (1997). Drug interactions with grapefruit juice. *Clin. Pharmacokinet.* **33**: 103-121.

2. Anastasio G.D., K.O. Cornell and D. Menscer (1997). Drug interactions: Keeping it straight. *American Family Physician.* **56**: 883-895.

3. Astrand B. (2009). Avoiding drug-drug interactions. *Chemotherapy.* **55(4)**: 215-20.

4. Benet L.Z., Izumi T., Zhang Y., J.A. Silverman and V.J. Wacher (1999). Intestinal MDR transport proteins and P-450 enzymes as barriers to oral delivery. *J. Controlled Release.* **62**: 25-31.

5. Boston Collaborative Drug Surveillance Program (1972). Adverse drug interactions. *JAMA* **220**: 1238-1239.

6. Degtyarenko K.N. and P. Fabian. 1999. Directory of P450-containing systems. http://www.icgeb.trieste.it/P450/p450Nom_Full.html#Animalia.

7. Durrence C.W. III, J.T. DiPiro, J.R. May, R.R. Nesbit, J.F. Sisley and J.W. Cooper (1985). Potential drug interactions in surgical patients. *Am. J. Hosp. Pharm.* **42**: 1553-1556.

8. Fish D.N (2001). Circumventing drug interactions. In: Piscitelli, S.C. and K.A. Rodvold, *eds.*, Drug interactions in infectious diseases. Humana Press Inc., Totowa, New Jersey, pp. 311-331.

9. Foisy M.M., K. Gough, C.M. Quan, K. Harris, D. Ibanez and A. Philips (1999). Hospitalizations due to adverse drug reactions and interactions pre- and post-HAART [abstractB215]. *Can. J. Infect. Dis.* **10** (suppl B): 24B.

10. Goldberg R.M., J. Mabee, L. Chan and S. Wong (1996). Drug-drug and drug-disease interactions in the ED: analysis of a high-risk population. *Am. J. Emerg. Med.* **14**: 447-450.

11. Gosney M. and R. Tallis (1984). Prescription of contraindicated and interacting drugs in elderly patients admitted to hospital. *Lancet* **1**: 564-567.

12. Grymonpre R.E., P.A. Mitenko, D.S. Sitar, F.Y. Aoki and P.R. Montgomery (1988). Drug-associated hospital admissions in older medical patients. *J. Am. Geriatr. Soc.* **36**: 1092–1098.

13. Hamilton R.A., L.L. Briceland and M.H. Andritz (1998). Frequency of hospitalization after exposure to known drug-drug interactions in a Medicaid population. *Pharmacotherapy.* **18**: 1112-1120.

14. Hanlon J.T., S.L. Gray and K.E. Schmader (2001). Adverse drug reactions. *In*: Delafuente J.C. and R.B. Stewart, *eds.*, Therapeutics in the elderly, 3rd edition, Harvey Whitney Books Co., Cincinnati, pp. 289-314.

15. Hansten P.D. and J.R. Horn (1999). Hansten and Horn's drug interaction analysis and management. Applied Therapeutics, Inc., Vancouver, WA.

16. Herr R.D., E.M. Caravati, L.S. Tyler, E. Iorg and M.S. Linscott (1992). Prospective evaluation of adverse drug interactions in the emergency department. *Ann. Emerg. Med.* **21**: 1331-1336.

17. Jankel C.A. and L.K. Fitterman (1993). Epidemiology of drug-drug interactions as a cause of hospital admissions. *Drug safety* **9**: 51-59.

18. Jankel C.A., J.A. McMillan and B.C. Martin (1994). Effect of drug interactions on outcomes of patients receiving warfarin or theophylline. *Am. J. Hospital Pharmacy* **51**: 661-666.

19. Jinks M.J., P.D. Hansten and J.L. Hirschman (1979). Drug interaction exposures in ambulatory patients. *Am. J. Hosp. Pharm.* **36:** 923-927.

20. Kashuba A.D. and J.S. Bertino Jr (2001). Mechanisms of drug interactions. *In:* Piscitelli, S.C. and K.A. Rodvold, *eds.,* Drug interactions in infectious diseases, Humana Press Inc., Totowa, New Jersey, pp. 13-38.

21. Kashuba A.D.M (2001). Metabolism interactions to improve systemic exposure. Program and abstracts of the 41st Interscience Conference on Antimicrobial Agents and Chemotherapy, Chicago, Illinois. Presentation 1280.

22. Khaliq Y., Gallicano K. and J. Sahai (2001). Introduction to drug interactions. *In*: Piscitelli, S.C. and K.A. Rodvold, *eds.*, Drug interactions in infectious diseases, Humana Press Inc., Totowa, New Jersey, pp. 9-11.

23. Leape L.L., T.A. Brennan, N. Laird, A.G. Lawthers, A.R. Localio, B.A. Barnes, L. Hebert, J.P. Newhouse, P.C. Weiler and H. Hiatt (1992). The nature of adverse events in hospitalized patients: results of the Harvard Medical Practice Study II. *NEJM* **324**: 377-384.

24. Lee A. and I.H. Stockley (2001). Drug-drug interactions. *In*: Van Boxtel, C.J. B. Santoso and I.R. Edwards, *eds.,* Drug benefits and risks: International textbook of clinical pharmacology, John Wiley & Sons Ltd., pp. 211-226.

25. Lee A. and I.H. Stockley (2003). Drug interactions. *In*: Walker, R. and C. Edwards, *eds.,* Clinical pharmacy and therapeutics, 3rd edition, Churchill Livingstone, London, pp. 21-32.

26. Levine R.R., C.T. Walsh and R.D. Schwartz-Boom (2005). Administration factors and drug effects. *In: Pharmacology: drug actions and reactions*, 7th edition, The Parthenon Publishing Group, London, 2005.

27. Li Wan, P.A. and W.Y. Zhang (1998). What lessons can be learnt from withdrawal from mibefradil from the market? *Lancet* **351**: 1829-1830.

28. Linnarsson R (1993). Drug interactions in primary health care: a retrospective database study and its implications for the design of computerized decision support system. *Scandinavian J. Primary Health Care.* **11**: 181-186.

29. Morgan E.T (1997). Regulation of cytochrome P450 during inflammation and infection. *Drug Metab. Rev.* **29**: 1129-1188.

30. Mayhew R, JM McKoy, T Ha Luu, I Lopez, M Frick, CL Bennett (2010). Adverse drug interactions: moving from perception to action. *Pharmacoeconomics.* **28(1)**: 19-22.

31. Puckett W.H. and J.A. Visconti (1971). An epidemiologic study of the clinical significance drug-drug interactions in a private community hospital. *Am. J. Hosp. Pharm.* **28**: 247-253.

32. Rabbaaa L., S. Dautrey, N. Colas-Linhart, C. Carbon and R. Farinotti (1997). Absorption of ofloxacin isomers in the rat small intestine. *Antimicrob. Agents Chemother.* **41**: 2274-2277.

33. Rupp M.T., M. De Young and S.W. Schondelmeyer (1992). Prescribing problems and pharmacists interventions in community practice. *Medical care.* **30**: 926-940.

34. Saitoh H., H. Fujisaki, B.J. Aungst and K. Miyazaki. 1997. Restricted intestinal absorption of some beta-lactam antibiotics by an energy dependent efflux system in the rat intestine. *Pharm. Res.* **14**: 645-649.

35. Sewer M.B. and E.T. Morgan. 1997. Nitric oxide-independent suppression of P450 2C11 expression by interleukin-1 beta and endotoxin in primary rat hepatocytes. *Biochem. Pharmacol.* **54**: 729-737.

36. Shapiro L.E. and N.H.Shear (2001). Drug Interactions/P450. *Curr. Probl. Dermatol.* **13**: 141-152.

37. Stockley I.H (1999). Drug interactions. A source book of adverse interactions, their mechanisms, clinical importance and management. 5th edition, Pharmaceutical Press, London.

38. Summers KH, Amy Puenpatom R, Rajan N, Ben-Joseph R, Ohsfeldt R (2011). Economic impact of potential drug-drug interactions in opioid analgesics. *J Med Econ.* **14**: 390-396.

39. Tinel M., M.A. Robin, J. Doostzadeh, M. Maratrat, F. Ballet, N. Fardel, J. Kahwaji, P. Beaune, M. Daujat and G. Labbe (1995). The interleukin-2- receptor down regulates the expression of cytochrome P450 in cultured rat hepatocytes. *Gastroenterol.* **109**: 1589-1599.

40. Tsuji A. and I. Tamai (1996). Carrier-mediated intestinal transport of drugs. *Pharm. Res.* **13**: 963-977.

41. Won CS, NH Oberlies, MF Paine. 2010. Influence of dietary substances on intestinal drug metabolism and transport. *Curr Drug Metab.* **11(9)**:778-92.

42. Zhang L., C.M. Brett and K.M. Giacomini (1998). Role of organic cation transporters in drug absorption and elimination. *Ann. Rev. Pharm. Tox.* **38**: 431-460.

<h1>CHAPTER 30</h1>

NATURAL PRODUCTS AND DRUG INTERACTION

Introduction

Natural product as well as their derivatives has historically been inestimable as a supply of therapeutic agents. For thousands of years, natural products have competed a really vital role in health care and prevention of various diseases. Natural products are generally outlined as herbs along with various supplements which include amino acids, minerals, vitamins and different products of natural origin. People usually consider these natural products as "healthy foods" and has developed a positive attitude that is, since it is natural therefore safe and beneficial also. However, though widespread but false perception about these substances is largely unregulated. So, despite of thinking the possible side-effects and interactions with other conventional drugs natural products are generally taken on a self-medication basis, without seeking any advice from pharmacist or a physician. Natural products and its interactions with standard drug therapy are among the serious problems in daily clinical practices since it interacts with same pharmacokinetic and pharmacodynamics principles. In conjunction with this, there's conjointly lack of skilled direction which can expose the buyer to numerous risks, together with those derived by interactions with standard medicine. For example, feverfew, garlic, ginkgo, ginger, and ginseng may vary bleeding time so it should not be used simultaneously with warfarin sodium. Also, ginseng could cause headache, tremulousness, and wild episodes in patients who are treated with phenelzine sulfate. Ginseng ought to additionally not be used with estrogens or corticosteroids as a result of attainable additive effects.

Natural Products

This class includes a range of products, such as herbs, vitamins, minerals, and probiotics. These products are also widely marketed, easily available to customer, and infrequently sold as dietary supplements.

From past few decenniums there is considerable rise in the interest of using these natural products as alternative or complementary therapy for various diseases. According to the 2007 National Health Interview Survey (NHIS), which has conducted a comprehensive survey for using complementary health approaches mostly by American citizen, they found that 17.7% of adults in America have used these natural products in the last year. These products are found to be the most populous complementary health approaches among people of all age groups, in which the natural products which are most commonly used among adults and children was fish oil/omega 3s constituting 37.4% and 30.5% followed by Echinacea that is 37.2%. The marketing and consumer use of herbs and dietary supplements (HDS) has risen dramatically in the USA over the past two decades. It is estimated that > 50% of patients with chronic diseases or cancers ever use HDS and nearly one-fifth of patients take HDS products concomitantly with prescription medications. Despite their widespread use, the potential risks associated with combining HDS with other medications are poorly understood by these consumers. Although many HDS users believe that HDS are safe HDS products have been reported to be associated with mild-to-severe adverse effects such as heart problems, chest pain, abdominal pain and headache. Because, a majority of patients often fail to disclose that they have taken HDS products to their healthcare providers, e.g., one study estimated only 30% disclosure patient-provider communication concerning the risks and benefits of HDS is critically important. Important online resources about HDS, including the website of National Center for Complementary and Alternative Medicine (NCCAM), and Office of Dietary Supplements. Few products have been studied in massive, placebo-controlled trials, but most of them failed to show certain effects. Various researches are on-going to determine whether others are effective and safe or not. While there are indications that some may be helpful, more needs to be learned about the effects of these products in the human body and about their safety and potential interactions with medicines and with other natural products.

Mechanism of Interaction

Natural products can interact with drugs as well as with other natural products by the same mechanisms as of other drugs, it means that they interacts with drug pharmacodynamically or pharmacokinetically or sometimes by both the mechanism.

1. Pharmacokinetic interactions affect drug action quantitatively by altering the route of drug or natural medicine absorption, distribution, metabolism, or elimination processes.

2. Pharmacodynamics interaction mostly alters the way by which natural products or any other drugs interact with their receptors thereby producing toxic or pharmacological actions.

Clinically necessary interaction seems to involve drug metabolism consequences mostly through cytochrome P450 isoenzymes, impairment of hepatic or renal function, and other probable mechanisms. Cytochrome P450 constitutes system of enzymes which are generously involved in the metabolism of huge number of drugs. Mostly these enzymes are present in liver and expressed all through GIT, but very less amounts in lung, kidney along with CNS. These cytochrome P450 enzymes belong to a super-family of heme-thiolate proteins which are widely distributed among all living kingdoms. The enzymes are involved in the metabolism of a plethora of chemically diverse, endogenous and exogenous compounds, including drugs, environmental chemicals and other xenobiotics. More than thirty human CYP isozymes have been identified and out of these thirty isozymes only six main enzymes that is, CYP1A2, CYP2C9, CYP2C19, CYP2D6, CYP2E1 and CYP3A4 attributes to greater than 90% of all the aerophilic breakdown of drugs. CYP3A4 is also one of the most profusely expressed enzymes that are exclusively involved in metabolism of around 50% of all clinically used drugs. The function of this enzymatic system is susceptible to various substrates which are present in our body and can be accordingly induced or inhibited depending upon the nature of substrate. The method of induction or inhibition of enzymes is wedged variety of things which includes: genetic polymorphism, age, nutrition, liver disease and exposure to endogenous chemicals. When drugs and natural products are taken at the same time they can interact in ways that diminish the effectiveness of the ingested drug or reduce the absorption of ingredient of the natural product. Additionally, vitamin and herbal supplements taken with prescribed medication can result in adverse reactions. The interactions can occur when the food intake affects the ingredients in a medication, preventing the medicine from working the way it should. Some constituents of the natural products can affect the way of metabolizing certain drugs by binding with drug ingredients, thus reducing their absorption or speeding their elimination. For example, the acidity of the fruit juice may decrease the effectiveness of antibiotics such as penicillin. It is believed that the P450 system evolved > 400 million years ago to enable animals to detoxify chemicals found in plants.

Following detoxification by cytochrome enzyme system, many substances are further metabolized in a process of various chemical reactions that generally involve conjugation reactions to render an intermediate substance produced from enzymatic reaction into a relatively stable polar molecule that can be easily excreted.

Here are the few examples and case studies of pharmacokinetic mechanism of herb-drug interactions, which alter drug's metabolic pathway. Herbs like aloe vera, cascara, rhubarb, senna etc. has laxative action is mainly used for treatment of diarrhea and it has been found that these herbs interfere with other drug which are absorbed intestinally mainly by accelerating up intestinal transit that causes decrease in absorption and finally, their therapeutic effect. Pharmacokinetic interactions usually occur by the alteration in the activity of drug metabolizing enzymes and other transporter proteins, especially cytochrome P450 (CYP) isoenzymes and P-glycoprotein (P-gp). The action of these enzymes and drug transporters can be accelerated or decelerated by both synthetic drugs as well as by the natural products. Drugs are mainly metabolised in the liver and if, there is any, sorts of interference in the function of enzyme that plays vital role in drug or natural product metabolism can consequently increase or decrease the plasma level of drug that ultimately impose toxic effects in patients. St. John's wort which acts as an inducer found to speed-up the metabolic rate of drug "indinavir" that leads to decrease in drug plasma concentration thereby decreasing the effectiveness of drug. Most of the drugs like those used for anxiety cardiac arrhythmia, depression, insomnia, coma and others are primarily metabolized in liver. Hence all these drugs those are susceptible to such type's interactions and should be taken with caution. Drug interactions due to alterations in elimination of drugs through the kidney can only occur if a drug is primarily eliminated from the body through the kidney. When the kidney function diminishes due to effect of drugs or any other natural products, then the amount of the drugs which can be eliminated by the kidneys is found to be increased. Few herbs have sedative effects, such as sage, nettle and kava are also found to elevate the sedative properties of other sleeping medications. Others have antiplatelet effect, like; ginkgo biloba, garlic, ginseng, and ginger which increases the risk of bleeding in patients taking traditional drugs with antiplatelet activity or blood thinners. Few more herbs are hypertensive, such as blue cohosh, ginger, licorice and bayberry which interfere with the standard drugs that is used for treating high blood pressure (Table 30.4).

Consequences of Interaction: Most of natural products interact with standard drugs to either produce side effects or to cause additive effects, but the main concern rises in order to observe cases where natural products produces side effects in elderly patients. Interaction between natural products and drug may lead to rise, fall or no change in action of a drug. Increase in action may lead to toxicity whereas decrease in action can lead to therapeutic failure of the drug. This ultimately leads to:

    (a) Prolonged period of stay in the hospital,

    (b) Rise in global morbidity and mortality,

    (c) Increase in economic and social burden on a country

Caution to use Natural Products or Herbal Medicine Product

Many people have the mistaken notion that, being natural, all herbs and foods are safe. This is not so. Most of the time, herbs and foods may interact with medications normally taken that may result in serious side effects.

    1. Always keeps a good practice to tell doctor or health practitioners what patients is taking so that physician can advise the patients regarding possible complications, if there is any.

2. One should also keep an eye for unusual symptoms. Very often, this may foretell the symptoms of a drug interaction.

3. Patients with high risk for drug interactions or taking drugs with a narrow therapeutic index should be monitored very closely for drug interactions

Cardiovascular Disorders

Cardiovascular disease (CVD) is the leading cause of death all over the world and according to WHO it will lead to around 24 million death by the year 2030, mostly from heart disease and stroke. So, as a major concern of global mortality most of the drug therapies are mainly belongs to cardiovascular system and used for treating cardiovascular disorders like hypertension, angina, irregular heartbeat, and high cholesterol. Now among, all hypertension is major contributory factor for overall mortality from CVD and prevalence is found to be about 50% in population of higher age groups that is in between 60-69 years with the further increase in prevalence beyond 70 year's age group. Thus, according to the third National Health and Nutrition Examination Survey (NHANES III), conducted in between 1992-1994, found that about 27% of the American adult is suffering from hypertension. The natural products which are biologically active have been used in china as therapeutic agents to treat CVD from millions of year. However, natural product ingredients are very complicated (usually hundreds of compounds) and yet to confirm the biological mode of action. Most common natural remedies which produces adverse events on the cardiovascular system includes, St. John's wort, motherwort, ginseng, gingko biloba, garlic, grapefruit juice, hawthorn, saw palmetto, danshen, echinacea, tetrandrine, aconite, yohimbine, gynura, licorice, and black cohosh. Among all these, St. John's wort is one of the 10 best-selling herbs in the United States. It is typically used to treat depression, anxiety, sleep disorders, the common cold, herpes, and the human immunodeficiency virus. It is used as a topical analgesic, and even as an enema for ulcerative colitis. Use of St. John's wort could potentially result in serious adverse reactions because of its effect on drug metabolism; it induces the hepatic cytochrome P450 system, particularly CYP3A4, an enzyme involved in oxidative metabolism of more than 50% of all prescription medications. Therefore, co-administration of this herb and drugs metabolized by CYP3A4 is avoided, as it may result in reduced bioavailability and effectiveness with subsequent recurrence of arrhythmia, hypertension, or other undesirable effects. Concomitant use of warfarin with St. John's wort decreases prothrombin time, which may result in sub-therapeutic anticoagulation and increased risk of thromboembolism.

Table 30.1 Commonly used natural products in cardiovascular diseases: application and possible drug interaction with standard therapy

Natural products	Application	Possible drug interaction
Co-Enzyme Q10	Anti-oxidant and free radical scavenger; used to treat heart failure, hypertension, and myopathies.	Decreased efficacy of chemotherapeutics and radiation. Procoagulant; lowers INR in patients on stable coumadin dose.
Gugulipid	Lipid-lowering through blocking nuclear hormone receptor, farnesoid X.	Decrease bioavailability of diltiazem and propranolol.
Hawthorn (Crataegus species)	Treatment of heart failure and arrhythmias.	Digoxin-like effects; potential interaction with digoxin
L-Carnitine	Involved in cellular energy production, supplement in nutritional deficiency, possible role in heart failure and myocardial infarction.	Limited data on drug interactions.
Motherwort	Traditionally used as cardiac debility, tachycardia, anxiety, insomnia, and amenorrhea.	Drug interaction with benzodiazipines; synergistic sedative effect and may result in coma.
Policosanol	Believed to inhibit cholesterol synthesis. Used in South America as hypocholesterolemic.	Limited data on Drug interaction
Red rice yeast	Typical HMG-CoA reductase inhibitor.	Drug interactions with macrolides, ketoconazole, protease inhibitors, verapamil, cyclosporine, and Others
Tetrandrine	Treatment of hypertension and angina Has vasodilative effect, due to inhibition of the L-type calcium channels	Drug interaction with other calcium channel blocker
Uzara Root (Xysmalobium undulatum)	Used for treating non-specific diarrhea.	Potential interaction with Digoxin

Central Nervous System

A large population across the globe utilizes herbal medicine in the hope of promoting health and to manage diseases related with central nervous system (CNS). The prevalence of CNS disorders were observed in UK was 625 per 1,00,000 population annually and 4,070 cases per 1,00,000 population in Banglore (India). When these natural products are co-administered with therapeutic drugs, it increase the risk of drug-herb interactions which may show synergistic effects and can leads to toxicity or inhibitory effects that leads to decrease in therapeutic effect.

Few clinical studies have observed the combined effect of these natural products and drugs in CNS. Patient cases have been reported where the combined use of St John's wort and selective serotonin re-uptake inhibitors caused symptoms characteristic of central serotonergic syndrome in the elderly patients characterized by confusion, agitation, hyperreflexia etc. This is mainly caused by inhibitory effect of St. John's wort on serotonin transporters in the CNS.

Ginseng benefit serum glucose control in diabetic patients, but also aids central nervous system complications in them. It has the potential to prolong bleeding time and therefore should not be used concomitantly with warfarin. Moreover, ginseng may cause headache, tremulousness, and manic episodes in patients treated with phenelzine sulfate, an antidepressant agent. Ginseng may interfere with the actions of estrogens or corticosteroids and may impede digoxin metabolism or digoxin monitoring.

St John's wort (*Hypericum perforatum*) is another medicinal herb used primarily for depression, sold over the counter (OTC). The herb is potentially able to stimulate P450 enzyme system specifically it induces CYP1A2 and CYP3A4, involved in the metabolism of clozapine (anti-psychotic agents). It has been observed that the induction of P-glycoprotein by St John's wort aggravated psychiatric deterioration of the patient. A clinical study showed amitriptyline, an antidepressant agent when co-medicated with St John's wort resulted in decreased plasma and urine concentration of the drug in 12 patients.

The potential effect phenytoin get reduced when administered with Shankhpushpi, herbal syrup. The drug specifically used in epilepsy. The use of the herb and drug concomitantly in disease state should be considered. The potential effect of Anise (*Pimpinella anisum L.; Apiaceae*) and its essential oil on CNS have been widely accepted but its interaction with the drugs administered in CNS ailments should be considered. It has been reported that co-administration of fluoxetine and imipramine with essential oil reduced the antidepressant activity of the drugs and enhance the motor impairment effects of midazolam. The intake of herbs with codeine significantly increases of analgesic effect. The herb also reported to minimize the pentobarbital induced sleeping time. So, finally it has been concluded that concomitant intake of aniseed essential oil preparations and drugs that act on CNS should be avoided due to potential herb–drug interactions.

Paullinia cupana seeds extract has been used in popular medicine as a stimulant of the central nervous system, in cases of physical and mental stress, and as an anti-diarrheic, diuretic, and anti-neuralgic. It has been strongly urged not to take concomitantly amiodarone, an antiarrhythmic agent with *Paullinia cupana.*

Conventionally PO (*peppermint oil- Menthal piperita*) is predominantly used in the treatment of various ailments including gastrointestinal and respiratory disorders. It has been reported that acute PO pretreatment in higher dose caused significant prolongation of pentobarbitone-induced sleeping time, while it was significantly shortened by chronic PO pretreatment at the same dose. Chronic administration of PO enhances Midazolam effect.

Kava (*Piper methysticum*) has traditional uses as a relaxing soporific and is used extensively in modern phytotherapy to treat a variety of ailments, in particular anxiety. Potential interaction of Kava with benzodiazepines causing increased sedation has been posited.

Table 30.2 Commonly used natural products in central nervous system: application and possible drug interaction with standard therapy

Natural product	Applications	Possible interactions
St. John's wort	Anti-depressant activity	Decreased plasma level of alprazolam
Kava	Sedative activity	Reduced efficacy of Levodopa, semi-comatose activity when interacts with Alprazolam
Psylium	Cholesterol reduction	Decreased plasma lithium concentration
Echinacea	Immunogenic effect	Increased (oral midazolam) or decreased (systemic midazolam) clearance
Evening primrose oil	Arthritis, skin disorders	interacts with fluphenazine leads to seizures
Ginseng	Anti-diabetic agent, stimulant	Sleeplessness, tremor and headache when interacts Phenelzine
Ginkgo	In dementia	When interacts Trazodone leads to Comtose

NSAIDs

Nonsteroidal anti-inflammatory drugs or simply NSAIDs are a class of drugs that characterized by having antipyretic, analgesic and anti-inflammatory properties. The drug is available over the counter in most of the countries. A data was collected in United States which unveiled that 30 billion over-the-counter NSAIDs get sold and the drug accounted for 70,000,000 prescriptions every year. So the feasibility to interact with various natural products is more in case of NSAIDs. So, it is indispensable to let know the physician concerning every drug which patients are taking including non -prescription drugs or any herbal products.

Known for its antioxidant and neuroprotective effects, the leaf extract of the commonly used herb, *Ginkgo biloba* is used for the treatment of a variety of conditions today, which include asthma, bronchitis, tinnitus, Alzheimer's disease and other dementias, decreased memory, sexual dysfunction and multiple sclerosis. When used with NSAIDs (aspirin, ibuprofen), ginkgo displays additive/synergistic antiplatelet and anticoagulant properties.

Saw palmetto (Serenoarepens), is the most widely used herbal drugs for the treatment of lower urinary tract symptoms (LUTS) and for benign prostatic hyperplasia (BPH). Use of *saw palmetto* with NSAIDs/anticoagulants is contraindicated because of its ability to inhibit the enzymes cycloxygenase and 5-lipoxygenase as it may predispose to serious bleeding.

Another immunomodulatory herb of choice is Echinacea, which is used as non-specific immune-stimulant for upper respiratory tract infections. The active components of the herbs are proven to be hepatotoxic and there is a possibility for potentiation of hepatotoxicity when it is co-administered with acetaminophen or other NSAIDs. There are reports of cases of breakthrough bleeding with oral contraceptives and gastrointestinal bleeding with non-steroidal anti-inflammatory (NSAIDS), when taken simultaneously with St John's Wart.

NSAIDs used to increase the absorption of an element known as chromium and cause its retention. The adverse drug reaction has been reported from chromium consumption such as anemia, thrombocytopenia, hepatic dysfunction. So, the patients should use this combination with caution, especially at higher doses. Similarly, evening primose *(oenothera)* oil may predispose patients to more severe adverse effects of NSAIDs. So, one should avoid their concomitant use.

Diabetes

Diabetes mellitus (DM) is a metabolic disorder caused because of insufficient or inefficient insulin secretary response and it is characterized by increased blood glucose levels (hyperglycemia). As per the prevalence about 382 millions of people have diabetes. The disease causes substantial morbidity, mortality, and long-term complications and remains an important risk factor for cardiovascular disease.

Gum guar has been found to be effective in hyperglycemic state. It has prolonging gastric retention potential which results in slow diffusion of the administered drugs and hence gum guar affects the absorption of drugs. Some studies proposed that gum guar reduced the absorption of metformin and glibenclamide (gliburide). Gum guar also found to enhance the insulinogenic and blood glucose lowering effect of glibenclamide.

Liquorice is traditionally used as expectorant, carminative and as a food ingredient. Apart from its conservative action, it has also found to effect blood glucose level and possible interferes with hypoglycemic therapy. Numerous of preliminary studies shown that ginseng may increase the risk for hypoglycemia and, therefore, concomitant use of ginseng with anti-diabetic medication may increase the risk for hypoglycemia.

Fenugreek (*Trigonella foenum-graecum*) is an herbal medication extracted from the dried seeds of a plant which native to mainly eastern part of the world. An amino acid i.e., 4-hydroxyisoleucine derived from the herb appeared to stimulate the secretion of insulin and decrease blood sugar levels. When the herb taken orally, it cause gas, bloating, or diarrhea. It may also increase the potency of certain medications like aspirin and other blood thinning drugs and also interacts with hormonal agents.

Garlic and karela also found to decrease the glucose level in a diabetic patient who was on chlorpropamide. This indicates the additive effect on glucose level, as both garlic and karela possess hypoglycaemic effects.

Ginger is used to relieve nausea, vomiting and vertigo and found to interact with anti-diabetics due to its hypoglycemic effect.

Table 30.3 Commonly used natural products in diabetes: application and possible drug interaction with standard therapy

Natural product	Application	Possible interaction
Gum guar	Effective in hyperglycemic condition	Prolonged retention of drugs in GIT
Liquorice	Expectorant, carminative	Interacts with hypoglycemic therapy
Ginseng	Anti-dibetic, stimulant	Hypoglycemia
Neem (Azadirachta indica)	Anti-bacterial, antimalarial, antifertility, hepato-protective and antioxidant effects	Hypoglycemia
Chromium	Blood sugar control	Hypoglycemia
Psyllium	Cholestrol reduction	Hypoglycemia

Table 30.4 Summarized the different natural products and its physiological and pharmacological role following concomitant use of drugs

Natural products	Physiological and pharmacological role	Precaution in clinical practice
Aloe	Laxative	Increases potential for potassium loss which may increase the risk of toxicity.
Alfalfa	Arthritis, asthma, dyspepsia, hyperlipidemia, diabetes.	Increases bleeding risk with warfarin.
Apple cider vinegar	Effective in the treatment of acid reflux disease and heartburn. Have antibiotic effects and useful in GI tract infections.	Interact with digoxin, insulin and diuretics.
Black cohosh (*Cimicifuga racemosa*)	Herbal antidote for such menopausal symptoms as hot flashes, recommended as an alternative to standard hormone replacement therapy (HRT), which can produce unwanted side effects. Has estrogenic, antihypertensive and hepatotoxic effects	Contains coumarin constituents- Increases potential for bleeding

Table 30.4 *Contd...*

Natural products	Physiological and pharmacological role	Precaution in clinical practice
Bilberry leaf (*Vaccinium myrtillus*)	For clear vision and light adjustment, anti-diabetic, strengthen the immune system, useful for relieving stress, inflammation, and anxiety. Also urinary tract antiseptic, as well as a daily dietary supplement.	Anthocyanoside components may decrease excessive platelet aggregation, Increases potential for bleeding.
Chondroitin sulfate	Enhance the effect of warfarin	Use with caution
Chromium	Its absorption and retention occurs leading to increased risk of adverse reactions from the chromium consumption (e.g., anemia, thrombocytopenia, hepatic dysfunction).	Use with caution especially at higher doses (600-2400 mcg/day).
Coenzyme Q-10	Decreases blood pressure	Use with caution and monitor blood pressure
Cod liver oil	Reduces platelet aggregation and increases fibrinolytic activity	Monitor signs and symptoms of bleeding.
Cranberry juice	Prevent urinary tract infection and GI ulcer	Use with caution as it interacts with aspirin.
Danshen	Treatment of coronary artery disease and menstrual abnormalities inhibits cyclic adenosine monophosphate phosphodiesterase	Concomitant use with warfarin increases prothrombin time. Also interact with digoxin.
Dong Quai	Based on animal studies, have anticoagulant effect. Also have photoreactive and photocarcinogenic effects.	Caution is advised for patients receiving chronic treatment with coumadin (warfarin)
Echinacea	Inhibits CYP3A4	Increases serum drug concentration of CYP3A4 substrates.
Ephedra (Ma Huang)	Thermogenic (fat burning) properties, anti asthmatic	Enhance thermogensis, elevation of BP, arrythmia, reduce effectiveness of steroids.
Evening primose oil (EPO)	Reduces platelet aggregation and increases fibrinolytic activity. Increase risk of seizures.	Use with caution and monitor for signs and symptoms of bleeding.
Feverfew	Reduces platelet aggregation and increases fibrinolytic activity	Use with caution and monitor for signs and symptoms of bleeding.

Table 30.4 *Contd...*

Natural products	Physiological and pharmacological role	Precaution in clinical practice
Garlic (*Allium sativum*)	Induces CYP3A4 activity. Reduces platelet aggregation and increases fibrinolytic activity	Avoid concomitant use with drugs metabolized by this system. Use with caution and monitor for signs and symptoms of bleeding.
Ginger (*Zingiber Officinale*)	Theoretical interaction based on the ability of ginger to decrease platelet aggregation.	Use with caution and monitor for signs and symptoms of bleeding.
Ginkgo (*Ginkgo biloba*)	Causes induction of 2C19	Avoid concomitant use with drugs metabolized by this system.
Ginseng (*Panax ginseng*)	Have hypoglycemic effects, Inhibit the metabolism of Nifedipine and also increases the risk of bleeding with anticoagulants	Monitor blood glucose in combination with antidiabetic or insulin products. Inhibits cyclic AMP phosphodiesterase activity Spontaneous bleeding, Also monitor B.P. with concurrent treatment.
Glucosamine	High dose chondroitin (2400 mg/d) combined with high dose glucosamine (3000 mg/d) may enhance the effects of warfarin.	Use with caution.
Grape fruit juice	Increases bioavailability of calcium channel blockers. BP and heart rate is doubled.	Use with caution.
Green tea	Catechins and caffeine may have antiplatelet activity; therefore, concomitant administration may increase the risk of bleeding.	Use with caution and monitor for signs and symptoms of bleeding.
Gynura	Associated with hepatic toxicity. inhibit angiotensin-converting enzyme activity	Use with caution
Hawthorn	Has synergistic effect with digitalis glycosides, β-blockers and other hypotensives.	Use concomitantly with caution. So, modification of drug dosage is required.
Horse chestnut (*Aesculus hipposcastanum*)	In treatment of varicose veins and haemorrhoids	Contains coumarin, aesculin, that can additively interact with blood thinners such as NSAIDs, potentially leading to increased bleeding tendency.

Table 30.4 *Contd...*

Natural products	Physiological and pharmacological role	Precaution in clinical practice
Irish moss	In the treatment of ulcers, gastritis	Use with caution. Possible interaction with other antihypertensives.
Kava (*Piper methysticum*)	Inhibit CYP1A2, 2C9, 2D6 and 3A4.	Use with caution.
Licorice root (*Glycyrrhiza glabra*)	Inhibit CYP1A2, 3A4, 2B1, 2B6 and also decreases potassium levels in body.	Avoid use with the drugs which are substrates of these enzymes.
Milk thistle (*Silybum marianum*)	In the treatment of liver, spleen and kidney problems	Reduce liver toxicity due to drugs. Use with caution.
Pau D' Arco	Napthaquinones have warfarin like action.	Contraindicated with anticoagulants.
Peppermint oil	Inhibits metabolism of nifedipine in human liver microsomes.	Use with caution.
Probiotics	Used in allergies, diarrhea, Inflammation, IBS,colitis.	Interact with antibiotics as well as immunosuppressant like cyclosporine.
Red clover (*Trifolium pratense*).	For the treatment of skin conditions, menopause, cough and other respiratory problems	May interact with blood thinners such as NSAIDs to augment the risk of bleeding.
Saw palmetto	Concomitant administration may increase the risk of bleeding. Also has antiestrogenic effect.	Use with caution and monitor for signs and symptoms of bleeding. Avoid use with hormonal preprations.
Soy	Concurrent use may result in decreased effectiveness of warfarin. Has estrogen like property.	Monitor INR closely when initiating or discontinuing soy milk or other soy supplements. Should consult with physician while taking any hormonal preparation with soy.
ST John's Wort (*Hypericum perforatum*)	Treatment of mild to moderate depression, anxiety, or sleep disorders.	Induces metabolism of endeavor-decreasing its effectiveness in AIDS therapy, potentiation of action of sedatives, cardiac arrhythmia. And risk of transplant rejection.

Table 30.4 *Contd...*

Natural products	Physiological and pharmacological role	Precaution in clinical practice
Tamarind (*Tamarindus indica*)	Used as a laxative. It is also indicated for stomachaches, and liver and gallbladder ailments.	Increases the bioavailability of aspirin, leading to gastrointestinal bleeding.
Turmeric (*Curcuma longa*).	High dose should not be given to patients taking platelet or anticoagulant drugs.	With caution in stomach ulcer or hyperacidity.
Yohimbine	MAO inhibitor Concomitant use can interfere with BP control. Decreases effect of ACE inhibitors It antagonizes the effect of clonidine	Use concomitantly with caution. Avoid concomitant use
SAMe (S-S-adenosylmethionine)	Concomitant use with TCAs, SSRIs, MAOIs may lead to an increase in serotonergic effects (e.g., serotonin syndrome)	Avoid concomitant use.
Sarsaparilla	Elimination of hypnotics is accelerated	Use with caution.
Valerian (*Valeriana officinalis*)	Increases liver enzymes. May increase the effect of other CNS depressants Concomitant use with loperamide may result in delirium with symptoms of confusion, agitation, and disorientation.	Avoid concomitant use. Caution patients to avoid driving or operating machinery.

Conclusion

Most of the population have the habit of taking natural medicines either in forms of herbs or any other formulations as a therapeutic cure. However, experts suggest that natural stuff does not mean that it is completely safe and beneficial, but have has the potential to interact with concomitant treatment. So, when a drug is mixed with food or another herb, each can alter the way the body metabolizes the other. Also there is a question mark regarding regarding efficacy and safety, as most of these natural products are not validated through scientific evidences. Additionally, these natural products are considered as "food products" so, they are not subjected to the similar surveillance and regulation as existing drug therapy. As a result, manufacturers are exempt from premarket safety and efficacy testing before the release of an herbal product and from any post-marketing surveillance. So, clinicians need to review the complete patient profile in order to make the most appropriate therapeutic recommendations. As the current information reveals that these interactions are variable and unpredictable. So, it appears reasonable to caution patient not to take anything at the same time they are on medication. The patient ought to tell regarding all his natural ingestion habits so physician will guide properly regarding the additional consequences. It's not solely the responsibility of patients however conjointly physician ought to raise each patient regarding the daily routine. Furthermore, physician should be aware of all the current interactions of drugs with natural products and should apply to their routine prescriptions which can minimize the hazard of drug interactions upto at least some extent. The regulatory and scientific organization should also organize programs to increase awareness of effect of natural products on the prescribed drugs. So, overall natural products and drug interaction can be minimised by awareness as well as by following stringent guideline to launch any natural product for remedies.

Suggested Readings

1. Abebe W (2002). Herbal medication: potential for adverse interactions with analgesic drugs. *Journal of clinical pharmacy and therapeutics.* **27(6):** 391-401.

2. Almeida JC and Grimsley EW (1996). Coma from the health food store: interaction between kava and alprazolam. *Annals of Internal Medicine.* **125(11):** 940-1.

3. American Society of Hospital Pharmacists (1989). ASHP guidelines on adverse drug reaction monitoring and reporting. *Am J Hosp Pharm.* **46:** 336-337.

4. Aslam M, Stockley I (1979). Interaction between curry ingredient (karela) and drug (chlorpropamide). *The Lancet.* **313(8116):** 607.

5. Barbenel D, Yusufi B, O'shea D, Bench C (2000). Mania in a patient receiving testosterone replacement post-orchidectomy taking St John's wort and sertraline. *Journal of Psychopharmacology.* **14(1):** 84-6.

6. Barnes PM, Powell-Griner E, McFann K, Nahin RL, editors (2002). Complementary and alternative medicine use among adults, United States.

7. Blendon RJ, DesRoches CM, Benson JM, Brodie M, Altman DE (2001). Americans' views on the use and regulation of dietary supplements. *Arch Intern Med* **161:** 805-10.

8. Bressler R (2005). Herb-drug interactions: Interactions between saw palmetto and prescription medications. *Geriatrics.* **60(11):** 32-4.

9. Chang GW, Kam PC (1999). The physiological and pharmacological roles of cytochrome P450 isoenzymes. *Anaesthesia* **54(1):** 42-50

10. Chattopadhyay R, Chattopadhyay R, Nandy A, Poddar G, Maitra S (1987). Preliminary report on antihyperglycemic effect of a fraction of fresh leaves of Azadirachta indica (Beng. Neem). *Bull Calcutta Sch Trop Med.* **35:** 29-33.

11. Coxeter P, McLachlan A, Duke C, Roufogalis B (204). Herb-drug interactions: an evidence based approach. *Current medicinal chemistry.* **11(11):** 1513-25.

12. Cupp MJ (1999). Herbal remedies: adverse effects and drug interactions. *American Family Physician.*

13. Dannawi M (2002). Possible serotonin syndrome after combination of buspirone and St John's Wort. *Journal of Psychopharmacology.* **16(4):** 401.

14. Eisenberg DM, Davis RB, Ettner SL, Appel S, Wilkey S, Van Rompay M, Kessler RC (1998). Trends in alternative medicine use in the United States, 1990-1997: results of a follow-up national survey. *JAMA.* **280(18):** 1569-75.

15. Ernst E (1999). Second thoughts about safety of St. John's wort. *Lancet* **354(9195):** 2014-6.

16. Fugh-Berman A, Ernst E (2001). Herb–drug interactions: review and assessment of report reliability. *British Journal of Clinical Pharmacology.* **52(5):** 587-95.

17. Galluzzi S. ZO, Binetti G., Trabucchi M., Frisoni G.B (2000). Coma in a patient with Alzheimer's disease taking low dose trazodone and gingko biloba. *J Neurol Neurosurg Psychiatry.* **68:** 679-80.

18. Gardiner P, Graham RE, Legedza AT, Eisenberg DM, Phillips RS (2006). Factors associated with dietary supplement use among prescription medication users. *Arch Intern Med* **166:** 1968-74.

19. Gayle Nicholas Scott (2002). Update on Natural Product-Drug Interactions. *Am J Health Syst Pharm.***59(4).**

20. Gonzalez FJ, Gelboin HV (1994). Role of human cytochromes P450 in the metabolic activation of chemical carcinogens and toxins. *Drug Metab Rev* **26(1-2):** 165-83.

21. Gonzalez FJ, Tukey RH (2006). Drug Metabolism. In: Brunton LL. Eleven edition: The pharmacological basis of therapeutics. Mc Graw Hill, pp-71-91.

22. Gordon JB (1998). SSRIs and St. John's wort: possible toxicity. *Am Fam Physician.* **57(5):** 950-3.

23. Gorski JC, Huang S-M, Pinto A, Hamman MA, Hilligoss JK, Zaheer NA, *et al.,* (2004). The Effect of Echinacea (Echinacea purpurea Root) on Cytochrome P450 Activity *in vivo. Clinical Pharmacology & Therapeutics.* **75(1):** 89-100.

24. Haller C KT, Bent S (2008). Dietary supplement adverse events: report of a one-year poison center surveillance project. *Journal of Medical Toxicology.* **4(2):** 84-92.

25. Hepler CD, Strand LM (1990). Opportunities and responsibilities in pharmaceutical care. *Am J Hosp Pharm* **47:** 533.

26. Hoffman BB (2006). Therapy of hypertension. In: Brunton LL. Eleven edition: The pharmacological basis of therapeutics. Mc Graw Hill, pp- 845-868.

27. Hui H, Tang G, Go VL (2009). Hypoglycemic herbs and their action mechanisms. *Chinese Medicine.* **4(1):** 11.

28. Izzo AA (2005). Herb–drug interactions: an overview of the clinical evidence. *Fundamental & clinical pharmacology.* **19(1):** 1-16.

29. Joseph Boullata (2005). Natural Health Product Interactions with Medication. *Nutr Clin Pract* **20:** 33

30. Joshi R, Medhi B (2008). Natural product and drugs interactions, its clinical implication in drug therapy management. *Saudi Med J* **28(3):** 333-339

31. Kalra BS (2007). Cytochrome P450 enzyme isoforms and their therapeutic implications: an update. *Indian journal of medical sciences* **61(2):** 102-16.

32. Kendler BS (1997). Recent nutritional approaches to the prevention and therapy of cardiovascular disease. *Prog Cardiovasc Nurs.* **12(3):** 3-23

33. Lantz MS, Buchalter E, Giambanco V (1999). St. John's wort and antidepressant drug interactions in the elderly. *Journal of geriatric psychiatry and neurology.* **12(1):** 7-10.

34. Lucinda G. Miller (1998). Herbal Medicinals: Selected Clinical Considerations Focusing on Known or Potential Drug-Herb Interactions. *Arch Intern Med* **158(20):** 2200-11.

35. Markowitz JS, Donovan JL, DeVane CL, Taylor RM, Ruan Y, Wang J-S, *et al.,* (2003). Effect of St John's wort on drug metabolism by induction of cytochrome P450 3A4 enzyme. *Journal of the American Medical Association.* **290(11):** 1500-4.

36. Mehta DH, Gardiner PM, Phillips RS, McCarthy EP (2008). Herbal and dietary supplement disclosure to health care providers by individuals with chronic conditions. *J Altern Complement Med* **14:** 1263-9.

37. Mendis S PP, Norrving B (2011). Global Atlas on Cardiovascular Disease Prevention and Control. WHO.

38. Miller MF, Bellizzi KM, Sufian M, Ambs AH, Goldstein MS, Ballard-Barbash R (2008). Dietary supplement use in individuals living with cancer and other chronic conditions: a population-based study. *J Am Diet Assoc* **108:** 483-94.

39. NIH's 2007 survey of Complementary and Alternative Medicine (CAM) http://nccam.nih.gov/health)

40. Palmer ME, Haller C, McKinney PE, *et al.,* (2003). Adverse events associated with dietary supplements: an observational study. *Lancet* **361:** 101-6.

41. Perlman B (1990). Interaction between lithium salts and ispaghula husk. *The Lancet.* **335(8686):** 416.

42. Prabhakar PK, Doble M (2011). Mechanism of action of natural products used in the treatment of diabetes mellitus. *Chinese journal of integrative medicine.* **17(8):** 563-74.

43. Samojlik I, Mijatović V, Petković S, Škrbić B, Božin B (2012). The Influence of Essential Oil of Aniseed (*Pimpinella anisum* L.) on Drug Effects in Central Nervous System. *Fitoterapia*. 83(8):1466-73.

44. Samojlik I, Petković S, MimicaDukić N, Božin B (2012). Acute and Chronic Pretreatment with Essential Oil of Peppermint (*Mentha piperita* L., Lamiaceae) Influences Drug Effects. *Phytotherapy Research*. **26(6):** 820-5.

45. Schelosky L, Raffauf C, Jendroska K, Poewe W (1995). Kava and dopamine antagonism. *Journal of neurology, neurosurgery, and psychiatry*. **58(5):** 639.

46. Shader RI, Greenblatt DJ (1985). Phenelzine and the dream machine-ramblings and reflections. *Journal of clinical psychopharmacology*. **5(2):** 65.

47. Sierra M, Garcia J, Fernandez N, Diez M, Calle A (2002). Therapeutic effects of psyllium in type 2 diabetic patients. *European journal of clinical nutrition*. **56(9):** 830-42.

48. Sievenpiper J, Arnason J, Leiter L, Vuksan V (2003). Variable effects of American ginseng: a batch of American ginseng (*Panax quinquefolius* L.) with a depressed ginsenoside profile does not affect postprandial glycemia. *European journal of clinical nutrition*. **57(2):** 243-8.

49. Spinella M, Eaton LA (2002). Hypomania induced by herbal and pharmaceutical psychotropic medicines following mild traumatic brain injury. *Brain Injury*. **16(4):** 359-67.

50. Tachjian A, Maria V, Jahangir A (2010). Use of Herbal Products and Potential Interactions in Patients with Cardiovascular Diseases. *J Am Coll Cardiol*. **55(6):** 515-525.

51. Tanaka E, Hisawa S (1999). Clinically significant pharmacokinetic drug interactions with psychoactive drugs: antidepressants and antipsychotics and the cytochrome P450 system. *J Clin Pharmacy ther* **24(1):** 7-16.

52. Tao WY, Xu X, Wang X, Li BH, Wang YH, Li Y, Yang L (2013). Network-pharmacology-based prediction of the active ingredients and potential targets of chinese herbal radix curcumae formula for application tocardiovascular disease. *J Ethnopharmacol* **145(1):** 1-10.

53. Tatro DS (1999). Drug interactions with natural products. *Drug Facts and Comparisons NEWS*. 34-38.

54. Timbo BB, Ross MP, McCarthy PV, Lin CT (2006). Dietary supplements in a national survey: prevalence of use and reports of adverse events. *J Am Diet Assoc* **106:** 1966-74.

55. Vivian JC (1996). Liability for drug-drug interaction. *U.S. Pharm*. **21:** 93-95.

56. Yeh GY, Eisenberg DM, Kaptchuk TJ, Phillips RS (2003). Systematic review of herbs and dietary supplements for glycemic control in diabetes. *Diabetes care.* **26(4):** 1277-94.

57. YN S (2005). Potential for kava and St John's wort with drugs. *J Ethnopharmacol.***100:** 108-13.

58. Yue QY, Bergquist C, Gerden B (2000). Safety of St John's wort (Hypericum perforatum). *Lancet* **355(9203):** 576-7.

59. Zaffani S, Cuzzolin L, Benoni G (2006). Herbal products: behaviors and beliefs among Italian women. *Pharmacoepidemiol Drug Saf.* **15(5):** 354-9.

60. Zhao J, Jiang P, Zhang WD (2010). Molecular networks for the study of TCM Pharmacology. *Brief Bioinform* **11(4):** 417-430.

CHAPTER 31

CLINICAL RELEVANCE TO DRUG INTERACTIONS

Introduction

Drug interaction is defined as "A measurable modification (in magnitude or duration) of the action of one drug by prior or concomitant administration of another substance". This interaction may occur between drug-drug (Rx, OTC, herbal), drug-food, drug-alcohol, drug-laboratory, drug-disease or drug-chemical. Clinically significant drug interactions are those where the therapeutic activity and/or toxicity of a drug is changed to such an extent that a dosage adjustment of the medication or medical intervention is required. There are certain core parameters to assess the clinical relevance of drug interactions likewise:

- Evidence of drug interactions.
- The clinical relevance of potential adverse reaction resulting from drug interaction.
- Risk factors; the drug interaction may be of specific importance in patients with special risk factors.
- Incidence of adverse drug reaction given the combination of drugs.

It has been observed that 6.5% of adverse drug reactions in USA were attributed to drug interactions (0.2% of these patients may have life-threatening interactions). The potential drug interactions have been observed to be 17% in surgical patients, 22% in patients in medical wards, and 23% in outpatient clinics.

Consequence of Drug Interaction

Drug interaction can lead to additive effect (1 + 1 = 2), synergistic effect (1 + 1 > 2), potentiating effect (1 + 0 = 2) or antagonism effect (1 − 1 = 0). The effect can induce an adverse as well as intended response. For example, the competition between penicillin and probenecid for renal elimination results in increased penicillin serum concentrations, and in the past was employed as a way to decrease the expense of penicillin therapy. Similarly, it has been suggested to combine cyclosporine with ketoconazole or grapefruit juice, and to increase the efficacy of retinoid therapy by concomitant treatment with inhibitors of retinoic acid 4-hydroxylation such as azole derivatives or vitamin D (cholecalciferol) analogues.

Unfortunately, most drug interactions occur in the form of adverse effects. In the use of commercially available drugs, and especially in the development of new drugs, the detection of drug interactions is one of the main challenges in clinical pharmacology.

Thus drug interactions can lead to:

- Early termination from clinical development
- Refusal of approval
- Severe prescribing restrictions or withdrawal of a drug from the market

In the development of new drugs, potential interactions between drugs with low therapeutic indices require careful consideration. Usually, such clinical testing is performed in healthy participants, and the tolerability of a drug in patients with hepatic or renal dysfunction can only be estimated from these data. However, clinical studies in patients with hepatic or renal dysfunction are usually conducted with low numbers of patients. The complexity of these considerations is exemplified by the fact that a constant inhibition of the metabolism of drug A by 50% can be less problematic with regard to the maintenance of a stable therapeutic concentration than an inhibition of 25% that varies from 10 to 70%. For most of these drugs, determination of plasma drug concentrations may reduce the risk of potentially hazardous interactions. However, not all of these drugs need to have plasma concentration monitoring during therapy. Adverse drug interactions occur especially in patients receiving drugs with a low therapeutic index (Table 31.1).

Table 31.1 Drugs with a low therapeutic index

Drug	Adverse effect
Antiarrhythmic (quinidine, procainamide)	Cardiotoxicity
Anticonvulsants	CNS toxicity
Antihistamines (terfenadine, astemizole)	Cardiotoxicity, QT-interval prolongation, ventricular arrhythmias
Cyclosporine	Nephrotoxicity, hypertension
Digoxin	Cardiotoxicity
Methotrexate	Hepatotoxicity, haematological toxicity
Oral anticoagulants (warfarin)	Haemorrhage
Theophylline	CNS toxicity

Usually, several factors are required for a theoretically predictable interaction to become clinically relevant. A study in 2422 patients over 25,005 days of therapy revealed 113 (4.7%) drug combinations with potential interactions but only 0.3% leading to detectable clinical manifestations, indicating that the recognition of clinically relevant drug interactions remains a challenge for every physician and healthcare professional who is responsible for patients receiving multiple drugs.

Factors that Enhance the Probability of Serious Drug Interactions

Several factors play roles in determining the chance of occurrence of drug interactions and leading to serious consequences. The risk is cumulative, and the relative impact of each factor at different time points of patient treatment i.e., from disease diagnosis to end of effect of drug is unknown. The factors are

- Polypharmacy
- Underlying renal or hepatic dysfunction, chronic diseases
- Drugs with narrow therapeutic index
- Drugs with sharp response curve (e.g., phenytoin, aminoglycosides, vancomycin)
- Debilitation/malnutrition/chronic immunosuppression
- Genetic predisposition (i.e., poor metabolizer, polymorphism)

Drug Interactions and Adverse Drug Reactions

Depending on the individual patient, the prevalence of adverse drug reactions varies from 0.3% to more than 80%, as observed in elderly patients who may take more than 20 different drugs simultaneously. Therefore, patients receiving multiple drugs, such as those with AIDS, diabetes mellitus or other chronic diseases, are at very high risk of developing adverse reactions caused by drug interactions. Such pharmacologically relevant drug interactions can occur at any step from absorption to elimination. Drug interactions occurring before absorption, such as precipitations caused by an incorrect mixture of several drugs, are termed drug incompatibilities.

Drug interactions can lead to different types of adverse drug reactions. There are many different classifications for adverse drug reactions. Adverse drug reactions are classified originally into two types: type A (pharmacological) and type B (idiosyncratic). The type A reactions characterize an augmentation of the recognized pharmacological activities of a drug. These are dose-dependent and are readily reversible on drug withdrawal, or even simply after dose-reduction. Similarly, the type B, or idiosyncratic adverse reactions, are bizarre type, which cannot be envisaged from the recognized pharmacological effects of the drug. There is lack of simple dose dependency, and their reproduction in animal models is not feasible. The incidence of type A reactions are more than the type B reactions accounting for over 80% of all reactions.

Type A reactions are commonly seen in patients on polytherapy, which is mostly found in geriatric practice. The likelihood of developing an adverse interaction increases with the number of drugs prescribed. Though this is more prevalent in elderly population, it is becoming increasingly frequent in younger patients with chronic diseases such as AIDS, where patients may be on 6-10 different drugs. According to an Australian study 4.4% of all adverse drug reactions resulting from drug interactions lead to hospital admission. Drug interactions pertaining to metabolic pathways of drugs may either be due to enzyme induction or enzyme inhibition. Induction of drug metabolising enzymes usually leads to increased degradation of the drug and thus enhances drug clearance. Most of the cases this results in loss of efficacy of the drug e.g., rifampicin induces glucuronidation of oral contraceptive pills and leads to failure of contraception. In some circumstances, the metabolite of the drug may be in higher concentration leading to metabolite related adverse drug effects e.g., meperidine has active metabolite nor-meperidine which causes CNS stimulation and seizure like side effects. On the other hand, inhibition of drug metabolising enzymes causes reduction in clearance of the affected drug, and their concentration increases in body. This is more likely to lead to type A adverse drug reactions particularly when the affected drug has a narrow therapeutic index. There are several examples with such drug interactions leading to regulatory cap on number of marketed drugs. Non-sedating antihistamine terfenadine interaction with the CYP3A4 inhibitors ketoconazole and erythromycin resulted in decreased conversion of terfenadine to its active metabolite (now marketed as fexofenadine). Adverse effects of terfenadine include interference with delayed rectifier potassium current, which leads to QT interval prolongation. Sometimes this is precipitated into torsades de pointes and sudden death. A similar type drug interaction occurs with cisapride and CYP3A4 inhibitors leading to banning of the former.

Another means of adverse drug interaction is described following the identification of the function of drug transporters in the disposition of drugs. Drug transport proteins, which are mainly located on membranes, have multitude effects including drug influx, drug efflux, while others can transport in both directions. Among the drug transporters P-glycoprotein (Pgp), which is encoded by the MDR1 gene, has been extensively studied. Pgp mainly acts as drug efflux transporter, and its over-expression has been significantly responsible for resistance of tumours to chemotherapy. Another example is digoxin toxicity induced by such as quinidine, verapamil, and amiodarone. Digoxin does not undergo biodegradation, however, inhibition of its efflux from the intracellular compartment of gut and kidney due to inhibition of Pgp by the above mentioned drugs can precipitate digoxin toxicity.

Since many type B adverse drug reactions are thought to be mediated by the formation of chemically reactive metabolites through metabolism by P450 enzymes (a process termed bioactivation), perhaps a relationship exists with the "internal dose", i.e., the concentration of the toxic metabolite formed in the body. Drug- drug interactions can lead to imbalance of the metabolizing enzyme and thus can precipitate the accumulation of toxic metabolite. For example there occurs increased incidence of isoniazid hepatitis with concomitant administration of rifampicin.

Polypharmacy, Elderly and Drug Interaction

As the age progresses, the prevalence of many diseases also increases. These include hypertension, osteoarthritis and prostatic hypertrophy. Drug therapy in the elderly is characterised by long duration of treatment and polypharmacy. As Drug treatment in elderly subject is often directed towards chronic conditions, so medicines tend to be continued for longer periods. This may be associated with several drug induced side effects, e.g., increased rates of gastrointestinal bleeding in patients taking non-steroidal anti-inflammatory drugs (NSAIDs). This type of problem emphasizes the need for reviewing repeat prescription and medication in the elderly. Polypharmacy in elderly is due to prevalence of many diseases simultaneously in the subject; these may be age-related or may co-exist due to impaired immunity status in the elderly. Again it may not be possible to achieve an adequate therapeutic response from the use of a single drug. Another reason for giving multiple numbers of drugs simultaneously is to counteract or minimise the risk of adverse effect occurrence. For example, potassium loss can be corrected with spironolactone or amiloride in patients who are receiving either a benzothiadiazine or loop diuretic. However, one of the most important predictors of adverse drug reactions is the total numbers of drugs given simultaneously.

Adverse drug reactions are common in the elderly. This is frequently a consequence of multiple drugs prescribing which leads to the occurrence of drug-drug interactions. Drug interactions represent a change in either the magnitude or duration of action of one drug caused by the presence of a second drug. This may enhance or reduce the efficacy of one or both of the drugs or a new effect may appear which is not seen with either of the drugs alone. Interactions may be pharmacokinetic or pharmacodynamic. The most important adverse interactions occur with drugs that have easily recognisable toxicity and a low therapeutic index.

Pharmacokinetic Drug Interactions

Absorption

Drug absorption is liable to be interfered by drug interaction among multiple drugs administered to the elderly subject. Drugs like anticholinergics (e.g., hydroxyzine), tricyclic antidepressants, morphine, isoniazid, chloroquine, phenytoin and aluminium hydroxide inhibit gastric motility leading to decreased drug absorbption in the gastrointestinal tract. There are instances where the total amount of drug absorbed is not reduced; however, the retarded reabsorption of certain drugs (e.g., analgesics) can result in significant change in the distribution of a drug between different body organs and lower their therapeutic concentrations (Table 31.2). In another situation, drugs such as metoclopramide and sodium bicarbonate increase gastric motility and may enhance the absorption rate. There is chemical interaction among drugs leading to chelation or insoluble complex formation, which also reduces drug absorption. For example, drugs like digoxin are converted into complexes in the gut by the simultaneous administration of agents such as antacids and cholestyramine. This reduces the extent of digoxin absorption by 20%-35%. Similarly high dose of metformin blocks vitamin B12 absoprtion and phenytoin can block folic acid absorption from gastrointestinal tract. However, clinical significances of many of these drug interactions are lacking. First pass metabolism is one potential step for drug interaction. Drugs which alter liver blood flow or compete for metabolism, affects the status of agents that undergo extensive first-pass metabolism. For example, in non-selective monoamine oxidase (MAO) inhibited subjects, the indirectly acting sympathomimetic amines like tyramine (found in cheese, tomatoes and chocolate), pseudoephedrine (in cough mixtures) and dopamine escape degradation in the intestinal wall and liver; thereby reaching into systemic circulation. They displace large amounts of noradrenaline from transmitter loaded adrenergic nerve endings and simultaneously MAO inhibition prevents noradrenaline breakdown leading to hypertensive crisis. Another example is propranolol administration, which reduces hepatic blood flow, thereby reduces first pass metabolism of drugs like glyceryl trinitrate.

Table 31.2 Drug interactions affecting drug absorption

Drug	Interacting drug	Effect of interaction
Amoxicillin	Amiloride	Decreased therapeutic effect of amoxicillin
Antihistamines	Other drugs	Decreased intestinal motility, decreased absorption of other drugs
Ketoconazole or itraconazole	Antacids, H_2 antagonists, didanosine	Increase in gastric pH decreased absorption of drugs
Azoles	Cyclosporin	Increased plasma cyclosporine
Calcium	Tetracycline	Reduced absorption of calcium
Corticosteroids	Cholestyramine	Decreased plasma corticosteroids
Ciprofloxacin, ketoconazole, itraconazole	Didanosine	Buffering agents included in didanosine formulations can reduce the bioavailability of other drugs
Dapsone	Didanosine	Decreased plasma dapsone
Digoxin	Tetracyclines, macrolides	Increased plasma digoxin with cardiotoxicity
Digoxin	Cholestyramine, colestipol	Reduced absorption of digoxin
Griseofulvin	Barbiturates	Decreased plasma griseofulvin
Penicillamine	Aluminium/magnesium-containing antacids, food, iron-containing drugs	Formation of chelates

Table 31.2 *Contd...*

Drug	Interacting drug	Effect of interaction
Penicillins	Atenolol	Decreased plasma atenolol
Penicillins, vitamin A, digoxin	Neomycin	Neomycin-induced malabsorption syndrome leading to reduced absorption of these drugs
Quinolones	Aluminium/magnesium-containing antacids, milk, zinc, iron	Formation of complexes of low solubility
Quinolones	Cholestyramine, colestipol	Reduced absorption of quinolones
Tetracyclines	Aluminium/magnesium-containing antacids, milk, zinc, iron	Formation of chelates with low plasma tetracyclines

Distribution

Drugs interactions may also affect the distribution of others within the body by influencing drug binding in plasma and tissues. Concurrent administration of two or more highly protein-bound drugs compete for binding to plasma proteins, thereby one may increase the free fraction or unbound portion of the other. Though this type of interaction seems to be of importance, in many cases they have been overstated. For example, the NSAIDs and warfarin, both are highly protein bound drugs. NSAIDs can displace warfarin from its binding site and increase its anticoagulant effect. But *in vivo* this effect is negligible; it is much more likely that warfarin metabolism is inhibited by NSAIDs. Similarly, sulfonylureas like tolbutamide is highly protein bound drug and it can be displaced from blood protein binding sites by NSAIDs. This can lead to a short-term increase in free (unbound) sulfonylurea and hence temporary hypoglycaemia. However, inhibition of tolbutamide metabolism by the NSAID was probably more important in causing such effect (Table 31.3).

Drug toxicities based on competition between drugs for binding sites is not of clinical concern for most therapeutic agents. Since drug responses, both efficacious and toxic, are a function of the concentrations of unbound drug, steady-state unbound concentrations will change significantly only when either drug input (dosing rate) or clearance of unbound drug is changed. Thus, steady-state unbound concentrations are independent of the extent of protein binding. However, for drugs with

(i) Narrow-therapeutic-index (e.g., phenytoin, tolbutamide, anticoagulants),

(ii) Low volumes of distribution (e.g., confined to the central compartment blood),

(iii) Long elimination half-life drugs (e.g., digoxin, clofazimine, chloroquine), and

(iv) In patients with albumin deficiency (e.g., liver cirrhosis, renal dysfunction and the elderly), a transient change in unbound concentrations occurring immediately following the dose of a competing drug could be of concern, such as with the anticoagulant warfarin.

A more common problem resulting from competition of drugs for plasma protein binding sites is misinterpretation of measured concentrations of drugs in plasma because most assays do not distinguish free drug from bound drug.

Table 31.3 Drug interactions based on displacement from protein binding sites

Drug A	Drug B (Displace Drug A from serum protein binding sites)
Diazepam	Phenytoin
Methotrexate	Sulfonamides, salicyaltes
Salicylates	Sufonylureas
Sulfonamides and Vitamin K	Bilirubin
Warfarin	Loop diuretic, valproate, indomethacin, phenytoin

Metabolism

Low-molecular-weight xenobiotics and drugs are usually cleaved to hydrophilic metabolites, facilitating biliary and/or renal elimination. This is achieved initially by a CYP isoenzyme, which produces highly reactive intermediate products. These metabolites are further cleaved to their corresponding organic acids by epoxide hydrolase, reductase and transferase enzymes. Inhibition or induction of drug metabolism is one of the most important mechanisms for drug-drug interactions. Interactions involving a loss of action of one of the drugs are at least as frequent as those involving an increased effect. There are many examples of one drug interfering with the metabolism of another by inhibition of the cytochrome P450 (CYP) enzymes in the liver (Table 31.4). The enzymes responsible for transforming drugs in humans belong to 6 CYP subfamilies, i.e., CYP1A, 2A, 2C, 2D, 2E and 3A. Each subfamily contains a number of different isoforms. It has been estimated that about 90% of human drug oxidation can be attributed to six of these, i.e., CYP1A2, CYP2C9, CYP2C19, CYP2D6, CYP2E1, CYP3A, and enzyme inhibition interactions have been reported with all. Each CYP isoenzyme may metabolise many drugs, and interaction of a single drug with CYP isoenzymes can be very complex. For example, the H2 antagonist cimetidine inhibits CYP2D6, CYP3A4, CYP1A2 and CYP2C9. Furthermore, drugs can modulate the activity of several CYP isoenzymes while being metabolised by another, as is the case for quinidine, which inhibits CYP2D6 while being a substrate for CYP3A4. Also, many β-blockers inhibit CYP2D6-dependent activity, but only a few of them are metabolised by this enzyme. So the potential for drug-drug interactions is high in patients taking several medications. For example, in a group of elderly male patients, cimetidine inhibited the metabolism of procainamide, giving rise to toxic plasma concentrations of the antiarrhythmic. Other drugs which are similarly affected by cimetidine are benzodiazepines, β-adrenoceptor blockers, tricyclic antidepressants, theophylline, phenytoin and oral anticoagulants. Although few of these drug-drug interactions are of clinical significance, caution is indicated when cimetidine is given concomitantly with drugs that have a narrow range of therapeutic concentration such as warfarin, theophylline and phenytoin. Other common inhibitors of one or more CYP isoenzymes include amiodarone, fluconazole, erythromycin, clarithromycin, sulphonamides, ciprofloxacin, omeprazole and paroxetine. Occasionally, clinically severe interactions occur as has been shown recently with combined administration of terfenadine and ketoconazole, erythromycin and itraconazole resulting in prolongation of the QT interval and torsades de pointes. At present, there is no evidence that CYP inhibition by these agents is affected by age.

Xenobiotic-metabolising enzymes also exhibit substantial genetic polymorphisms that can explain the variability of their basal activity and their inducibility in a population. Interestingly, these polymorphisms do not become clinically relevant until exposure to the relevant drug. This is the case for CYP2D6, where an exaggerated or even fatal response can occur because of failure of drug elimination (e.g., perhexiline, sparteine), or it may cause a lack of response because of a failure of prodrug activation (e.g., codeine is not converted to morphine).

Liver enzyme induction by one drug may lead to inactivation of a second drug. Well-recognised examples include the decreased efficacy of warfarin seen with barbiturate therapy and the reduced efficacy of dihydropyridine calcium-channel blocking drugs with carbamazepine therapy. The delay between the commencement of the enzyme-inducing agent and its full effect can take 7 to 10 days, making recognition of the interaction more difficult. However, in general terms, elderly individuals appear to be less sensitive to drug induction than younger individuals. For example, the distribution of hexobarbitol before and after treatment with rifampicin was studied in young and elderly volunteers. Rifampicin produced differential increases in hexobarbitol metabolism with 90- and 19-fold increases in the young and elderly volunteers, respectively (Table 31.5).

Combination of dapsone with rifampicin, which is recommended by the World Health Organization for treatment of lepromatous leprosy, increases the risk of these adverse effects. The combination of dapsone with ketoconazole, cimetidine or grapefruit juice may reduce the risk of dapsone toxicity, since these drugs inhibit CYP3A4.

Table 31.4 List of some drugs affecting enzymatic system of metabolism

Inducers	Inhibitors
Barbiturates	Allopurinol
Carbamazepine	Azoles
Dexamethasone	Chloramphenicol
Ethanol	Cimetidine
Grisofulvin	Ciprofloxacin
Glutethimide	Contraceptives
Phenytoin	Disulfiram

Table 31.4 *Contd...*

Inducers	Inhibitors
Rifampicin	Erythromycin
	Isoniazid
	Metronidazole
	Naringenin
	Propanolol
	Quinine
	Selective serotonin reuptake inhibitors
	Sulfonamides
	Trimethoprim
	Verapamil

Table 31.5 Pharmacokinetic drug interactions due to altered metabolism

Enzyme	Enzyme inducers	Enzyme inhibitors	Metabolism decreased of substrates
CYP1A2	Cabamazepine, chargrilled meat, methylcholanthrene, omeprazole, phenobarbital, rifampin, tobacco	Amiodarone, celecoxib, cimetidine, fluvoxamine, gyrase inhibitors (quinolones), tobacco compounds	Antipsychotics, clozapine, cyclobenzaprine, duloxetine, fluvoxamine, haloperidol, imipramine, naproxen, olanzapine, ondansetron, propranolol, tacrine, theophylline, tizanidine, triamterene, verapamil, (R)-warfarin, zileuton, zolmitriptan
CYP2B6	Artemisinin, cabamazepine, efavirenz, rifampin, nevirapine, phenobarbital, phenytoin	Clopidogrel, ThioTEPA, ticlopidine, voriconazole	Artemisinin, cyclophosphamide, bupropion, efavirenz, ifosfamide, ketamine, methadone, meperidine, nevirapine, propofol, selegiline, sibutramine, ThioTEPA
CYP2C9	Carbamazepine, nevirapine, phenobarbital, phenytoin, rifampicin, ST John's wart	Amiodarone, azoles, cimetidine, clpidogrel, cotrimoxazole, disulfiram, fluoxetine, isoniazid, metronidazole, omeprazole, paroxetine, sulfinpyrazone, tobutamide, tolcapone, valproate, zafirlukast	Angiotensin receptor blocker, carbamazepine, celecoxib, diclofenac, disulfiram, fluvastatin, flubiprofen, ibuprofen, naproxen, oral hypoglycemics, NSAIDs, phenytoin, piroxicam, retinoids, torsemide, valproic acid, (S)-warfarin, zafirlukast

Table 31.5 *Contd...*

Enzyme	Enzyme inducers	Enzyme inhibitors	Metabolism decreased of substrates
CYP2C19	Efavirenz, Rifampicin	Cimetidine, felbamate, fluoxetine, fluvoxamine, isoniazid, ketoconazole, lansoprazole, omeprazole, oral contraceptives, ticlopidine, voriconazole	Carisoprodol, citalopram, clopidogrel, clomipramine, clobazam, cyclophosphamide, diazepam, esomeprazole, fluoxetine, imipramine, lansoprazole, nelfinavir, omeprazole, phenytoin, pantoprazole, thalidomide, voriconazole
CYP2D6		Amiodarone, bupropion, diphenhydramine, fluoxetine, haloperidol, paroxetine, quinidine, terbinafine	antidepressants, antipsychotics, atomoxetine, β blockers, carvedilol, codeine, debrisoquine, desipramine, dextromethorphan, encainide, flecainide, fluoxetine, metoprolol, ondansetron, oxycodone, paroxetine, propafenone, propranolol, risperidone, tamoxifen, timolol, thioridazine, tramadol, venlafaxine
CYP2E1	Ethanol	Azoles, griseofulvin	Ethanol (increase metabolism cause disulfiram-like reaction occurs), paracetamol (Increased metabolism of paracetamol produces hepatotoxic hydroquinone metabolites)
CYP 3A4	carbamazepine, efavirenz, macrolides, nevirapine, phenytoin, phenobarbital, oxcarbazepine, primidone, rifampicin, St. John's wort	Amiodarone, azoles, cimetidine, clarithromycin, diltiazem, erythromycin, grapefruit juice, HIV protease inhibitors (indinavir), macrolide antibiotics (NOT azithromycin), naringenin, nifedipine, omeprazole, ritonavir, verapamil	Alfentanyl, alprazolam, antihistamines, astemizole, azoles, buspirone, calcium channel blockers, caffeine, carbamazepine, codeine, corticosteroids, cyclosporin, digitoxin, erythromycin, haloperidol, HIV protease inhibitors, oral contraceptives, statins (NOT pravastatin and rosuvastatin), midazolam, nevirapine, PDE 5 inhibitors, tacrolimus,

Table 31.5 *Contd...*

Enzyme	Enzyme inducers	Enzyme inhibitors	Metabolism decreased of substrates
			tamoxifen, terfenadine, triazolam, theophylline, vincristine, dapsone (Increased metabolism of dapsone to a strong oxidant hydroxylamine leading to methemoglobinemia)
Alcohol dehydrogenase		Large dose of ethanol	Abacavir (increase in abacavir plasma AUC by 41%)
Retinol dehydrogenase		Retinoids	Vitamin A
UGT (UDP glucuronosyl transferase)		Valproate	Lamotrigine, lorazepam, chloramphenicol, irinotecan, morphine

Elimination

Finally, drug-drug interactions may occur in the kidney resulting in altered drug elimination although is relatively rare. Five potential mechanisms exist for drug interactions in the kidney.

1. Increase in free drug concentration leads to an increase in drug excretion by glomerular filtration

2. Competitive inhibition of tubular secretion leading to increase in drug concentration

3. Competitive inhibition of tubular reabsorption resulting in an increase in drug excretion

4. Depending on the pKa of the drug, the change in urinary pH and/or flow rate may increase or decrease the drug excretion

5. Alteration of renal drug metabolism

The important step in drug elimination is tubular secretion, which is primarily affected by number of agents by competitive inhibition. Renal tubules have organic anion transporter protein (OATP), organic cation transporter protein (OCTP), P glycoprotein (P-gp) and others for transport of drug molecules across tubular membrane. Probenecid is one of the best recognised drugs which have high affinity for OATP and blocks active secretion/elimination of penicillin/ampicillin and methotrexate. Probenecid blocks uric acid reabsorption from renal tubules and salicylates block this uricosuric action of probenecid and sulfinpyrazone. Quinidine interferes with digoxin renal and biliary clearance by 40%-50% due to inhibition of ATP-dependent P-gp in over 90% of patients. This is also accompanied by displacement of digoxin from its binding sites in tissues by quinidine. Similar drug interactions have been reported with amiodarone and verapamil, leading to 70%-100% increases in serum digoxin concentrations. Non-competitive interference with drug secretion may also occur, e.g., prolonged thiazide like diuretic treatment causes a compensatory increase in proximal tubule reabsorption of sodium, resulting in increased lithium reabsorption. This interaction can result into serious lithium toxicity. NSAIDs can also reduce renal elimination of lithium by up to 60% (Table 31.6).

Table 31.6 Drug interactions due to interference of elimination

Drug A	Interacting drug B	Effect of interaction
Aciclovir, cidofovir, ganciclovir, foscarnet	Probenecid	Inhibition of renal elimination and increased plasma concentration of antiviral drugs
Amphotericin	Pentamidine (and other nephrotoxic drugs)	Disturbed renal function
Corticosteroids	Azoles	Increased plasma corticosteroids
Digoxin	Amiodarone, diltiazem, verapamil	Reduced clearance of A
Fluconazole	Thiazides	Increased plasma fluconazole
Lamivudine	Trimethoprim-sulfamethoxazole	Increases lamivudine plasma AUC by 43%
Lithium	NSAIDs, thiazide diuretics	Reduced clearance of A
Methotrexate	Cyclosporin, NSAIDs, Salicylates, probenecid, Penicillin	Reduced clearance of A due to cyclosporin Nephrotoxicity, decreased prostaglandin synthesis by NSAIDs, reduced renal clearance by others
Procainamide	Quinolones	Increased plasma procainamide
Tetracyclines	Urinary alkalinizers	Decreased plasma tetracycline concentrations

Pharmacodynamic Interactions

Drugs administered simultaneously or in close interval may be indifferent to each other or may influence each other's action. The influence may be antagonistic or synergistic type. In antagonistic pharmacological interaction, one may counteract or reduce other's intended therapeutic effects (Table 31.7). The interaction between non-specific β-adrenoceptor blocking drug propranolol and theophylline is antagonistic type. Propranolol may induce bronchoconstriction in a patient taking theophylline for asthma. Another example is interaction between NSAIDs and antihypertensives. NSAIDs lead to inhibition of prostaglandins in the juxtaglomerular apparatus of kidney. This reduces the natriuresis effect and tends to cause sodium retention; this nullifies the hypotensive effect of antihypertensives. Furthermore, NSAID usage posed to be an independent risk factor for hypertension in the elderly age group.

Drugs may interact in a way to facilitate or enhance their own action in a synergistic way. As for example nitrous oxide and halothane put their effect together to enhance the general anaesthetic effect. ACE inhibitors like enalapril when combined with diuretic like hydrochlorothiazide, there is supraadditive antihypertensive effect. Aminoglycoside antibiotic like gentamicin is combined with beta lactam antibiotic like penicillin to have a broad spectrum antibacterial coverage. However, the administration of one drug in combination with other or during the course of action of other drug, may not always lead to beneficial effect. There is chance of influence of one drug's effect upon other's pharmacodynamic response in direct or indirect way leading to noxious and unwanted response (Table 31.8). For example, digoxin toxicity is enhanced by hypokalemia. If a diuretic is co-administered with digoxin then diuretic induced hypokalemia may precipitate toxicity of digoxin. Similarly, verapamil and diltiazem have myocardial depressant effect, so co-administration of β-adrenoceptor blockers may lead to hypotension and atrioventricular block.

Though drug-drug interactions can occur in a number of ways which may or may not have a sound pharmacological explanation, it has been seen that only about 10% of potential interactions result in clinically significant events. Serious clinical consequences or death are rare pertaining to drug interactions, but mild clinical morbidity may be much more common. In the elderly subjects, non-specific complaints such as confusion, dizziness, depression, lethargy, weakness, incontinence and falling may indicate an underlying drug-drug interaction. In some cases, the pharmacokinetic or pharmacodynamic mechanisms may not fully explain the cause of the interaction and this enhances complexity. For example, treatment of epilepsy with antiepileptic drugs is often accompanied by antidepressants or antipsychotic drug treatment. This may be due to the coexistence of epilepsy with psychiatric disorders or may be to manage the side effect profile of one of the type of drug therapy which is administered on long term basis. Antiepileptic drugs have the propensity to cause cognitive dysfunction and agitative behaviour in epileptic patients. Similarly antidepressants and antipsychotic drugs are believed to lower the seizure threshold. Again, the potential for drug-drug interactions in psychiatric patients is high because multiple medications are given to treat co-morbid psychiatric disorders, to treat concomitant medical conditions, to manage the side effects of one drug or to handle the noncompliance in the subject. In particular, the tricyclic antidepressants have not only one type of pharmacodynamic response to treat the depression; rather they have the potential of sedation, seizure precipitation, antimuscarinic activity, hypertension, and cardiac arrhythmia precipitation. The selective serotonin uptake inhibitors (SSRIs) inhibit drug metabolizing isoenzymes, particularly, CYP2D6 and CYP3A4, which leads to elevation of plasma levels of several co-administered drugs like tricyclic antidepressants, clozapine, haloperidol, some benzodiazepines, carbamazepine, terfenadine, astemizole, and warfarin.

Table 31.7 Pharmacodynamic drug interactions that may lead to a reduced effect

Drug A	Interact with Drug B	Effect of Interaction
Abacavir	Tenofovir and lamivudine	This triple NRTI has high rate of early virological nonresponse seen in treatment-naive patients
Antihypertensives (e.g., ACE inhibitors, thiazides and β blockers)	NSAIDs	Reduced effect of A
Tenofovir	Didanosine and lamivudine	This triple NRTI has high rate of early virological nonresponse seen in treatment-naive patients
Warfarin	Vitamin K	Reduced effect of A
Zalcitabine	Lamivudine	Pharmacologic antagonism
Zidovudine	Stavudine	Pharmacologic antagonism

Table 31.8 Pharmacodynamic drug interactions that may lead to an enhanced effect

Drug A	Interacting drug B	Effect of interaction
ACE inhibitors	NSAIDs	Additive nephrotoxic, Hyperkalaemia
Acetyl-salicylic acid	NSAIDs	Peptic ulceration
Amitriptyline	Minocycline	Skin pigmentation
Amphotericin (intravenous)	Nucleoside analogues, intravenous pentamidine and other nephrotoxic drugs	Nephrotoxicity
Antihypertensive agents	Vasodilators (e.g., nitrates for angina) antipsychotics and some antidepressants	Postural hypotension
Atazanavir	Indinavir	Potential additive hyperbilirubinemia

Table 31.8 *Contd...*

Drug A	Interacting drug B	Effect of interaction
Azathioprine	Allopurinol	Pancytopenia
Azoles	Aciclovir	Potentiated antiviral effects
Cephalosporins (second generation)	Aminoglycosides	Increased nephrotoxicity
Corticosteroids (oral)	NSAIDs	Corticosteroid prevents healing of peptic ulcer
Cyclosporin	Colchicine	Severe gastrointestinal, hepatic, renal and neuro-toxicity
Didanosine, stavudine, zalcitabine	Ethambutol, isoniazid, vincristine, cisplatin, hydroxyurea, phenytoin and pentamidine	Severe peripheral neuropathy
Didanosine	stavudine and zalcitabine	Increased pancreatitis and peripheral neuropathy
Digoxin	Diuretics (loop and thiazides)	Diuretic induced Hypokalemia increases effect of A
Diuretics (potassium sparing)	ACE inhibitors, potassium supplements	Hyperkalemia, impaired renal function
Epinephrine (Along with local anaesthetics)	βBlockers	Hypertensive crisis
Erythromycin	Warfarin	Increased anticoagulation and haemorrhage
Ganciclovir	Zidovudine	Severe haematological complication
Methotrexate	Sulfonamides	Increased methotrexate toxicity
Methotrexate	Trimethoprim	Bone marrow suppression
Methotrexate	Cyclosporin	Increased nephrotoxicity
Phenothiazines and butyrophenones	Anticholinergic drugs (e.g. some antihistamines and tricyclic antidepressants)	Excessive anticholinergic effects (e.g. constipation, urinary hesitancy, dry mouth, confusion)

Table 31.8 *Contd…*

Drug A	Interacting drug B	Effect of interaction
Psoralen-ultraviolet A (PUVA) therapy	Photosensitizers such as astemizole, chlorothiazide, coal tar, griseofulvin, interferon (IFN α, β), retinoids (e.g., tretinoin, isotretinoin), methoxsalen, nalidixic acid, naproxen, quinolones (e.g., ciprofloxacin), terfenadine, tetracyclines (e.g., minocycline, doxycycline) and sulfonic derivatives	Photosensitisation
Quinolones	NSAIDs	Seizures
Retinoids	Tetracycline or minocycline	Pseudotumour cerebri, elevated intracranial pressure
warfarin	Aspirin, NSAIDs, clofibrate, antibiotic causing reduced gut flora (decreased Vitamin K synthesis)	Anticoagulant effect accentuated

Specific Group of Drugs and their Drug Interactions

Antifungals: Azoles and Echinocandins

Azole antimycotics inhibit C14 α desmethylase by binding to the hem group of CYP. C14 α desmethylase is required for the conversion of lanosterol into ergosterol. This molecular mechanism is in part responsible for the clinically relevant drug interactions of this class of antifungals. The extent of drug interactions, however, varies between the different azoles depending on their hepatic metabolism. Numerous drug interactions have been described and ketoconazole is used as a model substance for CYP3A4 inhibition in pharmacokinetic studies. Ketoconazole inhibits CYP3A4, CYP2C8, CYP2C9, and also is an inhibitor of P-glycoprotein (Pgp). Fluconazole inhibits hepatic CYP3A4 and CYP2C9, itraconazole is a strong inhibitor of CYP3A4, voriconazole enzyme inhibition comprises of CYP3A4 and CYP2C10, and posaconazole is an inhibitor of CYP3A4. Regarding other antifungals like echinocandins, caspofungin is not an inhibitor or a substrate of CYP enzymes or for P-glycoprotein (Pgp), Micafungin is reported to be a weak inhibitor of CYP 3A, and anidulafungin has no significant effect on CYP. So drug interactions can be expected to play a minor role in patients on echinocandins treatment. Some important drug interactions of itraconazole are depicted here (Table 31.9).

Table 31.9 Drug interactions of azoles and echinocandins

Drugs displaying enhanced levels during itraconazole therapy	Possible complications
HMG-CoA-reductase inhibitors (lovastatin, simvastatin, atorvastatin)	Rhabdomyolysis
Immunosuppressives (Cyclosporine A, tacrolimus, sirolimus, everolimus)	Over-immunosuppression, nephrotoxicity, CNS toxicity
Antihistamines (terfenadine, astemizole)	Cardiac arrhythmias
Midazolam, triazolam	Over-sedation
Warfarin	Bleedings
Quinidine	Arrhythmias, nausea
Calcium antagonists (felodipine, nifedipine)	Hypotension, edema
Anti HIV medication (ritonavir, indinavir, saquinavir)	Enhanced toxicity

Protease Inhibitors

It is a common practice to combine HIV protease inhibitors with a low dose of ritonavir to take advantage of that drug's remarkable capacity to inhibit CYP3A4 metabolism. Although the approved dose of ritonavir for antiretroviral treatment is 600 mg twice daily, doses of 100 or 200 mg twice daily are sufficient to inhibit CYP3A4 and increase the concentrations of concurrently administered CYP3A4 substrates. This allows a reduction in both drug dose and dosing frequency while increasing systemic concentrations. Combinations of amprenavir, fosamprenavir, or atazanavir with ritonavir are approved for once-daily administration. Lopinavir is available only in a coformulation with ritonavir that is designed to take advantage of this beneficial pharmacokinetic drug interaction.

Indinavir and nelfinavir appear to be much weaker inhibitors of the CYP3A4 than is ritonavir. Interestingly, the metabolism of indinavir in the intestine is strongly inhibited by ketoconazole, and the finding of an anti-rat CYP3A1 antibody in the intestine and liver induced by dexamethasone suggests the involvement of CYP3A isoforms in both organs. Non-nucleoside reverse transcriptase inhibitors (NNRTIs) also modulate the activity of CYP3A4 or are metabolised by this enzyme. Therefore, delavirdine should not be co-administered with rifampicin, rifabutin, didanosine and other CYP3A4 inducers. When NNRTIs are combined with saquinavir and indinavir, the serum concentrations of the protease inhibitors can increase because of competition for binding to CYP3A4. The dosage of indinavir may be reduced, but that of saquinavir does not have to be altered. Nevirapine is another NNRTI that is a strong inducer of CYP3A4, and should therefore not be co-administered with drugs that are substrates for this enzyme. Finally, it should be emphasised that most of the interactions that could occur with antiretroviral agents have not yet been well studied, and other interactions may be still be unrecognised (Table 31.10).

Table 31.10 Drug interactions of protease inhibitors

Parameter	Saquin-avir	Indin-avir	Riton-avir	Nelfin-avir	Ampren-avir	Fosampren-avir	Lopin-avir	Atazan-avir
Metabolism	CYP3 A4	CYP3 A4	CYP3 A4 > CYP2D6	CYP2 C19 > CYP3 A4	CYP3 A4	CYP3A4	CYP3 A4	CYP3A4
Auto-induction of metabolism	No	No	Yes	Yes	No	No	Yes	No
Inhibition of CYP3A4	+	++	+++	++	++	++	+++	++

Abbreviations: +, weak; ++, moderate; +++, substantial.

Antiepileptics

Concurrent administration of any drug metabolized by CYP2C9 or CYP2C10 can increase the plasma concentration of phenytoin by decreasing its rate of metabolism. Carbamazepine, which may enhance the metabolism of phenytoin, causes a well-documented decrease in phenytoin concentration. Interaction between phenytoin and phenobarbital is variable. Phenobarbital, phenytoin, and valproate may increase the metabolism of carbamazepine by inducing CYP3A4. Concurrent administration of carbamazepine may lower concentrations of valproate, lamotrigine, tiagabine, and topiramate. Carbamazepine reduces both the plasma concentration and therapeutic effect of haloperidol. The metabolism of carbamazepine may be inhibited by propoxyphene, erythromycin, cimetidine, fluoxetine, and isoniazid. Valproate primarily inhibits the metabolism of drugs that are substrates for CYP2C9, including phenytoin and phenobarbital. Valproate also inhibits UGT and thus inhibits the metabolism of lamotrigine and lorazepam. A high proportion of valproate is bound to albumin and the high molar concentrations of valproate in the clinical setting result in displacement of phenytoin and other drugs from albumin. Along with this inhibition of phenytoin metabolism by valproate exacerbates free concentration of phenytoin in blood. The concurrent administration of valproate and clonazepam has been associated with the development of absence status epilepticus; however, this complication appears to be rare. (Table 31.11)

The antiepileptic drugs not metabolised by CYP or UGT (UMP glucuronosyl transferase) are: gabapentin, lacosamide, levetiracetam, pregabalin, stiripentol, vigabatrin.

Table 31.11 AEDs and their main mechanisms of elimination and susceptibility to pharmacokinetic interactions

Type of AEDs	CYP3A4	CYP2C9	CYP2C19	UGT	Epoxide hydrolase
Substrate AEDs	Carbamazepine Tiagabine Zonisamide Ethosuximide Clonazepam Clobazam Felbamate	Phenytoin Phenobarbital Valproic acid	Phenytoin Phenobarbital Valproic acid Clobazam	Valproic acid Lamotrigine Oxcarbazepine Eslicarbazepine acetate Topiramate Stiripentol Rufinamide	10,11-epoxy-Carbamazepine
Enzyme inducing AEDs	Phenytoin Carbamazepine Phenobarbital Oxcarbazepine Eslicarbazepine acetate Topiramate Felbamate Rufinamide	Phenytoin Carbamazepine Phenobarbital	Phenytoin Carbamazepine Phenobarbital	Phenytoin Carbamazepine Phenobarbital Oxcarbazepine Lamotrigine	Phenytoin Carbamazepine Phenobarbital
Enzyme inhibiting AEDs	Stiripentol	Valproic acid Phenytoin Clobazam Stiripentol	Valproic acid Felbamate Oxcarbazepine Topiramate Zonisamide Clobazam Stiripentol	Valproic acid Topiramate	Valproic acid Topiramate

Table 31.12 Other drugs affecting commonly used AEDs. Examples from therapeutic drug classes of clinical importance

Therapeutic Drug Classes	Affected AEDs	Mechanism of Interaction and Clinical Consequence
Antidepressants and antipsychotics Haloperidol, risperidone, chlorpromazine, clomipramine, sertraline	Carbamazepine Valproic acid Carbamazepine, phenytoin, phenobarbital, valproic acid Carbamazepine, lamotrigine, phenytoin, valproic acid	Enzyme inhibition leading to increased serum concentrations of AEDs
Oral contraceptives	Lamotrigine, valproic acid (oxcarbazepine?)	Induction of metabolism (glucuronidation) and reduced serum concentrations of AEDs

Table 31.12 *Contd...*

Therapeutic Drug Classes	Affected AEDs	Mechanism of Interaction and Clinical Consequence
Antimicrobal drugs Macrolides (clarithromycin, erythromycin, troleandomycin) Rifampicin Isoniazid	Carbamazepine Lamotrigine Carbamazepine, Ethosuximide, Phenytoin, Valproic acid	Enzyme inhibition by antimicrobal drugs leading to increased serum concentrations of AEDs
Others		
Probenecid	Carbamazepine	Induction of metabolism and reduced serum concentrations of carbamazepine
Antacids Cimetidine	Gabapentin	Decreased absorption of gabapentin Reduction in excretion of gabapentin leading to a prolonged half-life
Salicylates and naproxene	Tiagabine	Displacement of tiagabine from plasma proteins leading to a decrease in the total serum concentration of tiagabine but unchanged free concentration

Psychotropic Medications

The patients with psychiatric problem are generally on polypharmacy or there is increased chance of self medication practice among them. This leads to occurrence of significant drug interactions in these subjects. Monoamine oxidase inhibitors (MAOI) interact with vasopressor agents in foods (tyramine, dopamine, histamine). These agents are generally deaminated rapidly by MAO; MAOIs prevent the breakdown of tyramine and other pressor agents. Thus significant intake of high-tyramine foods (aged cheeses, cured meats) by pts on MAOIs can precipitate hypertensive crisis. The metabolism of midazolam is significantly reduced by increasing the dose of concomitant CYP3A inhibitors like ketoconazole, itraconazole, clarithromycin, cimetidine, ranitidine and erythromycin therapy as represented by increase in midazolam AUC (area under curve).

Many medications/substances have serotonin activity. These serotonergic agents include SSRIs, selective serotonin-norepinephrine reuptake inhibitors (SNRIs) and most tricyclic antidepressants (TCAs) along with some analgesic agents such as meperidine. These combinations of an MAOI with a serotonergic agent may result in a life-threatening **serotonin syndrome.** This syndrome is thought to be caused by overstimulation of 5-HT receptors in the central gray nuclei and the medulla. Symptoms range from mild to lethal and include a triad of cognitive (delirium, coma), autonomic (hypertension, tachycardia, diaphoreses) and somatic (myoclonus, hyperreflexia, tremor) effects. Most serotonergic antidepressants should be discontinued at least 2 weeks before starting an MAOI. Fluoxetine, because of its long half-life, should be discontinued for 4-5 weeks before an MAOI is initiated. Conversely, an MAOI must be discontinued for at least 2 weeks before starting a serotonergic agent (Table 31.13).

Table 31.13 Interaction of psychotropic drugs

Psychotropic drugs (A)	Interacting drugs (B)	Effect of interaction
Monoamine Oxidase Inhibitors (MAOI's)	Decongestants (pseudoephidrine) Asthma (salbutimol) Foods rich in tyramine	Enhanced effects of drugs B
Monoamine Oxidase Inhibitors (MAOI's)	SSRIs (Paroxetine, sertraline, fluoxetine, fluvoxamine, citalopram), SNRIs (Venlafaxine, milnacipran, duloxetine, sibutramine), TCAs (Clomipramine, imipramine) Misc Antidepressant (Mirtazapine, trazodone, St. John's Wort), Opioids (Meperidine, fentanyl, methadone, tramadol, pentazocine, dextromethorphan), CNS stimulants/Psychedelics [Amphetamine, sibutramine, methylphenidate, cocaine, MDMA (ectasy), LSD], Triptans (Sumatriptan, zolmitriptan, rizatriptan, almotriptan, frovatriptan), Selegilene, Linezolid, Furazolidone, Chlorpheniramine, Brompheniramine	Serotonin syndrome
Tricyclic antidepressant	Charcoal	Charcoal absorbs drug A, reduce toxicity in overdosage
Selective serotonin reuptake inhibitors	Aspirin	Increased GI bleeding
Phenothiazines	Antacids	Reduce absorption of drug A → decreased effect
Risperidone	Carbamazepine	Induction of CYP3A4 by B cause decreased effect of A

Table 31.13 *Contd...*

Psychotropic drugs (A)	Interacting drugs (B)	Effect of interaction
Thioridazine	HIV Protease inhibitors	Increased plasma concentration of A can cause ventricular arrhythmias
Clozapine	CYP inhibitors: Ritonavir, Antidepressants, Cimetidine	Increased risk of agranulocytosis with clozapine
Lithium	Amiloride, Spironolactone, Thiazide diuretics, Angiotensin converting enzyme (ACE) inhibitors and Non-steroidal anti-inflammatory drugs	Decreased excretion of the drug A leading to toxicity
Alprazolam and Diazepam	Digoxin	Drugs A raise digoxin level
Diazepam and Triazolam	Cimetidine, contraceptives	Increased half-life and plasma level of A
Benzodiazepines	Antacids	Decreased absorption of A
Benzodiazepines	Disulfiram	Increased duration of action of sedatives
Benzodiazepines	Levodopa	Inhibition of antiparkinsonism effect
Benzodiazepines	Warfarin	Decreased prothrombin time
Benzodiazepines	Alcohol	Precipitate CNS depression, respiratory depression, hypotension, coma
Diazepam	Phenytoin	Diazepam displaces B from plasma proteins→increased effect of B
Diazepam	Isoniazid	Increased plasma diazepam
Diazepam	Propoxyphene	Impaired clearance of diazepam
Diazepam	Rifampin	Decreased plasma diazepam
Diazepam	Ketamine	Potentiate anaesthetic action, synergistic effect

Antimicrobial Agents

Beta-lactam antibiotics got eliminated from body by renal elimination through organic anion transporter. Synergistic effects of dopamine, dobutamine and furosemide occurs with beta-lactams in increasing renal elimination of these antibiotics by increasing renal blood flow. Macrolides are metabolised by and also inhibitors of CYP enzymes.

Erythromycin reduce metabolism of midazolam (oral/iv) and increases its bioavailability, C_{max}, AUC. So avoid or reduce midazolam dose by 50-75%. Clarithromycin decreases midazolam clearance. Minor changes in Pk of nitrazepam, diazepam and flunitrazepam are seen with macrolides. Erythromycin and clarithromycin increase AUC of cyclosporine by 75-215%, whereas roxithromycin and azithromycin safe as they do not perturb the metabolism to such extent. Similar drug interaction is also seen with tacrolimus. Bioavailability of felodipine is increased by erythromycin, and similar is the case with simvastatin, which require dose reduction by 50-80%. Alfentanil and theophylline clearance is decreased by erythromycin. But with clarithromycin and azithromycin, clearance of theophylline is not affected. Pharmaco-dynamic action of warfarin is enhanced with macrolides. Clarithromycin cause inhibition of CYP3A4 and P-glycoprotein thereby reduce clearance of verapamil and it also increases bioavailability of cisapride. The following is the list of some drugs which are affected by concomitant therapy with macrolides. (Table 31.14)

Table 31.14 List of drugs affected by macrolides

Azithromycin	Clarithromycin	Dirithromycin	Erythromycin	Roxithromycin
Cyclosporine, digoxin, lovastatin, rifabutin, theophylline, warfarin	Astemizole, carbamazepine, cimetidine, cisapride, cyclosporine, digoxin, fluoxetine, indinavir, laoratadine, midazolam, pimozide, rifabutin, ritonavir, saquinavir, terfenadine, verapamil, warfarin, zidovudine	Astemizole, cyclosporine, digoxin, oral contraceptives, theophylline	Astemizole, benzodiazepine, buspirone, carbamazepine, cisapride, clozapine, cyclosporine, digoxin, felodipine, fexofenadine, HMG-CoA inhibitors, methylprednisolone, tacrolimus, terfenadine, theophylline, vinblastine, warfarin	Cyclosporine, digoxin, theophylline

Drug-Drug Interaction Prevention: A Stepwise Approach

Drug interactions represent a challenge to clinicians for long time. Current knowledge regarding the drug interaction is inadequate and is constantly changing with the advancement of pharmacological knowledge and new drug discoveries. Thus successful management of this major concern of drug interaction requires familiarity with a variety of drug references and vigilant surveillance. Pharmacokinetic data regarding the drugs should be critically evaluated. Considering the current gaps in knowledge on pharmacokinetic and pharmacodynamic interactions between different medications and the potential for serious consequences, further human subject studies are required to better understand the underlying mechanism of drug interactions. A systematic and step wise approach ensures accurate answers based on available information.

1. Take a medication history: Proper history regarding the use of medications with their significant altered effect is to be noted before prescribing any new medication. The following points are to be considered:

   - Allergies associated with the subject,
   - Concomitant therapy of vitamins and herbs,
   - Any other drugs (old and current) and etc., (over the counter) medications being taken by the subject,
   - Any interactions noted with previous therapy,
   - History of drug dependence and abuse,
   - Family history of benefits or problems with any drugs

2. Remember high-risk patients

   - Any patient taking ≥ 2 medications
   - Patients treated with anticonvulsants, antibiotics, digoxin, warfarin, amiodarone, etc.

3. Check pocket drug reference/drug formulary

4. Consult pharmacists or drug info specialists

5. Check up-to-date computer program for drug interaction for e.g., Medical Letter Drug Interaction Program, www.epocrates.com and others

There is a distinct lack of evidence to support the touted benefits or cost-effectiveness of drug interaction software. Without sufficient evidence, large investments to support widespread implementation of these softwares in clinical practice are premature. The drug interaction literature itself is of insufficient quality to mandate against most drug combinations and the methods of presenting computerized decision support, including drug interactions, require further refinement. Although decreasing medication errors is a laudable goal, health information technology should be held to the commonly accepted and well under-stood current standards of evidence, which are based on randomized trials examining clinical patient outcomes. There is an urgent need for higher quality studies exploring drug interactions specifically, then a need for studies exploring the impact of software detecting and alerting clinicians at the point of prescribing of high clinical impact drug interactions.

Study Designs used to Determine Drug-Drug Interactions

Drug interactions are mostly studied based upon the pharmacokinetic parameters an i.e., concentration of substrate drug (S) is estimated while being administered with and without the interacting drug (I). Different types study designs can be used for this purpose, which include: (i) parallel group design where S is given to one group of subjects and S + I are given to other group of subjects, (ii) a randomized crossover design with a washout period i.e., only one group of subjects are treated with different drugs at different time interval. The sequence of drug administration in crossover design may be S followed by S + I, or S + I followed by S. For finding out the dose response relationship between drugs interacting with each other, factorial design can be used. Multiple dose regimens of one drug or both drugs are used and number of possible pairing between them is done. Dosing regimen selection depends on features related specifically to the substrate drug and the interacting drug. These factors include (i) pattern of use of S and I either acute or chronic use, (ii) narrow or broad therapeutic index of the drug, (iii) safety aspects of drugs, (iii) pharmacokinetic and pharmacodynamic properties of both the substrate drug and the interacting drug and (iv) drug metabolizing enzyme inhibition as well as induction. The dosing of substrate drug and interacting drug should be adjusted according to inhibiting/inducing capacity of drugs which will be appropriate to their clinical use, including the highest doses likely to be used clinically. Drug-drug interaction studies in appropriate patient populations have higher relevance and accuracy, providing they are feasible and can be conducted safely. Well documented case reports play a definite role in informing and guiding well-controlled further studies. *In vitro* studies, particularly for CYP450-mediated interactions, can be helpful in estimating the likely magnitude of any interaction and understanding its mechanism. The incidence of drug-drug interactions in clinical therapeutics will continue to increase and challenge prescribers; as well as drawing the interest of clinical pharmacologists.

Suggested Readings

1. Bellmann R (2007). Clinical Pharmacokinetics of Systemically Administered Antimycotics. *Current Clinical Pharmacology* **2:** 37-58.

2. Flexner C (2006). Antiretroviral agents and treatment of HIV infection. GOODMAN & GILMAN'S THE PHARMACOLOGICAL BASIS OF THERAPEUTICS. The McGraw-Hill Companies 11th Ed., chapter 50.

3. Important Drug Interactions in Dermatology. Drugs 2000 **59(2):** 181-192.

4. Johannessen SI and Landmark CJ (2010). Antiepileptic Drug Interactions - Principles and Clinical Implications. *Current Neuropharmacology* **8:** 254-267.

5. Pea F and Furlanut M (2001). Pharmacokinetic Aspects of Treating Infections in the Intensive Care Unit Focus on Drug Interactions. *Clin Pharmacokinet* **40(11):** 833-868.

6. Randat JM, Marchbank CR, Dudley MN (1992). Interactions of fluoroquinolones with other drugs: mechanisms, variability, clinical significance, and management. *Clin Infect Dis* **14:** 272-84.

7. Rawlins MD, Thompson JW (1991). Mechanisms of adverse drug reactions. In: Davies DM, ed., Textbook of Adverse Drug Reactions. Oxford: Oxford University Press, pp. 18-45.

8. Stanton LA, Peterson GM, Rumble RH, Cooper GM, Polack AE (1994). Drug-related admissions to an Australian hospital. *J Clin Pharm Therapeut* **19:** 341-7.

9. Stockley IH (1994). Drug interactions. Oxford: Blackwell Science, pp. 3-6.

10. Wright 1992. Drug Interactions. In: Melmon and Morrelli's Clinical Pharmacology 1992.

CHAPTER 32

ANTIBIOTIC PROPHYLAXIS IN SURGERY

Introduction

Postoperative surgical wound infection accounts for approximately 15% of all nosocomial infections. The majority of infections are detected within 7 to 10 days and up to 30 days postoperatively. Postoperative wound infections have an enormous impact on the quality of life of the patient and substantially increase the financial cost of patient care. Postoperative wound infection leads to increased pain at the wound site, wound dehiscence, sepsis and even death. More than 1 million surgical wound infections are reported from United States each year, increasing hospital stay by 1 week and increasing the cost of hospitalization by 20%.

Infection develops when endogenous flora are translocated to a normally sterile site. Seeding of the operative site from a distant site of infection can also occur (especially in patients with prosthesis or other implant). The process of surgical wound infection is complex and depends on interaction between host, local tissue and microbial virulence. Factors influencing the surgical wound infection include bacterial inoculum and virulence, host defense, perioperative care and intraoperative management. Measures intended to prevent surgical wound infection are targeted towards modification of the host and local tissue factor like proper cleansing of surgical wound, preoperative optimization of the co morbid illness, use of proper aseptic surgical technique and control of operative environment. Antibiotic prophylaxis to prevent surgical wound infection is one of the many preventive measures that prevent postoperative surgical wound infection.

The goal of prophylactic antibiotics is to reduce the incidence of postoperative wound infection. Antibiotic prophylaxis is shown to be effective in preventing post operative surgical wound infection and its impact has been clearly demonstrated in various studies. In prospective, randomized, double-blind trials comparing placebo with prophylactic antibiotic in clean-contaminated procedures, patients receiving placebo had postoperative surgical site infection rates of 24% to 87%. Antibiotic prophylaxis is associated with lower rates of postoperative surgical site infection ranging from 2% to 38%.

Why there is Need of Prophylactic Antimicrobial Therapy?

Wound infections occur when a critical number of bacteria are present in the wound at the time of closure. Prophylactic administration of antibiotics before surgery inhibits the growth of contaminating bacteria and their adherence to prosthetic implants, thus reducing risk of surgical site infection. Antibiotic agents directed against the invading microorganism may prevent infection by reducing the number of viable bacteria below the critical level. Postoperative infection has been reported in 9% to 30% of patients with uncomplicated appendicitis who did not receive prophylactic antimicrobials, while use of prophylactic antibiotic reduced the postoperative infection to 3% to 6% in these patients.

Though, antimicrobial prophylaxis prevents surgical wound infection, it should be remembered that other strong factors such as surgeons experience and his surgical technique, length of postoperative stay, hospital and operating room environment and underlying medical condition of the patient are important factors for prevention of surgical wound infection. Antibiotic prophylaxis should be regarded as one component of an effective policy for the control of surgical site infection.

Goal of Surgical Prophylaxis

Surgical prophylaxis with antimicrobial should achieve the following goals:

1. Prevent postoperative infection of the surgical site
2. Prevent postoperative infectious morbidity and mortality
3. Reduce the duration and cost of health care
4. Produce no adverse effects
5. Should have no adverse consequences for the microbial flora of the patient or the hospital
6. Should cause minimal change in patients host defense

To achieve this goal an ideal antimicrobial for surgical prophylaxis should have the following characteristics:

1. Effective against pathogens most likely to contaminate the wound
2. Does not induce bacterial resistance
3. Effective tissue penetration
4. Minimal toxicity
5. Long half-life
6. Cost effective
7. Narrow spectrum

Risk Factors for Surgical Site Infection

There are many risk factors for surgical site infection (SSI) which can be classified into patient factors, operation factors and surgical wound (Table 32.1).

Table 32.1 Factors for surgical site infection

Patient factors	Extremes of age
	Poor nutritional state
	Obesity (> 20% ideal body weight)
	Diabetes mellitus
	Smoking
	Coexisting infections at other sites
	Bacterial colonization
	(e.g., nares colonisation with *Staphylococcus aureus*)
	Immunosuppression
	(steroid or other immunosuppressive drug use)
	Prolonged postoperative stay
Operation factors	Length of surgical scrub
	Skin antisepsis
	Preoperative shaving
	Preoperative skin preparation
	Length of operation
	Antimicrobial prophylaxis
	Operating theatre ventilation
	Inadequate instrument sterilization
	Foreign material in surgical site
	Surgical drains
	Surgical technique including haemostasis, poor closure, tissue trauma
	Postoperative hypothermia

Wound Classification and Susceptibility of Infection

Surgical operations can be classified into four categories based on increasing incidence of infection

Table 32.2 Showing classification of wound and incidence of infection

Class	Definition	Susceptibility to infection
Clean	Operations in which no inflammation is encountered. There is no break in aseptic operating theatre technique Elective surgical procedures not involving respiratory, alimentary or genitourinary tracts.	< 2%

Table 32.2 *Contd...*

Class	Definition	Susceptibility to infection
Clean contaminated	Operations in which the respiratory, alimentary or genitourinary tracts are entered but without significant spillage.	2-10%
Contaminated	Operations where there is visible contamination of the wound. Examples include gross spillage from a hollow viscus during the operation or compound/open injuries operated on or within four hours.	10-30%
Dirty	Operations with presence of pus, where there is a previously perforated hollow viscus, or compound/open injuries more than four hours	> 30%

Recommendations

Clean wound: Clinical trials have proven that prophylactic antibiotic do not reduce postoperative surgical infection in clean procedures.

Clean contaminated wound: Antimicrobial prophylaxis based on best available evidence is recommended for the majority of clean-contaminated procedures.

Contaminated wound and dirty wound: Additional postoperative antibiotic coverage for few days is recommended in addition to the prophylactic dose.

Timing and Duration of Administration of Prophylactic Antimicrobial

Timing of administration of antibiotics for surgical prophylaxis is very critical. The timing of antibiotic administration should be adjusted to maximize prophylactic efficacy. Antimicrobial activity must be present at the wound site till the time of closure of wound. Thus, the drug should be given preoperatively (and repeated intra-operatively for prolonged procedures) to ensure that therapeutic levels are maintained throughout the procedure.

Recommendations

Several studies and randomized trials have been performed with regards to administration of antibiotic in surgical prophylaxis and their recommendations:

A single preoperative dose is as effective as 5 day course of postoperative therapy assuming an uncomplicated procedure.

Prophylactic antibiotics should be administered ideally within 30min to 2hr before the time of incision.

During prolonged procedures antibiotic should be repeated at intervals of one or two times the half life of the drug. This ensures adequate tissue levels of antibiotic throughout the duration of the procedure. However, re-administration of prophylactic antibiotic is recommended only in special circumstances like severe trauma, contamination secondary to rupture of viscus, major blood loss. Even in these circumstances antibiotic coverage should not exceed more than 24-48 hr.

What Antimicrobials should be used in Prophylaxis?

The basic principles for selection of antibacterial agents for treatment or for prophylaxis, depends on an understanding of following parameters:

1. Mechanisms of action, spectrum of activity, pharmacokinetics, pharmacodynamics, toxicities and interactions of particular drug.

2. Mechanisms underlying bacterial resistance.

3. Sensitivity of common microbes in particular area observed by clinicians (resistance pattern in the particular area).

4. Patient-associated parameters, such as infection site, other drugs being taken, allergies, and immune and excretory status, are critically important while selecting appropriate antibiotic for prophylaxis.

Recommendations

The antibiotic selected for antibiotic prophylaxis must cover the expected pathogen for that operative site.

The choice of antibiotic should take into account the local resistance pattern.

Cephalosporin's (such as cefazolin) are appropriate first line agents for most surgical procedures. For patients with documented allergy to cephalosporin's, vancomycin is a reasonable alternative for coverage of Staphylococcus. Metronidazole or clindamycin and an aminoglycoside may be used for coverage of anaerobic and gram-negative organisms, respectively. A quinolone, such as ciprofloxacin may also be effective for coverage of gram-negative organisms.

Broad-spectrum antibiotics should be avoided for surgical prophylaxis as it may lead to the development of antimicrobial resistance.

Single dose prophylaxis is as efficient as multiple dose for surgical prophylaxis without any additional benefits.

Kernodle and Kaiser in their review - Postoperative infections and antimicrobial prophylaxis, describe following regimen is to be used. These regimens are also supported by Mandle *et al.,* and many other authors.

Abdominal Surgery

1. Gastro-duodenal surgery in patients with hemorrhage, cancer, obstruction, or other high-risk features - Enteric Gram-negative bacilli, Enterococcus, anaerobes Cefazolin 1-2 gm IV preoperatively or Clindamycin 600 mg plus Gentamicin 120 mg IV preoperatively.

2. Gastric bypass - Enteric Gram-negative bacilli, Enterococcus - Cefazolin 1-2 gm IV preoperatively.

3. Colorectal surgery (emergency) - Enteric Gram-negative bacilli, Enterococcus, anaerobes Cefoxitin, Cefotetan, or Cefmetazole 2 gm IV preoperatively and q 4 hr for 3 doses Or Metronidazole 500 mg IV plus Gentamicin 1.7 mg/kg IV preoperatively and q 8 hr for 3 doses.

4. Colorectal surgery (elective) - Enteric Gram-negative bacilli, Enterococcus and anaerobes Neomycin 1 gm plus Erythromycin base 1 gm at 1, 2, and 11 PM on the day before surgery ± parenteral drugs as for emergency colorectal surgery.

In Cochrane review author found certain regimens appear to be inadequate in colorectal surgeries. E.g., Metronidazole alone, Doxycycline alone, Piperacillin alone, oral Neomycin plus Erythromycin on the day before operation. A single dose administered immediately before the operation (or short-term use) is as effective as long-term postoperative antimicrobial prophylaxis. There is no convincing evidence to suggest that the new-generation cephalosporins are more effective than first-generation cephalosporins.

Cardiac Surgery

1. Coronary artery bypass graft surgery, valve surgery or pacemaker insertion-*S. epidermidis*, *S. aureus*, Gram-negative bacilli and Enterococcus.

   Cefazolin 2 gm IV preoperatively and q 4-6 hr intraoperatively *or*
   Cefuroxime 1.5 gm IV preoperatively and q 4-6 hr Intraoperatively *or* Vancomycin 1 gm IV preoperatively.

Neurosurgery

1. Craniotomy, high-risk only (e.g., re-explorations, microsurgery, entry into sinuses or nasopharynx) - Vancomycin 1 gm IV plus Gentamicin 1.5 mg/kg IV preoperatively *or*
   Cefazolin 1 gm IV preoperatively.

2. CSF shunt placement-only in hospitals with high infection rates (15% to 20%) - Trimethoprim 160 mg IV plus Sulphamethoxazole 800 mg IV preoperatively and q 12 hr for 3 doses *or*

Vancomycin 10 mg plus Gentamicin 3 mg injected into a cerebral ventricle.

3. Penetrating trauma - Ceftriaxone or Clindamycin.

4. Skull fracture, CSF leak - Cefazolin or Clindamycin.

Orthopedic Surgery

1. Arthroplasty, including replacements - Cefazolin 1-2 gm IV preoperatively and q 6 hr for 3 doses *or* Cefuroxime 1.5 gm IV preoperatively and q 12 hr for 2 doses or Vancomycin 1 gm IV preoperatively.

   Closed fractures - Cefazolin 1 gm IV preoperatively and as a single postoperative dose.

2. Open fracture - Cefazolin 1 gm IV + Gentamicin 80 mg IV or Clindamycin 600 mg IV + Gentamicin 80 mg IV.

Vascular Surgery

1. Lower-extremity or abdominal arterial surgery or lower extremity amputation for ischemia -Cefazolin 1-2 gm IV preoperatively and q 6 hr for 24 hr *or* Vancomycin 1 gm IV preoperatively and 12 hr after the procedure.

Obstetric-Gynecologic Surgeries

1. Cesarean delivery, high-risk only (e.g., premature rupture of membranes) - Cefazolin 1 gm IV after clamping cord and q 6 hr for 2 doses.

2. Abortion, 2nd trimester instillation - Cefazolin 1 gm IV preoperatively and q 6 hr for 2 doses.

3. Abortion, 1st trimester in patients with a history of pelvic inflammatory disease, gonorrhea, or multiple partners -Penicillin G 1 to 2 million units IV preoperatively and 3 hr later *or* Doxycycline 100 mg PO before the procedure and 200 mg 1/2 hr afterward.

4. Hysterectomy, vaginal or Abdominal - Cefazolin 1 gm IV preoperatively and q 6 hr for 2 doses *or* Doxycycline 200 mg IV preoperatively.

Urologic Surgeries

1. Prostatectomy - Cefazolin 1 gm IV preoperatively or another drug selected based on susceptibility tests.

2. Penile prosthesis insertion - Cefazolin 1 gm IV preoperatively.

Otolaryngologic Surgery

1. Major head and neck surgery involving mucosa of the oral cavity or pharynx - Cefazolin 1-2 gm IV preoperatively and q 8 hr for 2 doses *or* Clindamycin 600-900 mg IV ± Gentamicin 1.5 mg/kg IV preoperatively and q 8 hr for 2 doses.

Ophthalmic Surgery

1. Extraction of lens, with or without insertion of prosthesis- Gentamicin, Tobramycin, or Neomycin-gramicidin-polymyxin B drops over 2-24 hr plus Cefazolin 100 mg subconjunctivally at the end of the procedure.

Antibiotic Resistance

Antibiotic resistance has emerged as major public health issue in recent years. A steady increase in antibiotic resistance continues despite introduction of newer antibiotics. Resistant bacteria are associated with increased patient morbidity and mortality. Prevalence of antibiotic resistance in any population depends on patient population receiving antibiotics and total antibiotic exposure. Increased antibiotic use leads to more antibiotic resistance as demonstrated by various studies.

Three uncontrolled observational studies have demonstrated that antibiotics for surgical prophylaxis are associated with increased incidence of antimicrobial resistance. Trials of patient exposure to a single dose of either ciprofloxacin or vancomycin for surgical prophylaxis showed an absolute increase in the number of people with resistant organisms following treatment compared to pre-treatment (4 *versus* 8%).

Preoperative care and choice of prophylactic antibiotic may need to be modified where patients are colonized with methicillin-resistant *staphylococcus aureus* (MRSA). Carriage of multiresistant organisms should be recognized as a potential risk factor for surgical site infection during high risk operations.

Recommendation: For prevention of antimicrobial resistance-

1. Optimize prophylactic antimicrobial use prior to surgical procedures.
2. Optimize choice and duration of empiric antimicrobial use. The duration of prophylactic antibiotic therapy should be single dose except in special circumstances.
3. Improve antimicrobial prescribing practices through educational and administrative means.
4. Establish a system that monitors and provides feedback regarding the occurrence of resistance.
5. Define and implement guidelines for antimicrobial use.

Conclusion

Cochrane review recommends the use of prophylactic antibiotics for patients at high and moderate risk for endocarditis, with immunodeficiencies, metabolic diseases, irradiated in the head and neck area and when, an extensive or prolonged surgery is anticipated.

For many surgical procedures, there is clear evidence supporting the use of antibiotic prophylaxis, administered in a timely manner, to prevent surgical site infections. Single-dose antibiotic prophylaxis appears to be at least as effective as multiple-dose regimens for a broad range of surgical procedures and may pose less risk to patients in terms of adverse events (e.g., *Clostridium difficile* colitis) and less risk to the population in terms of microbial resistance.

Future research will continue to address, what prophylactic regimens are most effective for various surgical procedures. Investigation should also focus on methods to improve compliance. The optimal strategies for implementation will likely vary from institution to institution.

Suggested Readings

1. Andreasen JO, Drbc O, Jensen SS, *et al.,* (2006). A systematic review of prophylactic antibiotics 246 in the surgical treatment of maxillofacial fractures. *J Oral Maxillofac Surg.* **64:** 1664-8.

2. Antibiotic Prophylaxis for Surgical Site Infection Prevention in Adults from Institute for Clinical Systems Improvement; Third Edition/September 2009.

3. Aznar R, Mateu M, Miro JM, Gatell JM, Gimferrer JM, Aznar E, *et al.,* (1991). Antibiotic prophylaxis in non-cardiac thoracic surgery: cefazolin versus placebo. *Eur J Cardiothorac Surg.* **5(10):** 515-8.

4. Bozorgzadeh A, Pizzi WF, Barie PS, *et.al.,* (1999). The duration of antibiotic administration in penetrating abdominal trauma. *Am J Surg.* **177:** 125-31.

5. Brook I (2007). Microbiology and principles of antimicrobial therapy for head and neck 236 infections. *Infect Dis Clin N Am.* **21:** 355-91.

6. Classen DC, Evans RS, Pestotnik SL, Horn SD, Menlove RL, Burke JP (1992). The timing of prophylactic administration of antibiotics and the risk of surgical-wound infection. *N Engl J Med.* **326:** 281-6.

7. Culver DH, Horan TC, Gaynes RP, Martone WJ, Jarvis WR, Emori TG, *et al.,* (1991). Surgical wound infection rates by wound class, operative procedure, and patient risk index. National Nosocomial Infections Surveillance System. *Am J Med.* **91(3B):** 152S-7S.

8. Dellinger EP (1991). Antibiotic prophylaxis in trauma: penetrating abdominal injuries and open fractures. *Rev Infect Dis.* **13(10):** S847-57.

9. Dellinger EP, Gross PA, Barrett TL, Krause PJ, Martone WJ, McGowan JE Jr, *et al.,* (1994). Quality standard for antimicrobial prophylaxis in surgical procedures. *Clin Infect Dis.* **18:** 422-7.

10. Dolin R (2000). New York, Churchill Livingstone, pp. 3186-3187 and from Antimicrobial prophylaxis in surgery. *The Medical Letter* 37, 1995: 79-82.

11. Donovan IA, Ellis D, Gatehouse D, *et al.,* (1979). One-dose antibiotic prophylaxis against wound infection after appendectomy:a randomized trial of clindamycin, cefazolin sodium and a placebo. *Br J Surg.* **66:** 193-6.

12. Ehrenkranz NJ (1981). Surgical wound infection occurrence in clean operations; risk stratification for interhospital comparisons. *Am J Med.* **70:** 909-14.

13. Fabian TC, Croce MA, Payne LW, *et al.,* (1992). Duration of antibiotic therapy for penetrating abdominal trauma: a prospective trial. *Surgery.* **112:** 788-95.

14. Goossens H, Ferech M, Vander Stichele R, Elseviers M (2005). Outpatient antibiotic use in Europe and association with resistance: a cross national database study. *Lancet.* **365(9459):** 579-87.

15. Gorbach SL, Condon RE, Conte JE Jr, *et al.,* (1992). Evaluat ion of new anti-infective drugs for surgical prophylaxis. Infectious Diseases Society of America and the Food and Drug Administration. *Clin Infect Dis.* **15(1):** S313-38.

16. Haley RW, Schaberg DR, Crossley KB, Von Allmen SD, McGowan JE Jr (1981). Extra charges and prolongation of stay attributable to nosocomial infections: a prospective inter hospital comparison. *Am J Med.* **70:** 51-8.

17. Harbarth S, Samore MH, Lichtenberg D, Carmeli Y (2000). Prolonged antibiotic prophylaxis after cardiovascular surgery and its effect on surgical site infections and antimicrobial resistance. *Circulation.* **101(25):** 2916-21.

18. Johnson JT, Myers EN, Thearle PB, *et al.,* (1984). Antimicrobial prophylaxis for contaminated 157 head and neck surgery. *Laryngoscope.* **94:** 46-51.

19. Johnson JT, Myers EN, Thearle PB, *et al.,* (1984). Antimicrobial prophylaxis for contaminated 157 head and neck surgery. *Laryngoscope.* **94:** 46–51.

20. Johnson JT, Wagner RL (1987). Infection following uncontaminated head and neck surgery. *Arch Otolaryngol Head Neck Surg.* **113:** 368-9.

21. Johnson JT, Yu VL, Myers EN, *et al.,* (1987). An assessment of the need for gram-negative 159 bacterial coverage in antibiotic prophylaxis for oncological head and neck surgery. *J 160 Infect Dis.* **155:** 331–3.

22. Kachroo S, Dao T, Zabaneh F, Reiter M, Larocco MT, Gentry LO, *et al.,* (2006). Tolerance of vancomycin for surgical prophylaxis in patients undergoing cardiac surgery and incidence of vancomycin resistant enterococcus colonization. *Annals of Pharmacotherapy.* **40(3):** 381-5.

23. Kernodle DS, Kaiser AB (2000), Postoperative infections and antimicrobial prophylaxis. In *Principles and Practice of Infectious Diseases,* edited by GL Mandell, JE Bennett. 5th edition. New York, Churchill Livingstone, pp. 3186-3187.

24. Levy M, Egersegi P, Strong A, Tessoro A, Spino M, Bannatyne R, *et al.,* (1990). Pharmacokinetic analysis of cloxacillin loss in children undergoing major surgery with massive bleeding. *Antimicrob Agents Chemother.* **34(6):** 1150-3.

25. Lorian V (1975). Some effects of subinhibitory concentrations of antibiotics on bacteria. *Bull N Y Acad Med.* **51(9):** 1046-55.

26. Lovato C, Wagner JD (2009). Infection rates following perioperative prophylactic antibiotics versus postoperative extended regimen prophylactic antibiotics in surgical management 207 of mandibular fractures. *J Oral Maxillofac Surg.* **67:** 827-32.

27. Luchette FA, Borzotta AP, Croce MA, *et.al.,* Practice management guidelines for prophylactic antibiotic use in penetrating abdominal trauma. Available online at: http://www.east.org.

28. Lves R, Cooper JD, Todd TR, Pearson FG (1981). Prospective, randomized, double-blind study using prophylactic cephalothin for major, elective, general thoracic operations. *J Thorac Cardiovasc Surg.* **81:** 813-7.

29. Mangram AJ, Horan TC, Pearson ML, *et al.,* (1999). Guideline for prevention of surgical site 238 infection. *Infect Control Hosp Epidemiol.* **20:** 250-69.

30. Mangram AJ, Horan TC, Pearson ML, Silver LC, Jarvis WR (1999). Guideline for Prevention of Surgical Site Infection, 1999. Centers for Disease Control and Prevention (CDC) Hospital Infection Control Practices Advisory Committee. *American Journal of Infection Control.* **27(2):** 97-132.

31. Marroni M, Cao P, Fiorio M, *et al.,* (1999). Prospective, randomized, double-blind trial comparing teicoplanin and cefazolin as antibiotic prophylaxis in prosthetic vascular surgery. *Eur J Clin Microbiol Infect Dis.* **18:** 175-178.

32. McKittrick LS, Wheelock FC Jr (1954). The routine use of antibiotics in elective abdominal surgery. *Surg Gyn Obstet.* **99:** 376-7.

33. Miles BA, Potter JK, Ellis E III (2006). The efficacy of postoperative antibiotic regimens in the open treatment of mandibular fractures: a prospective randomized trial. *J Oral Maxillofac*ial *Surg.* **64:** 576-82.

34. National Institute for Health and Clinical Excellence. Surgical site infection. 2008. 244 (Clinical guideline 74).

35. Nichols RL (1995). Surgical antibiotic prophylaxis. *Med Clin North Am.* **79:** 509-22.

36. Page CP, Bohnen JM, Fletcher R, *et al.,* (1993). Antimicrobial prophylaxis for surgical wounds. Guidelines for clinicalcare. *Arch Surg.* **128:** 79-88.

37. Righi M, Manfredi R, Farneti G, *et al.,* (1996). Short-term versus long-term antimicrobial 177 prophylaxis in oncologic head and neck surgery. *Head Neck.* **18:** 399-404.

38. Savoca G, Raber M, Lissiani A, Plaino F, Ciampalini S, Buttazzi L, *et al.,* (2000). Comparison of single preoperative oral rufloxacin *vs* perioperative ciprofloxacin as prophylactic agents in transurethral surgery. *Archivio Italiano di Urologia Andrologia.* **72:** 15-20.

39. Simo R, French G (2006). The use of prophylactic antibiotics in head and neck oncological 155 surgery. *Curr Opin Otolaryngol Head Neck Surg.* **14:** 55-61.

40. Simons JP, Johnson JT, Yu VL, *et al.,* (2001). The role of topical antibiotic prophylaxis in patients 171 undergoing contaminated head and neck surgery with flap reconstruction. *Laryngoscope.* **111:** 329-35.

41. Skitarelić N, Morović M, Manestar D (2007). Antibiotic prophylaxis in clean-contaminated head 179 and neck oncological surgery. *J Craniomaxillofac Surg.* **35:** 15-20.

42. Song and Glenny, *et al.,* Antimicrobial prophylaxis in colorectal surgery: a systematic review of randomized controlled trials, *British Journal of Surgery.* **85(9):** 1232-1241. Published Online: 13 Jan 2003.

43. Tornqvist IO, Holm SE, Cars O (1990). Pharmacodynamic effects of subinhibitory antibiotic concentrations. *Scand J Infect Dis Suppl.* **74:** 94-101.

44. Wagenlehner F, Stower-Hoffmann J, Schneider-Brachert W, Naber KG, Lehn N (2000). Influence of a prophylactic single dose of ciprofloxacin on the level of resistance of *Escherichia coli* to fluoroquinolones in urology. *International Journal of Antimicrobial Agents.* **15(3):** 207-11.

SECTION – III

CHAPTER 33

REGENERATIVE MEDICINE

Introduction

Regenerative medicine is the most growing research field that focuses on new approaches to the autologous repair and/or replacement of cells, tissues and/or organs. The concept of regenerative medicine was started in 1956 when a boy suffering from leukemia was treated with the first bone marrow transplant. The most important issue with this type of medicine is to protect the regenerative tissue from host's immune system. In the 1956 transplant, doctors used the bone marrow from patient's identical twin and got round this problem.

Tissue typing method was used to match donor's tissue to patients in late 1960s and early 1970s. This meant some other person, who are not related to patient can also donate. Much of the recent interest in regenerative medicine arises from developments in stem cell research, but there are also promising possibilities in gene therapy, biomedical and tissue-engineering. This chapter look at some of the important parts of these regenerative medicines.

The concept of organ transplantation is an old known phenomenon. Best known example is kidney transplantation, where patients with diseased, non-functioning kidneys receive a healthy kidney from another person. In today's scenario, the supply of organs for transplantation is much lower than the demand there is a very long waiting list worldwide, with many hundreds of patients dying annually before an organ becomes available.

Regenerative medicine is the technique in which we use cell transplantation beside the organ transplantation to create products that improve tissue function or heal tissue defects, replace diseased or damaged tissue, because donor tissues and organs are in short supply. In this process we want to minimize immune system response by using our own cells or novel ways to protect transplant. Depending on the particular disease to be treated, the stem cells may first have to be differentiated to the specific cell type needed for tissue or organ repair. For example, for the brain it would likely be necessary to turn stem cells into nerve cells of the right type before transplantation.

Different Types of Regenerative Medicine

1. Cell Therapies
2. Tissue Engineering
3. Gene Therapy

Cell Therapies

Stem cells are specialized cells that can renew themselves for long periods through cell division and are capable of becoming cells with a specialized function e.g., beating cells of heart and insulin producing cells of pancreas etc. In order to be able to divide without losing the stem cell pool for later use, a stem cell is capable of multiplying by dividing into two, but after each cell division at least one of the two daughter cells retains the original stem cell properties and the daughter cell becomes fully differentiated specialized cell.

Key Properties of Stem Cells

1. *Stem cells are unspecialized:* Stem cells does not have any tissue specific markers or tissue specific markers that allow them to perform a specific functions, they are not capable of performing a specified function along their neighboring cells for e.g., cannot transmit electrical signals to other cells, however; under appropriate signal undefined stem cells can give rise to defined cells. E.g., neurons.

2. *Dividing and renewing ability of stem cells:* Unlike defined cells such as blood cells, muscle cells which do not replicate under normal conditions, stem cells are capable of dividing. They can produce new copies for long period, which is known as proliferation. It is seen that while starting with a small number of stem cells if they are allowed to proliferate for months millions of stem cells are produced.

3. *Stem cells can give birth to defined stem cells:* Under appropriate signals stem cells can give rise to specialized cells this process is known as differentiation. Stem cells differentiate into specialized cells either upon receiving internal signals triggered by products of certain genes or external signals given by chemical secreted inside the population of stem cells, signals obtained from neighboring cells or the signal obtained from the cells microenvironment. Scientists have started unraveling the mystery of appropriate signals that trigger stem cell differentiation.

Types of stem cells: Depending upon the degree of specialization stem cells are classified upon three different types.

1. *Totipotent cells:* If a stem cell can form all cell types of the embryo and adult, including germ cells (eggs and sperms) and the extra-embryonic structures such as placenta, it is considered totipotent. A fertilized egg cell, for example, is totipotent. The total potential of a fertilized egg is about four days. Totipotent stem cells can differentiate into any cell in an organism including embryonic tissue.

2. *Pluripotent cells:* If a stem cell have the potential to differentiate into almost any cell in the body but is unable to form the extra-embryonic structures (such as parts of the placenta) then it is called pluripotent. Embryonic stem cells are pluripotent.

3. *Multipotent cells:* The stem cells found in specialized tissues of the fetus or adult are multipotent, meaning that they are able to form many but not all tissue cells of the body, or are unipotent, i.e., they are able to form just one cell type. For example; multipotent stem cells are brain cells and haematopoietic cells.

Type of stem cells	Differentiate into
Hematopoietic stem cells	Red blood cells, B lymphocytes, T lymphocytes, natural killer cells, neutrophils, basophils, eosinophils, monocytes, macrophages, and platelets.
Mesenchymal stem cell	Bone cells (osteocytes), cartilage cells (chondrocytes), fat cells (adipocytes), and other kinds of connective tissue cells such as those in tendons.
Neural stem cell	Nerve cells (neurons) and two categories of non-neuronal cells–astrocytes and oligodendrocytes.
Epithelial stem cell	Absorptive cells, goblet cells, Paneth cells, and enteroendocrine cells.
Skin stem cell	Keratinocytes, hair follicle and epidermis.

Categories of Stem Cells

1. Embryonic stem cells (ESCs)

2. Adult stem cells (ASCs)

3. Induced pluripotent stem cells (iPSCs)

Embryonic Stem Cells (ESCs): Embryonic stem cells usually develop from eggs that are fertilized *in vitro*. Embryonic stem cells (ES cells) are unique biological entities that have the ability both to reproduce themselves endlessly and to give rise to all specialised cell types of the body. The ability to create all cell types is called "pluripotency". This property is usually restricted to cells that only exist for a few days in the early embryo before formation of the initial body plan embryonic stem cells are said to be pluripotent. Human embryonic stem cells are derived from embryos that are typically four to five days old and are a hollow microscopic ball of cells called the blastocyst. The blastocyst includes three structures: The trophoblast, which is the layer of cells that surrounds the blastocyst; the blastocoel, which is the hollow cavity inside the blastocyst; and the inner cell mass, which is a group of approximately 30 cells at one end of the blastocoel. The innermost populations of cells make up the inner cell mass, from which the entire embryo is formed. The outermost cells forms the trophectoderm, which gives rise to parts of the placenta and umbilical cord. Cells from the inner cell mass have become pluripotent and can thus differentiate into all the cell types that are necessary for the makeup of the body but can no longer contribute, for example, to placenta tissue. In these cells, almost all genes are still ready to be used for differentiation in a specific direction. This pluripotent period lasts for only a short time, as cells quickly start to differentiate as development proceeds. Embryonic stem cells are usually produced in the laboratory by special treatment of cells removed from blastocysts. Production of human embryonic stem cells involves the use of blastocysts discarded from infertility treatments or diagnosed by genetic screening as carriers of a lethal disease gene. There are several proteins which regulate the pluripotency of ES cells. Some are as follows:

Adult Stem Cells (ASCs): This type of stem cells are an undifferentiated cells, which can renew itself, and can differentiate to yield the major specialized cell types of the tissue or organ. Most tissues and organs contain adult stem cells that can help repair tissue that is lost or damaged by daily use or after disease or injury. Tissues with a high turnover rate such as the gut, bone marrow and skin, are thought to have more stem cells than quiescent tissues like the brain and heart. True stem cells within a tissue manage its turnover, have the potential for self renewal and can differentiate to at least one cell type. Adult stem cells are unipotent or multipotent, and the spectrum of cell types they can form is generally limited to those usually present in the organ from which they derive for e.g., stem cells from the bone marrow can for instance form all cells that constitute the blood, but cannot form nerve cells, intestinal cells, or insulin-producing cells. Unlikely embryonic stem cells which are obtained from the inner cell mass of the blastocyst the origin of adult stem cells is unknown. Till dates adult stem cells have been identified in many organs and tissues. Adult stem cells are very small number of stem cells in each tissue. The adult tissues reported containing stem cells include brain, bone marrow, peripheral blood, blood vessels, skeletal muscle, skin, umbilical cord and liver. Few discoveries on adult stem cells also advocate on the new property of adult stem cells i.e., plasticity or trans-differentiation, which is the ability of adult stem cell to form specialized cell types of other tissues,

Differentiation pathways of different types of adult stem cells: Depending upon their area of origin adult stem cells differentiate *via* different mechanisms and therefore can have a characteristic shape specialized structure and function based on the tissue of origin. The following examples of differentiation pathways are as follows:

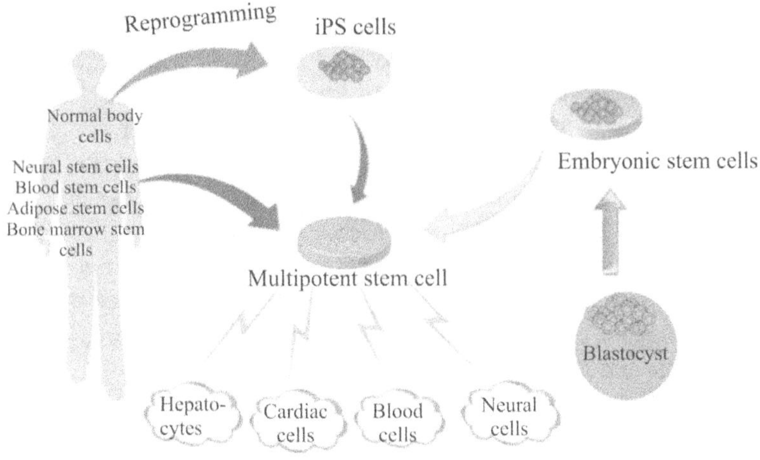

Sources of adult stem cells

Induced Pluripotent Stem Cells: Induced pluripotent stem cells (iPSCs) from somatic cells are revolutionizing the field of stem cells. They are obtained by reprogramming somatic stem cells of a patient through the introduction of certain transcription factors. The first iPSC reported were produced by transducing mouse fibroblasts with four retroviral vectors OCT4, SOX2, KLF4, and C-MYC .The first human iPSC (hiPSCs) were created using the same four retroviral vectors as described for mouse or OCT4, SOX2, LIN28, and NANOG. The hiPSC thus produced can be kept in culture indefinitely using a variety of undefined fibroblast feeder cells and fetal calf serum-based methods or defined mTESr/Matrigel-based protocols. The success of iPSC derivation has opened up a new era in research and treatment. The therapeutic potential of iPSC in regenerative medicine, cell-based therapy, and disease modelling and drug discovery is highly promising.

Following types of stem cells treatment is possible in present situation:

1. Allogenic stem cell treatment : Matched or unmatched
2. Syngenic stem cell transplant : Identical twin
3. Autologous stem cell transplant
4. Nonmyleoblastic stem cell transplant

Stem Cells for Therapeutic Options

(a) *Therapeutic potential of mesenchymal stem/stromal cells*: Mesenchymal stem cells are adult stem cells. In 1976, Friedenstein *et al.,* first identified mesenchymal stem/multipotent stromal cells (MSCs) when they isolated the cells from bone marrow by their tight adherence to the tissue culture plate. MSCs have also been referred to as "bone marrow stromal cells" because of their role in creating bone marrow niche for maintaining hematopoietic stem cell (HSC) functions and their use as feeder layers for HSCs. While MSCs are primarily isolated from bone marrow, it is now known that they exist in the connective tissues of many organs, such as adipose tissue, muscle, liver, lung, umbilical cord blood and amniotic fluid and amniotic membrane. MSCs are capable of self-renewal and differentiation into connective tissue cell types such as osteogenic, adipogenic, and chondrogenic cells. MSCs can also differentiate into connective vascular smooth muscle–like stromal cells in the bone marrow niche supporting HSC functions. More recently, it has been found that, under proper conditions, MSCs are capable of differentiating to non mesoderm lineages including muscle cells, neurons, and epithelial cells.

Tissue Engineering

Tissue engineering is a multidisciplinary/interdisciplinary field that applies the principles of biology and engineering to develop tissue substitutes to restore, maintain, or improve the function of diseased or damaged human tissues and forms part of the field of regenerative medicine. One of the goals of tissue engineering is to develop methods to construct organs in the laboratory that can subsequently be used in medical applications.

Now a days tissue engineering is very essential tool in the field of medicine as fewer livers available for transplant than there are patients waiting for new livers so that a strategy for construction of the organ must be developed using tissue engineering technique. Tissue engineering holds the promise of producing better organs for transplant and using tissue engineering techniques and gene therapy it may be possible to correct many otherwise incurable genetic defects.

Step 1 > Step 2 > Step 3 > Step 4 > Step 5 > Step 6 > Step 7

Tissue Engineering						
Start building material (e.g., extracellular matrix, biodegradable polymer)	Shape it as needed and seed it with living cells	Bathe it with growth factors	Cells multiply and fill up the scaffold and grow into three-dimensional tissue	Implanted in the body and cells recreate their intended tissue functions	Blood vessels attach themselves to the new tissue and the scaffold dissolves	The newly grown tissue eventually blends in with its surroundings

Due to the remarkable plasticity of MSCs (i.e., differentiation to cells of both ectodermal and endodermal nature, including cardiomyocytes, hepatocytes, neurons, skeletal muscle, pancreatic, epithelial cells, and epidermal-like cells), it has been suggested they can be used for treating a wide range of diseases, including heart disease, renal disease, liver disease, and neurologic diseases, some of which have been demonstrated to be feasible in animal studies. For example, bone marrow MSCs can differentiate into epithelial cells in the lung, liver, and skin in a mouse model. Transplantation of MSCs into infarcted hearts has been shown to improve cardiac function due to the enhanced.

Special features of biomaterials for cell therapy

- Biocompatible to prevent immune rejection or necrosis.
- Biodegradable and assimilable.
- Structural and mechanical properties to provide platform to growing tissues.
- Defined three-dimensional architecture.
- Materials may be metals, ceramic materials, natural materials, and synthetic polymers, or combinations.

Gene Therapy

In the 1980s, the human gene was sequenced and cloned due to the advances in molecular biology. After this researcher was looking for a unique method of easily producing proteins, such as the protein deficient in diabetics - insulin. Later they thought to utilize bacteria as protein production factory. Bacteria can easily harvest, and the product from them can be used for therapeutic purpose. Researcher thought the function of a gene inside the cell and took the logical step of trying to introduce genes straight into human cells, focusing on diseases caused by single-gene defects, such as cystic fibrosis, hemophilia, muscular dystrophy and sickle cell anemia, optic nerve disease, wound repair and regeneration, and cardiovascular disease. However, the transfer of the large segment of the DNA is much harder than the modifying simple bacteria in the gene therapy.

Type of gene therapy	Disease
Gene transplantation	To patient with gene deletion
Gene correction	To revert specific mutation in the gene of interest
Gene augmentation	To enhance expression of gene of interest

Gene therapy is a method for replacement or repair of the defective gene, responsible for disease development. In this process, the insertion of the desired gene into a nonspecific location within the genome at the place of a defective gene took place. The mechanism of homologous recombination is used to swap abnormal gene with a normal gene. Some selective reverse mutation is also important to make the abnormal gene normal. Gene therapy also involves the regulation of the gene expression by switching them on or off. In most gene therapy studies, a "normal" gene is inserted into the genome to replace an "abnormal", disease-causing gene. Vector is the most important part of the gene therapy which carries the desired gene to the patient's target gene. Genetically altered viruses are the most common used vectors to delivery therapeutic gene. Viruses have the capability to insert their genome into the host genome and researchers used this lethal mechanism for the betterment of the human by converting this experience into the gene delivery machine.

Disadvantages of Gene Therapy

- Most of our body cells are rapidly dividing; this nature of cell hinders the desirable outcome of the gene therapy because the stability of the inserted DNA compromised. Patients will have to undergo multiple rounds of gene therapy to overcome this problem.

- External viral entry can stimulate the immune system, thereby reducing effectiveness. The immune system's enhanced response to repeat invaders makes it difficult for many rounds of gene therapy.

- Viruses also present a different toxicity, immune and inflammatory responses, gene control and targeting issues. Also, there is the fear that the virus can get activated inside the host cell and can cause disease.

- Conditions arising from defect in one gene can be manageable by gene therapy but in some disease like Alzheimer's, arthritis, diabetes, etc. are caused by combined effects of variations in many genes making them difficult to treat by gene therapy.

Regenerative Medicine in Cancer

Tumors are functionally heterogeneous and hierarchical. They are composed of cells that can initiate tumors (tumor initiating cells or cancer stem cells) and cells that arise from CSCs but cannot initiate tumors. The frequency of CSC in a tumor is highly variable (often low). Cancer stem cells can (in many cases) be prospectively identified. Cancer stem cells may have different sensitivities to radiation or chemotherapy. Therefore, the concept of CSCs has significant clinical implications.

According to John Dick, leader of the team that discovered colon and leukemia CSCs

"It's like dandelions in the back yard: You can cut the leaves off all you want, but unless you kill the root, it will keep growing back"

Research on cancer stem cells with the help of regenerative medicine offers prospects for improvements in both cancer prognosis and treatment. Cancer stem cells show an intrinsic resistance to radiation and chemical therapy even if they represent a minority of cancer cells and they are likely to escape adjuvant therapy and underlie cancer relapse. Therefore, for the long term survival of the cancer patient, the development of therapies specifically targeted against CSCs shows a significant role in the regenerative medicine.

Regenerative Medicine in Cardiovascular Disorders

Cardiovascular disease remains the most potent killer in all developed and developing societies. Although, risk factor identification and modification, both through lifestyle and dietary changes and pharmacotherapies such as the statins, have had remarkable success in lowering mortality from myocardial infarction, heart failure persists at epidemic levels in our ageing as well as in young population. Therapeutic successes in the area of stem cell research have opened up many new avenues for treating cardiovascular diseases, especially, with respect to the prevention of the development of cardiac failure due to acute heart attack (acute myocardial infarction caused by sudden and prolonged oxygen starvation) or chronic coronary artery disease (gradual oxygen starvation due to cumulative narrowing of the coronary artery).

Regenerative Medicine in Bone Disorders

Bone marrow-derived cells can differentiate into cardiac specific cells (e.g., endothelial cells, smooth vascular muscle cells and cardiomyocytes), repair to damaged myocardium could be due to such trans-differentiation, as well as the migration and differentiation of resident cardiac stem cells in response to factors released by the newly introduced cells. Several clinical studies have confirmed that autologous bone marrow-derived stem cells taken from the patient herself/himself can repair the damaged heart, therefore, improving cardiac function, perfusion and metabolism in a number of cardiac disease states. Pharmaceutical stimulation of heart muscle growth from endogenous cardiac stem cells may offer a non-invasive method for myocardial repair. Cytokine-induced mobilization of stem cells from the bone marrow may offer an alternative method for myocardial regeneration, but the possibility of clinically relevant coronary re-narrowing currently weighs against such an approach.

The concept of skeletal stem cell is not original; it dates back to the late sixties. More recently, skeletal stem cells have risen to centre stage as a specific kind of post-natal stem cell, and have been renamed 'mesenchymal stem cells', contained in the fraction of the bone marrow that does not give rise to blood cells (called the stromal tissue). Skeletal stem cells (SSCs) give rise to bone, cartilage, fat, fibrous tissue, and hematopoietic stroma. The ability of SSCs to give rise to particular skeletal tissues has been tested, and can be exploited to regenerate bone and possibly other tissues in the future. Clinical trials testing the use of SSCs for bone repair are underway. SSCs make it theoretically possible to treat severe skeletal diseases that currently await a cure. SSCs and their progeny are functionally related to hematopoietic (blood-forming) cells.

Regenerative Medicine in Epithelia

Self-renewing tissues (such as blood and epithelia) contain a group of stem cells that are responsible for their production and continuous regeneration. The entire integrity of the tissue and its repair depend on these cells. Epithelium-derived stem cells have demonstrated their value in repairing congenital defects and injuries, some of which are completely beyond the reach of traditional tissue/cell grafting. The potential of epithelium derived stem cells is currently being tested for *ex vivo* gene therapy using stem cells, i.e., genetically repairing the patient's defect in his/her own cultured cells, before grafting them back in order to repair the lesion. The development of the epithelial stem cell into the tissue such as skin have been intensively studied and found that a type of adult stem cell from the epidermis (the outer protective layer of our skin, which possesses no blood vessels), and known as a "holoclone", has already shown great therapeutic promise.

A single epidermal holoclone can double enough times to produce the skin surface area of an adult human being (8×10^{10} cells). Under appropriate conditions, Human epidermal keratinocytes can be grown in the lab to give sheets of so-called stratified epithelium (the outer layer of our skin) by using human keratinocyte stem cells (which give rise to the tough layer of keratin in our skin.

Regenerative Medicine in Nervous System Disorders

Active research on stem cells in the developing and adult nervous system is now a day's gaining its importance. The realization of the maintenance of stem cells in the adult brain and the constant production of neurons has attracted increasing interest among the researchers. Neural stem cells are immature cells that have the potential to produce the main cell types of the central nervous system: neurons, astrocytes and oligodendrocytes. Another, key feature is their capacity to divide to give rise to new stem cells, i.e., self-renewal capacity, thus enabling the persistence and activity of the system over a long time. The neural stem cells also give rise to a variety of non-neural cells such as, muscle cells, cartilage cells, bone cells and pigment cells, few studies have demonstrated that neural stem cells mediate beneficial effects by positively supporting the resident cells either by secreting neurotrophic factors, which support the survival of neurons or have immunomodulatory effects. Understanding the development of the nervous system has helped direct the differentiation of stem cells for therapeutic applications. Neurons are generated from stem cells in discrete areas of the adult brain. Many neurological diseases have been suggested to help from cell transplantation, but most progress has been made in Parkinson's disease. Pharmaceutical stimulation of neurogenesis from endogenous stem cells may offer a non-invasive method for neural repair.

Regenerative Medicine in Vascular Disorders

Endothelium, the inner lining of the vessel wall plays a crucial role in the prevention of atherosclerosis and the initiation of new blood vessel formation after vessel blockage and oxygen starvation to a tissue (ischemia).The integrity of the endothelial monolayer appears to be maintained by circulating endothelial progenitor cells, which accelerate repair of the lining (re-endothelialisation) and limit atherosclerotic lesion formation. Circulating progenitor cells additionally home in on sites of injury, and contributes to new blood vessel formation. It is well established that integrity and functional activity of endothelial are crucially involved in the process of atherosclerotic lesion formation. Any injury to the endothelial cells induces a cascade of pro-inflammatory events that may lead to the destruction of the myocardium. Circulating bone marrow-derived cells can contribute to regenerate the endothelial monolayer after injury, and improve vascular. Patients with coronary artery disease show an impaired number and function of circulating endothelial progenitor cells. Infusion of progenitor cells from different sources (e.g., peripheral blood, bone marrow, vessel-associated cells, fat tissue, heart tissue etc.) has been shown to increase the recovery after ischemia (blood-starvation of a tissue). Several experimental studies showed positive results based on the experimental findings, clinical phase I trials were initiated in 2001 to test whether cell therapy may exert a beneficial effect in patients with acute myocardial infarction or peripheral vascular disease, primary clinical pilot trials indicated that infusion (by catheter-based technology) or injection of bone marrow-derived or circulating blood-derived progenitor cells improves the blood supply to the heart or to the legs in patients with ischemia. The consequences are improved heart function or longer pain-free walking distance, respectively. Large randomized, double-blind trials based upon the initial pilot studies confirmed the effect of cell therapy on the blood supply to the heart.

Regenerative Medicine in Diabetes

Diabetes develops as a consequence of β-cell loss and/or β-cell failure. The insulin producing β-cells cluster with the other pancreatic endocrine cells into small "mini-organs" called islets that constitute a mere 2-3 percent of the entire pancreas. Either destruction of β cells or unresponsiveness of β cells results in worsening of conditioning. Islet transplantation is a promising therapy for the treatment of diabetes, but there is the shortage of human islets. One of the attractive approaches to produce sufficient numbers of transplantable cells is to produce functional β-cells from stem and/or progenitor cells *in vitro*. An alternative approach would be to try to stimulate β-cell replication or neogenesis (*de novo* formation) *in vivo*. Many different approaches to produce new insulin producing β-cells have been or are being pursued which include a use of embryonic stem (ES) cells, bone marrow stem cells, adult pancreatic stem cells and trans-differentiation of adult stem cells into adult β-cells. The use of stem cells for the generation of insulin-producing β-cells is gaining interest. The current ongoing stem cells research, and in particular the recent developments regarding *in vitro* differentiation of ES cells, is encouraging, but the prospect of fully *in vitro* or *in vivo* differentiated β-cells is still for the future.

Regenerative Medicine in Skeletal Muscle Disorders

Diseases that specifically affect skeletal muscles are often associated with progressive destruction of the muscle fibers themselves, and in the most severe cases, progressive replacement of the muscle tissue with scar and fat. This leads to progressive and irreversible paralysis and ultimately death of the patient. As, the case in muscular dystrophies a diverse group of diseases; the most common and devastating of which is Duchenne Muscular Dystrophy (DMD), no effective treatment exists till date. Recently, only one myogenic progenitor cell (the precursor to the mature muscle fiber) had been clearly identified and partially characterized in post-natal skeletal muscle. Satellite cells are stem cells residing in muscles, identified in 1961 and so named because they occupy a position "satellite" to the muscle fiber, between the muscle membrane and the basal lamina that surrounds every fiber. In adult healthy muscle, these cells are in a resting phase, very small and with a condensed nucleus. If a muscle is injured, they are rapidly activated and begin to divide to create a progeny that repair damaged fibers and/or create new fibers to replace those that have degenerated. However, part of the progeny, does not differentiate, and resumes a place as satellite cells, thus ensuring the possibility of further regeneration in case of repeated damage. Stem cells from other tissues may have some value as a treatment, but their differentiation is a complex task and requires further studies. Stem cell research is likely to produce clearer and more comprehensive picture of the identity, biological features and lineage relationships of satellite cells and other non-standard muscle cell progenitors. Simultaneously, cell treatment protocols which will benefit from ongoing basic research are moving to large animal models, such as the dystrophic dog. This will set the stage for clinical trials in dystrophic patients.

Ethical and Legal Issues Associated with Regenerative Medicines

The creation and use of human embryonic stem cells still remain associated with ethical issues for parts of society in many countries. iPS cell technology, not requiring destruction of embryos but a simple skin sample, for example, has far more favourable status with respect to moral issues. However, this mainly refers to its derivation process. Once a pluripotent stem cell line has been made, the cells could potentially be differentiated towards "gamete cells" (sperm and eggs), and human embryos could even be produced if the gametes were really functional. This requires strict regulation and adequate control with respect to these uses, much like those already in place in most countries on the use of human embryonic stem cells, which of course have the same potential to become gametes. Privacy is an issue to consider for all sources of human stem cells, unless used for autologous transplantation where the donor of the cells is also the sole recipient. When embryos or adult cells (as for the derivation of iPS cell line) are used to derive cell lines that will be cultured indefinitely by a commercial company, the genome inside each of the cells remains identical to the genome of the original donor. Informed consent from the cell donor will always be required. This consent will need to deal with issues like anonymity of the cell line to be derived, the time period, as well as the range of applications the cells can be used for, and finally not-for-profit research applications versus commercial exploitation. Most "informed consent" documents result in the donor transferring the ownership of the cells to the organization that is carrying out further processing. Such legal and ethical issues should be strictly addressed before undertaking any type of stem cell research.

Regenerative Medicine a Vision of Future

The first decade of research on stem cells since in 1998 revolutionized the way we think about regenerative medicine. Stem cell therapy holds enormous potential for treating a wide range of genetic and sporadic degenerative disorders. For practical purposes, human embryonic stem cells are used in 13% of cell therapy procedures, while fetal stem cells are used in 2%, umbilical cord stem cells in 10%, and adult stem cells in 75% of treatments. To date, the most relevant therapeutic indications of cell therapy have been cardiovascular and ischemic diseases, diabetes, hematopoietic diseases, liver diseases and more recently, orthopedics, for example, more than 25,000 hematopoietic stem cell transplantations (HSCTs) are performed every year for the treatment of lymphoma, leukemia, immunodeficiency illnesses, congenital metabolic defects, hemoglobino-pathies, and myelodysplastic and myeloproliferative syndromes.

Suggested Readings

1. Ana P. Cotrim and Bruce J Baum (2008). Gene Therapy: Some History, Applications, Problems, and Prospects. *Toxicologic Pathology* **36:** 97-103.

2. Friedenstein AJ (1976). Precursor cells of mechanocytes. *Int Rev Cytol.* **47:** 327-359.

3. Hanna J, Cheng AW, Saha K, Kim J, Lengner CJ, Soldner F, Cassady JP, Muffat J, Carey BW, Jaensisch R (2010). Human embryonic stem cells with biological and epigenetic characteristics similar to those of mouse ESCs. *Proc Natl Acad Sci* **107:** 9222-9227.

4. Park K. I, Teng Y. D. and Snyder E. Y (2002). The injured brain interacts reciprocally with neural stem cells supported by scaffolds to reconstitute lost tissue. *Nat. Biotechnol.* **20:** 1111.

5. U.S. National Institutes of Health. Stem Cell Basics. Stem Cell Information. Available at http://stemcells.nih.gov/ info/basics/basics4.asp/. Accessed October 9, 2011.

CHAPTER 34

NANOMEDICINES

Introduction

Nanotechnology is a new arena of science that provides the tools and technology to work at atomic, molecular levels leading to creation of devices and delivery systems with fundamentally new properties and functions. Researchers in the biomedical field design nanocarriers for useful clinical applications and best therapeutic outcomes rather than fitting the particle dimension to the strict definition of nanotechnology. Its definition in core nanotechnology field, which restricts the "nano" to at least 1-100 nm in one dimension, nanocarriers in the biomedical field are often referred to as particles with a dimension a few nanometers to 1000 nm. Nanoparticles have the ability to deliver an ample range of molecules to varying areas of the body and for sustained periods of time. For a nanoparticle based delivery system, the key objectives are size of particles, surface properties as well as discharge of drugs or the active ingredients to accomplish highest efficacy. During the early 1980s, a number of delivery systems were formulated to get better the effectiveness of drug active agents and to reduce toxic side effects. During that time, micron sized particles or microparticles were formulated; but there was a size limit. Conversely, for the pharmaceutical industry, drug-loaded particles were comparatively less efficient due to rapid phagocytosis particularly after intravenous administration. Nowadays, this problem has been resolved through the surface modifications of the delivery particles. In this chapter, we highlight the different varieties and properties of nanoparticle based drug delivery systems and different promising pharmaceutical delivery systems. Further, we discuss the toxicological effects, commercial applications and future direction of nanoparticle based delivery systems.

Delivery technologies represent an important broader part of science, which engages multidisciplinary methodical improvement. Usually, delivery systems are associated with a carrier. In nanoparticle based delivery systems, the active compound is dissolved or entrapped or encapsulated in the carrier; in addition, the active compound could be adsorbed or attached to nanoparticle. Often the drug is attached with the nanosphere and encapsulated in nanocapsule. There are several advantages of nanoparticles as delivery systems. First, the particle size, particle morphology and surface charge of nanoparticles can be easily controlled. Second, controlled and sustained discharge of the active molecule in the time of the delivery and at the location of localization. Third, particle degradation properties can change with a modified carrier. Lastly, the site-specific delivery can be carried out in nanoparticle based delivery systems that can be used for various routes of drug deliveries like oral, nasal, parenteral, etc. Based on the importance, the development of nanoparticle based delivery systems is rapidly growing using proteins, natural polymers, synthetic polymers, and fullerenes.

Nanoparticles and Drug Delivery

Certain goals for research of nanotechnology in drug delivery include:

- More specific drug targeting and delivery
- Reduction in toxicity while maintaining therapeutic effects
- Greater safety and biocompatibility
- Faster development of new safe medicines

The main issues in the search for appropriate carriers as drug delivery systems pertain to the following topics that are basic prerequisites for design of new materials. They comprise knowledge on (i) drug incorporation and release, (ii) formulation stability and shelf life, (iii) biocompatibility, (iv) bio-distribution and targeting and (v) functionality. In addition, when used solely as carrier the possible adverse effects of residual material after the drug delivery should be considered as well. In this respect biodegradable nanoparticles with a limited life span as long as therapeutically needed would be optimal. The aims for nanoparticle entrapment of drugs are either enhanced delivery or uptake by, target cells and/or a reduction in the toxicity of the free drug to non-target organs

Nanocarriers being of submicron size have a very high surface to volume ratio, leading to increased dissolution rate. RES is usually responsible for the uptake of nanoparticles in the body. But, this uptake is related to properties of the nanocarriers such as size and the surface properties. Nanocarriers include a wide array of submicron system such as nanoparticles, nanocapsules, lipid complexes, polymeric micelles, and dendrimers (Table 34.1).

Table 34.1 Comparison of different nanocarriers

S. No.	System	Material	Drugs (Examples)	Advantages	Drawbacks
1	Nanocrystals	Dextran, Alginate	Amphoterecin B	For poorly soluble drugs	Limited stability
2	Carbon nanotubes	Carbon based carriers	Oligonucleotides	Increased internal volume	Tolerability
3	Silica NPs	Silica	Insulin	Protection to entraped drugs	Safety of in organic compound
4	Liposomes	Lipid in liquid state	Gene coding tyrosine hydroxylase	For amphiphilic, biocompatible	Limited stability
5	SLN	Solid Lipid	DNA	Cost effective, industrial scale up ease	Limited stability but more stable than liposomes
6	Polymeric Nps				
	(a) PLGA Nps	PLGA	MPLA	Ease of modification	Polymers may exibit cytotoxicity
	(b) Gelatin Nps	Gelatin	DNA	Good acceptibility	Lack of Large scale production
	(c) Chitosan Nps	Chitosan	GRA-1 Protein		
	(d) PLGA Nanospheres	PLGA	Calcitonin		
7	Polymeric Micelles	Pluronics	Taxol	Thermodynamic stbility	Selection of surfactant
8	Dendrimers	Branched Polymers	DNA/Genes	Ease of modification of various termini	Polymer dependent bioavailability biodistribution

MPLA: Mono phosphoryl liquids; PLGA: poly(lac tic-co-glycolic) acid

Nanocrystals and Nanosuspensions

Nanocrystals are aggregates of around hundreds or thousands of molecules that combine in a crystalline form, composed of pure drug with only a thin coating comprised of surfactant or combination of surfactants. Dispersion of drug nanocrystals in liquid media leads to so called "nanosuspensions" (in contrast to "microsuspensions" or "macro-suspensions").

Nanosuspensions of drugs are sub-micron colloidal dispersions of pure particles of drug, which are stabilized by surfactants. They are distinguished from nanoparticles, which are polymeric colloidal carriers of drugs, and from solid lipid nanoparticles, which are lipidic carriers of drugs. Nanosuspensions overcome delivery issues for these compounds by obviating the need to dissolve them, and by maintaining the drug in a preferred crystalline state of size sufficiently small for pharmaceutical acceptability.

Nanotubes

Carbon nanotubes (CNTs) or nanotubes, covalently bonded fullerenes, are used as molecular anchors (Figure 34.1). Fullerene, a hollow sphere or tube composed of carbon, can be used as a drug delivery system. Buckyball clusters are examples of fullerene which have been studied for drug delivery. These fullerenes have bigger inner volume which can be used as the active molecule container. Therefore, several molecules can be attached with this carrier which is readily taken up by the cell. CNTs are used in the drug delivery of several molecules, especially for cancer drugs. These can be applied as biological transporters as well an agent for some cancer cell destruction. *In vivo* distribution and tumor targeting of CNTs have been studied. Concerns about CNTs that prevents advancement in its drug delivery applications include lack of solubility, clumping and aggregation and 6.8 hr half-life. However, studies have demonstrated that functionalized CNTs are non-cytotoxic. CNT has fibrous contour which is needle-like and toxic property has been related with asbestos. One of the major concerns is that extensive application of CNT may lead to cancer especially lung cancer. However, to avoid excessive surface interactions, CNT can be used as nanocapsules shown its biocompatibility for intravenous drug delivery. Fullerenes are effective in tissue selective and intracellular targeting of mitochondria. Thus, these systems could be utilized further for targeting capabilities of biotech drugs such as genes, proteins and peptides.

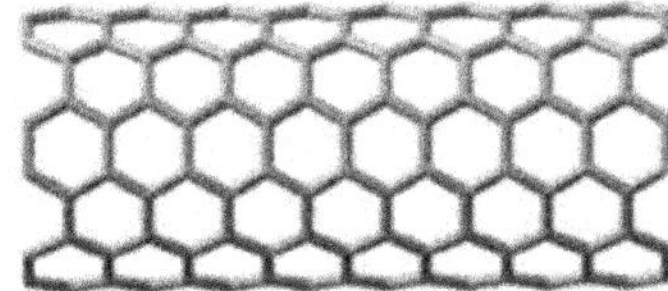

Fig. 34.1 Nanotubes: self-assembling lipid tubes.

Liposomes

Liposome, made of lipid bilayer, is an extensively explored drug delivery system. Its diameter varies from 20 nm to more than a few hundreds of nanometers and width of the phospholipid bilayer is about 4-7 nm (60) (Figure 34.2). Liposomes can be classified into three forms such as multilamellar vesicles (MLV), small unilamellar vesicles (SUV) and large unilamellar vesicles (LUV). MLV consists of a number of concentric bilayers in a particle and the diameter of this liposome may differ from hundred to thousands of nanometers. MLVs can be processed to produce unilamellar vesicles. According to size, unilamellar vesicles can be classified into two types such as small unilamellar vesicles (SUV) and large unilamellar vesicles (LUV). SUVs show a diameter lower than 100 nm, while LUVs have diameter bigger than 100 nm. In addition, there were several reports indicating the application of liposomes as dyes in textiles, pesticides for plants, food ingredients and cosmetics to the skin in areas other than drug delivery systems. Several drugs are in clinical trials, which use liposomal delivery systems. However, for targeted cancer drug and therapeutic protein delivery, liposome constructed with PEG (Polyethylene Glycol) is one of the sought after preferences for the delivery. It can increase the plasma stability and solubility property of the drug. Conversely, this increase properties help to decrease its immunogenicity and now PEGylated drugs in clinical practice. One example of PEGylated drug is Oncaspar (PEG-Lasparaginase) which familiar to treat acute lymphoblastic leukemia.

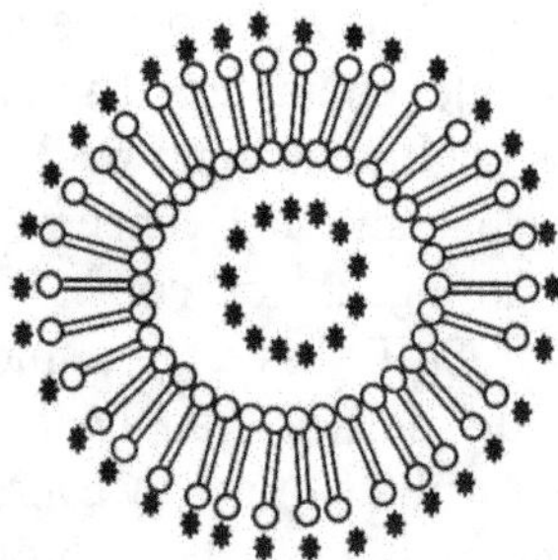

Fig. 34.2 Liposomes: concentric bilayered vesicles in which an aqueous volume is entirely enclosed by a membranous lipid bilayer.

Solid Lipid Nanoparticles (SLN)

SLN are the submicron colloidal carriers (50-1000 nm) composed of solid lipid dispersed either in water or in an aqueous surfactant solution (Fig. 34.3). These consist of solid hydrophobic core having a monolayer of phospholipid coating. The solid core contains drug dissolved or dispersed in the solid high melting fat matrix. SLN can improve the ability of the drug to penetrate through the blood-brain-barrier and is a promising drug targeting system for the treatment of central nervous system disorders. Controlled release of the incorporated drug can be achieved for upto several weeks. Further, by coating with or attaching ligands to SLNs, there is an increased scope of drug targeting. SLN formulations stable for even three years have been developed. This is of paramount importance with respect to the other colloidal carrier systems. Preparation of SLN is cost effective by high pressure homogenization method. It has the feasibility of incorporating both hydrophilic and hydrophobic drugs. The carrier lipids are biodegradable and hence safe.

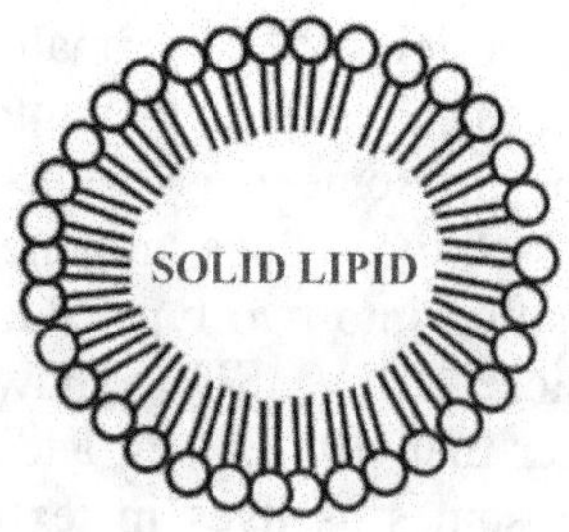

Fig. 34.3 Solid Lipid Nanoparticles (SLN): colloidal submicron carriers made from solid lipids.

Polymeric Nanoparticles

These nanoparticles are sub-nanosized colloidal structures composed of synthetic or semi-synthetic polymers that vary in size from 10-1000 nm.

Among the various approaches studied, reduction of particle size to a nanometer range and surface stabilization of nanoparticles with a layer of nonionic surfactants or polymeric macromolecules have proven to be one of the successful strategies. The presence of surfactants such as poloxamers (Pluronic1) and poloxamines (Tetronic1) on the particle surface strongly reduces opsonization and the inter-particulate attractive van der Waals forces, while increasing the repulsive barrier between two approaching particles. These nanoparticles vary in types of polymers, stabilizers, and surfactants used in their manufacturing process. Each excipient added may have a significant effect on drug absorption and distribution throughout the body, and persistence of the drug in the plasma. The drug loading can be accomplished by adsorption to the surface or encapsulation in the nanoparticle matrix [Fig. 34.4 (a and b)].

Once the polymeric nanoparticles reach the target tissue, the drug may be released by desorption, diffusion through the polymer matrix or polymer wall, or upon nanoparticle erosion. In most cases, especially with large molecular weight drugs, it appears that the release is dependent on the degradation of the nanoparticle matrix rather than diffusion.

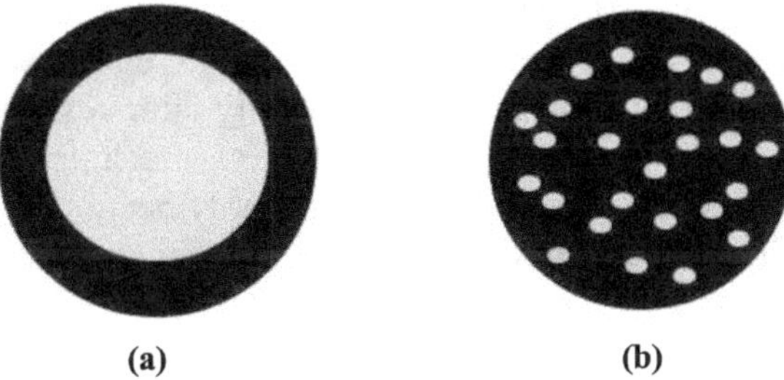

(a)   (b)

Fig. 34.4 (a) Nanocapsule: nanoparticles in which drug is encapsulated within the polymeric membrane. (b) Nanosphere: nanoparticles in which drug is dispersed within the polymeric membrane.

Polymeric Micelles

Polymeric micelles have received much attention in contemporary drug delivery research and they have tremendous potential utility to enhance the solubility of hydrophobic molecules and to achieve target-specific systemic delivery. Micelles are formed by self-assembly of amphiphilic AB diblock or ABA triblock copolymers in aqueous environment, which leads to unique characteristics such as nano size, thermodynamic stability, and their core-shell structure can mimic the naturally occurring transport systems and promote absorption and distribution of entrapped drugs. Due to their hydrophilic shell, micelles show low uptake by RES, protect the incorporated drug from rapid degradation, and decrease the clearance and elimination from the body. Because of their thermodynamic stability and narrow size distribution, they behave as single molecules, and the bio-distribution is dependent on molecular weight, especially in case of cancer chemotherapeutics.

Compared to liposomes, micelles (Fig. 34.5) are much smaller and can provide an alternative and more efficient way of passive as well as active targeting to the disease site in the body. Micellar administration has improved passive targeting of the drug due to prolonged circulation half-lives.

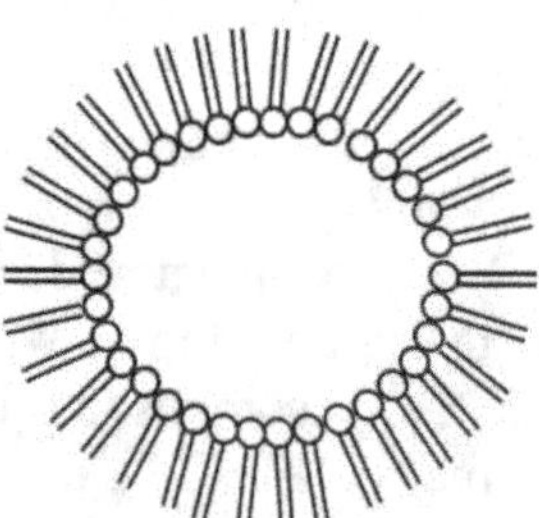

Fig. 34.5 Polymeric micelles: amphiphilic copolymers that self-associate in aqueous solution.

Dendrimers

Although self-assembling nanostructures, such as liposomes and micelles, are frequently used as drug-delivery systems, they can be unstable under shear force and other environmental effects, such as high dilution, especially after systemic administration. An alternative approach is either covalent or noncovalent attachment of drug molecules to dendritic macromolecules. As opposed to linear polymers, that have long chain of repeating units, dendrimers (Fig. 34.6) have a core functional group and different number of branches.

Many different types of dendrimer chemistry are available and the surface functional groups can be modified for covalent attachment of drugs and targeting ligands. In addition, noncovalent interactions of dendrimers with therapeutic molecules can occur through ionic, hydrogen bonding, and van der Waals interactions, resulting in encapsulation of the guest molecules. The size of these dendritic nanocarrier systems, based on different generations, is precisely defined between 5 and 20 nm.

Dendritic polymers with their regular and well defined unimolecular architecture, which can be further modified chemically either the core (to increase hydrophobicity) or shell (to increase hydrophilicity), is currently attracting considerable interest in drug solubilization and target specific delivery.

Poly(amidoamine) (PAMAM) dendrimers have been widely studied and used among the dendrimers so far. The PAMAM dendrimers could be modified with multiple functionalities such as drugs, genes, targeting molecules and imaging agents for the plentiful surface group.

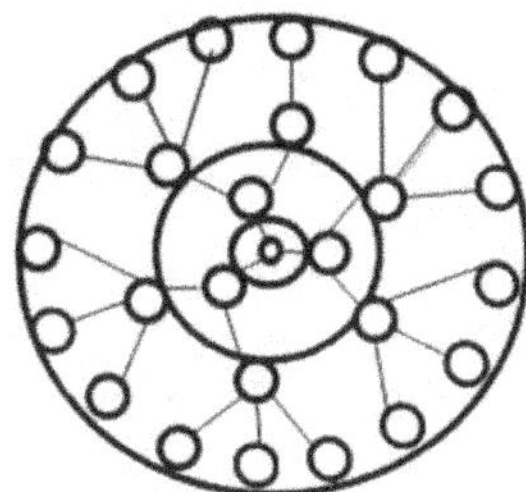

Fig. 34.6 Dendrimers: macromolecular molecules that consist of a series of
branches around an inner core.

Advantages of SLN over Polymeric Nanoparticles

SLN combine the advantages of polymeric nanoparticles, fat emulsions and liposomes while simultaneously avoiding their disadvantages, in particular,

(i)   SLN in the range of 120-200 nm are not taken up readily by the cells of the reticuloendothelial system and thus bypass liver and spleen filtration;

(ii) Drug release in controlled manner can be achieved for several weeks, and the drug targeting potential can be further enhanced by coating or attaching ligands to SLN;

(iii) SLN formulations are stable as long as for even 3 years, very important aspect with respect to the other colloidal carrier systems;

(iv) High drug loading efficiency as compare to polymeric nanoparticles;

(v)   Excellent reproducibility with a cost effective high pressure homogenization method as the preparation procedure. Differently from SLN, the preparation of polymeric nanoparticles can be performed either by polymerization of alkylcyanoacrylate monopolymers or by using the formed polymers;

(vi) Both hydrophilic and hydrophobic drugs can be incorporated;

(vii) The production processes avoid the use of organic solvents and

(viii) They can be produced easily on large scale and sterilization.

The scale up of polymeric nanoparticles is more complicated as it requires the use of solvents for solubilizing the polymers or monomers. In addition, there is a consistent lack of studies concerning the scale-up issues in the production of these systems. Sterilization of polymeric nanoparticles is hardly accounted for in the literature. However, general methods already considered for SLN and applied to other kind of particle can be considered useful.

SLN are prepared from biocompatible/biodegradable materials, thus better tolerability with respect to polymeric nanoparticles. The polymeric nanoparticle cytotoxicity is likely due to the burst release of degradation byproducts, directly related to the length of the polymer alkyl chains. Even if polymeric nanoparticle made of longer alkyl chain polymers are less toxic, they could adhere to cells, leading to a high local degradation product concentration. For brain targeting, less toxic, slow degrading polymeric nanoparticles should be more suitable, although their chronic administration would lead to 'waste disposal' in brain endothelial cells and/or other brain structures.

Cellular and Intracellular Targets for Drug Delivery

For drug delivery not only organ or cellular targeting is of importance but also the fate of the nanoparticles within the cells. Particles generally end intracellularly in endosomes or lysosomes followed by degradation. For activity of the encapsulated drugs release into the cytosol is needed. Chemical characteristics such as surface charge may also determine the fate of nanoparticles in cells. Surface functionalization of gold nanoparticles with PEG resulted in efficient internalization in endosomes and cytosol, and localized in the nuclear region. The hypothesis that the positive surface charge influenced the escape of the endosomes was supported by data obtained with negatively charged polystyrene nanoparticles which did not reach the cytosol but remained in the endosomal compartment of the smooth muscle cells used in this study.

Surface modifications of nanoparticles offer possibilities for medical applications like drug targeting in terms of cellular binding, uptake and intracellular transport. Carbohydrate binding ligands on the surface of biodegradable and biocompatible poly (D,L-lactic-co-glycolide) acid (PLGA) nanospheres were found to increase cellular binding. Such increased adherence may lead to an enhanced activity of the drug presented as or incorporated in nanoparticles. Coupling specific proteins such as antibodies to the nanoparticle surface may enable a more specific immunologically directed targeting of the particles.

Ultimate Target for Drug Delivery: The Brain

The brain is a challenging organ for drug delivery in several perspectives. Firstly, the incidence of degenerative diseases in the brain will increase with the ageing population. Secondly, the blood brain barrier (BBB) is the best well-known guard in the body toward exogenous substances. Generally pharmaceuticals including most small molecules do not cross the BBB. The endothelial barrier is specifically tight at the interface with the brain astrocytes and can in normal conditions only be passed using endogenous BBB transporters resulting in carrier mediated transport, active efflux transport and/or receptor mediated transport. However the barrier properties may be compromised intentionally or unintentionally by drug treatment allowing passage of nanoparticles. Physical association of the drug to the nanoparticles was necessary for drug delivery to occur into the brain. When nanoparticles with different surface characteristics were evaluated, neutral nanoparticles and low concentrations of anionic nanoparticles were found to have no effect on BBB integrity, whereas high concentrations of anionic nanoparticles and cationic nanoparticles were toxic for the BBB. The extent of brain uptake of anionic nanoparticles at lower concentrations was superior to neutral or cationic formulations at the same concentrations. So, nanoparticle surface charges must be considered for toxicity and brain distribution profiles. Especially coating of the nanoparticles with the polysorbate (Tween) surfactants resulted in transport of drugs across the blood brain barrier. The mechanism for transport was suggested to be endocytosis *via* the Low Density Lipoprotein (LDL) receptor of the endothelial cells after adsorption of lipoproteins form blood plasma to the nanoparticles. Additional, investigations revealed the role of apolipoprotein-E for transport of drugs across the BBB while apolipoprotein-E variants that did not recognized lipoprotein receptors failed in transporting the drug across the BBB. It was suggested that the recognition and interaction with lipoprotein receptors on brain capillary endothelial cells was responsible for the brain uptake of the drug.

Passage of the BBB may also be achieved by masking certain drug characteristics preventing or limiting binding to cellular efflux systems like p-glycoprotein, a cellular transporter associated with drug removal from cells. P-glycoprotein is one of the ATP dependent efflux transporters that have an important physiological role in limiting drug entry into the brain. In addition, p-glycoprotein also designated the multidrug resistance protein may be highly expressed in drug resistant tumor cells. Surfactant coated poly(butyl)cyanoacrylate nanoparticles have been used to deliver drugs to the CNS. The effect of entrapment of a cytotoxic drug paclitaxel (PX) in cetyl alcohol/polysorbate nanoparticles (PX NP) was evaluated in an *in situ* rat brain perfusion model. The results suggest that entrapment of paclitaxel in nanoparticles significantly increases the brain drug uptake and its toxicity towards p-glycoprotein expressing tumor cells (p-glycoprotein is an efflux transporter associated with drug removal from the cells). It was hypothesized that PX nanoparticles limit paclitaxel binding to p-glycoprotein and subsequent efflux from the cells, which consequently would lead to higher brain and tumor cell levels.

Uptake and Effects of Nanoparticles in the Brain

Two different mechanisms have been suggested for the uptake of nanoparticles to brain. Firstly, transsynaptic transport after inhalation through the olfactory epithelium, and secondly, uptake through the blood-brain barrier. The first pathway has been studied widely with model particles such as Au, MnO_2 and carbon, in experimental inhalation models in rats. The second pathway has been the result of extensive research and particle surface manipulation in drug delivery. The latter studies suggest that the physiological barrier may limit the distribution of some proteins and viral particles after transvascular delivery to the brain, suggesting that the healthy BBB contains defence mechanisms protecting it from blood borne nanoparticle exposure. When nanoparticles with different surface characteristics were evaluated, neutral nanoparticles and low concentrations of anionic nanoparticles were found to have no effect on BBB integrity, whereas high concentrations of anionic nanoparticles and cationic nanoparticles were toxic for the BBB. Nanoparticles have been shown to induce the production of reactive oxygen species and oxidative stress and this has been confirmed in the brain after inhalation of MnO_2 nanoparticles. Oxidative stress has been implicated in the pathogenesis of neurodegenerative diseases such as Parkinson's and Alzheimer's diseases. Evidence for the involvement of ambient air nanoparticles in these effects is presented by studies in biopsies from city dwellers. Alzheimer's like pathology was demonstrated in brain sections by increased markers of inflammation and AB42-accumulation in frontal cortex and hippocampus in association with the presence of nanoparticles. Also inhalation exposure of BALB/c mice to particulate matter showed activation of pro-inflammatory cytokines in the brain. Whether this is due to the fraction of combustion nanoparticles remains to be investigated.

Nanoparticle Toxicity

To use the potential of Nanotechnology in Nanomedicine, full attention is needed to safety and toxicological issues. For pharmaceuticals specific drug delivery formulations may be used to increase the so called therapeutic ratio or index being the margin between the dose needed for clinical efficacy and the dose inducing adverse side effects (toxicity). The Society of Toxicology defines toxicology as "the study of the adverse effects of chemical, physical and biological agents on people, animals and the environment". The ultra-small size and unique properties of nanomaterials have led to increasing concerns about their potential toxicity. Nanoparticles are known to exert oxidative stress as well as DNA damage and cell cycle arrest in human cells. The exact mechanisms of nanoparticle toxicity still remain a mystery (Fig. 34.7).

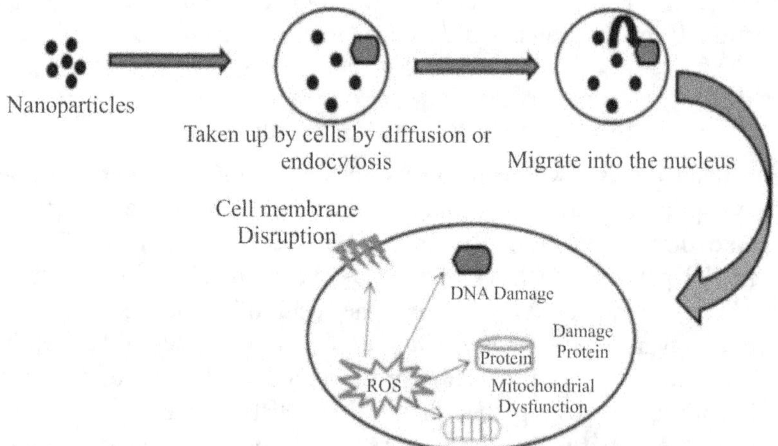

(NPs can enter into the cell by diffusion or endocytosis. Once inside the cytoplasm, they can interfere with energy production in mitochondria and promote the generation of reactive oxygen species (ROS). ROS may cross the nuclear membrane and cause DNA damage. DNA damage can be either repaired or lead to irreversible chromosome damage or cell death (apoptosis))

Fig. 34.7 Hypothetical mechanisms of nanoparticle cytotoxicity.

The toxic effects of nanomaterials depend not only on structural features of the particle itself but also on the nano-bio interface, i.e., their interaction with cellular structures and biomolecules. Other processes may also play a crucial role in nanotoxicity, such as the generation of radicals (causing oxidative stress), the induction or modulation of proinflammatory reactions, potential genetic mutations etc. Nanomaterials are developed for their unique (surface) properties in comparison to bulk materials. Since surface is the contact layer with the body tissue, and a crucial determinant of particle response, these unique properties need to be investigated from a toxicological standpoint. When nanoparticles are used for their unique reactive characteristics it may be expected that these same characteristics also have an impact on the toxicity of such particles. Although, current tests and procedures in drug and device evaluation may be appropriate to detect many risks associated with the use of these nanoparticles, it cannot be assumed that these assays will detect all potential risks. So, additional assays may be needed. This may differ depending on the type of particles used, i.e., biological versus non-biological origin.

Nanoparticles are attributed qualitatively different physico-chemical characteristics from micron-sized particles, which may result in changed body distribution, passage of the blood brain barrier, and triggering of blood coagulation pathways. In view of these characteristics specific emphasis should be on investigations in (pharmaco) kinetics and distribution studies of nanoparticles. What is currently lacking is a basic understanding of the biological behavior of nanoparticles in terms of distribution *in vivo* both at the organ and cellular level.

Effects of combustion derived nanoparticles in environmentally exposed populations mainly occur in diseased individuals. Typical pre-clinical screening is almost always done in healthy animals and volunteers and risks of particles may therefore be detected at a very late stage.

The use of nanoparticles as drug carrier may reduce the toxicity of the incorporated drug. In general the toxicity of the whole formulation is investigated while results of the nanoparticles itself are not described. So, discrimination between drug and nanoparticle toxicity cannot be made. So, there should be a specific emphasis on the toxicity of the "empty" non-drug loaded particles. This is especially important when slowly or non degradable particles are used for drug delivery which may show persistence and accumulation on the site of the drug delivery, eventually resulting in chronic inflammatory reactions.

Role of Regulatory Bodies in Nanotechnology

For the testing of nanomaterials as per international standards are still being developed. Until now, generally applicable criteria have been developed, and the corresponding validated tests will soon become available. Competent authorities are dependent on case-by-case decisions, using existing data to estimate the toxic potential of nanomaterials.

The next key steps needed to involve developing the appropriate methodology for quantifying and monitoring the exposure risk for consumers at the workplace and in the environment. There is currently no adequate data on the behaviour of nanomaterials in the food chain. Similarly, there are no routine monitoring methods for detecting nanoscale contaminants and residues in food products.

The Working Party on Manufactured Nanomaterial (WPMN) established by the Organisation for Economic Co-operation and Development (OECD) aims to provide a solid basis for assessing the toxic potential of nanomaterials. This program for the first time will carry out a comprehensive comparative evaluation of all endpoints relevant to toxicological assessments for standardized nanomaterials. It will also develop nano specific test guidelines. The Working Party is implementing its work through specific projects to further develop appropriate methods and strategies to help ensure human health and environmental safety. OECD strategies also include safety testing of a representative set of manufactured nanomaterials; co-operation on voluntary schemes and regulatory programs; co-operation on risk assessment; exposure measurement and exposure mitigation; and environmentally sustainable use of manufactured nanomaterials. The OECD has developed a global resource which collects research projects that address environmental, human health and safety issues of manufacture nanomaterials. This database helps to identify research gaps and assists researchers' in future collaborative efforts.

Since 2005, the Environmental Protection Agency (EPA) has received and reviewed over 100 new chemical notices under Toxic Substances Control Act (TSCA) for nanoscale materials, and that number is expected to increase over time. The Agency has taken a number of actions to control and limit exposure to nanomaterials. They have implemented regulations limiting the uses of nanoscale materials; requiring the use of personal protective equipment; limiting environmental releases; and requiring testing, to generate data on health and environmental effects.

Future Perspectives

Exciting opportunities for more improved therapeutic management of a disease can be provided by the use of Nanotechnology. A massive research attempts in this field has generated to develop new compounds for targeting brain in the treatment of neurodegenerative diseases which has led to the extreme growth in CNS drugs discovery in the recent years. It is particularly important to consider that the pharmaceutical sector is moving toward the development of high molecular weight products, which cannot cross the BBB and could get benefit from the use of nanocarriers. However, this field is still in the nascent stage. Considering the complexity of the brain, in-depth and comprehensive toxicological studies of brain targeting nanomedicines are required. A nanocarrier formulation should be evaluated both with and without its drug encapsulated. As many CNS diseases require chronic treatment, the chronic and cumulative effects of nanomedicine on brain tissues need to be clarified in addition to their acute toxicity.

Because damages to the brain are more difficult to evaluate than to other organs such as liver, heart or kidney, it will be useful to incorporate advanced diagnostic technologies such as magnetic resonance imaging, positron emission tomography and computed tomography scan to help with the evaluation of nanocarriers associated CNS toxicity.

The future of nanotechnology will depend on rational design of nanomaterials and tools based around a detailed and thorough understanding of biological processes rather than forcing applications for some materials currently in vogue.

Suggested Readings

1. De Jong WH, Borm PJA (2008). Drug delivery and nanoparticles: applications and hazards. *International Journal of Nanomedicine.* **3(2):** 133.

2. Moghimi SM, Hunter AC, Murray JC (2005). Nanomedicine: current status and future prospects. *The FASEB Journal.* **19(3):** 311-30.

3. Patel M, Souto EB, Singh KK (2013). Advances in brain drug targeting and delivery: limitations and challenges of solid lipid nanoparticles. *Expert Opinion on Drug Delivery.* **10(7):** 1-17.

4. Rawat M, Singh D, Saraf S, Saraf S (2006). Nanocarriers: promising vehicle for bioactive drugs. *Biological and Pharmaceutical Bulletin.* **29(9):**1790-8.

5. Wong HL, Wu XY, Bendayan R (2012). Nanotechnological advances for the delivery of CNS therapeutics. *Advanced Drug Delivery Reviews.* **64(7):** 686-700.

CHAPTER 35

COMPUTER AIDED DRUG DISCOVERY (CADD): A QSAR APPROACH

Introduction

Computer-aided drug design (CADD) using docking techniques and high throughput virtual screening, along with target/structure focusing combinatorial chemistry, has become a powerful tool in the multi-step process of drug discovery. As an emerging technology, CADD accelerates drug development by making use of the accumulated information of existing drugs and diseases, combined with inter-disciplinary inputs from other fields. This process extensively uses mathematical models and simulation tools based on the evaluation of potential risks from drug safety and the experimental design of new trials. The first successful story where CADD has been applied to design peptide-based HIV-proteinase inhibitors dates back to early 1990s. Similarly, CADD approaches have been successfully employed for the discovery of various novel enzyme inhibitors like inhibitors of thymidylate synthase, HIV-1 Protease, purine nucleoside phosphorylase, Fructose 1,6-Bisphosphatase and a proteinase inhibitor of viral main proteinase Mpro. Generally, it is believed that the drug discovery procedure involves three pre-clinical stages prior to actual clinical trials, specifically target selection, lead identification, and clinical candidate selection. It is expected that a characteristic drug discovery phase, from lead identification all the way through to clinical trials, can take up to 14 years with expenditure of about 800 million US dollars. Therefore, the design, development and commercialization of a drug is a tiresome, time-consuming and cost-intensive process. Taking into account both the possible benefits to human health and the colossal costs in time and funds of drug discovery, any tool or technique that boosts the competence of any stage of the drug discovery venture will be extremely valued. CADD is one of these tools which can be used to augment the effectiveness of the drug discovery method.

The primary step in the structure-based CADD is the determination of the three dimensional (3D) structure of a target protein or nucleic acid with the help of X-ray crystallography or NMR as well as homology modeling in case of protein targets. By means of recently constructed protein and nucleic databases, novel computational methods utilize the 3D structural information of the unliganded target to design completely new lead compounds *de novo*. In this way, large virtual combinatorial library of compounds can then be screened computationally before attempting expensive actual synthesis and biological studies. The potential to rapidly and precisely dock large numbers of candidate molecules into the binding site of a target macromolecule is a key module of lead generation in structure-based drug design. The most broadly used computational docking methods are the programs DOCK, ADAM, AutoDOCK, FlexX and SLIDE.

With the rapid growth of biological and chemical information, CADD now plays a significant role to explore the novel molecular entities. Present focus includes enhanced design and organization of data sources, formation of programs to create enormous libraries of pharmacologically exciting compounds, development of innovative algorithms to measure the effectiveness and selectivity of lead molecules, and design of predictive tools to recognize possible ADME/Tox issues.

Data Sources

Data accessibility is significant for the achievement of a drug discovery and development drive. Large amounts of organic molecules, biological sequences and associated information have been amassed in scientific literature. These data are assembled and piled in an ordered manner in a variety of databases. Traditionally, the chief resource of biologically active compounds used in drug discovery programs have been natural products, isolated from plant, animal or fermentation sources. During the past decade, thousands of drug molecules have been constantly developed. Therefore, it's extremely essential to handle these valuable chemical data with the assistance of Chemical Databases (Table 35.1). Here we list some of the most important small molecule databases used in CADD.

PubChem

It is a database of chemical molecules and their activities against biological assays. The database is maintained by the National Center for Biotechnology Information (NCBI), a part of the National Library of Medicine (NLM), which in turn is component of the United States National Institutes of Health (NIH). Its main focus is on the chemical, structural and biological properties of small molecules, predominantly their relevance as diagnostic and therapeutic agents. PubChem is structured as three correlated databases namely; PubChem Substance, PubChem Compound, and PubChem BioAssay. PubChem also provides a fast chemical structure similarity search tool.

Available Chemicals Directory (ACD)

One of the major structure-searchable collections of commercially offered chemicals globally is provided by Accelrys Available Chemicals Directory (ACD). The directory comes with the pricing and supplier information for over 7 million unique chemicals, including 3D models, from 940 suppliers. Accelrys ACD is considered as the Gold Standard for the supply of chemicals to various pharmaceutical, biotechnology, chemical, and agrochemical companies globally.

ZINC

It is a freely available database of compounds for virtual screening. ZINC contains over 13 million purchasable compounds in various 3D formats annotated with biologically significant properties (molecular weight, calculated Log P and number of rotatable bonds) which are ready for docking. ZINC is mainly developed for target based virtual screening (docking), however, it is also used for ligand based virtual screening and other computational drug discovery approaches.

KEGG LIGAND

This database is a combination of various different sections namely;

- *COMPOUND* - provides information about metabolites and other chemical compounds (17,628 entries)
- *GLYCAN* - provides information about glycan structures (10,978 entries)
- *REACTION* - meant for the compilation of substrate-product relations indicating metabolic and other reactions (8,458 entries)
- *RPAIR* - provides information about Reactant pair alignments (12,599 entries)
- *RCLASS* - provides information about Reaction class (2,324 entries)
- *ENZYME* - used for the information about enzyme molecules (5,419 entries).

Drug Bank

This database is a unique bioinformatics and cheminformatics warehouse that merges complete drug (i.e., chemical, pharmacological and pharmaceutical) data with widespread drug target (i.e., sequence, structure, and pathway) information. Drug bank contains detailed information on about 6827 drug entries including 1431 FDA-approved small molecule drugs, 134 FDA-approved biotech drugs, 83 nutraceuticals and 5211 experimental drugs. Moreover, these drug entries are linked to about 4434 non-redundant protein (i.e., drug target/enzyme/transporter/ carrier) sequences.

ChemDB

It is a chemical database, which contains practically 5 million commercially available compounds as leads for the discovery of drugs and other useful molecules. The data is openly available over the web for download and for targeted searches using different types of search methods. The chemical data comprises predicted or experimentally verified physicochemical properties, like 3D structure, melting temperature and solubility.

ChemIDPlus

With the help of this database a user is able to search the NLM ChemIDplus database of over 370,000 chemicals. The database can be searched by using compound identifiers such as Chemical Name, CAS Registry Number, Molecular Formula, Classification Code, Locator Code, and Structure or Substructure. Other searchable parameters include search and display by Toxicity indicators such as Median Lethal Dose (LD_{50}), by Physical/Chemical Properties such as LogP, and by Molecular Weight.

CLiBE

A database for helping the analysis of Drug Binding Competitiveness. It includes information regarding the Computed Ligand-Receptor Interaction Energy and other traits such as energy components; ligand classification, functions and properties as well as Ligand structure. At present, the database contains 67,184 entries, in which there are 5,978 unique ligands and 2,258 distinct receptors.

The NCI Drug Information System 3D Database

A collection of 3D structures for over 400,000 drugs which was built and is maintained by the *Developmental Therapuetics Program Division of Cancer Treatment*, National Cancer Institute. The database is an extension of the *NCI Drug Information System*.

1. **Protein Data Bank (PDB):** It is the chief source of structural data for biological macromolecules. As of May 2011, there are 73,503 biological macromolecular structures deposited in PDB. The PDB database contains information regarding experimentally-determined structures of proteins, nucleic acids, and complex assemblies.

2. **Therapeutic Target Database (TTD):** A warehouse which gives information about the well-known and explored therapeutic protein and nucleic acid targets, the targeted disease, pathway information and the corresponding drugs directed at each of these targets. Moreover, the database is linked to various other significant databases that contain information about target function, sequence, 3D structure, ligand binding properties, enzyme nomenclature and drug structure, therapeutic class, clinical development status. Currently, TTD contains 2,025 targets, including 364 successful, 286 clinical trial, 44 discontinued and 1,331 research targets, and 17,816 drugs, including 1,540 approved, 1,423 clinical trial and 14,853 experimental drugs (14,170 small molecules and 652 antisense drugs with existing structure or oligonucleotide sequence).

3. **Drug ADME Associated Protein Database:** A database for assisting the search for drug Absorption, Distribution, Metabolism, Excretion associated proteins. It contains information about known drug ADME associated proteins, functions, similarities, substrates/ligands, tissue distributions, and other properties of the targets. Currently, this database contains 321 protein entries.

4. **Drug Adverse Reaction Target (DART):** The Drug Adverse Reaction Database (DART) provides broad information about adverse effect targets of drugs illustrated in the literature. Additionally, proteins concerned in adverse effect targets of chemicals not yet established as ADR targets are also incorporated as potential targets. This database gives physiological function of all targets, binding drugs/agonists/antagonists/activators/inhibitors, IC_{50} values of the inhibitors, resultant adverse effects, and type of ADR induced by drug binding to a target. DART is also cross linked to other databases that facilitates the access of information about the sequence, 3-dimensional structure, function, and nomenclature of each target along with drug/ligand binding properties, and related literature.

5. **PROCARB:** Many carbohydrate-binding proteins are being considered as targets for new medicines, especially extracellular lectins which account for most of the molecular targets that are being investigated in current drug discovery program. PROCARB is a single resource where all the relevant information about a pair of interacting protein and carbohydrate is available in addition to a number of pre-computed features of these carbohydrate-binding proteins like solvent accessibility, secondary structure, and hydrogen bonding information. PROCARB consists of 604 protein-carbohydrate complexes with at least one but possibly more carbohydrate molecule(s) in each complex. The database also contains the three-dimensional structures of different types of glycoproteins (both N- and O-linked), with unknown structures by using homology modelling. This module of PROCARB consists of 26 N-linked and 20 O-linked modelled structures.

QSAR

Drug discovery is a complex, expensive and very time-consuming exercise as, there is no single systematic way to automatically discover a drug even when the disease and targets have been well understood. There may be millions of candidate molecules if *in-silico* filtering is not performed. Experiments cannot be performed on such large number of drug candidates due to prohibitive costs both in terms of time and money. Quantitative structure-activity relationship (QSAR) studies form the center stage, when a protein (typically an enzyme) is the target and there is a need to find a suitable molecule, which can control (inhibit) the activity of its target.

The basic principle of such a study is the structure dependence of chemical activity. QSAR has existed much longer than the first popularity of computers because chemical structure has always been able to explain at least some aspects of chemical properties. However, with the availability of powerful computers and high quality databases of molecular libraries and interactions have made QSAR an essential component of drug discovery today.

QSAR based (*in-silico*) analysis may be better regarded as an exercise to screen or filter drug candidates, before they are subjected to more intensive calculations such as docking or an experimental measurement of activity *(in-vitro)* and finally under real conditions *(in-vivo)*. Many times, this step will pick up a dozen of drug candidate from a library of millions of well-studied molecules. Traditional QSAR is specific to a particular target or enzyme and all the screening is performed on drug candidates (ligand molecules). These ligand molecules are very diverse and in order to screen them suitably, we need to describe their structure as well as chemical nature. This leads to the issue of finding descriptors of molecular properties of ligands and drugs. Hundreds of molecular properties or descriptors are used to represent molecules. Moreover, when physicochemical properties or structures are expressed by figures, one can outline a numerical relationship, or quantitative structure-activity relationship among the two. The arithmetical expression can then be used to predict the biological response of other chemical structures.

Mathematically-Activity = f (physiochemical properties and/or structural properties)

These properties may be purely geometric, topological, electromagnetic, classical and quantum-mechanical. Often, predicting activity of a protein-ligand combination if the descriptors of the ligand are known carries out this screening. Regression techniques such as Principal Component Analysis (PCA), Neural Network and Multivariate correlation are the major techniques used for this purpose.

QSAR Methods

- 1D-QSAR- Affinity correlates with global molecular properties like pKa, logP, etc.
- 2D-QSAR- Affinity correlates with structural patterns like connectivity indices, chemical connectivity, 2D-pharmacophores, etc. The 3D-representation of these properties is not considered.
- 3D-QSAR- Affinity correlates with the three-dimensional structure, non-covalent interaction fields surrounding the molecules.
- 4D-QSAR- Additionally including multiple representations of ligand conformation/orientation in 3D-QSAR.
- 5D-QSAR- As with 4D, but with explicitly representing different induced-fit models.
- 6D-QSAR- As with 5D, but with different solvation models.

Molecular Descriptors

Molecular descriptors are used in QSAR for a unique representation and identification of ligand molecules, which are likely to be drug candidates, and may be classified as Constitutional descriptors (e.g., molecular weight, number of atoms, number of H-bonds), Topological descriptors]e.g., total structure connectivity index, Pogliani index), Functional group counts (e.g., terminal primary C(sp3), total secondary C(sp3), total tertiary C(sp3)], Charge descriptors (e.g., maximum positive charge, maximum negative charge) and Molecular properties (e.g., unsaturation index hydrophilic Factor). Many more descriptors may be calculated and comprehensive lists can be found elsewhere. A broad review of molecular descriptors is also presented by Karelson (2000). Some of the molecular descriptors are used in QSAR based studies are described below:

Constitutional Descriptors

Constitutional descriptors such as molecular weight, van der Waals volume, electronegativities, polarizability, number of atoms, non-H atoms, number of H-bonds, multiple bonds, bond orders, aromatic ratio, number of rings, number of double and triple bonds, aromatic bonds, 3 different types of (n-membered) rings, benzene-like rings. Constitutional descriptors are extensively used in QSAR analysis e.g., these were used to describe herbicidal properties of a fluorovinyloxyacetamide set of compounds. The top model elucidated more than 83% of data variance, stressing the importance of mean atomic Sanderson electronegativity, molecular polarizability as well as the number of O and F atoms and aromatic bonds, to describe herbicidal properties.

Topological Descriptors

Topological descriptors such as total structure connectivity index, Pogliani index, ramification index, polarity number, average vertex distance degree, mean square distance index (Balaban), (Balaban), Molecular Topological Index (MTI), square reciprocal distance sum index, quasi-Wiener index (Kirchhoff number), spanning tree number, hyperdistance-path index, reciprocal hyper-distance-path index, detour index, hyper-detour index, reciprocal hyper-detour index, distance/detour index, all-path Wiener index, Wiener-type index from Z weighted distance matrix (Barysz matrix), molecular electrotopological variation, E-state topological parameter, Kier symmetry index eccentricity, mean distance degree deviation, unipolarity, centralization, variation. E.g. QSAR models for 157 epipodophyllotoxins were generated using multiple topological descriptors of chemical structures, including molecular connectivity indices (MCI) and molecular operating environment descriptors.

Path/walk Counts

Path/walk counts such as molecular walk counts, total walk count, self-returning walk counts, molecular path counts, molecular multiple path counts, total path count, conventional bond-order ID number, Randic ID number, Balaban ID number, ratio of multiple path count over path count, difference between multiple path count and path count. Path/walk Randic shape indices of order m (PWm) are calculated by summing the ratios of the atomic path counts over atomic walk counts of order m for all atoms, and dividing the sum by the number of non-hydrogen atoms (Randic, 2001). Recently, Sharma *et al.*, (2011) have highlighted the role of path/walk 4-Randic shape index (PW4), in a QSAR study on 2-(4-Methylpiperazin-1-yl) quinoxalines as human histamine H4-receptor ligands. In their analysis, the sign of regression coefficient of this descriptor shows positive influence on the activity and a higher value of this descriptor would be in favor of the activity.

Connectivity Indices

Connectivity indices such as connectivity indices, average connectivity indices, valence connectivity indices, average valence connectivity indices, solvation connectivity indices, modified, reciprocal distance Randic-type index, reciprocal distance squared Randic-type index. In a QSAR study of Camptothecin (CPT) derivatives as inhibitor of DNA Topoisomerase-I, it was shown that connectivity index in addition to electron affinity, mol. wt. & ether group count highly contribute to inhibitory activity of CPT derivatives.

Information Indices

Information indices such as information index on molecular size, total information index of atomic composition, mean information index on atomic composition, mean information content on the distance equality, mean information content on the distance magnitude, mean information content on the distance degree equality, mean information content on the distance degree magnitude, total information content on the distance equality, total information content on the distance magnitude, mean information content on the vertex degree equality, mean information content on the vertex degree magnitude, graph vertex complexity index, graph distance complexity index (log), Balaban U index, Balaban V index, Balaban X index, Balaban Y index Basak indices of neighbourhood symmetry.

2D Autocorrelations

2D autocorrelations Broto-Moreau autocorrelations of a topological structure, Moran autocorrelations, Geary autocorrelations. The 2D autocorrelation descriptors were used to elucidate the factors that stabilize the G-quadruplex structure and consequently the inhibition of telomerase by using a QSAR approach on a dataset of 546 inhibitors of telomerase activity.

Edge Adjacency Indices

Edge adjacency indices edge connectivity index of order 0, edge connectivity index of order 1 eigenvalues from edge adj. matrix weighted by edge degrees, eigenvalues from edge adj. Matrix weighted by dipole moments, eigenvalues from edge adj. matrix weighted by resonance integrals spectral moments from edge adj. matrix, spectral moments from edge adj. matrix weighted by edge degrees, spectral moments from edge adj. matrix weighted by dipole moments, spectral moments from edge adj. matrix weighted by resonance integrals. The eigenvalues were described as one of the most frequent descriptors in a QSAR model which describe the importance of the shape, i.e., the scaffold 6-fluoroquinolone moiety (1,4-dihydro-4-oxo-3-pyridinecarboxylic acid) for activity.

Eigenvalue-Based Indices

Eigenvalue-based indices Lovasz-Pelikan index (leading eigenvalue), leading eigenvalue from Z weighted distance matrix (Barysz matrix), leading eigenvalue from mass weighted distance matrix, leading eigenvalue from van der Waals weighted distance matrix, leading eigenvalue from electronegativity weighted distance matrix, leading eigenvalue from polarizability weighted distance matrix. The application of Lovasz-Pelikan index descriptor along with Average valence connectivity index chi-5 justifies the use of these two parameters in all the QSAR modelling of antimycobacterial activity of 3-formyl rifamycin SV derivatives.

Geometrical Descriptors

Geometrical descriptors 3D-Wiener index, 3D-Balaban index, 3D-Harary index average geometric distance degree, D/D index, average distance/distance degree gravitational index G1, gravitational index G2 (bond-restricted), radius of gyration (mass weighted), span R, average span R. Geometrical descriptors like 3D petijean shape index (PJI3), Gravitational index, Balaban index, Wiener index, etc., are the major factors that affect protein tyrosine kinase inhibitory activity of compounds and have positive effects on the protein tyrosine kinase inhibitory activity.

Functional Group Counts

Functional group counts terminal primary C(sp3), total secondary C(sp3), total tertiary C(sp3), total quaternary C(sp3), ring secondary C(sp3), ring tertiary C(sp3), ring quaternary C(sp3) aromatic C(sp2), unsubstituted benzene C(sp2), substituted benzene C(sp2), non-aromatic conjugated C(sp2), terminal primary C(sp2), aliphatic secondary C(sp2), aliphatic tertiary C(sp2), allenes groups, terminal C(sp), non-terminal C(sp) cyanates (aliphatic), cyanates (aromatic), isocyanates (alip-hatic), isocyanates (aromatic), thiocyanates (aliphatic), thiocyanates (aromatic), isothiocyanates (aliphatic), isothiocyanates (aromatic). E.g., a QSAR model proposed by Gupta et al., 2010 suggests that the aromatic bonds and, number of ring quaternary (sp3) structures are conductive for HIV- 1 inhibitory potency of DABOs derivatives.

Charge Descriptors

Charge descriptors maximum positive charge, maximum negative charge, total positive charge, total negative charge, total absolute charge (electronic charge index - ECI), mean absolute charge (charge polarization), total squared charge, relative positive charge, relative negative charge, sub-molecular polarity parameter, topological electronic descriptor, topological electronic descriptor (bond restricted), partial charge weighted topological electronic descriptor, local dipole index. A 4D-QSAR study on anti-HIV HEPT analogues showed that charge descriptors provide better modeling efficiency.

Molecular Properties

Molecular properties unsaturation index hydrophilic factor, Ghose-Crippen molar refractivity topological polar and non-polar surface area. The Refractotopological State Index for atoms promises to be helpful in quantitative structure-activity relationships studies, particularly in those concerning dispersive atomic interactions with active sites. The index has a direct structural understanding since, it expresses the atomic role of a significant physico-chemical property (molar refractivity) correlated to dispersive forces in biologically active sites and in addition, contains topological information about the chemical structure of the atomic environment.

Tools to Calculate Molecular Descriptors

Dragon: Dragon is commercial software for the computation of molecular descriptors. These descriptors can be used to calculate molecular structure-activity or structure-property relationships, as well as for similarity study and high-throughput screening of molecule databases. In its latest version i.e., Dragon 6, it calculates about 4885 molecular descriptors and includes various new molecular descriptors such as CATS 2D, Klein TDB autocorrelations, atom-type E-state indices, ETA descriptors, P_VSA descriptors, ring descriptors, several indices from different 2D and 3D matrices, drug-like and lead-like filters. [http://www.talete.mi.it/products/dragon_description.htm].

HyperChem

HyperChem is another commercially available sophisticated molecular modeling environment that is known for its quality, flexibility, and ease of use. HyperChem has a range of features, ideal for chemists in drug discovery. One of the most important features is QSAR Properties that allows calculation and estimation of a variety of molecular descriptors commonly used in Quantitative Structure Activity Relationship (QSAR) studies. Some of the properties which can be estimated using QSAR Properties are Atomic charges, Van der Waals and solvent accessible surface area, Molecular volumes, Hydration energy, Log P, Refractivity, Polarizability, Mass, etc. [http://www.chemistry-software.com/hyperchem/]

PaDEL-Descriptor

PaDEL-Descriptor is software for calculating molecular descriptors and fingerprints. The software currently calculates 797 descriptors (663 1D, 2D descriptors, and 134 3D descriptors) and 10 types of fingerprints. These descriptors and fingerprints are calculated mainly using-The Chemistry Development Kit. Some additional descriptors and fingerprints were added, which include atom type electrotopological state descriptors, McGowan volume, molecular linear free energy relation descriptors, ring counts, count of chemical substructures identified by Laggner, and binary fingerprints and count of chemical substructures identified by Klekota and Roth. It is free and open source, has both graphical user interface and command line interfaces, can work on all major platforms (Windows, Linux, MacOS), supports more than 90 different molecular file formats, and is multithreaded. [http://padel.nus.edu.sg/software/padeldescriptor]

PreADMET

It is a web-based application for predicting ADME data and building drug-like library using *in silico* method. PreADMET program resides entirely on a Web server, and can be accessed by browsers such as Netscape or Internet Explorer. The application is written mainly in PHP, a scripting language commonly used for Web application which communicates with the browser through a CGI interface. The PHP code in turn uses a set of C-program that implement much of the functionality of PreADMET. It consists of four main parts as following: Molecular Descriptor Calculation, Drug-likeness Prediction, ADME Prediction and Toxicity prediction. [http://preadme.bmdrc.org/]

Open 3D QSAR

It is an open-source tool aimed at pharmacophore exploration by high-throughput chemometric analysis of molecular interaction fields (MIFs). Open3DQSAR can generate steric potential, electron density and MM/QM electrostatic potential fields; furthermore, it can import GRIDKONT binary files produced by GRID and CoMFA/CoMSIA fields (exported from SYBYL with the aid of a small SPL script). The main output is arranged as human-readable plain ASCII text, while a number of additional files are generated to store data and to export the results of computations for further analysis and visualization with third party tools. In particular, Open3DQSAR can export 3D maps for visualization in PyMOL, MOE, Maestro, SYBYL, and can generate graphical statistic output ready to be imported into gnuplot. [http://www.open3dqsar.org/?Home]

BlueDesc (Molecular Descriptor Calculator)

A key step in classical quantitative structure-activity/property relationship (QSAR/QSPR) modeling is the encoding of a chemical compound into a vector of numerical descriptors. Although, most of the available chemoinformatic software packages provide routine for the calculation of descriptors, but they are not easy to use in most cases. This simple command-line tool converts an MDL SD file into ARFF and LIBSVM format for machine learning and data mining purposes using CDK and JOELib2. A ready-to-use (executable JAR), 100% Java tool, which includes JOELib2 (GNU GPL) and the CDK (LGPL), sources and the GNU GPL. It computes 174 descriptors taken from both libraries. **Works on 3D structures only.** Output is ARFF (WEKA) and libSVM format. [http://www.ra.cs.uni-tuebingen.de/software/bluedesc/welcome_e.html]

ADRIANA.Code

It comprises a unique combination of methods for calculating molecular structure descriptors on a sound geometric and physicochemical basis. These descriptors can be used for a wide range of applications in all areas of chemistry, in particular in drug design. Lead discovery and optimization, diversity assessment of compound libraries and prediction of ADME/Tox properties are some of the problems that have been addressed and successfully solved with descriptors from ADRIANA.Code. Input file formats are MDL SDFile (incl. Molfile), Daylight SMILES and CTX file. Output file format are MDL SDFile, CSV, TSV and SONNIA.
[http://www.molecular-networks.com/products/adrianacode]

GenerateMD

It is an application program for the generation of various *molecular descriptors* including chemical (topological) fingerprints, namely ChemAxon Chemical Fingerprint and ECFP, as well as 2-dimensional pharmacophore fingerprints, reaction fingerprint and structural keys of molecular structures. These descriptors can be used to characterize molecules and search through large compound libraries with respect to chemical, structural as well as pharmacological properties.
[http://www.ambinter.com/jchem/doc/user/GenerateMD.html]

MODEL (Molecular Descriptor Lab)

Molecular descriptors represent structural and physicochemical features of compounds. They have been extensively used for developing statistical models, such as quantitative structure activity relationship (QSAR) and artificial neural networks (NN), for computer prediction of the pharmacodynamic, pharmaco-kinetic, or toxicological properties of compounds from their structure. MODEL is accessible free of charge for academic use.
[http:// jing.cz3. nus.edu.sg/cgi-bin/model/model.cgi].

MolconnZ TOOLKIT

Molconn-Z is commercially available software for 2D molecular descriptors comparison. Researchers have found MolconnZ's ability to rapidly generate over 300 descriptors invaluable for evaluating their databases of existing compounds as well as their databases of potential new compounds. Use of the MolconnZ molecular descriptors along with database tools, statistical and component analysis provides valuable methods for Bioinformatic Similarity Analysis. [http://www.molconn.com/products.html]

Statistical Methods to Build QSAR Models

After the descriptors of molecules have been calculated, redundant descriptors are removed using Statistical or chemometric techniques that outline the mathematical foundation for building a QSAR model.

Among the growing pool of diverse statistical methods existing in the literature, Linear Regression analyses are considered as easiest interpretable methods indicated for QSAR study. These regression methods build a statistical model to symbolize the relationship of one or more independent variables (a) with a dependent explicative variable (b). The model can be employed to predict (b) from the data of (a) variables, which can be either quantitative or qualitative. Simple linear regression, multiple linear regression (MLR), and stepwise multiple linear regression are some of the variants of linear regression. However, these methods have now been replaced by multivariate chemometric methods which try to explain an extended set of variables by means of reduced number new latent variables possessing the maximum amount of information relevant to the problem. These latent variables are orthogonal and hence can be used in multiple linear regressions. This method includes Principal component analysis (PCA), Partial least square analysis (PLS), Principal component regression (PCR), etc. Additionally, the non-linear methods also called as pattern recognition methods based on the principle of analogy are used for the detection of the distance or closeness within large amount of multivariate data. These methods search for structural features such as the presence or absence of certain groups, number of a certain type of atom, or mass spectral-fragmentation so that new compounds can be classified as similar or dissimilar to the members of the existing classes. Examples of pattern recognition methods include Cluster analysis, artificial neural networks (ANNs) and k-nearest neighbor (kNN) method. Table summarizes all the various types of statistical methods. Since describing each method in details is beyond the scope of this chapter, as an example we have only summarized MLR method here.

The main steps in MLR based QSAR analyses are as follows:

Data Set

The data set used in the investigation will mainly depend upon the type of investigation. For example, Wang *et al.,* (2010) used 82 estrogen receptor (ER) ligands, primarily represented by 2-arylnaphthalene and 2-arylquinoline derivatives, which were collected from the literature. For QSAR analysis, negative logarithm of IC_{50} values, i.e., pIC_{50} (M), were generated. Moreover, molecular descriptors correlating with the selectivity (S) of binding affinity of ligands between ERα and ERβ were considered. Similarly, in another study a dataset of 261 nucleoside analogues comprising 96 actives and 165 inactives and measured in a single, consistent cytotoxic assay were assembled. The 96 actives included the compounds with $IC_{50} < 200$ μM, while the inactives included compounds with $IC_{50} \geq 200$ μM.

The structures of ligands could be constructed by using Fujitsu Scigress Explorer Ultra v7.7.0.47 http://www.dl4all.com/soft-ware/113790-fujitsu-scigress-explorer-ultra-v77047. html] or Hyper-Chem [http://www.hyper.com/] software. However, the chemical structures of known drugs could be retrieved through any of the databases described earlier in section 2a. The 3-D structures of selected ligands are cleaned up and subjected to energy minimization using Molecular Mechanics (MM2) for optimizing the molecules up to its lowest stable energy state.

Descriptor Generation

A large number of molecular descriptors are available and used. The numerical descriptors are responsible for encoding key characteristics of the structure of the molecules and can be categorized as electronic, geometric, hydrophobic, and topological characters. The molecular descriptors for each compound can be calculated using the various available tools like HyperChem or Dragon program packages. Table 35.1 lists some of the widely used tools to calculate various descriptors.

Table 35.1 List of some widely used tools to calculate molecular descriptors.

S. No.	Tools name	Authors	Web address	Methods
1	Dragon	Tetko *et al.,* 2005	http://www.talete.mi.it/products/dragon_description. Htm	computation of molecular descriptors
2	HyperChem	Hyperchem 8.0	http://www.chemistry software.com/hyperchem/	Quantum chemical calculations, molecular mechanics, and dynamics
3	PaDEL-Descriptor	Yap CW., 2011	http://padel.nus.edu.sg/software/padeldescriptor/	calculating molecular descriptors and fingerprints
4	PreADMET	Lee *et al.,* 2003	http://preadme.bmdrc.org/	Molecular Descriptor Calculation, Drug-likeness Prediction, ADME Prediction and Toxicity prediction
5	Open3D QSAR	P. Tosco, T. Balle, 2011	http://preadme. bmdrc.org/	Chemometric analysis of molecular interaction fields
6	BlueDesc	Georg Hinselmann	http://www.ra. cs.unituebingen. de/software/bluedesc/welcome_e.html	QSAR/QSPR modeling
7	ADRIANA. Code	commercial	http://www. molecular networks.com/ products/adrianacode	Calculate molecular descriptors
8	GenerateMD	commercial	http://www.chemaxon.com/jchem/doc/user/GenerateMD .html	Molecular descriptors based on 2D structure and fingerprints

Table 35.1 *Contd...*

S. No.	Tools name	Authors	Web address	Methods
9	MODEL	Z.R. Li *et al.,* 2007	http://jing.cz3.nus.edu.sg/cgi-bin/ model/model.cgi	Calculate molecular descriptors based on 3D structure of a molecule
10	Molconn-Z	commercial	http://www.molconn.com/products.html	2D molecular descriptors comparison
11	PRODRG	A. W. Schüttel-kopf and D. M. F. van Aalten, 2004.	http://davapc1.bioch.dundee.ac.uk/prodrg/	Generates coordinates and molecular topologies

Table 35.2 List of widely used QSAR tools.

S. No.	Tools name	Authors	Web address	Methods
1	Molconn-Z	commercial	http://www.molconn.com/products.html	2D molecular descriptors comparison
2	Codessa pro		http://www.codessa-pro.com/	
3	Dragon	Tetko *et.al.,* 2005	http://www.talete.mi.it/products/dragon_description.htm	computation of molecular descriptors
4	PreADMET	Lee *et al.,* 2003	http://preadme.bmdrc. org/	Molecular Descriptor Calculation, Drug-likeness Prediction, ADME Prediction and Toxicity prediction
5	CORINA	Commercial	http://www.molecular-networks.com/products/ corina	Convert 2D structures into 3D
6	HQSAR	Hurst T, Heritage T, 1997	http://tripos.com/index.php?family=modules,SimplePage,,,&page=HQSAR	Fragment-based structure-activity relationships
7	QSAR with CoMFA	Commercial	http://tripos.com/index.php?family=modules,SimplePage,,,&page=QSAR_CoMFA	Molecular descriptors, and performs statistical analyses

Statistical Analysis using MLR

MLR is also known as the linear free-energy relationship (LFER) method and represents an extension of the simple regression analysis to more than one dimension. MLR creates QSAR equations by performing model multivariable regression computations to classify the dependence of a drug property on several or all of the descriptors under analysis. The likelihood of possible correlation is verified through the values of multiple correlation coefficient (r), Student's t-value; Fisher's F ratio, standard deviation (s), and through independent tests like the leave-one-out (LOO) method. MLR models have been frequently used as mathematical equations which can relate chemical structure with the inhibitory action. Recently, a multiple linear regression (MLR) procedure was used to model the relationships between molecular descriptors and the antibacterial activity of the benzimidazole derivatives.

In any multiple linear-based QSAR method, it is desirable that the variables included in the model are not interrelated to each other. Highly correlated variables clearly contain redundant information that might be more effectively encoded by a single variable. Further, and most importantly from the view point of a QSAR model, correlated independent variables lead to multicollinearity, which can cause problems in interpreting the individual estimated coefficients. One very useful and informative approach of avoiding multicollinearity is known as orthogonal descriptors technique suggested by Randic (Randić 1991).

Validation of QSAR Models

Validation of the final model with compounds, which are not part of the training set, is crucial but necessary step to ensure generalization, and also of great relevance to future QSAR studies. The reliability of a QSAR model depends on how well the model can predict the activity of compounds outside the training set rather than how well the model reproduces the biological activity of compounds included in the model. The good quality QSAR model also depends on many other factors, such as the quality of biological data, the choice of descriptors and statistical methods. Any QSAR modelling should ultimately lead to statistically robust models capable of making accurate and reliable predictions of biological activities of new compounds.

For validation of QSAR models, different strategies are usually adopted namely:

Internal validation or Cross validation (CV)

This procedure is repeated n number of times until all compounds have been excluded and predicted once, i.e., Leave-one-out (LOO) method. Analogously, leaving more than one molecule of the dataset at a time is termed as leave-n-our or leave-many-out CV method.

Correlation coefficient (r)

It is a measure of the degree of linearity of the relationship. In an ideal situation the correlation coefficient approaches unity, but in real situation, any value above 0.9 is acceptable due to the complexity of biological data. Correlation coefficients for the variables in a dataset are compiled in a correlation matrix, which shows the relationship of one descriptor with another. The increase in r caused by adding new variable signifies over-fitting of the data.

The coefficient of multiple determinants is known as Pearson's correlation coefficient (r^2), which is the squared correlation coefficient and informs about how well the model reproduces the experimental data. However, an r^2 close to 1 does not mean that the model perfect; the addition of any new descriptor to the model induces an ever-increasing of r^2, even if the newly added descriptor does not contribute to the model.

Bootstrapping

Another technique, that can be used along with cross-validation to evaluate the robustness and the statistical confidence of the QSAR model. It involves simulating a large number of datasets which are of the same size as original dataset. Since, this method demands heavy computation power with relatively smaller gains as compared to cross-validation, the technique is not very attractive.

Randomization or y-scrambling

A rigorous alternative to cross-validation and bootstrapping in which the biological activity values are re-assigned arbitrarily to different molecules in the same data set, and a new regression is performed. The randomization test analyses the ability of the statistical model to derive real structure-activity relationships.

Table 35.3 List of some statistical method for QSAR study.

Statistical Method		Study	Authors
Linear Regression Analysis (RA)	Simple linear regression	Quantitative structure-activity relationships for the toxicity of selected shale oil components to mixed marine bacteria	Warne MS. *et al.*, 2011
		Design and synthesis of anti-MRSA benzimidazolylbenzene-sulphonamides. QSAR studies for prediction of antibacterial activity	González-Chávez MM. *et al.*, 2011
	Multiple linear regression (MLR)	*In silico* Comparative Study and Quantitative Structure-activity Relationship Analysis of Some Structural and Physiochemical Descriptors of Elvitegravir Analogs	Satpathy R, Ghosh S. - 2011
		In Silico prediction of estrogen receptor subtype binding affinity and selectivity using statistical methods and molecular docking with 2-arylnaphthalenes and 2-arylquinolines	Wang Z. *et al.*, 2010
	Stepwise multiple linear regression	Prediction of biliary excretion in rats and humans using molecular weight and quantitative structure-pharmacokinetic relationships	Yang X. *et al.*, 2009
		Comparative QSAR studies of CYP1A2 inhibitor flavonoids using 2D and 3D descriptors	Roy K, Roy PP. - 2008
	Principal component analysis (PCA)	Dibenzazecine compounds with a novel dopamine/5HT2A receptor profile and 3D-QSAR analysis	Hamacher A. *et al.*, 2006

Table 35.3 *Contd...*

Statistical Method		Study	Authors
Multivariate data analysis		An integrated approach to epitope analysis II: A system for proteomic-scale prediction of immunological characteristics	Bremel RD, Homan EJ. 2010
	Principal components regression (PCR)	A QSAR study of HIV protease inhibitors using theoretical descriptors	Basak SC. *et al.*, 2010
		QSARs for 6-azasteroids as inhibitors of human type 1 5alpha-reductase: prediction of binding affinity and selectivity relative to 3-BHSD	Bakken GA, Jurs PC. *et al.*, 2001
	Partial least square analysis (PLS)	Quantitative structure-pharmacokinetic parameters relationships (QSPKR) analysis of antimicrobial agents in humans using simulated annealing k-nearest-neighbor and partial least-square analysis methods	Ng C. *et al.*, 2004
	Genetic function approximation (GFA)	QSAR studies on chalcones and flavonoids as anti-tuberculosis agents using genetic function approximation (GFA) method	Sivakumar PM. *et al.*, 2007
		Quantitative structure-activity relationship studies on 1-aryl-tetrahydroisoquinoline analogs as active anti-HIV agents	Chen KX. *et al.*, 2008
	Genetic partial least squares (G/PLS)	3D-QSAR investigation of synthetic antioxidant chromone derivatives by molecular field analysis	Samee W. *et al.*, 2008
		Statistical deconvolution of enthalpic energetic contributions to MHC-peptide binding affinity	Davies MN. *et al.*, 2006
Pattern recognition	Cluster analysis	Characterization of diversity in toxicity mechanism using *in vitro* cytotoxicity assays in quantitative high throughput screening	Huang R. *et al.*, 2008
		A structure-odour relationship study using EVA descriptors and hierarchical clustering	Takane SY, Mitchell JB. 2004

Table 35.3 *Contd...*

Statistical Method		Study	Authors
	Artificial neural networks (ANNs)	Computational neural network analysis of the affinity of lobe line and tetrabenazine analogs for the vesicular monoamine transporter-2	Zheng F. *et al.,* 2008
		Prediction of genome wide conserved epitope profiles of HIV-1: classifier choice and peptide representation	Xiao Y, Segal MR. 2005
	k-nearest neighbor (*k*NN)	Development of quantitative structure-binding affinity relationship models based on novel geometrical chemical descriptors of the protein-ligand interfaces	Zhang S. *et al.,* 2006
		Modeling liver-related adverse effects of drugs using k-nearest neighbor quantitative structure-activity relationship method	Rodgers AD. *et al.,* 2006

Table 35.4 Image, molecular/chemical formula of drug, drug name, receptor name for which the drug was made and the author reference.

Image	Molecular formula of drug	Drug name	Receptor	Reference
	$C_{12}H_9F_3N_2O_2$	Leflunomide	Dihydroorotate dehydrogenase	Shun-Lai Li *et al.,* (2011) 3D-QSAR Studies on a Series of Dihydroorotate Dehydrogenase Inhibitors: Analogues of the Active Metabolite of Leflunomide. *Int. J. Mol. Sci.* **12:** 2982-2993.
	$C_{32}H_{31}BrN_2O_2$	TMC207	Diarylquinoline	Jerome Guillemont *et al.,* (2011). Diarylquinolines, synthesis pathways and quantitative structure–activity relationship studies leading to the discovery of TMC207. *Future Med. Chem.* **3(11):** 1345-1360

Table 35.4 *Contd…*

Image	Molecular formula of drug	Drug name	Receptor	Reference
	$C_6H_4N_2O_5$	2,4-Dinitrophenol (DNP)	Cathepsin B	Zhigang Zhou *et al.*, (2010). QSAR Models for Predicting Cathepsin B Inhibition by Small Molecules: Continuous and Binary QSAR Models to Classify Cathepsin B Inhibition Activities of Small Molecules. *J Mol Graph Model.* **28(8):** 714–727.
	$C_{13}H_{14}O_4$	1'-acetoxy-chavicol acetate	Myeloid leukemia cells	Takashi MISAWA *et al.*, (2008). Structural Development of Benzhydrol-Type 1_-Acetoxychavicol Acetate (ACA) Analogs as Human Leukemia Cell-Growth Inhibitors Based on Quantitative Structure–Activity Relationship (QSAR) Analysis. *Chem. Pharm. Bull.* **56(10):** 1490-1495

Suggested Readings

1. Accelrys Available Chemicals Directory (ACD)

2. Adam BL, Qu Y, Davis JW, Ward MD, Clements MA, Cazares LH, Semmes OJ, Schellhammer PF, Yasui Y, Feng Z, Wright GL Jr (2002). Serum protein fingerprinting coupled with a pattern-matching algorithm distinguishes prostate cancer from benign prostate hyperplasia and healthy men. *Cancer Res.* **62(13):** 3609-14.

3. Adam BL, Vlahou A, Semmes OJ, Wright GL Jr (200). Proteomic approaches to biomarker discovery in prostate and bladder cancers. *Proteomics.* **1(10):** 1264-70.

4. Anand K, Ziebuhr J, Wadhwani P, Mesters JR, Hilgenfeld R (2003). Coronavirus Main Proteinase (3CLpro) Structure: Basis for Design of Anti-SARS Drugs. *Science.* **300(5626):** 1763-7.

5. Appelt K, Bacquet RJ, Bartlett CA, Booth CL, Freer ST, Fuhry MA, Gehring MR, Herrmann SM, Howland EF and Janson CA (1991). Design of enzyme inhibitors using iterative protein crystallographic analysis. *J Med Chem.* **34(7):** 1925-34.

6. Archdeacon TJ (1994). Regression and explained variance. In: *Correlation and Regression Analysis: a Historian's Guide;* Archdeacon, T.J., Ed.; Univ of Wisconsin Press: USA, pp. 178-196.

7. Axford J (1997). Glycobiology and medicine: an introduction. *R Soc Med.* **90(5):** 260–264.

8. Bak A, Polanski J (2006). A 4D-QSAR study on anti-HIV HEPT analogues. *Bioorg Med Chem.* **14(1):** 273-9. Epub 2005 Sep 26.

9. Basak SC, Gieschen DP, Magnuson VR and Harriss DK (1982). Structure activity relationships and pharmacokinetics: a comparative study of hydrophobicity, van der Waals' volume and topological parameters. *IRCS Med. Sci.* **10:** 619.

10. Basak SC, Raychaudhury C, Roy AB and Ghosh JJ (1981). Quantitative Structure-Activity Relationship (QSAR) studies of bioactive agents using structural information indices. *Ind. J. Pharmacol.* **13:** 112.

11. Berk RA (2003). Simple Linear Regression. In: Regression Analysis: A Constructive Critique; Berk, R.A., Ed.; SAGE Publications Ltd: London, pp. 21-38.

12. Berk RA (2003). The Formalities of Multiple Regression. In: Regression Analysis: A Constructive Critique; Berk, R.A., Ed.; SAGE Publications Ltd: London, pp. 103-110.

13. Berman HM, Westbrook J, Feng Z, Gilliland G, Bhat TN, Weissig H, Shindyalov IN, Bourne PE (2000). The Protein Data Bank. *Nucleic Acids Res.* **28(1):** 235-42.

14. Beuth J, Ko LH, Pulverer G, Uhlenbruck G and Pichlmaier H (1994). *Int. J. Med. Microbiol. Virol. Parasitol. Infect. Dis.* **281:** 324-333.

15. Buzko OV, Bishop AC, Shokat KM (2002). Modified AutoDock for accurate docking of protein kinase inhibitors. *J Comput Aided Mol Des.* **16(2):** 113-27.

16. Carlson HA, McCammon JA (2000). Accommodating protein flexibility in computational drug design. *Mol Pharmacol.* **57(2):** 213-8.

17. Carrasco-Velar R, Padrón JA, Gálvez J (2004). Definition of a novel atomic index for QSAR: the refractotopological state. *J Pharm Pharmaceut Sci.* (www.ualberta.ca/~csps) **7(1):** 19-26.

18. Castillo-González D, Cabrera-Pérez MA, González MP, Durán-Martínez A, Saíz-Urra L and Teijeira M (2007). Telomerase inhibitory activity by stabilization of G-quartet: A QSAR approach using 2D autocorrelation descriptors. The Eleventh International Electronic Conference on Synthetic Organic Chemistry, November 1-30.

19. Chen JH, Linstead E, Swamidass SJ, Wang D, Baldi P (2007). ChemDB update-full-text search and virtual chemical space. *Bioinformatics Applications Note.* **23(17):** 2348-2351.

20. Chen X, Ji ZL, Zhi DG, Chen YZ (2002). CLiBE: a database of computed ligand binding energy for ligand-receptor complexes. *Comput Chem.* **26(6):** 661-6.

21. Congreve M, Murray CW, Blundell TL (2005). Structural biology and drug discovery. *Drug Discov Today.* **10:** 895-907.

22. Deeb O, Singh J, Varma RG, and Khadikar PV (2007). Topological modeling of antimycobacterial activity of 3-formyl rifamycin SV derivatives. ARKIVOC (xiv) 141-162.

23. DiMasi JA, Hansen RW, Grabowski HG (2003). The price of innovation: new estimates of drug development costs. *Journal of Health Economics.* **22:** 151-185.

24. Dixit KS, Mitra SN (2002). Bioinformatics in Drug Discovery. *CRIPS.* **3:** 2-6.

25. Dowell RD, Jokerst RM, Day A, Eddy SR, Stein L (2001). The Distributed Annotation System. *BMC Bioinformatics.* 2:7

26. Erickson J, Neidhart DJ, VanDrie J, Kempf DJ, Wang XC, Norbeck DW, Plattner JJ, Rittenhouse JW, Turon M, Wideburg N, et al., (1990). Design, activity, and 2.8 A crystal structure of a C2 symmetric inhibitor complexed to HIV-1 protease. *Science.* **249(4968):** 527-33.

27. Ernst B & Magnani JL (2009): From carbohydrate leads to glycomimetic drugs. *Nature Reviews Drug Discovery.* **8:** 661-677.

28. Fassihi A and Sabet R (2008). QSAR Study of p56lck Protein Tyrosine Kinase Inhibitory Activity of Flavonoid Derivatives Using MLR and GA-PLS. *Int. J. Mol. Sci.* **9:** 1876-1892.

29. González MP, Helguera AM, Medina R, and Ruiz RM (2004). QSAR with Constitutional Descriptors for the Herbicidal Properties of Fluorovinyloxy-acetamides, *Internet Electron. J. Mol. Des.* **3:** 200-208.

30. Good AC, Ewing TJ, Gschwend DA, Kuntz ID (1995). New molecular shape descriptors: application in database screening. *Comput. Aided Mol. Des.* **9:** 1-12.

31. Goodsell DS, Morris GM, Olson AJ (1996). Automated docking of flexible ligands: applications of AutoDock. *J Mol Recognit.* **9(1):** 1-5.

32. Goto S, Okuno Y, Hattori M, Nishioka T, Kanehisa M (2002). LIGAND: database of chemical compounds and reactions in biological pathways. *Nucl. Acids Res.* **30:** 402-404.

33. Gozalbes R, Doucet JP, Derouin F (2002). Application of topological descriptors in QSAR and drug design: history and new trends. *Curr Drug Targets Infect Disord.* **2(1):** 93–102.

34. Gupta L, Patel A, Karthikeyan C and Trivedi P (2010). QSAR studies on dihydro-alkoxy-benzyl-oxopyrimidines (DABOs) derivatives, a new series of potent, broad-spectrum non-nucleoside reverse transcriptase inhibitors. *Journal of Current Pharmaceutical Research.* **01:** 19-25.

35. Hansch C, Leo L. and Hoekman D (1995). Monograph: Exploring the QSAR. Hydrophobic, Electronic, and Steric Constants, Heller S. R., Ed. ACS, Washington, DC.

36. Hawkins CA, Watson C, Yan Y, Gong B, Wemmer DE (2001). Structural analysis of the binding modes of minor groove ligands comprised of disubstituted benzenes. *Nucleic Acids Res.* **29(4):** 936-42.

37. Helguera AM, Rodríguez-Borges JE, García-Mera X, Fernández F, Cordeiro MN (2007). Probing the anticancer activity of nucleoside analogues: a QSAR model approach using an internally consistent training set. *J Med Chem.* **50(7):** 1537-45.

38. Hindle SA, Rarey M, Buning C, Lengaue T (2002). Flexible docking under pharmacophore type constraints. *J Comput Aided Mol Des.* **16(2):** 129-49. http://accelrys.com/products/databases/sourcing/available-chemicals-directory.html.

39. Hyde RM, Livingstone DJ (1988). Perspectives in QSAR: computer chemistry and pattern recognition. *J Comput Aided Mol Des.* **2(2):** 145-55.

40. Ji ZL, Han LY, Yap CW, Sun LZ, Chen X, Chen YZ (2003). Drug Adverse Reaction Target Database (DART): Proteins related to adverse drug reactions. *Drug Saf.* **26(10):** 685-90.

41. Karelson M (2000). Molecular Descriptors in QSAR/QSPR. John Wiley & Sons, New York.

42. Keseru GM (2001). A virtual high throughput screen for high affinity cytochrome P450cam substrates. Implications for *in silico* prediction of drug metabolism. *J Comput Aided Mol Des.* **15(7):** 649-57.

43. Kier LB & Hall LH (1999). The Kappa Indices for Modeling Molecular Shape and Flexibility. In: Topological Indices and Related Descriptors in QSAR and QSPR, Devillers, J. and A.T. Balaban (*Eds.,*). Gordon and Breach Science Publishers, The Netherlands, pp: 455-489.

44. Klebe G (2006). Virtual ligand screening: strategies, perspectives and limitations. *Drug Discov Today.* **11:** 580-94.

45. Knegtel RM, Bayada DM, Engh RA, von der Saal W, van Geerestein VJ, Grootenhuis PD (1999). Comparison of two implementations of the incremental

construction algorithm in flexible docking of thrombin inhibitors. *J Comput Aided Mol Des*. **13(2):** 167-83.

46. Knox C, Law V, Jewison T, Liu P, Ly S, Frolkis A, Pon A, Banco K, Mak C, Neveu V, Djoumbou Y, Eisner R, Guo AC, Wishart DS (2011). DrugBank 3.0: a comprehensive resource for 'omics' research on drugs. *Nucleic Acids Res*. 39 (Database issue):D1035-41.

47. Kuhlman J (1997). Drug research: from the idea to the product. *International Journal of Clinical Pharmacology and Therapeutics*. **35:** 541.

48. Kuntz ID (1992). Structure-based strategies for drug design and discovery. *Science*. **257:** 1078-1082.

49. Kuntz ID, Blaney JM, Oatley SJ, Langridge R, Ferrin TE (1982). A geometric approach to macromolecule-ligand interactions. *J Mol Biol*. **161(2):** 269-88.

50. Labute P (2000). A widely applicable set of descriptors. *J Mol Graph Model*. **18(4-5):** 464-77.

51. Maizell RE, How to find Chemical Information, 3rd edition, Wiley, New York.

52. Malik A, Firoz A, Jha V, and Ahmad S (2010). PROCARB: A Database of Known and Modelled Carbohydrate-Binding Protein Structures with Sequence-Based Prediction Tools. *Adv Bioinformatics*. **2010:** 436036.

53. Malik A, Singh H, Andrabi M, Husain SA, Ahmad S (2007). Databases and QSAR for cancer research. *Cancer Inform*. **2:** 99-111.

54. Marzilli LG, Saad JS, Kuklenyik Z, Keating KA, Xu Y (2001). Relationship of solution and protein-bound structures of DNA duplexes with the major intrastrand cross-link lesions formed on cisplatin binding to DNA. *J Am Chem Soc*. **123(12):** 2764-70.

55. Minovski N, Vračko M, Solmajer T (2011). Quantitative structure-activity relationship study of antitubercular fluoroquinolones. *Mol Divers*. **15(2):** 417-26. Epub 2010 Mar 14.

56. Mizutani MY, Tomioka N, Itai A (1994). Rational automatic search method for stable docking models of protein and ligand. *J Mol Biol*. **243(2):** 310-26.

57. Montgomery JA (1993). Purine nucleoside phosphorylase: a target for drug design. *Med. Res. Rev*. **13:** 209-228.

58. Muegge I, Oloff S (2006). Advances in virtual screening. *Drug Discov Today Tech*. **3:** 405-11.

59. Myers S & Baker A (2001). Drug discovery - an operating model for a new era. *Nature Biotechnology*. **19:** 727-730.

60. Ooms F (2000). Molecular Modeling and Computer Aided Drug Design. Examples of their Applications in Medicinal Chemistry. *Current Medicinal Chemistry*. **7:** 141-158.

61. Osterberg F, Morris GM, Sanner MF, Olson AJ, Goodsell DS (2002). Automated docking to multiple target structures: incorporation of protein mobility and structural water heterogeneity in AutoDock. *Proteins*. **46(1):** 34-40.

62. Peterangelo SC (2004). Seybold, P. G. Synergistic interactions among QSAR descriptors. *Int. J. Quant. Chem.* **96:** 1-9.

63. Pirard B & Pickett SD (2000). Classification of kinase inhibitors using BCUT descriptors. *J Chem Inf Comput Sci.* **40(6):** 1431-40.

64. Podunavac-Kuzmanović SO, Cvetković DD, Barna DJ (2009). QSAR Analysis of 2-Amino or 2-Methyl-1-Substituted Benzimidazoles Against *Pseudomonas aeruginosa*. *Int. J. Mol. Sci.* **10:** 1670-1682.

65. Raevskyv RO (1999). Molecular structure descriptors in the computer-aided design of biologically active compounds. *Russ. Chem. Rev.* **68:** 505.

66. Randić M (1991). Correlation of enthalphy of octanes with orthogonal connectivity indices. *J. Mol. Struct.* **233:** 45-59.

67. Randić M (1991). Orthogonal Molecular Descriptors. *New J. Chem.* **15(7):** 517-525.

68. Randić M (1991). Resolution of Ambiguities in Structure-Property Studies by Use of Orthogonal Descriptors. *J. Chem. Inf. Comput. Sci.* **31:** 311-320.

69. Randic M (2001). Novel shape descriptors for molecular graphs. *J Chem Inf Comput Sci.* **41(3):** 607-13.

70. Reddy MR & Erion MD (2005). Computer Aided Drug Design Strategies Used in the Discovery of Fructose 1,6-Bisphosphatase Inhibitors. *Current Pharmaceutical Design*. **11:** 283-294.

71. Rucker C, Rucker G, Meringer M (2007). y-Randomization and its variants in QSPR/QSAR. *J. Chem. Inf. Model.* **47:** 2345-2357.

72. Shao J (1996). Bootstrap model selection. *J. Am. Stat. Assoc.* **91:** 655-665.

73. Sinaÿ P (1999). Sugars slide into heparin activity. *Nature.* **398(6726):** 377-8.

74. Song CM, Lim SJ, Tong JC (2009). Recent advances in computer-aided drug design. *Briefings in bioinformatics*. **10(5):** 579-591.

75. Street AG & Mayo SL (1999). Computational protein design. *Structure.* **7(5):** R105-9.

76. Sun LZ, Ji ZL, Chen X, Wang JF, Chen YZ (2002). ADME-AP: a database of ADME associated proteins. *Bioinformatics.* **18(12):** 1699-700.

77. Todeschini R & V.Consonni V (2009). Molecular Descriptors for Chemo-informatics, (2 volumes), WILEY-VCH, Weinheim (Germany), 1257 pp.

78. Varney MD, Appelt K, Kalish V, Reddy MR, Tatlock J, *et al.,* (1994). Crystal structure-based design and synthesis of novel C-terminal inhibitors of HIV protease. *J. Med. Chem.* **37(15):** 2274-84.

79. Verma J, Khedkar VM, Coutinho EC (2010). 3D-QSAR in Drug Design - A Review. *Current Topics in Medicinal Chemistry.* **10:** 95-115.

80. Veselovsky AV, Ivanov AS (2003). Strategy of computer-aided drug design. *Curr Drug Targets Infect Disord.* **3(1):** 33-40.

81. Vigers GP, Rizzi JP (2004). Multiple active site corrections for docking and virtual screening. *J Med Chem.* **47(1):** 80-9.

82. Wang Y, Chiu JF and He QY (2005). Proteomics in Computer-Aided Drug Design. *Current Computer-Aided Drug Design.* **1:** 43-52.

83. Wang Z, Li Y, Ai C, Wang Y (2010). *In Silico* Prediction of Estrogen Receptor Subtype Binding Affinity and Selectivity Using Statistical Methods and Molecular Docking with 2-Arylnaphthalenes and 2-Arylquinolines. *Int. J. Mol. Sci.* **11:** 3434-3458.

84. Wildman SA & Crippen GM (2002). Three-dimensional molecular descriptors and a novel QSAR method. *J Mol Graph Model.* **21(3):** 161-70.

85. Xiao Z, Xiao YD, Feng J, Golbraikh A, Tropsha A, Lee KH (2002). Antitumor agents. 213. Modeling of epipodophyllotoxin derivatives using variable selection k nearest neighbor QSAR method. *J Med Chem.* **45(11):** 2294-309.

86. Xue L & Bajorath J (2000). The analysis of structure-anticancer and antiviral activity relationships for macrocyclic pyridinophanes and their analogues on the basis of 4D QSAR models (simplex representation of molecular structure). *J Chem Inf Comput Sci.* **40(3):** 801-809.

87. Yadav D, Khan F, and Srivastava S: Docking and QSAR Studies of Camptothecin Derivatives as Inhibitor of DNA Topoisomerase-I. Available from Nature Precedings <http://dx.doi.org/10.1038/ npre.2011. 5773.1> (2011).

88. Zhu F, Han B, Kumar P, Liu X, Ma X, Wei X, Huang L, Guo Y, Han L, Zheng C, Chen Y (2010). Update of TTD: Therapeutic Target Database. *Nucleic Acids Res.* 38(Database issue): D787-91.

CHAPTER 36

ELECTRONIC PRESCRIBING (eRx)

Introduction

In the present era, technology is playing an important role in human life to improve the quality of life and care. Henceforth, the advances came in medical field. There are several changes made in the treatment pattern and drugs to be prescribed, but as the advances gave the facilities, it also induced some potential hazards results as medication adverse effects and errors. Hence, to reduce the prescription errors and the adverse effects related to the drug treatment, modern techniques have contributed to give electronic prescription (e-prescription or eRx) and trying to substitute five-thousand year-old prescription technology i.e., pen and paper. Physician in developed countries thought that eRx reduces their liability and hence, they can give more focused medical care. Recent, study including 400 physicians observed that 85% of physicians think e-prescribing is a compatible and good idea, 81% said that it reduced medication errors, and 65% thought it would save time.

Need of Electronic Prescribing (eRx)

In developing countries, most of prescriptions are pen and paper based, which is an error prone process. These errors are predominately due to illegible handwriting, poor communication by phone and fax, multiple intermediaries, and duplication of data entry, wrong dosing, missed drug-drug or drug-allergy reactions, resulting in serious patient risk and adverse drug events (occurring in 5 to 18% of ambulatory patients). In a typical physician practice, physicians and pharmacists/dispensers spend a lot of time in handling phone calls and extra work from prescription issues. Elderly patients with complex health problems are at the greatest risk, because they see multiple different physicians and deal with complex medication lists. With approximately, more than 3 billion prescriptions written every year, this constitutes one of the largest paper-based processes in the India and developed countries. However, the writing of prescriptions can be streamlined and efficient by using an e-prescribing system. It is estimated by the Institute of Medicine (IOM) that approximately 7,000 deaths and 1.5 million injuries occur each year in the United States due to medication errors resulting a cost of $2 billion per year. Physicians write more than 4.5 billion prescriptions each year, out of which less than 20 percent is by electronic prescribing in the United States.

Electronic prescribing has been shown to dramatically decrease medication errors and improves efficiency, when it can create a prescription electronically and receive automated decision support during script creation.

Definitions

Electronic prescribing (e-prescription or eRx): The transmission, using electronic media, of prescription or prescription-related information between a prescriber, dispenser, pharmacy benefit manager, or health plan either directly or through an intermediary, including an eRx network. Electronic prescribing includes, but is not limited to, two-way transmissions between the point of care and the dispenser. (Faxes do not qualify as electronic prescribing).

Electronic prescribing event: For the purposes of this measure, an electronic prescribing event includes all prescriptions electronically prescribed during a patient visit.

Electronic prescribing system: A qualified eRx system is one that is capable of ALL of the following:

- Generate a complete active medication list incorporating electronic data received from applicable pharmacies and pharmacy benefit managers (PBMs), if available.

- Select medications, print prescriptions, electronically transmit prescriptions, and conduct all alerts (defined below).

- Provide information related to lower cost, therapeutically appropriate alternatives (if any).

- Provide information on formulary or tiered formulary medications, patient eligibility, and authorization requirements received electronically from the patient's drug plan (if available).

Benefits of eRx

Better ways to treat patients

- Patients benefit from increased safety, efficiency and better compliance due to lower co-pays.
- It displays patient's prior and present information in order to treat them properly. This data includes medication history, eligibility determination, and formulary coverage from the insurer, including co-pay information, prior authorization requirements and clinical decision support (including drug interactions, drug-allergies, etc.).

- It indicates if the patient is eligible for care in regards to the patient's insurance policies.
- The software serves as a decision-support tool for doctors as it makes doctors aware of patient-medication histories, patient's allergies and pharmacy-fill histories.
- It can check for appropriate dosages and duplicate forms of therapy.
- Reduction in new prescription rates which may indicate reduction in accumulation of multiple medications.
- Patient satisfaction in a process that results in fewer errors and less waiting time.
- It will also have clinical pharmacology drug reference information, including drug monographs, interaction reports and a drug identifier tool.
- *Offers True Provider Mobility*: Full mobility can be attained when using a wireless network to write or authorize prescriptions anytime from anywhere.
- Patient information protected by strict privacy and security measures.

> *The eRxs can give alerts to physicians to warn about possible undesirable or unsafe situations, including potentially inappropriate dose or route of administration of a drug, drug-drug interactions, allergy concerns or warnings and cautions by pop-up window.*

Efficient Communication of Doctor with Pharmacies

- A doctor can access renewal requests from pharmacies.
- Renew medications for multiple patients.
- Write a prescription from an often-used 'favorite' list.
- Can send eRx to a patient's pharmacy of choice (including mail-order pharmacies).
- Avoidance of unnecessary phone calls for clarification between physicians and pharmacies.
- Helps pharmacy to process electronic scripts in their system without data re-entry.

Benefits of Doctor

- Securely share patient data with other treating physicians and send/receive referrals.
- It helps physicians to address administrative duties in an efficient and timely manner.

Research and Rational Drug use

- Easier data collection of physician prescribing patterns aid in research (e.g., Rhode Island is the first state in the U.S. to begin tracking swine flu outbreaks using eRx data).
- Improved formulary compliance for health plans, pharmacy benefit managers and employers.

Electronic Prescribing (eRx) Incentive Program in Developed Countries

Medicare Improvements for Patients and Providers Act of 2008 (MIPPA) authorizes a new and separate incentive program for eligible professionals (EPs) who are successful electronic prescribers as defined by MIPPA in the United States. This new incentive program (began on 1st January 2009) is separate from quality reporting incentive program under the Physician Quality Reporting Initiative (PQRI), which was formed after the Tax Relief and Health Care Act of 2006. Eligible professionals do not need to participate in PQRI to participate in the Electronic Prescribing (eRx) Incentive Program.

A successful individual eRx prescriber is eligible to receive an incentive payment equal to 2.0% of their total estimated Medicare Part-B Physician Fee Schedule (PFS) allowed charges for covered professional services furnished during that same reporting period. For this the following criteria are to be fulfilled: must generate and report one or more eRxs associated with a patient visit, a minimum of 25 unique visits per year. Each visit must be accompanied by the eRx G8553-code attesting that during the patient visit at least one prescription was electronically prescribed. Electronically generated prescriptions not associated with a denominator eligible patient visit do not count towards the minimum of 25 different eRx events. Additionally, 10% of an eligible professional's Medicare Part-B charges must be comprised of the codes in the denominator of the measure to be incentive eligible.

Note: The eRx Incentive Program requirements and measure specifications for the current program year may be different from the eRx Incentive Program requirements and measure specifications for a prior year. EPs are responsible for ensuring that they are using the eRx incentive documents for the correct program year. Beginning in 2012, Centers for Medicare and Medicaid Services (CMS) will impose penalties on physicians who aren't prescribing electronically in the United States.

Implementing Electronic Health Record, e-prescribing is Challenging, but Beneficial over Time

The European Commission investigated the qualitative socio-economic impact of interoperable Electronic Health Record *(EHR)* and e-prescribing systems in Europe, the U.S. and Israel. According to their recommendation, "Decisions to invest in EHR and e-prescribing systems should (involve the adoption of) strategies that fit their local or regional setting and be designed to succeed by meeting clearly identified, measurable needs".

The socio-economic gain to society from interoperable EHR and e-prescribing systems eventually exceed the costs, it can take an average of nine years to realize a cumulative net benefit.

How to Implement Electronic Prescribing

There are several private eRx software provider and depends on the hospitals/institute need and policies. The steps are as follows:

1. Decide whether you wish to choose stand-alone eRx software or a full EHR system which includes e-prescribing functionality (EHR system is costlier than eRx soft ware).

2. Choose an eRx software vendor. The e-prescribing vendor will need to utilize a company which supplies the electronic prescribing network (hub or gateway for transmissions). There are a few different eRx networking companies. Among the industry leaders are Surescripts (http://surescripts.com/), RxHub (http://www.rxhub.net/index.html), and ProxyMed (http://www.proxymed.com/).

3. Install an internet connection; high speed is highly recommended.

4. Purchase hardware such as desktop PC's, laptops, and other accessories.

Disadvantages

Unfortunately, the economic benefits are not evenly distributed. Payors receive the major benefit, but incur no cost in buying or implementing the systems. As a result, providers are concerned about the cost of buying, installing, implementing and supporting a system, and the current lack of reimbursement for costs, time, and resources. They are also concerned about the increase in user time that results in initial reduced productivity, as well as the increased time required to review warnings, alerts and recommendations. In addition, electronic prescribing is still not considered a routine standard of practice.

Strategies to Improve eRx use

Economic Incentives

It includes grants and loan programs, reimbursement for utilization, pay-for-performance programs, reductions in malpractice insurance premiums and group discounts from healthcare IT suppliers.

Policy incentives and programs: It includes accreditation programs, certification of inpatient and ambulatory healthcare set up and electronic prescribing systems, national e-prescribing standards, further, refinement of tax exemptions to allow other organizations to help defray these costs.

Educational campaigns: These are to increase awareness for physicians, pharmacists and the public to increase demand.

Evidence Supporting the Criterion of the Quality Measure

eRx is still is in the infancy stage. A number of pilot studies and observations have been performed. Overall evidence suggests reduction of adverse drug events, reduction of unnecessary utilization, and improved patient safety, but still there is need of high quality evidence. Some of the evidences are as follows:

- Roland *et al.,* (1985). Evaluation of computer assisted repeat prescribing program in a general practice. *British Medical Journal* (Clin Res Ed). **291(6493):** 456-458. The study showed that Electronic Medical Records with electronic prescribing saved provider time and reduced costs.

- Corley (2003). Electronic prescribing: a review of costs and benefits. *Topics in Health Information Management.* **24(1):** 29-38. Cost savings was estimated from reduction of adverse drug events following implementation of electronic prescribing.

- Teich *et al.,* (2004). Electronic prescribing: Toward maximum value and rapid adoption. eHealth Initiative, Washington, D.C. in 2004. It suggested that electronic prescribing could improve safety, quality, efficiency, and cost of medical care.

- Hillestad *et al.,* (2005). Can electronic medical record systems transform health care? Potential health benefits, savings and costs. *Health Affairs* **24(5):** 1103-1117. This study reported that two-thirds of the approximately 8 million adverse drug events that occur in the outpatient setting would be avoided through the widespread use of computerized order entry (CPOE).

- Middleton (2005). The value of health information technology in clinical practice. Pennsylvania eHealth Initiative, Harrisburg. Dr. Middleton discusses the value of ambulatory computerized order entry (ACPOE). A model was developed based on data derived from HIT implementation in the Partners Healthcare System. When applied nationally, this model predicts a potential savings of $44 billion and the prevention of 2 million adverse drug events per year.

- Bell & Friedman (2005). E-Prescribing and the Medicare Modernization Act of 2003. *Health Affairs.* **24(5):** 1159-1169. This article discusses the potential impact that e-Prescribing could have on improving patient safety by decreasing adverse drug events as well as the cost benefits. Version 2.0 11/13/09 Page 4 of 4.

- Shekelle P, Morton S, Keeler E (2006). Costs and benefits of health information technology. Evidence Report/Technology Assessment, AHRQ. 132. Electronic prescribing is widely believed to improve accuracy of the prescription process and thereby reduce potential for medical errors and increase health care quality.

- Schade *et al.,* (2006). e-Prescribing, efficiency, quality: Lessons from the computerization of UK family practice. *Journal of American Medical Informatics Association.* **13(5):** 470-475. Computerized prescription system is reported to have favorable impact in health practice.

Suggested Readings

1. http://www.cms.hhs.gov/ERxIncentive/06_E-Prescribing_Measure.asp#TopOfPage

2. http://www.eprescriptionservices.com/

3. http://www.cms.hhs.gov/pqri

4. http://www.getrxconnected.org/aad

5. http://www.aad.org/pm/hit/eprescribing/

6. http://www.cms.hhs.gov/erxincentive/

7. http://www.cms.hhs.gov/ERxIncentive/Downloads/Claims-BasedReportingPrinciplesforeRx111309(2).pdf

8. Pat Hale. Electronic Prescribing Update. HIMSS fact sheet. The Healthcare Information and Management Systems Society (HIMSS). http://www.himss.org

CHAPTER 37

MEDICATION RECONCILIATION

Introduction

Medication safety is a challenging job in the healthcare system in India as well as abroad, due to frequent occurrence of medication errors and Adverse Drug Events (ADEs). Medication errors and ADEs are common occurrences, but preventable during patient's intervention. Surveys have estimated that 40% of the medication errors are due to the inadequate reconciliation during the admission, transfer and discharge of patients which further leading to the harm in about of 20% of the cases. Medication reconciliation is a formal process and integral part for creating the most complete and accurate medication list to improve medication safety among patients. By medical reconciliation, we can compare a list of the patient's current medication with the list in the patient record or medication orders. Medication reconciliation refers to a process that seeks to assure that the medications, which a patient is supposed to take, are the same as what they are actually taking. Hence, it is stressed to make it as the essential process among healthcare providers at various patient care transitions, so as to decrease medication errors, which are responsible for adverse drug events. To reduce errors and harm associated with loss of medication information, as patients transfer among community-based and hospital providers, medication reconciliation is an effective process. According to National Coordinating Council (NCC) on medication error reporting and prevention defines adverse drug events as any preventable event that may cause or lead to inappropriate use or patient harm, while the medication is in the control of the healthcare professional, patient, or consumer.

Among the important contributors of adverse drug events, medication discre-pancies are an important among hospitalized and recently discharged patients and for this reason, the Joint Commission designated inpatient medication reconciliation as a National Patient Safety Goal in 2005. This reconciliation is being done to avoid medication errors such as omissions, duplication, dosing errors or drug interactions.

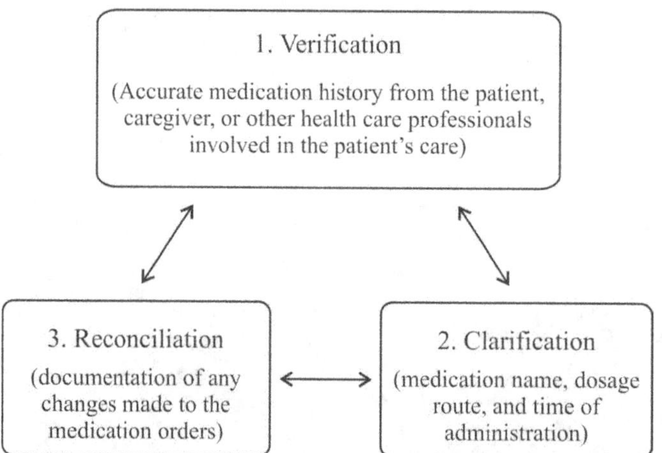

Reasons for the Necessitating Medication Reconciliation

Various reasons for the need of the medication reconciliation includes patient, physician and nurses factors along with patient's health records handling. Among patient factors, the various reasons are lack of knowledge of their medications, work burden on the physician and the nurses and lack of integrations of the health records.

This constitutes five steps which are as follows:

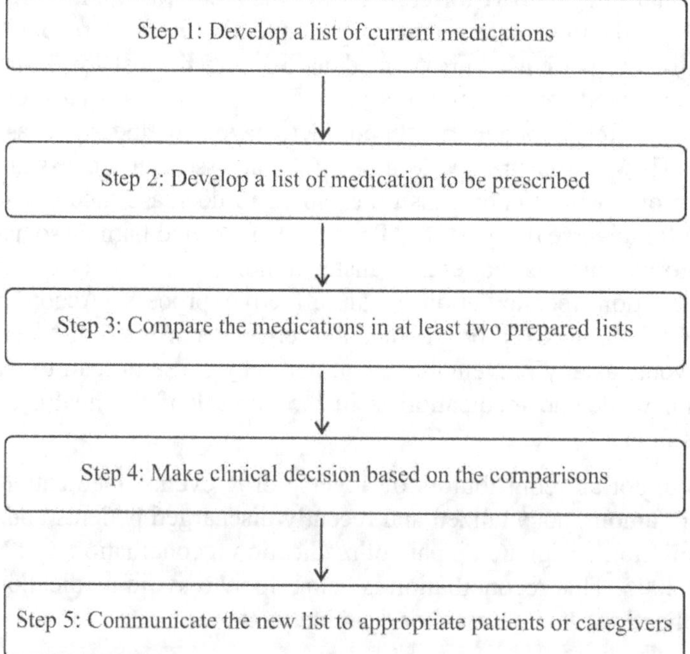

Medication Information

A list of all prescribed medications should be prepared for the medication reconciliation. Medication means, it involved all the prescription/non-prescription medications, herbals, vitamins, nutritional supplements, over the counter drugs, vaccines, diagnostic and contrast agents, radioactive medications, parental nutrition, blood derivatives and intravenous solutions.

Medication Reconciliation helps to avoid Errors

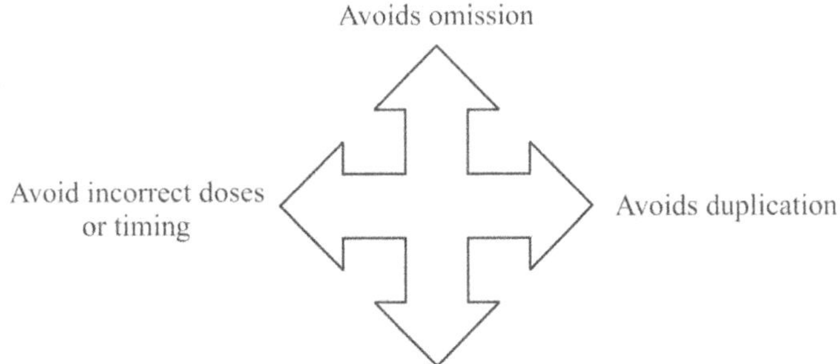

Different Types of the Medication Errors that can be Reduced through Effective Medication Reconciliation

- Discontinued medications that are continued in error in the hospital and upon discharge
- Omitting a medication
- Failure to restart a medication that has been placed on hold
- Failure to discontinue contraindicated home medications
- Failure to resolve discrepancies in dosages or route

Assigning Responsibility for Each Step of the Three-Step Process is Crucial to Success

There comes the collaborative role of nurses, pharmacists and the physician, which includes gathering the information about medication and then comparing the medication order to the history and/or current medication list for transfers and discharge. Lastly, resolving any discrepancies that exist between the medication history (or current medication list for transfers and discharge) and the medication orders, can also be done by the nurse, the physician and/or the pharmacist.

Medication History and Documentation

The basic step of medication reconciliation is to record and analyse accurately patients prescribed or non-prescribed medications history. All the prescription medications, over the counter and herbal medications on the history form, should be documented, along with the dose, route, frequency, when was the last dose and why the patient is taking it. Afterwards, place the medication list in a readily accessible, consistent location in the medical record.

Comparing Medication History and Orders

Nurse or a pharmacist compares the medication history and the physician orders and note the omissions, (*a medication that appears on the history but not on the order and has no documented reasons for discontinuation*), or changes in dose, frequency or route. On admission, follow the steps above to collect the patient's history. On transfer and discharge, medication history taken on admission and the current list of medications, often referred to as the medication administration record (MAR) and compare this to the physician orders.

Resolving Discrepancy

Ethically, it becomes a moral responsibility to resolve the discrepancy with an order or provide an explanation for the omission. It constitutes the process in which the physician can be notified by phone, computer or page to resolve the discrepancies. Documentation to resolve the discrepancy will either be an explanation on the reconciliation form or in another location designated in the chart or a new physician order.

Approaches to Medication Reconciliation

Paper Based

Simplest and fastest, but associated inaccuracy along with high cost and increased time consumption. Apart from this, it also relies on the patients memory which can be unreliable, handwriting problem, difficult to understand the prohibited abbreviations, along with incomplete knowledge regarding drug interactions, allergy. Too long process and incomplete prescription data are the different problems being faced by the pharmacists and physicians.

Computerized Monitoring System

It has been seen that this system has the potential to prevent the adverse drug events by 28 to 95%. Electronic medication reconciliation solutions are being marketed but with the limitations that they tend to emphasize only on the one aspect of the medication reconciliation process like they decrease the pharmacy errors etc. The medication reconciliation solution is a web-based application which automates the process of creating, managing, and reconciling a patient's list of medications at every stage of their movement through the hospital. It integrates data from the HIS and outside prescription history data with tools for drug identification and interaction checking, providing comprehensive management of the patient medication list.

e-Prescription

It is an electronic technique of prescription being developed for safe and fast prescriber's ability for an accurate, error-free and understandable prescription which may be directly send to a pharmacy from the prescriber. Now a day, it is found more accurate prescriptions, finding the appropriate medication, simple eRx refill processes and drug information for physicians and patients as compared to paper based prescription method and hence, improved patient safety.

Medication Reconciliation at Transition Points

1. *Admission:* It involves comparing the home medication to physician admission orders.
2. *Intrahospital transfer:* It involves comparing the medication history and current medication lists to physician transfer medication orders.
3. *Discharge:* It involves comparing the admission reconciliation list and current medication lists to physician discharge medication orders.

Steps in Medication Reconciliation in a Hospitalized Patient

- Obtaining and verifying the patients medication history
- Documenting the patients medication history
- Writing orders for the hospital medication regimen
- Creating a medication administration record

Steps in Medication Reconciliation at Discharge

- Determining the post discharge medication regimen
- Developing discharge instructions for the patient for home medications
- Educating the patient
- Transmitting the medication lists to follow up physician

Evidence of Outcome of Related to Inadequate Medication Reconciliation

In the outpatient's settings, it has been found by Ernst and colleagues that during prescription renewal, medication discrepancies was found in the 26.3% of patients. Similarly, Miller *et al.,* had reported that during patient records of an ambulatory family practice, 76% of patients had prescribed medications, 87% of the charts had incomplete or no documentation of those medications. When medical reconciliation process, by introducing a chart was done, which enlisted all the medications ordered, found that 82% of charts had complete prescription medication documentation.

In acute inpatient settings, a study conducted by the Bayley *et al.,* identified the common discrepancies in medication history from ambulatory to inpatient care were omission of the medication orders, altered doses or incomplete allergy histories. Apart from this, different studies documented 38% discrepancy rate in newly hospitalized patient and the most common discrepancy was omission of medication and with the introduction of the medication reconciliation process, there was a reduction in discrepancies from 70% to the 15%.

In ICU settings, Pronovost *et al.,* found that there is a need to change the discharge orders in 94% of the cases and implementations of the paper based medication tracking system, the error rate of the discharge medication orders was reduced to zero.

Similarly at discharge, Moore *et al.,* demonstrated that 42% had one or more errors in the discharge medication order, mostly they were not restarted, which include most commonly the cardiovascular drugs (36.4%), then gastrointestinal (27.3%) and then pulmonary medications (13.6%).

Evidence Regarding the usefulness of the Medical Reconciliation

In a study conducted by Whittington J, it was reported that a series of interventions, including medication reconciliation, introduced over a seven-month period, successfully decreased the rate of medication errors by 70% and reduced adverse drug events by over 15%.

In another study, conducted by Michels RD, the utilization of pharmacy technicians to initiate the reconciling process by obtaining medical histories for the scheduled surgical population reduced potential adverse drug events by 80% within three months of implementation.

A successful reconciling process also reduces work and re-works associated with the management of medication orders. After implementation, nursing time at admission was reduced by over 20 minutes per patient. The amount of time that pharmacists were involved in discharge was reduced by over 40 minutes.

Barriers of Medication Reconciliation

- It could be considered as an additional work by the staff, hence developing the forms and the system to ensure that the process is completed reliably each time will require some time. It has been shown in the long run, reconciling medications saves time for physicians, nurses, and pharmacists apart from reduction in the opportunity for errors and the associated adverse events that can lead to harm.

- Physician may object and say "Isn't this the physician's job?" As a whole it is a team process and all disciplines must be involved and complete portions of the process, similarly the patient can also play a key role in facilitating the verification and clarification steps.
- Fear of change, all change is difficult.
- Communication breakdown, organizations have not been successful when they failed to communicate with staff about the importance of reconciling medications, as well as the ongoing teaching of new staff.
- Physician and staff "partial buy-in".

In order to enlist support and engage staff, it is important to share baseline data as to how reliable the existing process is in reconciling medications.

Steps to be taken Encourage Implementations of the Medical Reconciliation Process

Properly define the steps in the medication reconciliation process, which includes collection of medication history along with the clarifying the medications and dosages and them reconcile and document any changes.

Healthcare professionals should be adequately given proper training along with the proper designing of the education programs for the medication reconciliation process implementations. Standardized forms to be used and time for completion frame and regular monitor check to keep while implementing this whole process.

Suggested Readings

1. Bartick M, Baron D (2006). Medication reconciliation at Cambridge Health Alliance: experiences of a 3-campus health system in Massachusetts. *Am J Med Qual.* **21:** 304-6.

2. Bayley KB, Savitz LA, Rodiquez G, *et al.,* (2005). Barriers associated with medication information handoffs. In: Advances in patient safety: from research to implementation Vol. 3. Rockville, MD: Agency for Healthcare Research and Quality; 2005. AHRQ Publication No. 050021-3.

3. Cornish PL, Knowles SR, Marchesano R, *et al.,* (2005). Unintended medication discrepancies at the time of hospital admission. *Arch Intern Med.* **165:** 424-9.

4. Ernst ME, Brown GL, Klepser TB, *et al.,* (2001). Medication discrepancies in an outpatient electronic medical record. *Am J Health Syst Pharm.* **58:** 2072-75.

5. Gleaso KM, Groszek JM, Sullivan, *et al.,* (2004). Reconciliation of discrepancies in medication histories and admission orders of newly hospitalized patients. *Am J Health Syst Pharm.* **61:** 1689-95.

6. Haig K (2006). Medication reconciliation. *Am J Med Qual.* **21:** 299-303.

7. JCAHO, 2005 National patient safety goals. Available at: http://www.jointcommission.org/PatientSafety/NationalSafetyGoals/05_npsga.htm

8. Michels RD, Meisel S (2003). Program using pharmacy technicians to obtain medication histories. *Am J Health-Sys Pharm.* **60:** 1982-1986.

9. Miller LG, Matson CC, Rogers JC (1992). Improving prescription documentation in the ambulatory setting. *Fam Pract Res J.* **12:** 421-9.

10. Moore C, Wisnivesky J, Williams S, *et al.,* (2004). Medical errors related to discontinuity of care from an inpatient to an outpatient setting. *J Gen Intern Med.* **18(8):** 646-51.

11. Pronovost P, Hobson DB, Earsing K, *et al.,* (2004). A practical tool to reduce medication errors during patient transfer from an intensive care unit. *J Clin Outcomes Manag.* **11:** 2633.

12. Pronovost P, Weast B, Schwarz M, *et al.,* (2003). Medication reconciliation: A practical tool to reduce the risk of medication errors. *J Crit Care.* **18(4):** 201-5.

13. Rogers G, Alper E, Brunelle D, *et al.,* (2006). Reconciling medications at admission: safe practice recommendations and implementation strategies. *Jt Comm J Qual Saf.* **32:** 37-50.

14. Rozich JD, Howar d RJ, Justeson JM, *et al.,* (2004). Patient safety standardization as a mechanism to improve safety in healthcare. *Jt Comm J Qual Saf.* **30(1):** 5-14.

15. Rozich JD, Resar RK (2001). Medication safety: One organization's approach to the challenge. *JCOM.* **8(10):** 27-34.

16. Rozich JD, Resar RK, *et al.,* (2004). Standardization as a mechanism to improve safety in health care: impact of sliding scale insulin protocol and reconciliation of medications initiatives. *Joint Commission Journal on Quality and Safety.* **30(1):** 5-14.

17. Schnipper JL, Kirwin JL, Cotugno MC, *et al.,* (2006). Role of pharmacist counseling in preventing adverse drug events after hospitalization. *Arch Intern Med.* **166:** 565-71.

18. Using medication reconciliation to prevent errors (2006). *Jt Comm J Qual Patient Saf.* **32:** 230-2.

19. Whittington J, Cohen H (2004). OSF Healthcare's journey in patient safety. *Quality Management in Health Care.* **13(1):** 53-59.

CHAPTER 38

TOOLS FOR PATIENT SAFETY: PHARMACOVIGILANCE, BIOVIGILANCE, MATERIOVIGILANCE

Introduction

In the contemporary world of health management; drugs, biologicals, medical devices, transplant of organs, tissues and cells play an important role in management of disease of the patient. Efficacy and safety of all these interventional substances is tested rigorously through clinical trials before their market authorization. Post marketing surveillance in these areas is referred to as Pharmacovigilance, Biovigilance and Materiovigilance which aims at patient safety.

Drugs have been a boon for mankind since their advent in curbing the ailments though not fully but to a great extent. Drugs are indispensible part of the disease management because of pharmacological actions elicited by them to offer health benefits to the consumers. Apart from the series of the beneficial effects, possibility of adverse effects with every drug cannot be ignored. No drug in the entire armamentarium of drugs is believed to be devoid of the adverse drug reactions. According to WHO, adverse drug reaction is defined as "A response to a drug which is noxious and unintended; and occurs at doses normally used in man for the prophylaxis, diagnosis or therapy of disease, or for modification of physiological function".

Adverse drug reactions (ADR) contribute to 6.7% of hospital admissions and may also contribute to significant life threatening events. In an Indian study, it was found that 6.89% hospital admissions are attributable to ADRs and the average hospitalization cost incurred per patient was INR 6197/- (USD 150).

ADRs can be classified in several ways. According to Rawlins and Thompson classification, they can be of either type A (Augmented) or type B (Bizarre) Augmented ADRs are due to extension of active pharmacologic properties of drug. Type B ADRs also known as bizarre are either unpredictable or idiosyncratic. Some important types of ADRs are tabulated below:

Table 38.1 Types of adverse drug reactions

1	**A:** Dose related	Extension of pharmacologic effect	Prazosin induced Hypotension
2	**B:** Non dose related	Idiosyncratic reactions	Stevens Johnson Syndrome secondary to Diclofenac
3	**C:** Continuing	ADR remaining for longer time	Osteonecrosis of the jaw with bisphosphonates
4	**D:** Delayed effect	Occur after lag time	Leucopoenia after weeks after a dose of Lomustine
5	**E:** At the **End** of treatment	When drug is withdrawn	Insomnia after withdrawal of Diazepam
6	**F:** Failure	Ineffective treatment	Antibiotic resistance
7	**G:** Genetic	Involvement of genetic risk Factors	Haemolytic anaemia due to sulphonamides in G6PD deficient persons

Pharmacovigilance

Pharmacovigilance is the science and activities relating to the detection, assessment, understanding and prevention of adverse effects or any other drug-related problem where an adverse drug reaction is a response which is noxious and unintended and which occurs at doses normally used in man for the prophylaxis, diagnosis, or therapy of disease as for the modification of physiological function. The safety of medicine is under constant evaluation throughout the drug development cycle. In this process, clinical trials are conducted under controlled conditions and therefore are incapable in identifying infrequent or late emerged adverse drug reactions. Only long term surveillance of drug use can evaluate chronic toxicity after its use in diversified population like children, elderly or pregnant women along with effects in co-morbid conditions. Such post marketing surveillance is the objective of Pharmacovigilance and pivots the pathway for regulatory bodies in making the decision over the fate of the drug in market. Several times because of emergence of safety issues drugs even need to be withdrawn from the market. Market has witnessed several such withdrawals of drugs because of their safety concern. The important examples of such drugs are thalidomide (1960), Ticrynafen (1982) because of hepatitis, Alpidem (1996), Pemoline (2005), because of suicidal risks and Efalizumab (2009) because of progressive multifocal leucoencephalopathy. Few recent examples are Sibutramine (2010) and Rosiglitazone (2010).

It is crucial to ascertain the safety of drug in every country because of diversity in several factors. Like drugs used, drug processing, drug delivery systems, races, genetics, diet, tradition of people, use of traditional and herbal medicines. The word pharmakon means "drug" in Greek and vigilare means "to keep watch" in Latin giving rise to term Pharmacovigilance.

Birth of Pharmacovigilance

Collection of data of adverse drug reactions dates back to early 19th century especially for vaccines but systematic and stringent system for collection of adverse drug reactions started only after the Thalidomide Tragedy in 1960s. Thalidomide was first marketed in the late 1950s as a sedative and was used in the treatment of morning sickness in pregnant women. Extensive marketing of the drug was started in 1956 for respiratory infections. Later on, use of thalidomide was extended to indications like morning sickness, insomnia. More than 10,000 pregnant women who consumed thalidomide gave birth to offsprings having phocomelia. Majority of the children born with this congenital abnormality were in Germany.

In 1961, USFDA started systematic formal collection of reports on adverse drug reactions and set a gold standard. USFDA has started a Kelsey award since 2010 after the name of Frances Oldham Kelsey who stopped the sale of thalidomide in the United States.

Sources of Data in Pharmacovigilance

Information from many sources is used for detecting signal in pharmacovigilance in order to ensure the safe use of drugs. Sources of ADR data are depicted in figure below

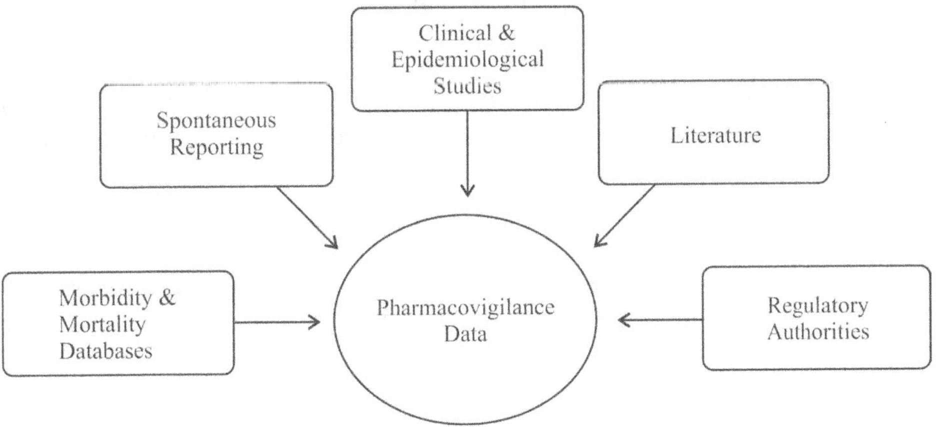

Spontaneous reporting is the backbone of pharmacovigilance to generate sufficient data for risk benefit ratio analysis of any drug.

Spontaneous Reporting

Spontaneous reporting is the most widely used method of pharmacovigilance, but weakest form of evidence for causation. 'Spontaneous reports' are so-called because they arise during a clinician's normal diagnostic appraisal of a patient, the clinician drawing the conclusion that a drug may be implicated in the causality of the clinical event. It is voluntary report from the health care professionals or medicine consumer regarding undesirable drug reaction in patients. Either clinician, clinical pharmacologists or pharmacist, dentist, nurses can report the ADRs. Then further this report is sent to the information collection centre within their health care facility or to the nearest pharmacovigilance centre. Apart from this, ADRs due to medication errors, suspected drug-drug, drug-food supplement or due to blood or blood components and vaccines are also reported. Relevant details regarding patient's demographic characteristics, details of ADRs, suspected medication details, laboratory data and history, seriousness of the reactions, outcome and reporter are captured in report. A report should contain four basic elements represented by four essential D's:

- Details of patient
- Details of ADR
- Details of suspected drug/drugs
- Details of reporter

All these essential segments of a form are highlighted in the ADR reporting form.

Suspected adverse drug reaction reporting form in India is available on official website of Indian Pharmacopoeia Commission and Central Drugs Standard Control Organization.

ADR reporting forms of various countries are approximately similar in terms of their content but differ slightly from each other in identity, for example in United Kingdom yellow card is used for reporting of ADRs, blue card is used in Australia but all of them seek similar information from reporter. Causality assessment of collected ADR reports is performed by using different causality assessment scales like WHO causality assessment scale, Naranjo's scale, Jones scale, European ABO system, Bayesian system.
Causality assessment determines the level of association of occurrence of ADR and administration of drug.

Medwatch in USA, yellow card in UK and blue card in Australia demonstrate the success story of spontaneous reporting. Indian regulatory has also developed suspected adverse reaction reporting form which is in harmony with forms of other counties. Spontaneous reports are submitted to regulatory bodies in two ways:

1. *Expedited Reporting:* **Regulatory bodies of different countries expect the market authorization holders to submit the serious ADR reports on priority basis and for this purpose a short period is kept as dead line which is 15 days in most of the**

countries. Reports not fitting into the bracket of expedited reporting become the part of periodic reports.

2. *Periodic Reporting:* Non-serious and serious expected ADR reports are reported in a compiled repot at some interval. Such reports are referred to as Periodic Safety Update Reports (PSUR). PSUR in many countries is these days referred to as the Periodic Benefit Risk Evaluation Report (PBRER).

Advantages of Spontaneous Reporting are as following:

1. It covers the large population of patients.
2. Simple and cost effective method.
3. It helps in detecting rare, serious adverse events and ADRs.
4. Hypothesis generation and signal detection.
5. Post marketing surveillance based upon spontaneous reports data is a powerful tool for detecting adverse events signals of direct clinical impact.
6. Feasibility in carrying out in hospitals, outpatient department and community pharmacy settings.

Limitations of Spontaneous Reporting

1. *Under reporting:* There has been a paradigm shift over last decade in the volume of reports as people are becoming more vigilant and conscious but still underreporting of ADRs is still a challenge to be met. Possible reasons of under reporting include fear of litigation, overburden of work, ignorance, diffidence and lethargy on the behalf of physician.
2. The recognition of ADRs is quite subjective and sometimes inaccurate in nature.
3. Bias can occur in spontaneous reporting as it touches the various spheres of population and reporters.
4. Authenticity of reports is sometimes questionable.

In India recently, Pharmacovigilance program of India was started in July 2010 to collect the spontaneous reports from health care professionals. ADR monitoring centres (AMCs) are identified in medical colleges of India which are coordinated by Indian Pharmacopeia Commission as National Coordination Centre. ADR data is collected at AMCs which undergoes the quality check and causality assessment by the experts at the ADR Monitoring Centre (AMC).

Valid reports are entered into vigiflow, a gateway to global database called as vigibase which is maintained and owned by Uppsala Monitoring Centre (UMC). ADR reports entered through vigiflow are reviewed by the quality check committee at National Coordination Centre in Indian Pharmacopoeia Commission. Information on the reports can be retrieved by the Indian regulatory from the database for decision making. Such flow of reports from reporter to global database is depicted in the figure below:

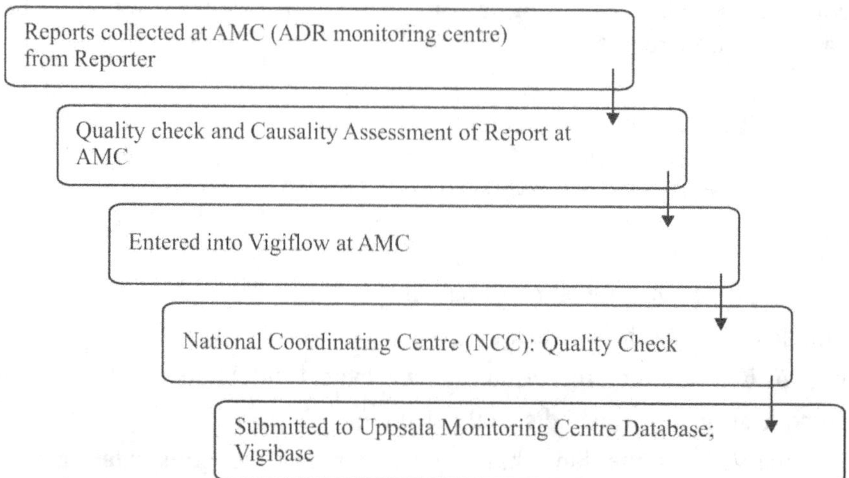

MAH's are required to submit the ADR reports in the form of PSUR's to Drug Controller General of India i.e., DCGI at interval of six months for the initial two years and thereafter annually for the next two years.

Data Management in Pharmacovigilance

It is essential to maintain good quality data so that raw data can be transformed into a meaningful representation of source data and should be appropriate for analysis. The pharmacovigilance data processing constitutes data collection, followed by its entry in computerized database like Adverse Event Reporting System (AERS), Adverse Reactions Information System global (ARISg) and Argus. WHO Adverse Reaction Terminology (WHOART), (Medical dictionary for regulatory activities) Med DRA are dictionaries meant to serve as a basis for rational coding of adverse reaction terms. The advantage of using these terminologies is to maintain the consistency in the storage and processing of data. The data is then carefully stored and properly maintained followed later to make the decision.

International Status of Pharmacovigilance

Pharmacovigilance in USA

In USA, the apex drug regulatory agency USFDA regulates the process of pharmacovigilance. Spontaneous reporting is done through Medwatch in two distinct formats i.e., Medwacth 3500, Medwatch 3500 A. Medwacth 3500 is meant for reporting of ADRs by, Medwatch 3500 A. Medwatch 3500 is used by healthcare professionals, consumers, and patients for voluntary reporting whereas 3500 A is used for mandatory reporting applicable on IND reporters, manufacturers, distributors, importers, user facilities personnel. Individual Case Safety Reports (ICSR's) are submitted to USFDA either through expedited or periodic reporting depending upon the type of reaction. Suspected-Unexpected Serious Adverse Reaction (SUSAR) reports are sent through expedited reporting within 15 calendar days of first notice of the case. Rest of the cases is submitted through periodic reports.

Pharmacovigilance in United Kingdom

Yellow Card reporting system is the principal reporting system which was started in 1964 by committee headed by Sir Derrick Dunlop after the alarming incidence of thalidomide disaster. This receives reports of healthcare professionals and patients can also report suspected adverse drug reactions secondary to medicines and vaccines. Yellow card scheme is one of the most successful programs across the world. In UK, Medicines and Healthcare products Regulatory Agency (MHRA) is the government body responsible for pharmacovigilance activities. All serious cases irrespective of their expectedness are reported on expedited basis in United Kingdom. MAH's are required to submit PSUR's at 6 months interval for first two years after placing the product in market and annually for next 2 years followed by three yearly submission in subsequent period.

Pharmacovigilance in European Union

European Medicines Agency (EMA) is the agency which coordinated the pharmacovigilance data management, exchange amongst European member countries. The European Medicines Agency (EMA) does not directly accept adverse drug reaction reports from healthcare professionals, patients or consumers rather they are expected to report the cases to their respective national authorities. Following table enlists the national competent authorities of various countries of European economic area.

Country	National Competent Authority
Austria	Austrian Medicines and Medical Devices Agency
Belgium	Federal Agency for Medicines and Health Products
Bulgaria	Bulgarian Drug Agency
Czech Republic	State Institute for Drug Control
France	Agence nationale de sécurité du médicament et des produits de santé
Germany	BfArM
Greece	National Organization for Medicines
Iceland	Icelandic Medicines Agency
Ireland	Irish Medicines Board
Norway	The Norwegian Medicines Agency
Slovakia	State Institute for Drug Control
Spain	Agencia Española de Medicamentos y Productos Sanitarios
Sweden	Medical Products Agency
United Kingdom	Medicines and Healthcare products Regulatory Agency

WHO- Uppsala Monitoring Centre

The World Health Organization started international drug monitoring programme in response to thalidomide disaster. Since 1978, the programme has been carried out by Uppsala Monitoring Centre (UMC) in Sweden. Uppsala Monitoring Centre is an organization which collates the data from all member countries and mines it to generate the signal for decision making on the fate of marketed drugs. The foremost aim of UMC is to support good decision-making regarding the benefits and risks of treatment options for patient taking medicines and help the regulatory bodies of various countries in making the decision over drugs.

Supporting effective communication of the most focused, up-to-date scientific information among various stakeholders is also priority of UMC. Apart from that, providing tools for data entry, management, retrieval, reference and research. Education and training in setting up and running national pharmacovigilance programmes, as well as in using the UMC Tools.

Important Terminologies in Pharmacovigilance

Adverse Event (AE)

Any untoward medical occurrence, that may present during treatment with a pharmaceutical product but which, does not necessarily have a causal relationship with this treatment.

Adverse (Drug) Reaction (ADR)

A response which is noxious and unintended and occurs at doses normally used in humans for the prophylaxis, diagnosis, or therapy of disease, or for the modification of physiological function. An adverse drug reaction, contrary to an adverse event, is characterized by the suspicion of a causal relationship between the drug and the occurrence, i.e., judged as being at least possibly related to treatment by the reporting or a reviewing health professional.

Data Mining

Process of extraction of potentially interesting patterns from large data sets, often based on statistical algorithms. A related term with essentially the same meaning is 'pattern discovery'. In pharmacovigilance, the commonest application of data mining is so called disproportionality analysis, for example using the Information Component (IC).

Dechallenge

The withdrawal of a suspected drug from a patient; the point at which the continuity, reduction or disappearance of adverse effects may be observed. Dechallenge may be of two types i.e., positive or negative depending upon change in outcome of ADR after stopping the drug. If the ADR recovers after stopping the drug then dechallenge is taken as positive else, it is said to be negative.

Rechallenge

When a suspected drug is re-administered to a patient after its previous withdrawal, it is called rechallenge. It may be positive of negative. When ADR reappears on rechallenge then rechallenge is said to be positive and in absence of occurrence of the same ADR on rechallenge, it is called as negative rechallenge.

Serious Adverse Drug Reaction

A serious adverse drug reaction is any untoward medical occurrence that at any dose and its outcome is any of the following:

- Death
- Inpatient hospitalization or prolongation of existing hospitalization
- Persistent or significant disability/incapacity
- Life-threatening condition
- Congenital abnormality
- Intervention required to preventing permanent impairment or damage or any other medically important condition considered serious by the medical professional judging the case.

Severe Adverse Drug Reaction

Severe means intensity of an event or reaction which usually is graded as mild, moderate or severe in the increasing order of intensity of the reaction.

This is worthwhile to mention that severity of the reaction should never be confused with seriousness of reaction. Severe and serious adverse drug reactions should be cautiously discriminated.

Any reaction having higher intensity or severity may be of relatively minor medical significance such as statins induced headache may have a high degree of pain but it may not be serious. Seriousness is based on patient/event outcome i.e., if its outcome matches with any of the criterion for serious reaction described above.

Signal

Reported information on a possible causal relationship between an adverse event and a drug, the relationship being unknown or incompletely documented previously. Usually more than a single report is required to generate a signal, depending upon the seriousness of the event and the quality of the information. The publication of a signal usually implies the need for some kind of review or action.

Biovigilance

Biovigilance may be defined as detection, gathering and analysis of information regarding the untoward and unexpected events of blood transfusion and transplantation of cells, tissues and organs. Biovigilance is the term describing the systems that collect, analyze and report on identifiable risks with the outcomes in the transfer of biologic materials between individuals. However, biovigilance systems are not created solely for information acquisition, but are intended to serve as the benchmark for drafting the policy and practice guidelines for patient safety. Biovigilance encompasses safety surveillance of blood, organ, tissue, and cellular therapy. Surveillance of blood or blood products transfusion related reactions come under purview of haemovigilance; a flourishing discipline in patient safety. Biovigilance targets the safety of both donors and recipient in case of organ, tissue, cell transplantations. Haemovigilance is a component of biovigilance established well in many countries. Haemovigilance and its network with various implications are described here in detail.

Haemovigilance

Blood transfusion is an evitable part of health management in every arena of the globe. Blood transfusion is done in 85 million people all around the world annually. Blood transfusion is life saving but still pose a risk of adverse reactions in few patients. To monitor and take preventive measures a newer safety concept known as Haemovigilance was born in 1990s with a lead from Japan to be the first country to start monitoring of adverse events secondary to blood transfusions. France was second to start haemovigilance system followed by several European countries. Haemovigilance is defined as detection, gathering and analysis of information regarding untoward and unexpected effects of blood transfusion. It encompasses a set of surveillance procedures covering the whole transfusion chain (from the collection of blood and its components to the follow-up of recipients), intended to collect and assess information on unexpected or undesirable effects resulting from the therapeutic use of labile blood products, and to prevent their occurrence or recurrence. The term Haemovigilance was originally coined by French people in 1991. Haemovigilance is derived from the Greek word *Haema* which means "blood" and latin word *vigilans* which means "watchful". Pharmacovigilance and haemovigilance are having the same objective of safeguarding the patients by monitoring the adverse reactions.

But there are certain differences between the two (Table 38.2)

Table 38.2 Differences between the pharmacovigilance and haemovigilance

Characteristic	Haemovigilance	Pharmacovigilance
Age	Too young, started in 1993 only	As old as thalidomide disaster which happened in 1960s
What should be reported	Only serious adverse reactions in most of the countries	Every reaction because of ADR irrespective of its seriousness should be reported

Table 38.2 *Contd...*

Characteristic	Haemovigilance	Pharmacovigilance
Scope	Reports the adverse reactions due to blood or blood products	Deals with the adverse reactions of drugs
Reporting requirement	Mandatory for HCP's in some countries (e.g., Italy, France)	Voluntary for HCP's in all countries

Birth of Haemovigilance

Humanity has witnessed revolutionary changes secondary to some disasters or scandals. Pharmacovigilance came into existence in response to the thalidomide disaster. Pharmacovigilance flourished well since its inception and became an inevitable part of healthcare system across the globe. Likewise haemovigilance was born in France because of major scandal revolving around HIV tainted blood in early nineties. It became mandatory to report serious adverse events due to blood transfusions. The importance of haemovigilance was then realized by many nations and almost all European Union countries established a haemovigilance system. Countries outside the Europe have also caught the pace steadily.

Need of Haemovigilance

In Cameroon, for instance, in an estimate on 40,000 transfusions side-effects linked to transfused whole blood (mainly fever and urticaria) were observed in more than 50% of the recipients: such data underline the importance of recipient follow-up and the need for corrective and preventive measures. For the challenge of the quality of transfusion and the development of haemovigilance in Africa, an appropriate system of evaluation should lead to intervention with the actors of the processes of elaboration and use of cellular blood products, with a method to improve the organization, the products, the prescription, the protocols, and the transfusion acts.

Haemovigilance in India

After the importance of monitoring of adverse reactions due to drugs was a haemovigilance program as an integral part of Pharmacovigilance Program of India (PvPI) at a national level was launched on December 10, 2012 with a road map of 5 years, i.e., year 2012-17, with four phases, i.e., initiation phase, expansion and consolidation phase, expansion and maintenance phase, and optimization phase.

Haemovigilance program has been launched with the following objectives:

- Monitor transfusion reactions
- Create awareness among health care professionals
- Generate evidence-based recommendations
- Advise Central Drugs Standard Control Organization (CDSCO) for safety related regulatory decisions
- Communicate findings to all key stakeholders
- Create national and international linkages

The Medical Colleges enrolled under haemovigilance program collects data in respect of adverse reactions associated with blood transfusion and blood product administration in Transfusion Reaction Reporting Form (TRRF). This data is collated and analyzed to identify trends and recommend best practices and interventions required to improve patient care and safety. These recommendations are to be forwarded to national coordinating Centres, PvPI for onward transmission to Drugs Controller General (India), Central Drugs Standard Control Organization (CDSCO). These recommendations can be used to formulate safety related regulatory decisions on blood and blood products transfusion that will be communicated to various stake holders.

International Status

In France, haemovigilance was created by law and notification of transfusion incidents is a legal obligation.

In Japan, a nation-wide network made up of medical representatives in each blood centre in charge of communication with medical institutions was established in 1992. Under law physicians are requested to report suspected cases of transfusion-associated adverse effects or infection. India is the first amongst SARC countries to start the haemovigilance.

In 1998, as a collaborative initiative five countries i.e., Belgium, France, Luxembourg, Portugal and Netherlands started European Haemovigilance Network. To establish a consistency and uniformity in this arena of health care International Haemovigilance Network came into existence which now has 28 member countries. Government of India is also committed to be a part of that and it has been mentioned under the mission of haemovigilance program of India to be a part of this international collaboration to safeguard the health of people undergoing the transfusion.

Country	Haemovigilance started in year	Comments
Japan	1993	First to establish haemovigilance
France	1994	First to start in Europe and spearhead the academic events on HV
United Kingdom	1996	Serious Hazards Of Transfusion (SHOT) run by professional body
Hong Kong	2001	Voluntary reporting
USA	2006	Late starting as compared to other developed countries
New Zealand	2005	Reporting of transfusion related adverse events is voluntary
Italy	2009	Mandatory reporting
India	2012	Extension of Pharmacovigilance Program of India (PvPI) to ensure safety on use of blood/blood products

Though, it took huge time but indeed we progressed from practice of transfusion of animal's blood to human beings to the sentience of reporting adverse reactions due to blood transfusions even with advanced techniques.

Materiovigilance

A medical device is an instrument, implant, apparatus, *in vitro* reagent, or similar or related article that is used to diagnose, prevent, or treat disease or other conditions, and does not achieve its purposes through chemical action within or on the body. The term "medical device" refers to the products ranging from therapeutic medical devices with local applications like tissue cutting; wound covering to advanced medical equipment and diagnostic medical devices. Examples of medical devices include heart valves, cardiac stents, catheters, drug-eluting stents, intraocular lenses, bone cements, scalp vein sets, silicone implants etc. Medical devices vary widely in type and complexity and used in critical conditions also. Therefore safety profile of medical devices should be of paramount importance. The adverse events related to the use of medical devices should be monitored and analysed to ensure the patient safety.

Materiovigilance is a system of identifying, collecting, reporting and estimating undesirable occurrences and reacting to them, or safety corrective actions related to medical devices. Materiovigilance includes activities of collecting, estimating, understanding and reacting to new findings of risks arising from the use or application of medical devices, particularly of harmful effects on patients/users or health care professionals, interaction with other substances or products, contraindications, falsifications, reduced efficiency, malfunctions or technical defects.

The materiovigilance was started in the United States by implementation of the Food and Drug Administration Modernization Act 1970.

Reporting of adverse events secondary to use of medical devices may contribute in reducing the future occurrence of such events. Materiovigilance i.e., post marketing surveillance of medical devices has been initiated in most of the countries including India. To harmonize the reporting of events under materiovigilance; Global Harmonization Task Force (GHTF) was constituted by USA, European union, Australia, Japan, Canada in 1992. Parallel to the Adverse drug reactions, reporting of adverse events due to medical devices mandatory for manufacturers and importers and voluntary for patients or healthcare professionals.

Conclusive Remarks

Patient safety is of paramount importance in healthcare management. Despite the several benefits offered by the drugs, biologicals and medical devices for the patient, possibility of adverse events secondary to their use cannot be denied. System of monitoring has been developed in response to the disasters like inception of pharmacovigilance after

Thalidomide Tragedy. Monitoring of adverse events started in developed countries decades ago but developing countries should not be dependent on extrapolating the data from other countries data by ignoring the genetic differences, lifestyle differences in various populations. Every country should become proactive in monitoring the patient safety by collecting the adverse events secondary to drugs, biologicals and medical devices to ensure the safety instead of waiting for the disasters to happen.

Suggested Readings

1. Davies DM, Rawlins MD, Thompson JW (1991). Mechanisms of adverse drug reactions. In: Davies DM, ed. Textbook of adverse drug reactions. Oxford: Oxford University Press, pp. 18-45.

2. De Vries RR, Faber JC, Strengers PF (2011). Board of the International Haemovigilance Network Haemovigilance: an effective tool for improving transfusion practice. *Vox Sang.* **100(1):** 60-7.

3. Debeir J, Noel L, Aullen J, Frette C, Sari F, Mai MP, *et al.,* (1999). The French haemovigilance system. *Vox Sang.* **77(2):** 77-81.

4. Faber JC (2002). Haemovigilance around the globe. *Vox Sang.* **83(1):** 71-6.

5. Ferner PE, Aronson JK (2005). National difference in publishing papers on adverse drug reactions. *Br J Clin Pharmacol.* **59(1):** 108-12.

6. ICH Guideline E2D; Post-approval Safety Data Management: Definitions and Standards for Expedited Reporting. Available from http://www.ich.org/products/guidelines/efficacy/article/efficacy-guidelines.html

7. Lazarou J, Pomeranz BH, Corey PN (1998). Incidence of adverse drug reactions in hospitalized patients: a meta-analysis of prospective studies. *J Am Med Assoc.* **279:** 1200-5.

8. Medhi B, Sewal RK (2012). Ecopharmacovigilance: An issue urgently to be addressed. *Indian J Pharmacol.* **44:** 547-9.

9. Pruett T L, Blumberg EA, Cohen DJ, Crippin JS, Freeman RB, Hanto DW, *et al.,* (2012). A Consolidated Biovigilance System for Blood, Tissue and Organs: One Size Does Not Fit All. *American Journal of Transplantation.* **12(5):** 1099-1101.

10. Tayou Tagny C, Mbanya D, Tapko JB, Lefrère JJ (2008). Blood safety in Sub-Saharan Africa: a multi-factorial problem. *Transfusion.* **48:** 1256-61.

11. WHO Technical Report No 498: International Drug Monitoring, The Role of National Centres (Geneva 1972) [Internet]. 1972 [Updated 2010 Oct 28; Cited 2010 Dec 21]. Available from www.who-umc.org/graphics/9277.pdf.

12. WHO. Safety of Medicines. A guide to detecting and reporting adverse reactions. Why health professionals need to take action. Available from: http://apps.who.int/medicinedocs/en/d/Jh2992e.

13. Wilke RA, Lin DW, Roden DM, Paul B. Watkins, David Flockhart, *et al.,* (2007). Identifying genetic risk factors for serious adverse drug reactions: current progress and challenges. *Nat Rev Drug Discov.* **6(11):** 904-16.

14. Williamson LM, Cohen H, Love EM, Jones H, Todd A, Soldan K (2000). The Serious Hazards of Transfusion (SHOT) initiative. The UK approach to haemovigilance. *Vox Sang.* **78(2):** 291-5.

CHAPTER 39

BIOLOGICS AND BIOSIMILARS

Introduction

Nowadays, biological products often represent the cutting edge of medical science and research. These products are derived from living material (plant, animal or microorganism) usually based on protein and/or nucleic acid used for the treatment of diseases in humans. Biologics have relatively large molecular weight and high structural complexity compared with biologically active substances typically made by chemical synthesis. Also, known as biologics, these products replicate natural substances such as enzymes, antibodies, or hormones in our bodies.

Biological products are used as other drugs for the treatment, prevention or cure of several deadly diseases in humans. In contrast to chemically synthesized drugs, which have a well-defined formula and can be thoroughly characterized, biological products are derived from living organism and have a very complex structure and function. Most of the biologic products are complex mixtures that cannot be easily identified or characterized. Biological products differ from conventional drugs in that they tend to be heat-sensitive and susceptible to microbial contamination. This requires sterile processes to be applied from initial manufacturing steps.

A biological is "a structurally complex compound such as a virus, therapeutic serum, toxin, antitoxin, vaccine, blood, blood component or derivative, allergenic product, or analogous product applicable to the prevention, treatment or cure of a disease or condition of human beings" Gene-based and cellular biologics, at the forefront of biomedical research today, may make it possible to treat a variety of medical conditions, including illnesses for which no other treatments are available. Research continues to develop more biologics that will help treat medical conditions or add to existing treatment options.

Biological Medicinal Products

Biological medicines (also called "biopharmaceuticals") are comprised of proteins such as hormones (growth hormone, insulin, erythropoietin), enzymes that are naturally produced in the human body, or monoclonal antibodies, but also blood products, immunological medicinal products such as sera and vaccines, allergens, and advanced technology products such as gene and cell therapy products.

The Public Health Services (PHS) Act 42 U.S.C. § 262(i) states that "A biological is a structurally complex compound such as a virus, therapeutic serum, toxin, antitoxin, vaccine, blood, blood component or derivative, allergenic product, or analogous product applicable to the   prevention, treatment or cure of a disease or condition of human beings". By statute, viruses, therapeutic sera, toxins and antitoxins, vaccines, blood, blood components or derivatives, allergenic products, any analogous products are included in the list of biological products. The term "Analogous products" makes the definition of biologics very broad. In the above given definition the components of "Analogous products" is not defined which makes the definition very unclear.

A virus is interpreted to be a product containing the minute living cause of an infectious disease and includes but is not limited to filterable viruses, bacteria, rickettsia, fungi, and protozoa.

A therapeutic serum is a product obtained from blood by removing the clot or clot components and the blood cells.

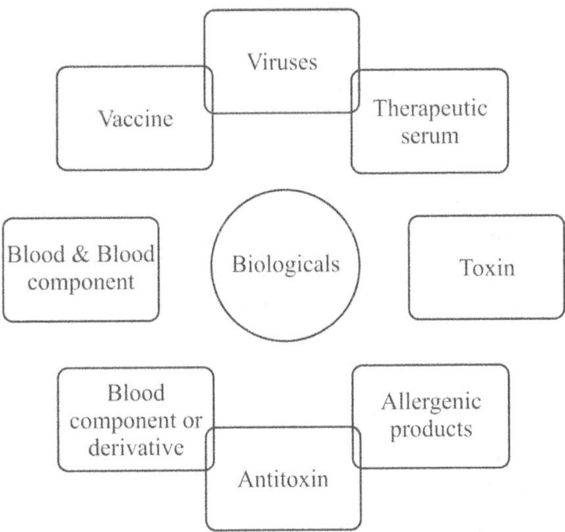

Fig. 39.1 Components of biological medicines.

A toxin is a product containing a soluble substance poisonous to laboratory animals or to man in doses of 1 millilitre or less (or equivalent in weight) of the product, and having the property, following the injection of non-fatal doses into an animal, of causing to be produced therein another soluble substance which specifically neutralizes the poisonous substance and which is demonstrable in the serum of the animal thus immunized.

An antitoxin is a product containing the soluble substance in serum or other body fluid of an immunized animal which specifically neutralizes the toxin against which the animal is immune.

Regulation of Biologics

Biologics include medical products made from living sources, such as humans, animals, plants, and microorganisms are included in biologics. Today, the FDA's Centre for Biologics Evaluation and Research (CBER) regulates biologics to ensure the safety, purity, potency, and effectiveness of these products, helping to get treatments on the market for known diseases and to protect against threats of emerging infectious diseases and bioterrorism.

The categories of therapeutic biological products regulated by Centre for Drug Evaluation and Research (CDER) (under the Federal Food Drug and Cosmetics Act (FDCA) and/or the Public Health Service Act (PHSA), as appropriate include the following:

- Vaccines
- Blood and blood components
- Allergenic patch tests and extracts
- Human Immunodeficiency Virus (HIV) and hepatitis tests
- Gene therapy products
- Cells and tissues for transplantation

Mechanism of Action

Like all other medicines, biological medicines work by interacting with the human body to produce a therapeutic outcome, but the mechanisms by which they do this may vary from product to product and across indications. Biopharmaceuticals can be tailor-made to fit the desired target. Therefore, the role of the physicians in treatment of patients with these complex medicinal products is particularly important.

Components of Biological Vaccines

As said above, there is no consistent definition which can define the word biological therapeutic, but most people working in this field consider biologics to include proteins (natural or recombinant), synthetic polypeptides, blood products, genetic compounds (oligonucleotides), and whole cells and tissues for transplantation. Vaccines are also classified as biological therapeutics, although many countries have placed vaccines under a separate set of guidelines and regulations. In Canada, compounds considered to be biological therapeutics (including vaccines) are listed within Schedule D of the Food and Drugs Act.

A suspension containing live, attenuated, modified, or killed microorganisms (or their toxins), or tumor antigens, which when administered into the body stimulates the body's immune system to produce antigen-specific antibodies known as vaccine.

Monoclonal Antibody (mAb)

An antibody is a protein used by the immune system to identify and neutralize foreign objects like bacteria and viruses. Each antibody recognizes a specific antigen unique to its target.

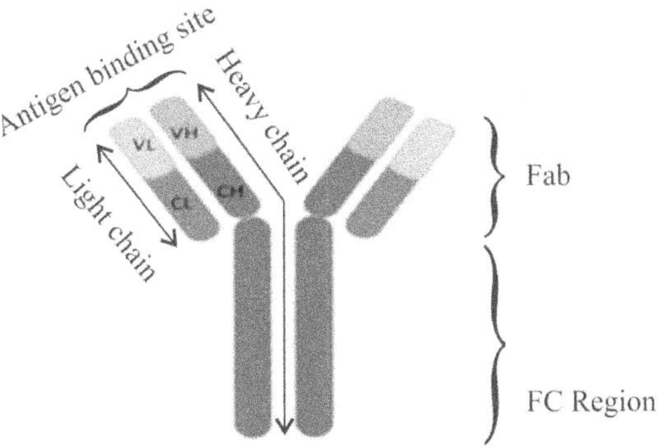

Fig. 39.2 Antibody structure.

Monoclonal Antibodies (mAb) are antibodies that are identical because they were produced by one type of immune cell, all clones of a single parent cell. Given (almost) any substance, it is possible to create monoclonal antibodies that specifically bind to that substance; they can then serve to detect or purify that substance. This has become an important tool in biochemistry, molecular biology and medicine.

Types of mAb	Specific features
Murine source mAbs	• Rodent's mAbs with excellent addinities and specificities. • Generated using conventional hybridoma technology. • Clinical efficacy compromised by HAMA (Human Anti Murine Antibody) response, which lead to allergic or immune complex herpersensitivities.
Chimeric mAbs	• Chimers combine the human constant regions with the intact rodent variable regions. • Affinity and specificity unchanged. Also cause human antichimeric antibody response (30% murine resource)
Humanized mAbs	• Contained only the CDRs of the rodent variable region grafted onto human variable region framework

In 1975, Kohler and Milstein introduced the monoclonal antibody production by somatic cell fusion or hybridoma technology (got Nobel Prize in 1984). Overall: The technique involves fusing a normal antibody producing B cell with a myeloma cell to produce a hybrid cell or hybridoma. The hybridoma would possess the immortal growth properties of the myeloma cell while secreting the antibody produced by the B cell. The resulting hybridoma could be cultured indefinitely thus providing large amounts of homogeneous antibody for research purposes.

Polyclonal antibodies are antibodies that are derived from different cell lines.

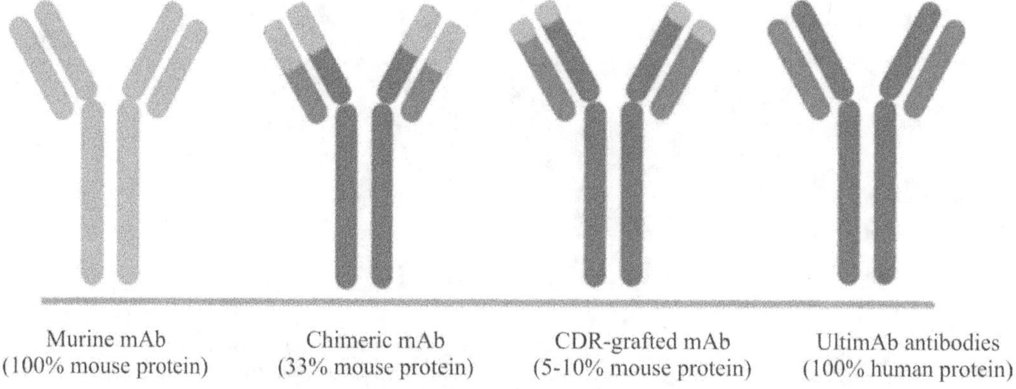

Fig. 39.3 Evolution of therapeutic antibodies

For the production of the monoclonal antibodies, first mouse is immunized with an antigen and then the spleen of that mouse is removed after the production of antibodies in its body against that antigen. Antibody producing B cell is dissociated with the spleen cells and fused with continuously dividing mouse myeloma cell line because B-cells will not divide in culture.

The spleen cells are fused with mouse myeloma cells to become a continuous hybridoma cell line. Many different antibody clones can be produced by a continuous hybridoma cell line with multiple B-cell clones. The population of hybridoma cells producing many antibodies is cloned in 96-well plates and each single B-cell clone of cultured cells produces one antibody. One mouse spleen can give many different antibodies to different epitopes on the same antigen. Monoclonal antibodies are raised in either tissue culture media, called supernatant, or generated from hybridoma cells injected into the peritoneal cavity (abdominal cavity), called ascites fluid.

Blood and Blood Components

"Any therapeutic substances derived from human blood, including whole blood, labile blood components and plasma-derived medicinal products" are come under the definition of blood products according to WHO.

Coagulation factors derived from either human plasma or culture media from genetically engineered cells for replacement therapy to treat patients with congenital deficiencies (e.g., hemophilia) lies in the list of biological product.

Potential Benefits of Therapy

- Effective in controlling bleeding episodes that are life threatening

Potential Risks of Therapy

- Infections due to adventitious agents

- Development of neutralizing antibodies due to modifications in the molecule

- Allergic reactions to impurities

Allergenic Patch Tests and Extracts

Allergen patch tests and allergenic extracts are only two type of allergenic products licensed for use which is regulated by The Center for Biologics Evaluation and Research (CBER).

Allergenic Patch Tests

Allergenic patch tests are diagnostic tests applied to the surface of the skin. Patch tests are used by physicians to determine the specific causes of contact dermatitis. Contact Dermatitis (CD) is a common skin disorder seen by allergists and dermatologists and can present with a spectrum of morphologic cutaneous reactions. Contact dermatitis is most common skin problem for which 5.7 million physician visits per year are made. In a large population-based survey of public health issues, it was found that all age groups are affected with CD, with a slight female preponderance.

Redness, edema, papules, vesiculation, weeping, crusting, and pruritus are the general characterization of CD. Exposure to UV light most commonly causes a phototoxic or sunburn type of reaction and less commonly a photoallergic reaction when the UV light interacts with chemical agents (i.e., fragrances, PABA, plants, parsnips, figs, or several ingested drugs) inducing photosensitization of various forms.

Patch testing is the gold standard for identification of a contact allergen. Although occlusive patch testing is them most common technique, but in some special type of cases technique like open, prophetic (provocative), repeated insult, photopatch, and atopy patch tests are also available.

These patches are composed of either natural substances or chemicals like; rubber, nickel etc. that can cause CD.

Allergenic Extracts

In the diagnosis and treatment of allergic diseases such as allergic rhinitis ("hay fever"), allergic sinusitis, allergic conjunctivitis, bee venom allergy and food allergy, allergenic extracts plays very crucial role. Some natural substance like; pollen, animal hair, food can elicit the immune response of human body in the susceptible individuals and they can be used as allergenic extracts. Food extracts are only used to diagnose food allergies, but other allergenic extracts may be used for both diagnosis and treatment of allergic disease.

Gene Therapy Products

There are about 25,000 genes inside the every human body. Each gene is responsible for the production of all the enzymes, hormones, antibodies and other proteins needed to make the body functional. Due to defect in any gene or missing gene that particular protein is absent in the body and cause disease. Biotechnology with bioinformatics plays an important role to guide biopharmaceutical scientist to determine which gene or protein is not functional or absent, so that they can develop new treatments across a range of therapeutic areas.

The biological products are so complex in structure that they cannot be characterized and the process is also so complex and sensitive according to their structure.

RNA interference therapeutics is an exciting new frontier for the development of novel therapies for patients, especially patients with genetic disorders. There are several RNAi therapies in clinical trials which have demonstrated potential in treating certain neuromuscular disorders, such as Duchenne Muscular Dystrophy (DMD). DMD is a genetic disorder impacting 1 in 3,500 newborn boys and is the most severe form of muscular dystrophy in childhood. One RNAi targeted therapeutic in development seeks to restore the function of dystrophin. Early clinical trials of the drug have demonstrated significantly improved dystrophin expression as well as improvement in DMD patients ability to walk.

Cells and Tissues for Transplantation

According to FDA, "autologous, allogeneic, or xenogeneic cells that have been propagated, expanded, selected, pharmacologically treated, or otherwise altered in biological characteristics *ex vivo* to be administered to humans and applicable to the prevention, treatment, cure, diagnosis or mitigation of disease or injuries" is known as somatic cell therapy.

Tissue engineering applies the principles of engineering and life sciences with the aim to generate biological substitutes that restore, maintain or improve the function of damaged or affected tissues and organs. For the development of autologous transplants (from patient's own cells), primary cells are isolated and expanded by appropriate cell-culture techniques until sufficient cell numbers are available for either the colonization of a matrix scaffold structure or for cell therapy.

Stem cells and stem cell-derived products

- Hematopoietic, mesenchymal, embryonic, umbilical cord blood, etc.

Cancer vaccines and immunotherapies

- Dendritic cells, activated T-lymphocytes (TIL, LAK), B-lymphocytes, monocytes, cancer cells chemically modified or unmodified.

Potential benefits of therapy

- Potential for much greater potency
- Applicable to a wide range of very difficult to treat diseases
- Potential for fewer adverse effects than conventional therapies
- More targeted

Potential risks of therapy

- Tumorigenicity
- Cellular contaminants
- Adventitious agents
- Safety of reagents
- Sterility
- Product stability
- Product variability

Biologicals *Vs* Small Molecule Drugs

Chemically-based drugs are made by using organic chemistry. In this process, addition and mixing of known small, chemically manufactured active substances, using a series of controlled and predictable chemical reactions are done. For example, a 180 Da weighted small molecule acetylsalicylic acid (ASA), aspirin's active ingredient can be trapped in a tablet and due to its simple structure, small size it can easily penetrate the cell membrane. In contrast, Biologics are made by the process of Genetic Engineering. In this process harvesting the substances produced and secreted by constructed cells done. Biologics are molecularly heterogeneous products. Biologics may not be completely characterized using physicochemical methods. Biological molecules are molecules with high molecular weight up to 150 KD.

Biologics bind to specific cell receptors that are associated with the disease process. Monoclonal antibodies are specialized in recognizing a very specific structure on the cell surface. Used in cancer therapy, they bind selectively – for example to the receptors of cancer cells, making it possible to mark and fight specific abnormal cells. Healthy cells are usually not attacked in this process, so that biologics often cause fewer side effects than classic chemotherapy.

Table 39.1 Differences between biological and classical drugs

Phenomena	Biological drugs	Classic drugs
Regulatory authority	Regulated under PHC act	Regulated under FDC act
Molecular weight	High	Low
Molecular characterization	Less characterized	Well characterized
Active ingredients	Complex mix heterogeneous proteins and impurities	Unique, well defined
Composition	Dozens of atoms	Millions of atoms
Structure	Can be described by chemical formula	Cannot be described by chemical formula
Dose response	Non-linear	Linear
Mechanisms of action	Multiple	Specific
Production	Chemical synthesis by scientists	Biological synthesis by 'organisms', e.g., bacteria, mammalian cell culture
Process steps	Sensitive to minor changes, products generally very sensitive to the manufacturing process	Highly reproducible, products that do not depend extensively on the manufacturing process
Immunogenicity (The ability to induce and immune response)	Potential formulation of antibodies, difficult to predict.	Rate

Manufacture of Recombinant Biological Products

Principle

The manufacture of biological medicinal products is quite different from the process of manufacturing of the chemical based classic drugs. In list of biological products, there are products like; vaccines, immunosera, immunoglobulins (including monoclonal antibodies), antigens, hormones, cytokines, allergens, enzymes. Each and every product is different from each other so that the manufacturing process of individual product involves certain specific considerations according to the nature of the products.

Unlike conventional medicinal products, which are synthesized using chemical and physical techniques, the production of biological products involves cells, tissues and living organism. In the production of biological products, involvement of microorganism, human and animals is also there. Several biotechnological techniques are used to manufacture these products.

Personnel

All personnel employed in areas where biological products are manufactured and tested should train in such a way that every personnel get adequate knowledge about hygiene and safety.

Persons responsible for production and quality control of biological products should be well qualified in the relevant areas like immunology, microbiology, chemistry, pharmacology, virology etc. They should have enough hands on experience to perform all the experiments.

For the biological products safety the health status of every personnel is very important. Every personnel should be screened for any infectious disease and should be vaccinated properly according to their working areas.

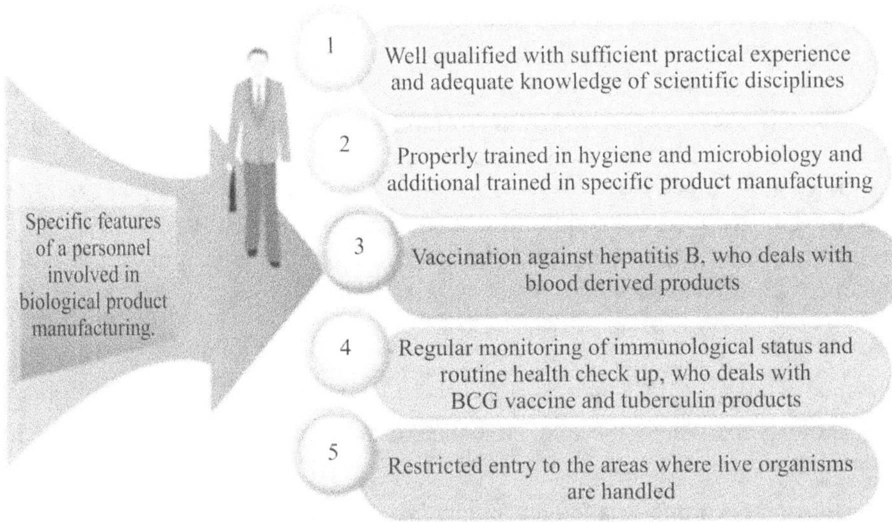

Fig. 39.4 Specific features of the personnel involved in biological product manufacturing.

All the personnel who are concern with cleaning, maintenance or quality control should be closely monitored for any change in their health and appropriate record should be kept.

In the production unit of live or attenuated vaccine like BCG or tuberculin, the working personnel's health should be under continuous monitoring system and the routine immunological and chest X-ray should be done. All the personnel should be vaccinated against hepatitis B who is dealing with blood or plasma derived products.

The entry of personnel should be restricted in the areas where the live microorganism or toxins are handled.

Biological Products and Animal Cells

Safety is the primary concern for the biological products because the central issue regarding these products have always been "Is the product derived from cell substrate not going to harm in any case to humans?" It took a long time to find out an appropriate cell substrate to manufacture biological products.

Phenotypic Characteristics of Animal Cells

Before using any cell for the production of biological compound, that cell should be phenotypically characterized. In literature, a large number of these characteristics have been defined, but out of them few are the most important characteristics like; life and tumorigenic potential of cell and chromosomal condition of the cell.

With regard to life potential, one type of cell have finite life such as human diploid cell and other one is cell derived from tumor tissue which have infinite life potential. Some time the cells with infinite life potential do not show its characteristics when it is grown *in vitro*. The test assay to detect the tumorigenicity is also an important part of this process. It took a long time to develop such a sensitive assay that can correctly detect the tumorigenicity and do not give the false negative result. In chromosomal condition, cell can be divided in to two classes: diploid cell and heteroploid cell. Diploid cell contain the normal number of chromosome, but heteroploid cell contain abnormal number of chromosome with several structural abnormalities.

Use of Animals

Animals are the main production house for the biological compounds, for example monkeys (polio vaccine), horse and goat (snake antivenom), rabbit, mice and hamster (rabies vaccine).

There are some unique challenges in the production of the biological product like development, manufacture, and quality control testing. Quality control for biologics is often based on animal tests, rather than on chemical-based *in vitro* assays that are used to release small molecule drugs onto the market. The quality control of most of the sera and vaccine are done in animals, e.g., BCG vaccine (guinea pig), pertussis vaccine (mice), pyrogenicity (rabbits). The use of live organisms/cultures in the production of biologics introduces regulatory concerns related to batch-to-batch variability and the potential introduction of culture contaminants. Therefore, potency and safety testing are typically required for each individual batch of a biologic in order to maintain quality control. Regulatory authorities may also require re-testing of individual lots by government laboratories.

Some time for the generation of fewer antibodies or similar structure no animal is used, in that case yeast and ribosomal display method is used.

Quarters for animal which are used in the production of the biological products should be separated from production and quality control area. The health status of the animal which is used in the production and used in the safety testing and quality control should be monitored and recorded. Personnel working with these animals should be well qualified and proper clothing and hygiene facility should be provided.

Table 39.2 Animals used in biological product production and type of tests

Animal	Vaccine	Type of Test
Monkey	Attenuated Poliomyelitis (oral)	Neurovirulence
Moust	Rabies Pertusssis Tetanus	Potency
Hamster	SPF Chicken Embryo Measles vaccine	
Rabbit	Rubbela vaccine (Live)	
Gerbil	Attenuated Hemorrhagic fever with renal syndrome vaccine (Live)	
Guinea pig	Diphtheria Tetanus BCG Tubercylin	Potency, absence of toxin Potency, absence of toxin Dermal reativity Sensitisation

Since, the production of biological products involves large number of animal, replacement, reduction and refinement have become a global focus for the development, manufacture and testing of biologics. For example, in the US, biologics testing has been identified by the Interagency Coordinating Committee on the Validation of Alternative Methods (ICCVAM) as one of their four highest priorities for the development of alternative methods. In Canada, CCAC policy requires that scientific use of animals should employ the most humane methods on the smallest number of appropriate animals required to obtain valid information. Therefore, the re-evaluation and the development of newer methodologies for biologics that implement replacement, reduction and refinement alternatives are particularly important.

Potential Pharmacology/Toxicology Issues for Biological Products

- Examples of cross-cutting concerns
  - Picking the relevant animal model
  - Dosing, safety
  - Biodistribution
  - Toxicity, tumorigenicity
  - Immunogenicity (rejection/elimination)
- Some unique concerns for cell/gene therapy products
  - Insertional mutagenesis
  - Alteration of germline
  - Long-term toxicity
  - Migratory potential

- Some unique concerns for protein products
  - Immune-mediated problems
    - Immune complexes
    - Obfuscation of toxicity
    - Allergy
  - Species specificity

FDA's and Biologicals

Public Health Service Act (PHSA) is the FDA's regulatory authority for the approval of biologics. According to Federal Food, Drug, and Cosmetic Act (FD&C Act), most biological products also meet the definition of "drugs" so that they are also regulated under this act.

Similarly, some medical devices used to produce biologics are regulated by Center for Biologics Evaluation and Research (CBER) under the FD&C Act's Medical Device Amendments of 1976.

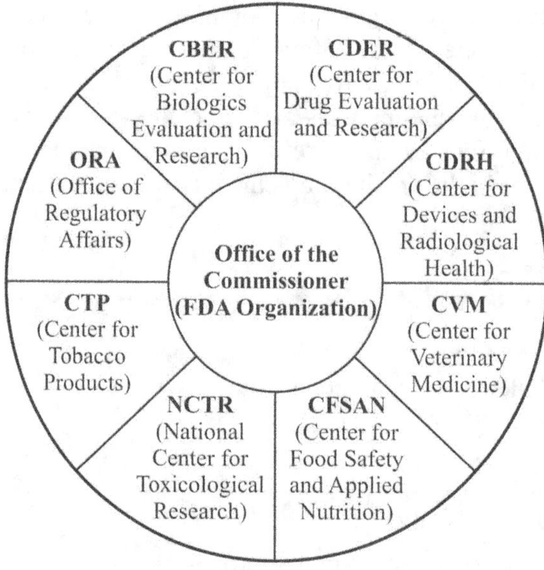

Fig. 39.5 Organization of FDA.

Biosimilars

Biotechnology has given us the way for the development of treatments for a variety of serious diseases in the form of biological and biosimilar medicine. Worldwide, many million patients have already benefited from these approved biological medicines. Most of the deadly diseases like; cancers, heart attacks, stroke, multiple sclerosis, diabetes, rheumatoid arthritis and autoimmune diseases are either preventable or treatable with the help of these medicines.

In 1980, the first biological medicinal product was approved which was produced by DNA recombinant techniques. Till the end of 2013, the exclusive rights (patents and other data protection) for several biological medicinal products have reached their expiration and many more will expire in the coming decade. Consistent with this expiry, the need of similar biological medicinal products, or biosimilar medicinal products ("biosimilars") felt by the pharmaceutical industry and in 2006, first biosimilar was approved and marketed (Omnitrope (somatropin) by EU).

Biological Medicine EMA Guidance: Biosimilar sponsor is to *"generate evidence substantiating the similar nature, in terms of quality, safety and efficacy, of the new similar biological medicinal product and the chosen reference medicinal product authorized in the Community"*.

USFDA (BPCIA*) definition: a follow-on biologic means:

"The biological product is highly similar to the reference product, notwithstanding minor differences in clinically inactive components"; and *"No clinically meaningful differences exist between the biological product and the reference product in terms of the safety, purity, and potency"*.

WHO definition: *"Similar Biotherapeutic Products"* is a biotherapeutic product that is similar in terms of quality, safety and efficacy to an already licensed biotherapeutic product.

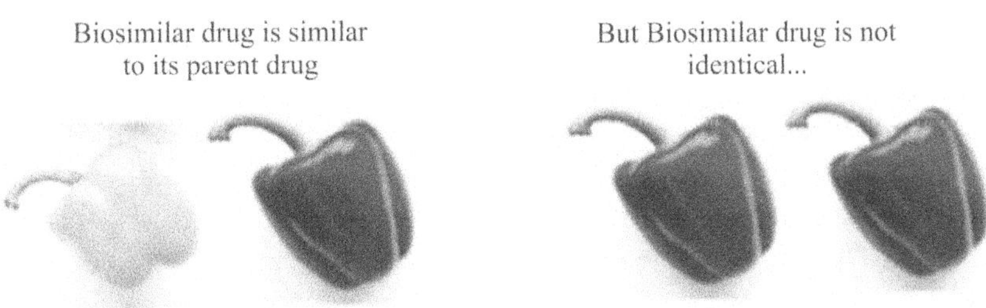

Biosimilar drug

How Biosimilar Differ from the Reference Product

Biosimilar drug is similar to its reference drug or parent drug but it is not identical. There are some parameter by which we can differentiate between biosimilar and its parent drug:

Manufacturing process: Manufacturing process of biosimilar will have variation from the manufacturing process of the reference product.

Structure and folding: As the manufacturing process of biosimilars is different so that the structure and folding of the biosimilar may be different from its reference drug.

Biosimilar products are very complex in structure and the available analysis techniques cannot yet fully characterise such complex molecules so it is not possible to prove biosimilar is the same or different from the original. In the production of biosimilars live organism are used so the risk of contamination of other molecules is always there. Variation in clinical effect and side effects from its reference drug only can be defined after the clinical trial of the product.

Table 39.3 Differences between generic and biosimilar drugs

Charactristics / Drugs	Production	Active product	Formulation	Clinical effect
Generic	Simple and consistent	Same	Variable	Can be assumed
Biosimilar	Complex and variable	Differeent	Variable	Can be assumed

Cancers, anemia and immunological diseases are becoming a big challenge for the next generation. Treatment of these diseases through chemically originated drug is very expensive and the side effects are very sever. Monoclonal antibodies and therapeutic proteins can be a less expensive option than the originator biologics.

Global biologics sales have grown to more than $100 billion. As an increasing number of biologics face patent expiration, biosimilars offer a major opportunity for drug developers. By 2020, patents will expire on twelve biologics with global sales of more than $67 billion.

Future Prospect

Producing natural substances of human body outside the body is the most challenging task, which was fulfilled by biological products. Production of natural substances using natural recourses like human, animals and microorganism or by the bioengineering methods helped a lot to fight the life threatening diseases.

Some diseases still exist with no treatment. Today's gene and cellular based treatment is the most promising treatment option to fight against such type of diseases and in future these treatment option will be in front row of the biomedical research as lots of advances are still expected.

In the 21st century, safety and quality will be the biggest challenges for the regulatory authorities as new therapies such as xenotransplantation (the transplantation of animal cells, tissues or organs into a human) are the next target of biomedical research. Beside the scientific and regulatory issue, legal and ethical issues are also challenging for the regulators.

Suggested Readings

1. Generics and Biosimilars Initiative (GaBi), June 2012. US $67 billion worth of biosimilar patents expiring before 2020. Available at: http://www.gabionline.net/biosimilars/general/US-67-billion-worth-of-biosimilar-patents-expiring-before-2020

2. Good manufacturing practices for pharmaceutical products. In: WHO Expert Committee on specifications for pharmaceutical preparations. Thirty-Second Report. Geneva, World Health Organization, 1992 (WHO Technical Report Series, No. 823), Annex 1.

3. http://3rs.ccac.ca/en/testing-and-production/tp-testing/biologics-and-vaccines.html

4. http://www.ema.europa.ed/docs/en/GB/document/library/scientific/guideline/2009/09/WC.

5. http://www.fda.gov/AboutFDA/Transparency/Basics/ucm194516.htm

6. http://www.fda.gov/BiologicsBloodVaccines/DevelopmentApprovalProcess/BiologicalApprovalsbyYear/ucm180879.htm

7. http://www.fda.gov/biologicsbloodvaccines/ucm133705.htm

8. http://www.law.cornell.edu/uscode/text/42/262

9. http://www.rspca.org.uk/ImageLocator/LocateAsset?asset=document&assetId=1232715021222&mode=prd

10. Laboratory biosafety manual, 2nd ed. Geneva, World Health Organization, 1993.

11. Parexel Biopharmaceutical R&D Statistical Sourcebook, 2011/2012.

12. Quality management for chemical safety testing. Geneva, World Health Organization, 1992 (Environmental Health Criteria, No 141).

13. WHO Expert Committee on Biological Standardization, Fortieth Report, Geneva, World Health organization, 1990 (WHO Technical Report Series, No, 800).

SECTION – IV

CHAPTER 40

BIOLOGICAL PASSPORT

Introduction

"Biological passport" is a term which define as a record of biological tests over a period of time of a sports person (Figure 40.1). This term is most commonly used for professional athletes in whom results of their biological markers are collated over a span of time. The results of the biological markers can further be used for doping test. There is no extra requirement of doping test in case of biological passports. The values of the markers can be evaluated to be present in the permissible limit of the tests. If any value is outside the limits of the continuous monitoring results can be an indication of doping. It will indirectly help in identifying the abuse substances in the body of an athlete. Nowadays, the term biological passport has been commonly used as Athlete passport, however, biological markers (Figure 40.1) had already been used since decades in the history of doping. The first biological marker was the ratio of testosterone over epitestosterone (T/E) to analyze anabolic steroids in urine samples during 1980s. Therefore, the concept of athlete passport came after the use of biological markers to detect doping in athletes. It also provides a proficient alternative to guarantee fairness in privileged sports.

The new paradigm in anti doping began in 1980s after the introduction and availability of substances which are similar to those formed by body of the human. These include "big 3"- erythropoietin, testosterone and growth hormones. Athletes started abusing these identical substances like recombinant human erythropoietin and autologous blood. As these substances are identical to the endogenous hormones in the human body and further boost them by combining with them, their detection in human body becomes very tedious process. The athletes used to exploit doping substances to trigger various physiological changes to enhance their performance in their respective fields. The term doping is defined as the use of the substances which enhances any kind of activity performance of humans. The importance of these substances mainly arises in the performance of a sportsman and is common in reference to the steroids or their precursors. In brief, numerous classes of agents used to come under the category of doping substances like anabolic drugs, stimulants, ergogenic aids, adaptogens, nootropics, human biomolecules, blood boosters, analgesics, sedatives, anxiolytics and gene doping (relatively newer term) etc.

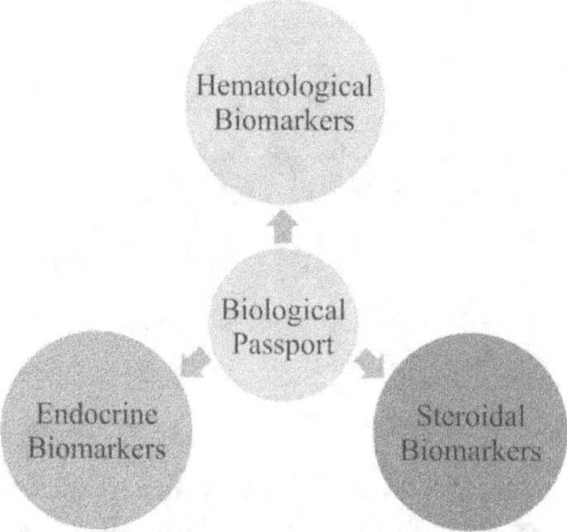

Fig. 40.1 Biological Passport comprised of majorly three categories of biomarkers over the sports activity of a sports person.

Doping is considered to be unethical and against the moral of human beings as it leads to illegal enhancement of one's performance towards his sportsman spirit. But then the question arises about the legal and illegal ways of increasing performance of an athlete. If doping is an offence then, how the enhancement of performance by taking any dietary supplements are justified. It is really not easy to differentiate between ethical and unethical ways of performance enhancing agents. The moral culprit should be identified. Usually the banned substances are found to be synthetic in origin and they artificially boost the performance of an athlete. However, unsurprisingly, various natural substances like EPO are also banned. Moreover, various techniques like blood doping which does not involve any synthetic substances are also banned by the anti-doping authorities. The anticipated effect of the agent may be the problem because blood doping leads to increase in stamina of the athlete by increasing red blood cell supply which can also be achieved by other means that may be permitted by the agencies. On the contrary, several synthetic enhancements like streamlined clothing, running shoes and cycling helmets etc. are also permitted. Hence, the moral outrage of doping should be discussed and explained in detail for the fair rules of games. Moreover, the advantage of doping to an athlete also encourages other athletes to dope too. The enhancement of natural limits of human nature by artificially extending the limits should be banned. Therefore, doping is considered to be an odd with the quintessence of a sport.

The doping is not only a boon to an athlete but it is also very detrimental to the health of an athlete. The prevalence of doping is increasing day by day. It has been found that approximately 30% of the athletes participated in world championships 2011 had used banned substances in their careers. Moreover, it has been noticed that Russian state had also sponsored their whole Russian track and field team for doping. As a result Olympic games 2016 had banned the whole team.

Athletes also tried to prevent the risk of detection of doping substances from their body by changing their behavior etc. Unfortunately, it leads to unnecessary encouragement of new doping methods which will be difficult to detect eg. changing route of administration, dose etc. This makes the detection criteria for an organization very critical. The agencies like World Anti-Doping Agency (WADA), United States Anti-Doping Agency (USADA), National Anti-Doping Agency (NADA), etc. are the organizations which are controlling the doping in sports. These agencies aim to avert athletes from doping by examining the athletes by performing battery of tests.

WADA was an initiation of a Canada based international Olympic committee. It was first established in November, 1999 by Dick Pound. It mainly focused on launching and ascertaining various rules and codes for all the sports played around the world. This organization mainly works with an aspiration to make the sports doping free all over the world. The main objectives was to encourage the athletes to play their games in a fairly manner with sportsmen spirit and high morals. They persuade them to avoid using performance-enhancing drugs or methods.

The steroid trafficking Act of 1989 was introduced in November 1, 1989 by US Senator Joseph Biden. This bill aimed to control the use of steroids by allocating anabolic steroids to Schedule II controlled substances and further restricting the illegal use of steroids. USADA had initially started a nine member non-profit organization on October 1, 2000. Among them, five were former Olympic athletes and other four were nominated from independent companies around the world. It has been found that steroids and performance enhancers have been used in all organizations of sports across the world. So, this agency has the rights to perform anti-doping tests in athletes playing across the nation. Moreover, it has been observed that steroids or performance enhancers are being used widely across the world in all sports organizations. An anti-steroid campaign named Play Asterisk Free was launched in February 2011 by the combined efforts of United States Olympic Committee and the Ad Council to aim at youth involved in sports. This campaign was initially instigated in 2008 underneath the heading of "Don't Be An Asterisk!". The USADA also released proof against cyclist Lance Armstrong in October 2012 to substantiate their doping claim.

World Anti-doping code was prepared with the aim of harmonizing anti-doping set of rules worldwide in all the sports. It comprises of the list of all the substances and methods to be avoided by the sportsmen around the world. It was implemented in 2004 in Athens, Greece before the Olympic games by sports organizations followed by a revision in 2007 and 2009. Amendments in the code were further approved in 2013 elucidating about the first offence and lenience to the anti-doping cooperative athletes. The final code came into effect on 1ˢᵗ January, 2015.

Various types of criticism also aroused regarding the validation of the anti-doping tests. They argued about the closed system followed by anti-doping agencies. Professor Donald A. Berry criticized the statistical validation of the battery of tests followed in anti-doping tests.

The Athlete Biological Passport

The concept of Athlete Biological Passport (ABP) came into regulations to identify the variations in performance of the athletes in concordance to the variations caused by doping in results of key biomarkers through the long term monitoring of such biomarkers. The system of ABP mainly depends on the principle of long term monitoring of the selected biological parameters which may directly or indirectly disclose the doping effects on the body. This approach will help the anti-doping organizations to engender the longitudinal profile of an individual athlete in order to come across any type of fluctuations which indicates the use of performance enhancers by the athletes.

The longitudinal profile of an individual athlete is created on the basis of various statistical tools which used to utilize the data from previous samples to calculate the possible individual range or reference array for future sampling. The interpretation of the data is done as per the reference limits of each athlete. Any variations in the data from the reference range results in signal generation for doping or any pathological condition. Same data can also be helpful in recognizing the athletes with abnormal profiles for conducting other targeted conventional anti-doping tests. During anti-doping rule violation cases, the ABP data may also be used as substantial evidence of doping.

Assumptions of the Athlete Biological Passport

The speculations of the athlete biological passport mainly emphasis on the individualization and prolonged monitoring of the doping substances in all the sports personnel. The main grey area to attain athlete compliance as per anti doping roles is the certainty of detection. This will help in accomplishing the aim of clean competition. Various factors are involved in attaining the certainty in detection of doping substances. The prolongation of the detection window mainly occurs due to presence of long lasting metabolites of the doping substances with prolonged half lives and continued advances in the detection methods.

Variables to be Monitored in the Athlete Biological Passport

Initially, WADA has only introduced hematological module for ABP followed by introduction of steroidal module as second module in 2013 and became operational from

January, 2014. The concept of ABP had replaced the approach of "population reference" to the approach of "intra-individual" which further direct to an extra refined evaluation of the anti-doping compaign.

The Concept of the Athlete Biological Passport

The most important element in achieving athlete compliance with anti-doping rules is the certainty of detection. Thus, scientific research plays a mission critical role in achieving clean competition. Many factors contribute to the advances in detection. The advances in the ability to detect prohibited substances and identification of long-lived metabolites continue to lengthen detection windows. The ABP aims to detect these changes through its 3 modules i.e. hematological, steroidal and endocrine modules.

Hematological module: A series of tests are performed from each athelete for the haematological profiling. The individual limits for each athelete is established based on the profiles of the various tests conducted. The approach known as the "indirect" detection is followed in which comparison of each sample is done with the individual's own "normal" haematological levels. The variations in the samples that are found to be statistically significant are further assessed for blood manipulation. The potential biomarkers identified for the purpose of detection are erythropoietic stimulants, blood transfusions, Hb concentration and reticulocyte levels.

The Analyses of Blood Samples and Examination of Results is Done in Three Steps

- The analysis of each sample is carried out by a laboratory that is accredited and approved by WADA. The analysis of blood samples should be done in accordance with the haematological module of ABP. The list of the laboratories conducting these tests can be obtained from website of the WADA. The results of these biological tests are required to be uploaded into Anti-Doping Administration & Management System (ADAMS).

- The Adaptive Model is a mathematical probability model which is used for the identification of unusual results of an athlete. This model keeps in check the athlete's passport. In this model, the longitudinal results of the interesting markers are calculated by assuming the normal physiological condition of an athlete while conducting the doping test.

- The report generated by the Adaptive Model is known as Atypical Passport Finding (ATPF). ATPF identifies the marker values which are outside the intra-individual range. The results obtained from these tests can be identified as solo or a profile of marker values.

- An ATPF is subjected to additional investigations based on the results of the tests. Firstly, the athlete's profile is sent to an independent expert in Lausanne by the independent Athlete Passport Management Unit (APMU). The selected expert must have thorough understanding of one or more fields of clinical haematology, sports medicine, clinical haematology and exercise physiology. The profile of an athlete is meticulously reviewed by the expert and then the feedback is sent to the APMU for final decision. The compliance to WADA standards are ensured by cross checking of results of all the tests carried out under haematological module of ABP by ADAMS. Moreover, WADA is constantly involved in reviewing of these results and thus assuring the full confidentiality and transparency.

Steroidal module: The anti-doping laboratories reported anabolic androgenic steroids as the most repeatedly banned substance for many years. Manfred Donike proposed the concept of T/E value to prevent testosterone misuse in 1980s. T/E value is a ratio of glucuroconjugated testosterone (T) to epitestosterone (E). A ratio higher than 6 was highly considered an abuse of testosterone considering the exception of abnormal physiological or pathological condition. However the authority of the T/E ratio was questioned due to introduction of various different supplementary testosterone formulations as well as the testosterone precursors. For this reason, other inactive metabolites (etiocholanolone, androsterone, and androstanediols) were included inorder to expand the steroid profile. Later in 2000, with the advancement of technology various other techniques like gas chromatography/combustion/isotopic ratio mass spectrometry (GC/C/IRMS) analyses were considered to be the ultimate direct detection tools. Then, GC/C/IRMS analysis became the gold standard in 2004, and is performed on all samples with abnormal metabolite concentration.

Analysis and Examination of Urine Sample

- The endogenous steroid data of an individual is followed over time. It was observed that the deviation of T/E values was not more than 30% of the individual mean value, except for the menstruating women and the women on oral contraceptives. Therefore, steroid profiles are mainly targeted to identify those athletes which are most likely going to manipulate their data. These individuals are further exposed to number of specific tests involving GC/C/IRMS analysis.

- The extensive scientific research and longitudinal steroid profiles help in precise detection of parameters that predict the testosterone abuse and related substances. This detailed analysis revealed that various factors like heterogeneous (e.g., age, gender and genotype) and other confounding factors adds to the data variation.

- The nonstandardized analytical procedures conducted for steroid analyses in various anti-doping laboratories are also the cause of steroidal passports for its mediocrity. Thus it became necessary to introduce the standardized protocols, such as the WADA technical documents.

- The sorting and integration of all the information from the urine steroid profile data is currently managed by ADAMS to produce the so-called steroidal passport, which is further assessed by the adaptive model to calculate individual limits.

- If the data in the steroidal profile falls out of the individual range, then that particular sample is marked and supplementary analysis are required. On the basis of results conducted by the particular laboratory, they are further analyzed (e.g. IRMS analysis) as per the ATPF generated by the steroidal module of the Adaptive Model.

Endocrine module: Various growth hormones (GH) are detected via the endocrine module. The function of growth hormone is to stimulate the growth of the cell and its regeneration. GH abuse in sports was indentified in early1980s, with the extraction and purification of "cadaver GH" from pituitary glands. There are various reasons for which which human growth hormone is used as a doping agent. Firstly it reduces body fats (lipolysis), secondly it leads to increase in muscle mass (anabolic effect), and thirdly it also has tissue repairing effect (recovery). The Insulin like growth factor -I (IGF-I) promotes the anabolic effect of GH by increasing the protein turnover and promoting muscle synthesis. In order to further enhance performance, GH is used synergistically with other performance-enhancing drugs by the atheletes.

In 1985, in an era of recombinant DNA technology, the first hormone to be produced was GH. The anti-doping test came into existence in the mid-2000s. The test was based on the degeneration pattern of GH isoforms synthesized by recombination technology. During the same time, various other useful biomarkers of GH were discovered that can be used for doping. This includes markers, such as IGF binding protein 1 (IGF)-1 and (IGFBP-3) which are the markers of action of GH on the liver and markers like procollagen III peptide which predicts the action of GH on tissue collagen turnover. During the Olympic games of 2012, growth hormone doping was tested through the GH-2000 detection test.

Analysis and Examination of Growth Hormones

- The markers are evaluated for several confounding factors, such as age, gender, e exercise, connective tissue injury, sporting discipline and social background. Interestingly, it was found that all these biomarkers showed low intra individual variations therefore by using one's own reference will increase the reliability of the methods (direct and indirect) used in detection of growth hormone doping.

- The implementation of these endocrinological biomarkers requires additional studies as there is no available data of the variations that arises after following the strict procedures of the ABP.

- The endocrine module employs various techniques for testing the target hormone levels. For eg: isoform immunoassay and chromatography-mass spectrometry is used to detect GH and its isoforms. Therefore, it enables the detection of violation of anti-doping regulations.

- The knowledge gathered from both steroidal and hematological modules serves as the basis to understand the role of endocrine module in implementation of ABP.

Table 40.1 Summary of different modules of Athlete biological passport

S. No.	Modules	Biomarkers
1.	Hematological module	Haemoglobin, red blood cell count, haematocrit, reticulocyte percentage, mean corpuscular volume, mean corpuscular haemoglobin, red cell distribution with standard deviation, immature reticulocyte fraction, off-hr score, abnormal blood profile score
2.	Steroidal module	Testosterone, epitestosterone, androsterone, etiocholanolone, testosterone to epitestosterone ratio, androsterone to etiocholanolone ratio, androsterone to testosterone ratio, 5α-androstane-3α,17β-diol, 5β-androstane-3α,17β-diol, 5α-androstane-3α,17β-diol to 5β-andro-stane-3α,17β-diol ratio, 5α-androstane-3α,17β-diol to 5β-androstane-3α,17β-diol ratio
3.	Endocrine module	Growth hormone and its isoforms, insulin like growth factor-1, insulin like growth factor binding protein-1, insulin like growth factor binding protein-3, procollagen III

Achievements in Anti-doping Research

Advancement of techniques: In almost every field of science, the measurement technology serves the basis of new advances and understanding. Antidoping science also follows the same basis. The recent advancement in MS, such as the improvement in mass analyzers with significantly increased ion storage and high mass resolution and scanning capabilities have brought revolution n in the detection methods of routine testing as well as detection of prohibited substances. The techniques like tandem and high mass resolution MS which are empowered to detect lower limits of detection have opened new areas of research. The limits of detection are decreased with the advancement in interface efficiency between techniques like liquid and gas chromatography and mass spectrometry. Finally, for an efficient separation speed and resolution, advanced chromatographic techniques like ultrahigh performance LC and two-dimensional GC and LC, are used.

Advancement in Methodology for Detection of Prohibited Substances

- The development of "dilute and shoot" methods in the urine analysis has augmented laboratory efficiency, by providing a method to rapidly detect a wide range of substances in one instrumental round.

- The discovery of long half life metabolites of the doping agents proved to be a boon to the anti-doping compaign. It was initially found in case of 17-alkylated steroids whose sulfate metabolites had very long half life. It was followed by detection of menadienone metabolite in urine after 19 days of intake. Moreover, a window period of 28 days was reported in case of 17-epistanozalol-N-glucuronide which is a metabolite of stanazolol.

- Longitudinal monitoring was made more meaningful by Sottas et al. with the use of bayesian network to include confounding factors. He introduced a evolution from population to individual-based statistics.

- The response of minor metabolites of testosterone and dehydroepiandrosterone (DHEA) like 4-hydroxy-androstenedione, 6α-hydroxy-androstenedione, 16α-hydroxyandrostenedione and16α-hydroxy-DHEA has shown to be more sensitive than current steroid profile. Therefore, new research opportunities are implemented that can also detect minor metabolites of steroids.

- The exogenous administration can be detected based on the difference between the 13C and 12C content and the mole fraction of the endogenous and exogenous testosterone in the metabolic pool.

- Lasne and de Ceaurriz introduced a technique known as isoelectric focusing in the year 2000 to detect rhEPO in urine. Isoelectric focusing separates various glycoforms of native and rhEPO.

- The recent mass spectrometers with enhanced sensitivity like LC-MS/MS can even detect receptor binding sites. Therefore the differences in the glycosylation at the binding sites of rhEPO and native EPO can be detected.

- In case of allogenic blood transfusion, a flow-cytometric test based on surface markers of red blood cells is found to be evidence in establishing a doping breach.

- The variations in the form of manipulation in athlete's blood levels can be minimized by comparing the parameters of detection in a new sample versus the previous sample. When an athlete is on performance enhancers, a steady profile cannot be maintained thus making him more prone to detection through doping control.

Challenges for Anti-doping Community

- Athletes obtain the drugs from the sources that make compounds "for research use only." There might be the metabolic fate and long term side effects of such drugs which are not yet published and reported by a pharmaceutical company. Many times, these companies do not share the information with anti-doping agencies regarding their confidential reference materials. Therefore, anti-doping laboratories are needed to develop methods and perform *in vitro* studies to detect the effects of the doping agents.

- The funding is a biggest challenge faced by scientific anti-doping agencies around the world due to continuous advances in the technologies involved in anti-doping. The cost of the new technology and the transference to the laboratories accredited by WADA- is highly expensive. For eg. The cost required to run a flow cytometer for detection of allogenic blood transfusion is very high due to involvement of various validation procedures and personnel training.

- The concern of requiring human subject approval for the conduction of anti-doping studies in healthy population inorder to establish decision limits for naturally occurring compounds is challenging.

- There are certain studies which require approval from FDA prior to human subjects' approval which leads to major delays in development of novel approaches for the detection of doping materials. For example, prior to obtain a human subjects' approval for an efficacy and safety study of inert gas like xenon, an investigational new drug exemption from the FDA is required.

- Athletes express concerns that reference range of the population studies are not applicable to the highly trained and privileged athletes. But on the other hand, very few athletes agree for donating their blood samples for research purposes. The response of participation of athletes in research studies is modest.

- The centralized storage of the samples is required to assist various clinical studies for detecting designer drugs. The present scenario is lacking in maintaining centralized sharing of theses samples.

- Another important challenge in the field of anti-doping is the procurement of reference materials required for identifying the prohibited substances.

- The collection and shipping charges of blood samples are very high.

Suggested Readings

1. Bowers LD, Bigard X. Achievements and Challenges in Anti-Doping Research. Med Sport Sci. 2017; 62: 77-90.

2. Cawley AT, Keledjian J. Intelligence-based anti-doping from an equine biological passport. Drug Test Anal. 2017; 9(9): 1441-1447.

3. Robinson N, Sottas PE, Schumacher YO. The Athlete Biological Passport: How to Personalize Anti-Doping Testing across an Athlete's Career? Med Sport Sci. 2017; 62: 107-118.

CHAPTER 41

DRUG IN LEGAL ASPECTS

Definition of Drug

Drug is defined as all medicines for internal or external use of human beings or animals and all substances intended to be used for or in the diagnosis, treatment, mitigation or prevention of any diseases or disorder in human beings or animals, including preparations applied on human body for the purpose of repelling insects like mosquitoes. So, from the above definition, it is clear that the term drug covers a wide spectrum of products with varying application. Some of the terms like misbranded, spurious and adulterated drugs which the reader vitally needs to be aware for the comprehension of drug regulation are presented in the following paragraphs.

Cognizance of Important and oft Repeated Terms in Drug Regulation

If a drug is not labeled in the prescribed manner (or) coloured/ coated to conceal and deceive so as to produce increase therapeutic appeal than what it really possesses, (or) if it's label or material accompanying the drug bear statements making false claim about the properties of the drug, then that drug is a **misbranded drug**.

If the drug is kept in a container composed of poisonous, deleterious substances (or) prepared, packed or stored in insanitary conditions (or) if it as a whole or part contain filthy, putrid or decomposed substance which is supposed not be present (or) if it contains harmful or toxic substances (or) contain reduced quality and strength of Active Pharmaceutical Ingredient (than which is claimed by the drug label), then the drug is a **adulterated drug.**

If a drug is imported in a name impersonating another drug (or) if it is an imitation of or substitute for another drug so as to deceive the consumers (or) if the label contains claim of company which does not exist in reality (or) if it is substituted wholly or part by another drug (or) if it claims to be a false product of a company but the claimed product is not in its portfolio, then the drug is a spurious drug.

Understanding the Gravity of Situation with a Practical Example

Misbranded, adulterated and spurious drugs portrays a formidable concern to the Government as well as people involved in the healthcare sector because it becomes very difficult to weed these drugs form that of the standard quality drugs. They often get mingled to a great extent with legitimate drugs that many a times, it is mistaken to be legitimate. It results in significant wastage of resources spent in healthcare along with loss of time.

Let us cite an example, for letting the readers decipher the gravity of the situation. A treatment course is planned with the drug Liposomal Amphotericin B for a patient who has acquired invasive fungal infection during the course of hospital stay. The weight of the patient is 60 Kg and the therapeutic dose to be administered is 4 mg/kg for a period of 14 days. The cost of single vial of Liposomal Amphotericin B (containing 50 mg) is hypothetically taken as Rs 4000/-. On the basis of above information, the cost for the treatment of fungal infection alone is Rs. 2,80,000/- and this amounts to a huge economic requirement for an average middle-class person. If at the end of treatment due to administration of misbranded/ adulterated/ spurious drug, there occurred failure of cure, then it would lead to further momentous amalgamation of triad of misery namely - sorrow, loss of wealth and loss of time. Thus, misbranded, adulterated and spurious drugs hit the economy, time as well as emotions of the society. It's like a cruzer blade which pierces the healthcare architecture and garners agony cum anguish by creating more failures than successes.

Central Drugs Standard Control Organization (CDSCO)

The CDSCO (Central Drugs Standard Control Organization) is the central drug authority who is vested with the duty of drug regulation under the Drug and Cosmetics Act, 1940. (2) Its vision is to promote and protect public health in India. Drug Control General of India (DCGI) is the chief authority of CDSCO. The current DCGI is Dr.S.Eswara Reddy and the former DCGI was Dr. G.N. Singh. Under CDSCO, there are 6 zonal offices, 4 sub-zonal offices, 13 port offices and 7 laboratories (as on July 2018). It forms the apex organisation for drug regulatory activities in India.

CDSCO has central and state division. Regulation of manufacturing, sale and distribution at the state level are taken care by the respective state authorities (lead by the respective State Drug Controllers), whereas the approval of new drugs, approval for the conduct of clinical trial, laying down norms regarding the standard of drugs, exercising control over the import of drug and supervision/coordination of state regulatory authorities are the function of central authorities (lead by the DCGI). CDSCO is constituted under the Ministry of Health, Government of India.

When genetically manipulated product or biologics come for review to CDSCO for conducting clinical studies then Genetic Engineering Approval Committee constituted by the Department of Biotechnology and Ministry of Environment additionally comes into play. But even for these products, the final go (or) no-go decision lies with CDSCO.

Important Acts and Agency Relating to Drug Regulation in India

The sale import and manufacturing of drugs in India is regulated by the Drugs and Cosmetics Act (1940). The Act has undergone series of amendments since its enactment in 1940. As described earlier, CDSCO is the highest regulatory agency under this Act. The D and C Act 1940 contain many schedules which are laying rules for different activities pertaining to drug regulation. Schedule M is for specifying the requirement of factory premises for manufacture of drugs. Schedule T lays GMP specifications for AYUSH medicines (Ayurveda, Siddha, Unani and Homeopathy). Schedule Y is for legislative requirements for conduct of clinical trial. The drugs are classified into Schedule X (narcotics), Schedule H and L (injectable, antibiotics and antibacterial) and Schedule C and C1 (biological product -serum and vaccine). The recent amendment of Drugs and Cosmetics Act (2011), enforces registration of Clinical Research Organisation (CRO) for the purpose of conducting Clinical Trials (CT) (Schedule Y1). Department of AYUSH is the regulatory authority for manufacture and marketing of herbal drugs.

Drugs and Magic Remedies (Objectionable Advertisement) Act (1954) was enacted for controlling drug advertisements in India, and under this proclamation of magic remedies for drugs is an offence. For the regulation of Narcotic and Psychotropic drugs, the important act is the Narcotic Drugs and Psychotropic Substances Act (1985). Medical Devices Rules(2017), brings in DCGI as the Central Licensing Authority (CLA) for medical devices. The medical devices are divided into 4 categories namely A to D (C and D are directly under the DCGI licensing whereas A and B are under the licensing of State Drug Controllers).

Regulation of Drug Prices

In India, the drug pricing regulation is looked after by the Department of Pharmaceutical - National Pharmaceutical Pricing Authority. It comes under the Ministry of Chemicals and Fertilizers. There is a list of drugs released as Drug Price Control Order for which maximum sale price is fixed. The latest DPCO released in 2013 contain 384 drugs. The readers should know that the retails price of the formulation is not arbitrarily set but it is calculated based on a formula which takes into consideration information such as material cost, conversion cost, cost of packing material, packing charges, excise duty and Maximum Allowable Post-Manufacturing Expenses into consideration.

Indian Pharmacopoeia Commission

Drug are compared by assessing their standard/quality with the respective reference standards present in pharmacopeia. These standards are set individually for every country. For India, we have the Indian Pharmacopoeia Commission (IPC) as the authority which spearheads the activities pertaining to creation and maintenance of Indian Pharmacopoeia (IP) as well as the National Formulary of India (NFI). IPC is an autonomous institution under the Ministry of Health and Family Welfare, Government of India. It also sets the standards for devices and technologies used in healthcare field, though additional approvals need to be obtained from other departments in that case. RN Chopra Committee was the pioneer in first preparing the list of material and drugs which were used in India as early as 1944. The first edition of Indian Pharmacopoeia was launched in 1955.

Radiopharmaceuticals

Radiopharmaceuticals are regulated and governed by AREB (Atomic Energy Regulatory Board). AREB is under the Department of Atomic Energy, Government of India. Even for radiopharmaceuticals, the final decision and overseeing is with CDSCO. There are 4 guidelines related to radiopharmaceuticals released by AREB; Regulatory Inspection and Enforcement in Nuclear and Radiation Facilities (2002), Security of Radioactive Material During Transport (2008), Nuclear Medicine Facility (2011), Radioisotope Handling Facilities (2015)). But considering the developed countries, the guidelines are sparse and there is an urgent requirement for new guideline enactment.

Regulation within Pharmaceutical Company and ICH

The regulatory affairs are the division within the pharmaceutical company concerned with regulatory works. It acts as a link between the company and regulatory body. A mandate of regulatory affairs is to be updated with latest rules in different geographical region in which the company is operating. The International Council for Harmonisation of Technical Requirements for Pharmaceuticals for Human Use (ICH) is for bringing together scientific and technical aspects of drug registration in different country. Its mission is to have development of high-quality medicines in a resource efficient manner.

Functions of the Drug Regulatory Authorities

The function of the drug regulatory authority includes

1. **Authorization for marketing a drug product:** This is foremost important job of drug regulatory authority. Think about this hypothetical scenario which would unfold if the drug regulation practices are not in place. A researcher undertakes a study in an animal model of stroke and found efficacy with an investigational drug (improved neurological scores). Based on the study results, he has started selling his drug directly to the patients through pharmacy stores near his home. So, with no

drug regulation, patient would be directly exposed to unregulated, unscientific and harmful drugs - culminating in patients facing serious consequences. These are kept in check by the stringent practices of regulation which are in place for authorization and for marketing a drug product.

2. **Monitoring the ways in which the advertisements are made for the drugs:** Pharmaceutical industry is a multi-billionaire sector and there is a huge competition among the players in competing with each other in bringing about their products in the forefront. Without the regulations in place for controlling drug promotion every company would foreseeably market their drug as a wonder-drug for curing illnesses and propel minute-to-minute advertisement in social media & television channels claiming out-of-box efficacy and null side effect.

3. **Setting up laboratory for testing quality of drugs:** For understanding this, think about the claims which are commonly uttered by the Physicians and patients

> *"Generic drug is of lower quality than branded drugs"*
>
> *"The quality of hospital supply is lesser than that of drugs which are procured from pharmacy."*
>
> *"My patient gets cured when he is prescribed brand drugs (some selected brand) and other brands seldom work."*
>
> *"My experience says that that brand drug will not work."*

These claims are unscientific in the current modern era of healthcare. The generic drug gets approved only after conducting proper bioequivalence studies. Experience is not taken as the factor and valid scientific study gets the limelight in proving a claim. The regulatory authorities have however provided measures for testing quality of drugs. Physician or any person can send drug samples which they feel as suspicious to Drug Testing Laboratories (for testing purpose). Regional Drug Testing Laboratories have been set up in almost every state. Samples can be sent for legal as well as routine testing to these centers. It is important to know that if you need a sample to be taken for legal testing, then the sample should be collected directly by the Drug Inspector. Legal testing means based on the result of the quality test, if the drug is found to be Not of Standard Quality (NSQ), spurious or misbranded, then legal action of varying spectra (extending from closing the manufacturing unit/company to issuing official warning) can be undertaken.

4. **The provision of information regarding the drug:** When the drug is marketed a huge amount of information is provided by the company to the drug regulatory authority. Much of these information's cannot be incorporated into the drug labels. Hence, it is imperative that a cross section of the claims be made available in the regulatory body's official portal so that public as well as the healthcare community access the information when required. In addition, many-a-times specific and special information about the safety of the drug in pregnancy, lactation,

renal/hepatic impairment are also provided. The regulatory authority possesses powers to bind the pharmaceutical company to undertake additional studies and make them provide time-bound explanation as and when new information surfaces (harnessing queries) about the drug.

1. **Issuing licenses to pharmaceutical manufacturers and importers, so as to regulate "who can do what?" in the country:** Then comes issuing licenses to distributors whose profile is to take the manufactured and imported drug to the retail and wholesale outlets. The licenses are also issued to retail and wholesale outlets. These licenses help in curbing the outlets - found selling misbranded or spurious drugs and helps in implementing key rules like requirement of prescription for dispensing drugs other than OTC drugs (Over the Counter).

2. **Inspection of the premises in which the licenses were issued:** this include manufacturing, distribution channels as well as outlets.

3. **Monitoring of adverse drug reaction:** The Regulatory body issues update report about any new adverse drug reaction arising out of treatment with the drug.

4. **Clinical trial:** authorization, sanction and indirect supervision.

5. Promotion of rational drug use and its supervision.

6. Making sure that the regulatory work does not unjustifiably hinder the access to medicine.

7. Arranging of meetings between different technical board for making key decisions. An example is CDSCO regularly arranges meetings with Drug Consultative Committee (DCC) and Drugs Technical Advisory Board (DTAB).

History of Drug Regulation

International Perspective

In US, the death of soldiers due to the supply of adulterated and spurious drugs from the Europe during the US-Mexico war serves as the sowing seed for incarnation of Import Drugs Act of 1848. The enacted Act made it mandatory for quality checking in imported drugs but had key pitfalls like failure of provision to address substandard domestic products. Subsequently, the United States Pharmacopoeia was made official for testing the quality of imported drugs against the respective reference standards. In 1901, the vaccine tragedy which consisted of death of 14 children due to contamination in diphtheria vaccine stocks raised eyes in US over the then existing Import Drugs Act (United States(US) - 1848), and mandated changes to be made to the Act to include wider zones of drug regulation into the purview. The Biologics Control Act (US - 1902) was created as an aftermath enforcing separate manufacturing facility for vaccines, specific labeling requirement and establishment of distribution channels. The post of Director of Drug Laboratory of the Bureau of Chemistry which is akin to the current DCGI was created as early as 1903.

In 1905, American Medical Association (AMA) came with a move which required companies to demonstrate proof for the claim of efficacy made in their drug product (will be reviewed by expert) so as to qualify for advertising in AMA related journals. This is similar to the current century clinical trial data review required for approving and giving market status to a drug. This program was voluntary and not legally bound. Then the original Food Drugs Act was enacted and passed in the year 1906 in US making mandatory the labelling of ingredients and contents of drug. The pitfall of this law is that it outlaws false labelling statement made in drug label but acquits drug makers making false medical statements. In order to overcome this, Sherley Amendment was made in 1912.

The next disaster which turned heads of the regulators for more stringent drug regulation law is the Elixir tragedy. The Elixir of Sulfanilamide which was marketed as a sweet tasting liquid for pediatric use lead to the death of 107 children. SE Massengill company, which marketed the drug could not be convicted under serious offences using the Pure and Food Drugs Act (1906) (this demonstrates the weakness of the then prevalent law) and the only crime which was purported on them was mislabeling of the solution as Elixir. The Food and Drug Administration (akin to CDSCO of India) was formed in the year 1930, but since the birth of FDA occurred with the Pure Food and Drugs Act (US - 1906), FDA celebrates 1906 as its foundation year. Following elixir tragedy, the Food, Drugs and Cosmetics Act was then created in the year 1938 which required proof of safety and requirement of regulatory agency (Food and Drug Administration (FDA)) authorization for marketing. This was the forerunner of the Drugs and Cosmetics Act (1940) of India. Then the Durham Humphrey Amendment was then made in US 1951, which brought about the discrimination between the drug which could be sold without prescription and those which need a prescription for sale. The chloramphenicol incident of 1952 propped up in US, and it essentially gave rise to the program of voluntary reporting of adverse drug reaction by the FDA (two years later).

One of the biggest disasters which brought about the global spotlight on drug regulation is the Thalidomide tragedy of 1962 in Western Europe. The babies of the pregnant women who were taking Thalidomide for pregnancy induced nausea and vomiting suffered from severe congenital anomaly known as phocomelia (condition of malformation of arms and legs). Almost 10000 children were affected in Europe. Following this incident, the 65/65/EC directive was passed by the European Economic Commission which mandated the process of drug approval for the purpose of marketing in Europe. The main goal of 65/65/EEC being protection of public health and enabling free movement of products among EU member countries.

Every pharmacologist should know about Dr Frances Oldham Kelsey a medical officer at the FDA who played a major role in prevention of occurrence of thalidomide disaster in America. When the drug manufacturers of Thalidomide, William S. Merrell petitioned for granting marketing approval in US, the then FDA regulatory official Oldham Kelsey demanded for more information on drug safety. Though she was initially taunted as bureaucrat for her ruthlessness, everyone ultimately realized her valuable vigilance which was responsible for saving American people from a big impending disaster. This incident also highlights the importance of drug regulation and aura of work of drug regulatory authorities. *Kefauver-Harris Amendment* was made in the US which mandatorily required company to prove that their drug had efficacy and greater safety before granting drug approval. Filing of INDA (Investigational New Drug Application) was also made compulsory.

Other significant historical Acts include the Over the Counter Drug Review (US - 1972), Orphan Drug Act (US - 1983) for promoting research in treating rare diseases, Drug Price Competition and Patent Term Restoration (US - 1984) for promoting generics & for provision of addition 5 years patent period for brand drug company. The Prescription Drug Marketing Act (US - 1988) was the forerunner for bringing about provision of granting licenses for distribution and wholesale of drugs by the drug regulatory authority. The Act essentially bans diversion of drugs other than legitimate channels. Concentration procedure (EU - 1987) is for assessing products and technology innovation related to biologics, blood and blood related products for granting marketing authorization. Pediatric Rule (US - 1998) was for drug safety and efficacy in children.

Indian Perspective

The Poisons Act (India - 1919) was the forerunner act for initial drug regulation in India. Though it is meant only for substance specified as poisons, it regulated rules for possession and sale of substance including clear labelling as well as audit of vendors who sell those substances. This was followed by the Dangerous Drugs Act (India - 1930) which regulated the cultivation of opium plant as well as possession and other activities related to opium. Both the above-mentioned act was later replaced by the Narcotics and Psychotropic Substances Act (India - 1985).

Indian Patent Act (1970) was the prime act for patent protection in India, under which only process patent was allowed in India and product patent was not allowed. Process patent refers to patent in the methodology implied in the manufacturing of drug. This can be better understood with an example. Suppose company named 'A' invented a drug X and applied for patent in India and was subsequently granted patent. Another company 'B' manufactured the same drug X using the same process as that of company 'A' within the patent period, then this becomes a patent infringement and the company 'B' will be facing legal consequences - if sued by company 'A'. Another company 'C' manufactured the same drug 'X' using an entirely new methodology, then the company 'C' is legally protected and has not any patent law of India. Even if company 'A' wishes, it cannot sue the company 'C'. There are both pros and cons due to this Act. The pro being application of reverse engineering by local companies leading to production of cheap drug and moving forward in endowing India as a hub of exporting pharmaceutical products to the world. The con being opposition from big pharmaceutical company which claim loss of capital of money invested in discovering and manufacturing the drug. But due to increased pressure from the global community, India then signed the Patent Cooperation Treaty (PCT 1999) and enforced product patent in India from 2005. Compulsory licensing was then introduced. Compulsory licensing is the granting of license (by the Government) to a company to manufacture a drug without the consent of the patent holder (when a health requirement arises).

Recent Developments in Drug Regulation

1. In 2016, the CDSCO banned 349 irrational FDC in India and revoked the licenses of miscreant pharmaceutical manufacturers. The pharmaceutical company then moved to the Delhi High Court which uplifted the ban. The Government then moved to the supreme court. The supreme court then asked to constitute a sub-committee of DTAB and looked into the matter. The committee then investigated the matter and recommended the banning of 343 drugs. The recommendation is currently in draft stage.

2. In 2016, a draft guideline for biopharmaceuticals was released in by CDSCO and Department of Biotechnology. Some salient point includes recognition of innovator product as reference biologic, approval for parallel submission to two different committee (namely CDSCO and Review Committee on Genetic Manipulation (RCGM)), fixing the lower limit as 100 for clinical trial evaluating bio-pharmaceuticals and fixing 200 as the minimum sample size for post marketing evaluation (phase IV trials).

3. A nationwide survey on spurious drugs (including random assessment of 47,012 drug samples drawn from market) was conducted between 2014- 2016. In this survey, it was known that 3.16% of drug was of Not of Standard Quality and 0.0245% was of spurious standards.

4. As on April 2018, CDSCO is in the process of preparation of guidelines for stem cells and nanomaterials manufacturing in India.

5. In 2018, the Expert committee constituted by CDSCO had earmarked a minimum fine of Rs 20 lakh for each patient affected by faulty implant (ASR XL Acetabular System) manufactured by the DePuy Orthopaedics (subsidiary of multinational pharmaceutical giant Johnson & Johnson pharmaceuticals).

6. In 2018, the Government issued a ban on the manufacture of oxytocin due to the abuse in cattle. The rights to manufacture of oxytocin was given only to a single company (Karnataka Antibiotics and Pharmaceuticals Ltd (KAPL)). However, due to apprehension of shortage of oxytocin, the ban on oxytocin was temporarily uplifted later.

Suggested Readings

1. Bhuiyan PS, Rege NN. ICH Harmonised Tripartite Guideline: guideline for good clinical practice. 2001; Available from: https://tspace.library.utoronto.ca/handle/1807/23547

2. Bren L. Frances Oldham Kelsey. FDA medical reviewer leaves her mark on history. FDA Consum. 2001 Mar; 35(2): 24-9.

3. CDSCO [Internet]. [Cited 2017 May 30]. Available from: https://cdscoonline.gov.in/CDSCO/homepage

4. Chandramouli R. Pharmaceutical Pricing in India: A Pharmacoeconomic Perspective. Journal of Pharmaceutical Research. 2015 Aug 1; 0(0): 35-35.

5. Dey S, Kumar M. Oxytocin ban put on hold till September | India News - Times of India [Internet]. The Times of India. 2018 [cited 2018 Sep 13]. Available from: https://timesofindia.indiatimes.com/india/oxytocin-ban-put-on-hold-till-september/articleshow/64830926.cms

6. Gupta YK, Ramachandran SS. Fixed dose drug combinations: Issues and challenges in India. Indian J Pharmacol. 2016 Jul; 48(4): 347-9.

7. The A.I.R. Manual: Criminal Procedure Code, section 241 to Drugs and Magic Remedies (Objectionable Advertisements) Act, 1954. All India Reporter; 1959. India.

8. Indian Pharmacopoeia Commission. Indian Pharmacopoeia 2014 (4 Vol Set). Indian Pharmacopoeia Commission; 2013.

9. Jain PK. Commentaries on The Narcotic Drugs and Psychotropic Substances Act, 1985 (61 of 1985) with Rules and Notifications (central & State Goverments) Including Preventive Laws & International Conventions Relating to Narcotics. Prashaut Publication; 1989. 761 p.

10. Kondratas RA. Biologics control act of 1902. The early years of federal food and drug control. 1982; 8-27.

11. Krantz JC Jr. New drugs and the Kefauver-Harris amendment. J New Drugs. 1966 Mar; 6(2): 77-9.

12. Roy S. Govt seeks to define stem cells as drug, regulate use in therapy - Times of India [Internet]. The Times of India. 2018 [cited 2018 Sep 13]. Available from: https://timesofindia.indiatimes.com/india/govt-seeks-to-define-stem-cells-as-drug-regulate-use-in-therapy/articleshow/63776306.cms

14. Torbenson M, Erlen J. A Case Study of the Lash's Bitters Company—Advertising Changes after the Federal Food and Drugs Act of 1906 and the Sherley Amendment of 1912. Pharm Hist. 2003; 45(4): 139-49.

15. Walch A. A Spurious Solution to a Genuine Problem: An In-Depth Look at the Import Drugs Act of 1848 [Internet]. 2002 [cited 2019 Jan 9]. Available from: https://papers.ssrn.com/abstract=2695100

16. Young JH. Pure Food: Securing the Federal Food and Drugs Act of 1906. Princeton University Press; 2014. 336 p.

CHAPTER 42

DRUG-EXCIPIENT INTERACTIONS

Drug excipients are defined as any substance added to the pharmaceutical dosage form other than active pharmaceutical ingredients (APIs) to build the desired form/shape. They are inserted to aid manufacturing, administration and absorption of the drug in the body. Earlier, they were usually categorized as "inert", however nowadays found to interact with API both chemically and physically leading to compromised quality or efficacy of the medicine. The choice of addition of an excipient to a pharmaceutical formulation has become an area of concern in the present scenario. The guidelines regarding the use of excipients should be revised periodically in view of the various issues regarding safety and efficacy of the formulated medicine. Excipients assist in designing a formulation by providing a wide range of properties to obtain a desired finished product. This chapter reviews the role of excipients in formulation development and challenges associated with their direct use as well as in combination with the APIs. A brief about various guidelines about the rationale of use of excipients and their interactions will also be discussed.

According to the International Pharmaceutical Excipients Council (IPEC), an excipient is defined as any substance required to be added to the formulation during manufacturing process supplementary to the active drug or prodrug to obtain a finished pharmaceutical dosage form. The IPEC Federation being a global organization promotes quality in pharmaceutical excipients. It represents five existing regional IPECs - IPEC-America, IPEC Europe, IPEC Japan, IPEC China and IPEC India. They integrate to endorse the vital use of excipients in formulating a medicine to provide safe and efficacious treatment to patients.

Commercially available excipients afford a range of various functions as a processing aid to the final product like lubricity, flowability, compressibility and compatibility. The US Pharmacopeia–National Formulary (USP-NF) classify excipients into categories of binders, disintegrants, lubricants, diluents, emulsifying–solubilizing agents, glidants, sweetening agents, antimicrobial preservatives, coating agents etc. The examples of agents belonging to above said categories are given in Table 42.1. An ideal excipient should be inert, chemically stable, non-reactive with the API, low equipment and process sensitivity, well characterized, have pleasant organoleptic properties, and compatible with industry and regulatory agencies (Fig. 42.1). A restricted selection of excipients with these preliminary attributes in market poses a great challenge to design a formulation.

Table 42.1 A list of Pharmaceutical Excipients used in pharmaceutical preparations

Types of Excipients	Examples
Fillers	Plant cellulose & Dibasic calcium phosphate. Vegetable fats & oils are used in soft gelatin capsules. Lactose, Mannitol, Sorbitol, Calcium carbonate, and Magnesium stearate are used as filler.
Solvents and co-solvents	Solvent: Glycerol ,propylene glycol, ethanol Co-solvent- sorbitol, glycerol, propylene glycol
Binders	Solution binders dissolved in a solvent e.g.; water or alcohol Dry Binders added to powder e.g.; Cellulose, methyl cellulose, Polyvinyl pyrrolidone, Polyethylene glycol.
Disintegrants	Polyvinylpyrrolidone, carboxymethyl cellulose and sodium starch glycolate
Antiadherants	Magnesium stearate, talc & starch
Glidants	Fumed silica, talc, & magnesium carbonate
Coating Agents	Film coating, sugar coating, compression coating
Sorbents	Natural sorbents: peat moss, sawdust, feathers & anything else natural that contains carbon. Synthetic sorbents: polyethylene and nylon.
Preservatives	Methyl & Ethyl parabens, Propyl paraben, Benzoic acid & its salts, Sorbic acid and its salts.
Chelating agents	EDTA: Ethylene diamine tetra-acetate used for estimation of metals ions. EDTAH4: Ethylene diamine tetraacetic acid used for softening water. Calcium Disodium Edetate: used in treatment of heavy metal poisoning mostly caused by lead. Disodium Edetate
Humectants	Inorganic humectants: Calcium chloride is example. It has compatibility problems and corrosive in nature, so not frequently used in cosmetics. Metal organic humectants: Sodium lactate has limited use in cosmetics because of compatibility problems, corrosive nature and pronounced taste. Organic humectants: Glycerol, ethylene glycol, polyethylene glycol, diethylene glycol, triethylene glycol, propylene glycol, dipropylene glycol, glycerin, sorbitol, mannitol, glucose.

Table 42.1 *Contd...*

Types of Excipients	Examples
Lubricants	Polyethylene glycol, Magnesium stearate, Stearic acid and its derivatives.
Antioxidants	BHT (Butylated Hydroxy Toluene), BHA (Butyl Hydroxy Anisol), Sod. Sulfite
Surface active agents	1. Anionic surfactant (the hydrophilic region is negatively charged i.e. an anion) Sodium lauryl sulphate: used as excipient on disolved aspirins. 2. Cationic surfactant (hydrophilic region is positively charged i.e. a cation), Cetyl trimethyl ammonium bromide (cetrimide) - is an effective antiseptic agent against bacteria and fungi. 3. Non-ionic surfactants: Tween 80 (polyoxyethylene sorbitol monooleate)- Polysorbate 80 is an excipient that is used to stabilize aqueous formulations of medications for parenteral administration. 4. Amphoteric surfactant: Lecithin
Buffering agents	Most of buffering system based on carbonate, citrates, gluconates, lactates, phosphates, or tartrates
Viscosity imparting agents	Hydroxy ethylcellulose Hydroxy propylmethylcellulose Methyl cellulose Polyvinyl alcohol Polyvinyl pyrrolidone
Flavouring agents	Clove oil, citric and syrup, glycerin, rose oil, orange oil, menthol
Colouring agents	1. White: Titanium dioxide 2. Blue: Brilliant blue, Indigo carmine 3. Red: Amaranth Carmine 4. Yellow: saffron 5. Brown: caramel
Sweetening agents	Sucrouse, Saccarine, Aspartame, Sorbitol

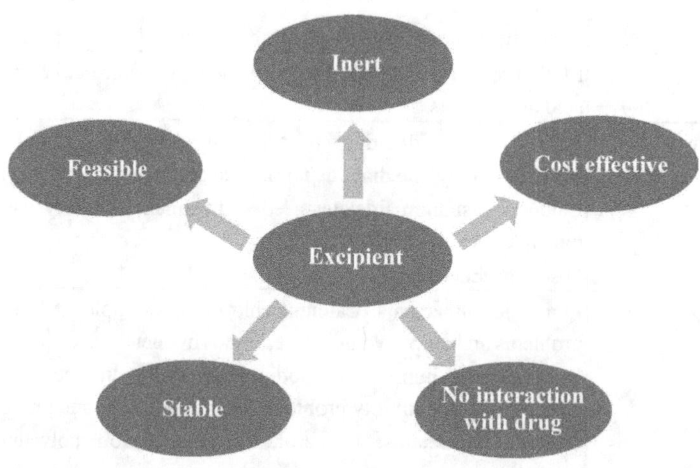

Fig. 42.1 Characteristics of an ideal excipients.

Excipients can also be classified into compendial and noncompendial materials. The composition of compendial excipients is used to be consistent with monographs published in compendia such as USP–NF. They are better characterized and possess all the previously stated desirable properties. However, non-compendial excipients are also used in pharmaceutical formulations but compendial materials are well recognized as preferred excipients. Utilization of noncompendial materials in pharmaceutical formulations is maintained by Type IV drug master files in regulatory dossiers like new drug applications, abbreviated new drug applications, and investigational new drug applications. Manufacturers of the excipients maintained these files to assure the quality, consistency and safety of these excipients during manufacturing of the final formulation. Non-compendial excipients are used to be present in approved drug formulations signifying the recognition of these excipients in the major markets by various agencies like USFDA etc. Formulators can get details about the safety and quality of the excipients from the manufactures and toxicology experts. The information may also be obtained from references like Food Chemicals Codex, Code of Federal Regulations and FDA Inactive Ingredients Guide. The list of food ingredients which are generally considered to be safe is also available in 21 CFR parts 182 and 184.

Efficient Pharmaceutical Development

Enhancement of the efficiency of an already approved medicine can be done by improving the properties of its formulations. The formulations should be patient compliance with minimal side effects, affordable in terms of cost effectiveness and availability. The quality and safety of the formulation can be maintained by vigilantly selecting sufficient number of excipients from a well organized excipient formulary. The establishment of an excipient formulary can help in gearing up the process of better understanding about the safety profile of excipients and improving drug-excipient interactions. This in turn will also improve first and second vendor relationships (identification and qualification). The excipient formulary also helps in proficient use of available assets, reducing development time, harmonizing specification, economic manufacturing and worldwide acceptance.

Selection of an ideal excipient plays an important role in the developmental phase of a formulation. It mainly emphasis on enviable characteristics of an excipient like consistency, regulatory acceptance, functionality, cost effectiveness, availability etc. Excipients (e.g., gelatin, starch) obtained from natural animal sources raised concerns of transmissible spongiform encephalopathy/bovine spongiform encephalopathy/genetically modified organism (TSE/BSE/GMO). A letter of verification is required from a vendor for consumer protection in order to support non-GMO or TSE/BSE implication of these natural materials. Prionics-check certification for ingredients from animal sources can also be obtained from vendors.

Drug Excipient Interactions

Excipients used to play a critical role in formulating a medicine by helping in maintaining its efficacy, safety, and stability in its respective form and also ensuring perfect delivery of their committed benefits to the patients. Optimal utilization of excipients aids the pharmaceutical manufacturing by assisting drug formulation innovation, reducing drug development cost, and enhancing functionality capability. However, excipients can also undergo physical or chemical interactions with the active drug which can compromise with the quality of the formulation. Their interactions may cause formation of some toxic products or causes degradation of the active drug. Excipients may contain some impurities or residues which in turn causes degradation of the active drug. Various unwanted effects of the excipients may also leads to serious consequences of the formulation. There are many modes of drug decomposition by chemical or physical interactions.

Modes of Drug Degradation

Medicinal agents perpetually have structural features to interact with receptors or to facilitate metabolic handling. As expected these agents are vulnerable to degradation (and interaction with other materials). They undergo various reactions like hydrolysis/dehydration, oxidation, isomerisation/epimerization, decarboxylation, rearrangement, photolysis and polymerization. These reactions are usually sensitive to temperature and high temperature used to accelerate them under various sets of humidity (low and high) conditions. Hydrolytic reactions can be accelerated by exposure to both elevated temperature as well as variable pH ranges. Oxidative degradation of formulations commonly occurs as a result of auto-oxidation. Photolytic reactions are propagated by absorption of photons from exposure to different light sources. Table 42.2 lists types of degradation reactions with examples of medicinal agents vulnerable to such modes of degradation. Degradation reflects susceptibility to environmental stresses like temperature, humidity, light and drug–drug interactions. Some of the excipients possess indispensible functional groups for drug interactions and residues to catalyze degradation processes. In some of the times, the new molecules are generated as a result of inherent changeable property of an excipient. The modifications in the property of an excipient also trigger the breakdown of various chemical processes.

Table 42.2 Different modes of drug degradation

S. No.	Type of Reactions	Description	Examples
1.	Hydrolysis	Functional groups such as amides, esters, Lactams or lactams in any drug moiety are more prone to hydrolytic degradation than other groups. Due to ubiquitous nature of water, it is a very frequent mode of degradation of the medicinal formulations. Utilization of water as a vehicle in turn also facilitates microbial growth.	Methyl dopa, Procaine, Penicillins

Table 42.2 Contd...

S. No.	Type of Reactions	Description	Examples
2.	Oxidation	Oxidative mechanisms are multifaceted, involving removal of an electropositive atom, radical or electron or, conversely, addition of an electronegative moiety. Oxidative reactions can be catalyzed by oxygen, heavy metal ions and light, leading to free radical formation. Free radicals react with oxygen to form peroxy radicals which in turn react with oxidizable compounds to generate additional free radicals to generate further reactions. The functional groups like Aldehydes, alcohols, phenols, alkaloids, unsaturated fats and oils are used to be susceptible to oxidation.	Calcitonin, Ascorbic acid, isoprenaline
3.	Isomerization	Isomerization involves conversion of a chemical into its optical or geometric isomer. Isomers may have different pharmacological or toxicological properties. For example, the activity of levo (L) form of adrenaline is 15-20 times greater than for the dextro (D) form.	Tetracycline, Vitamin A, Adrenaline
4.	Photolysis	Reactions such as oxidation-reduction, ring alteration and polymerization can be catalyzed or accelerated by exposure to sunlight or artificial light. Energy absorption is greater at lower wavelengths and, as many as drugs absorb UV light; degradation by low wavelength radiation is common. Exposure to light almost invariably leads to discoloration even when chemical transformation is modest or even undetectable.	Riboflavin, Folic acid, Nifedipine
5.	Polymerization	Intermolecular reactions can lead to dimeric and higher molecular weight species. Concentrated solutions of ampicillin, an amino-pencillin, progressively form dimer, trimer and ultimately polymeric degradation products	Ceftazidime, Ampicillin

Mechanism of Drug-Excipients Interactions

Although there is no precise mechanism of drug- excipient interaction is known till date. However, several mechanisms are well documented in the literature. Generally, drug-excipients interaction used to occur more frequently than other interactions like excipient-excipient interactions. Drug-excipients interaction can be either favorable or injurious, which can be further classified into physical and chemical interactions.

However, physical interactions are relatively common but quite difficult to detect. These interactions do not employ any type of chemical changes. They are commonly used in aiding manufacturing of the dosage forms in order to modify the drug dissolution rates. Though, many of the unintended physical interactions usually cause troubles in manufacturing process of a formulation. Physical interaction can be classified as beneficial or harmful to product performance. They can occur by various types of mechanisms like complexation, adsorption, solid dispersion etc. The detail of these physical interactions with its favorable and harmful effects is shown in Table 42.3.

Table 42.3 Types of physical interactions

Types	Description	Favorable	Harmful
Complexation	Complexing agents used to bind with the drugs reversibly to form a complex which can be soluble or insoluble. The soluble complexes are beneficial by increasing the bioavailability of the formulation. The insoluble complexes slows down the dissolution rate of the drug from its formulation and thus results in lower absortion in the body. Complexation also results in damaged formulation.	The use of cyclodextrin with poorly water soluble drugs improves their bioavailability	An insoluble complex is formed by interaction of calcium carbonate with tetracycline resulting in reduced dissolution and absorption of tetracycline.
Adsorption	Excipients used to adsorb the drug on their surface and increase the surface area of the drug for dissolution resulting in enhance bioavailability. However, the same process could also sometimes make the drug unavailable for dissolution in the body fluids which in turn reduces its bioavailability.	Kaolin increases bioavailability of indomethacin in the body.	Magnesium stearate reduces antibacterial activity of cetyl pyridinium chloride Microcrystalline cellulose also leads to incomplete release of novel k-opioid agonists from the capsules.
Solid Dispersion	Solid dispersion also improves the dissolution and bioavaila-bility of the hydrophobic drugs. It also sometimes leads to reduction in dissolution of the drug.	Solid dispersion of drugs like norfloxacin, nifedipine, piroxicam and ibuprofen using PEG results in their improved bioavailability.	Povidone and stearic acid reduces the dissolution rates of the drugs from the capsules.

Chemical interactions involve formation of unstable compounds by mutual interaction between APIs and excipients in the formulation. Numerous reports of interactions between chemical drugs and excipients are reported in literature. Usually, chemical interactions should be avoided as they elicit deleterious effect on the formulation. Table 42.4 lists various examples of chemical interactions between drug and excipients.

Table 42.4 Examples of Chemical reactions

Chemical moiety	Examples
Aldehydes	Cherry flavor excipient causes famotidine–benzaldehyde adduct formation
	Benzyl Alcohol Oxidation in parenteral formulations
	Amine containing compounds causes vanillin reaction
	Polysorbate 80 and PEG 300 leads to formation of BMS-204352 adduct impurity
	Phenylephrine Reaction used to react with formaldehyde and 5-HMF
	Cyclic heptapeptide causes oxidation of benzaldehyde
Transesterification	Transesterification Reactions between Two Parabens and Sugar Alcohols
	Ester and Amide Formation between Citric Acid and 5-Aminosalicylic Acid
	Reaction of Citric Acid with 6-Aminocaproic Acid
	Ester Formation of Cetirizine with Sorbitol and Glycerol
	Transesterification Reaction of Glycerin and Methylphenidate
	Buprenorphine Degradation in Presence of Citric Acid
Sulfate Adduct in the Parenteral Formulation	Sulfonate adduct formation by reacting dexamethasone sodium phosphate with sodium bisulfite under heat conditions
Magnesium Stearate	Benzilic Acid Rearrangement of Tacrolimus Due to Magnesium Stearate
	Stearoyl Rearrangement of Norfloxacin
	Metal Induced Degradation of Fosinopril Sodium Due to Magnesium Stearate
	Reaction of Duloxetine with HPMCAS
Maillard Reaction	Reaction of Fluoxetine with Lactose
	Reaction of Cetirizine with Hydroxy Propyl Cellulose
	Ceronapril Degradation in Presence of Mannitol and Dibasic Calcium Phosphate Dihydrate
	Olanzapine Stress Studies with Lactose Monohydrate and Lactose Anhydrous
	Condensation Products between Lactose and Hydrochlorothiazide
	Pregabalin Degradation Products in Presence of Lactose
	Acyclovir Degradation Products in Presence of Lactose
	Degradation of Desloratadine in Presence of Starch and Maltose
	Amlodipine Besylate and Lactose Adduct Formation
Peroxides	Peroxide Impurities in Povidones- Formation of N-Oxide in Raloxifene Hydrochloride
	Peroxide Degradation-Fluphenazine Deaconate

Biopharmaceutical interactions generally occur on administration of the medication. On administration of the drug, the body fluid influences the rate of absorption of the medicine. All the excipients used to interact physiologically with the API in the body of the patients. The examples of various biopharmaceutical interactions are stated as follows:

(a) **Enteric coat premature breakdown:** The polymers of enteric coating like cellulose acetate phthalate and hydroxylpropyl cellulose acetate phthalate, are highly soluble at basic pH. Although the enteric coated formulation are meant to release in intestine, however, antacids used to raise the pH of the stomach leading to premature breakdown of the enteric coat in stomach and releases APIs in the stomach itself, resulting in degradation of drug in the stomach. The premature breakdown of the enteric coat of NSAID's may lead to gastric bleeding type side effects.

(b) **Interactions due to adjunct therapy:** Antibiotics like tetracycline used to form complex with calcium and magnesium ions. These ions act as excipients in various types of .34formulations which in turn may be administered along with tetracycline as adjunct therapy. The complex formed by their interaction cannot be absorbed from the gastrointestinal tract.

(c) **Increased gastrointestinal motility:** Several excipients like sorbitol, xylitol, used to increase the gastrointestinal motility and thus reduce the contact time for absorption of drugs like metoprolol etc. Similarly, novel k-opioid agonist got adsorbed by microcrystalline cellulose leading to its partial release from the capsules.

Selection of Suitable Excipients

The decision of selection of a suitable excipient for a formulation is vital in both nonclinical and clinical studies. The formation of a final product mainly depends on the characteristics of the excipients used. The selection of excipients depends upon the need of the type of formulation. Some formulations are for extended release and effects absorption, distribution and tolerance of the product. Improper selection of excipients may impart negative effect on the evaluation of a formulation and consequently leading to interruption of the developmental process. Information regarding tolerability and local reactions is used to be available for experimental animals like mice, rats, rabbits, dogs and nonhuman primates, however, information particularly to guinea pigs is limited. Moreover, the criteria for selection of excipients become more critical in life saving formulations like vaccines, parentrals etc. Excipients are added to the vaccines either for stabilization or to prevent microbial contagions. Various excipients are supplementary to the manufacturing process of a finished product. Several excipients like egg protein, gelatin, latex, yeast, antibiotics and monosodium glutamate are used to be added in the developmental process of a vaccine.

Many of the vaccines of viruses required embryonated chicken eggs (e.g., influenza vaccines) or tissue culture–adapted chicken embryo fibroblasts (e.g., measles and mumps vaccines) for its growth. Egg albumin from eggs or tissue culture media is often added into influenza vaccines. Individuals with allergy to egg are at a greater risk for anaphylactic shock and should be administered precautionary. Gelatin is used vaccines like MMR, varicella, shingles, and rabies to protect them from deleterious effects of effects of heat and cold. Utilization of gelatin also leads to anaphylaxis and allergic reactions because of its origin from bones and connective tissues of animals like cows and pigs. Poorly hydrolyzed gelatin is more prone to these allergic reactions. The process of manufacturing of syringe plungers, vial stoppers, and injection ports utilize natural rubber which may enclose various allergens during the manufacturing process. Even though the latex related allergic reactions are rare but severe latex allergy case occurred with hepatitis B vaccine used to cause emergency conditions. Antibiotics are frequently used to prevent contamination in the production of bacterial and viral vaccines. Antibiotics like neomycin, polymyxin B, gentamicin, streptomycin etc. are added into the final product of vaccines. The use of these antibiotics can also lead to contact dermatitis at the site of injection. Although these reactions are not contra indicatory for the use of vaccines but individuals susceptible to these reactions should be well aware of these risks. Use of another excipient monosodium glutamate leads to a syndrome commonly known as *Chinese restaurant syndrome,* or *MSG symptom complex.* Symptoms like hives, abdominal cramps, nausea, vomiting, and diarrhea are very common in this condition. The incidence as well as mechanism of this adverse effect is not known.

Incompatabilities between Drug and Excipients

The therapeutic efficacy and safety of a drug depends upon the interactions (both physical and chemical) between drugs and its excipients. Most of the excipients are added to the formulation for their beneficial effects. However, these excipients also produce deleterious effects by degrading the formulation by affecting chemical and physical nature of the drug products. The safety and bioavailability of the drug product also get altered by interaction with the excipients. Various small molecules present in APIs interact with pharmaceutical excipients and leads to drug excipient incompatibilities resulting in degradation of finished drug product. Examples of these incompatibilities are summarized in Table 42.5.

Table 42.5 Common API and excipient(s) incompatibilities

S. No.	API	Excipient (s)
1.	Atenolol	Ascorbic acid, citric acid, butylated hydroxyanisole
2.	Clenbuterol	Maize starch, pregelatinized starch, sodium starch glycolate, Avicel PH 101 ®
3.	Ca-Phosphomycin	Sodium dioctylsulfosuccinate
4.	Glimepiride	Plasdone
5.	Hydralazine HCl	Sodium edetate, sodium bisulfate

Table 42.5 *Contd...*

S. No.	API	Excipient (s)
6.	Ketprofen	Palmitic acid
7.	Lapachol	Cetostearyl alcohol, methyl paraben, glyceryl monostearate
8.	Lipoic acid	Methyl paraben, propyl paraben, acetylated lanolin, butylated hydroxyl toluene
9.	Na_2–Phosphomycin	Succinic acid
10.	Promethazine hydrochloride	Pearlitol SD200
11.	Saproxetine maleate	Talc
12.	Temazepam	Precirol® ATO 5d
13.	Tetracycline	Calcium and Magnesium salts
14.	Tetrahydrocannabinol	Vitamin E succinate-processed films

The incompatibilities between API-excipients are the major concerns in formulation development. Most commonly reported interactions are the acid base interaction and Maillard reactions. There occurs the maximum utilization of excipients such as lactose and magnesium stearate in case of oral solid dosage forms. There occurs an increased chance of Maillard reaction between lactose as a diluents and amine containing APIs. The varied functional groups involved in drug excipient interactions summons the number of incompatabilities. Caution should be taken to avoid the same. The APIs susceptible to hydrolytic reactions should never be used with stearate containing tablet lubricants. Moreover, the excipients like DCPD should also be avoided with acidic drugs. A carboxyl group containing drugs like ibuprofen show electrostatic interactions with ammonium groups of Eudragit polymer. Therefore the use of Eudragit RL should be avoided as it affects the release profile of APIs. The APIs containing hydroxyl groups should also be used with utmost care. Some of the excipients like HPMCAS forms ester bond with APIs containing succinic or acetic acid. As we know that many of the incompatabilities used to occur at virtual states like high temperature, increased excipient and API ratio, elongated time interval etc. which cannot be met with the actual storage conditions of the finished product. Still this informative data is useful for determining any type of instability issues during commercialization of both marketed as well as new formulations. Understanding of the solid state reactions in a pharmaceutical system can be helpful to avoid the incompatabilities and to improve the stability of the finished products.

Impurities or Residues Present in Excipients

Residues or impurities present in the pharmaceutical excipients can cause significant degradations of the finished formulations. Multicomponent composition of the excipients made them prone to presence of various types of impurities or residues which are found to be detrimental to the finished product. No doubt many of the components are innocuous or even desirable for the formation of the finished product of a drug.

Awareness about the potential mechanisms behind the formation of residues in the excipients will help in better understanding of the risks associated with it in the finished products. It will also aid smooth functioning of the manufacturing process of the required type of the formulation. These impurities of a specific excipient depending upon its use as well as other formulation and processing factors, can affect the quality, safety and efficacy of a formulation. They can deteriorate the finished product even if present in trace amounts especially in case of highly potent drugs. The examples of various types of residues present in different types of excipients provided in Table 42.6.

Table 42.6 List of residues in different types of excipients.

Excipients	Residues
Povidone, crospovidone, polylobate	Peroxides
Magnesium stearate, fixed oils, lipids	Antioxidants
Lactose	Aldehydes (furfuraldehyde), lactose phosphate, reducing sugars
Benzyl alcohol	Benzaldehyde
Polyethylene glycol	Aldehydes, peroxides, formic acid
Microcrystalline cellulose	Lignin, hemicelluloses, free radicals, water
Starch	Formaldehyde, aldose
Talc	Heavy metals
Dibasic calcium phosphate dehydrate	Alkaline residues
Stearate lubricants	Alkaline residues
Hydroxy propyl methyl/ethyl celluloses	Glyoxal
Tween 80	Formaldehyde

Mitigation Strategies

1. Alterations in the properties of the API and API/Excipient Ratio
2. Addition of antioxidants and stabilizers can protect both excipients as well as drug products
   (a) Initiation inhibitors
   (b) Terminators of free radicals
   (c) Antioxidants as reducing agents
   (d) pH modifiers
3. Alteration in the drug product manufacturing process
4. Modification of the Drug Product Packaging
5. Change in Excipient Source
6. The packaging of the excipients can also be modified
7. Raw Material Specifications can be revised

Methods to Overcome Issues Regarding Drug Excipient Interactions

There are several approaches which can be proposed to satisfy the requirements of a drug-excipient compatibility screen. Mainly these approaches are computational and require an inclusive database of reactive functional groups in both APIs and excipients. It involves comprehensive knowledge about excipients as well as their potential impurities. It helps in rapid analysis of the interactions with minimal botheration. On the other hand, these approaches have their own intrinsic risks.

Another commonly employed method is binary mixture compatibility testing. In this method, binary (1:1 or modified) mixtures of the drug and excipient are stored under stressed conditions. These mixtures are prepared either as compacted or as slurries. The stressed conditions can be achieved by isothermal stress testing (IST) and get analyzed using a stability-indicating method like high performance liquid chromatography (HPLC).

Binary mixtures can also be screened by some other thermal methods like differential scanning calorimetry (DSC). Nowadays, DSC is used as a main technique to screen binary mixtures in the present scenario. The ability of DSC to rapidly screen the incompatibilities of the excipients resulting from the appearances disappearances or shifts of peaks makes this approach more commendable than others. This method involves low consumption of the samples. However, being a very conclusive and smart technique, the complications begin during analysis of its data. Another drawback of this technique is the exposure of the sample to high temperatures (300°C) which is not possible for the finished product. Therefore, the results of this technique can be often confusing and uncertain and should be carefully interpreted. So, the results should always be confirmed with IST in which the samples of drug-excipient are stored at high temperature for particular time period (usually 3-4 weeks) in order to hasten the process of degradation and interaction of drug with excipients. The samples are monitored for any physical change. The contents can be determined quantitatively. This technique is somewhat cumbersome and time consuming. Combined use of both DSC and IST is preferred for the choice of an excipient for the formulation. Various techniques like hot stage microscopy and scanning electron microscopy could also be used in combination with DSC to determine the nature of an evident incompatibility. These techniques are beneficial for studying the morphology of the drug/excipients as well as the characteristic physical transformations to determine the nature of incompatibilities. An authoritative result would also be obtained by using HPLC or HPLC-MS/MS. In the same way, isothermal micro calorimetry is also a well accepted method for detecting changes in the drug-excipient mixtures in the solid state during changes in heat flux.

Conclusion

Selection of the proper excipient during manufacturing of a formulation is an area of chief importance. The interactions between drug and excipients should be well understood before choosing the excipient for a particular formulation. Guidelines should be regularly updated for proper selection of the excipient and to maintain the quality and safety of the materials used as excipients. Understanding about the possible mechanisms involved in the excipient and drug incompatabilities would lead to better management of the risks or undesirable effects associated with them. Strategies should be made to overcome these risks either by modifying the processes or types of excipients used. There should be mutual cooperation and collaboration between excipient manufacturers and end users of the excipients to avoid residual impurities. Therefore, various newer techniques used be employed to overcome these issues at initial stages.

Suggested Readings

1. Bharate SS, Bharate SB and Bajaj AN. Interactions and incompatibilities of pharmaceutical excipients with active pharmaceutical ingredients: a comprehensive review. J. Excipients and Food Chem. 2010; 1 (3): 3-27.

2. Hotha KK, Roychowdhury S, Subramanian V. Drug-Excipient Interactions: Case Studies and Overview of Drug Degradation Pathways. American Journal of Analytical Chemistry, 2016, 7, 107-140.

3. Narang, A.S. Boddu. Excipient Applicatiions in Formulation Design and Drug Delivery. S.H.S (Eds.) 2015, XL, 681 p. 161.

4. Wu Y, Levons J, Narang AS, Raghavan K, Rao VM. Reactive Impurities in Excipients: Profiling, Identification and Mitigation of Drug–Excipient Incompatibility. AAPS PharmSciTech, 2011; 12 (4): 1248-1263.

CHAPTER 43

NUTRACEUTICALS

Introduction

About 2000 years ago, a Greek scientist, Hippocrates known as father of medicine introduced a phrase "let food be medicine". This term receives today a lot of interest by scientist working on food and consumers who realized that some foods are beneficial for health. The word nutraceuticals originated from Nutrition + Pharmaceuticals in 1989 by Stephen Defelice. According to him nutraceuticals are the food materials which offers health benefits related to prevention or treatment of disease. In 1999 Zeisel, considered nutraceuticals as those nutrients which is a part of normal diet by providing one or more active ingredients. In 1998, Browser reported that nutraceuticals are substances capable of providing medical and health benefits, with the prevention and treatment of diseases. In 2015, Merriam Webster Dictionary mentioned that nutraceuticals are food stuffs that provide beneficial health effect adding together its fundamental nutritional importance. According to ENA, 2016 nutraceuticals are nutritional food materials that offer therapeutic value, for prevention and treatment of diseases. One old phrase "an apple a day keeps the doctor away" is now changed as "one nutraceuical a day keeps the doctor away". The term "nutraceuticals" is evolving and the nomenclature varies across the countries. e.g., Canada named them as natural and non-prescription health products, the USA called them as dietary supplements and Japan named them as "foods for special health use". India also named these components in to 3 segments i.e. functional/ fortified food, functional beverages and dietary supplements. This shows that, different countries had different categories for defining "health supplements and nutraceuticals". According to our literature survey the global nutraceuticals market was estimated at US$ 169.32 billion in 2014 and is growing at a CAGR (Compounded Annual Growth Rate) of 6.5%. In 2014 North America was dominating the global nutraceuticals market followed by APAC and Europe. However, rise in the health conscious population, and increasing disposable income of consumers, a significant growth was witnessed by the APAC region. Due to a strong demand for dietary supplements in India its market is expected to double in size to US$ 4 billion by 2020.

Classification of Nutraceuticals: Nutraceuticals can be categorized in numerous ways depending upon their applications. Nutraceuticals can be classified according to food accessible in the market place (**Fig. 43.1**)

1. **Traditional nutraceuticals:** Natural food nutrients present in different foods. E.g. resveratrol in grapes, naringenin in orange, curcumin in haldi, lycopene in tomatoes. These nutraceuticals can be further categorized in to a) Chemical constituents: phytochemicals nutrients and herbals b) Probiotic microorganisms c) Nutritional enzymes: microbial enzymes, plant enzymes, animal enzymes.

2. **Non-traditional nutraceuticals:** These are Synthetic food material, prepared by biotechnological techniques. These can be further categorized in to a) fortified nutraceuticals b) recombinant nutraceuticals.

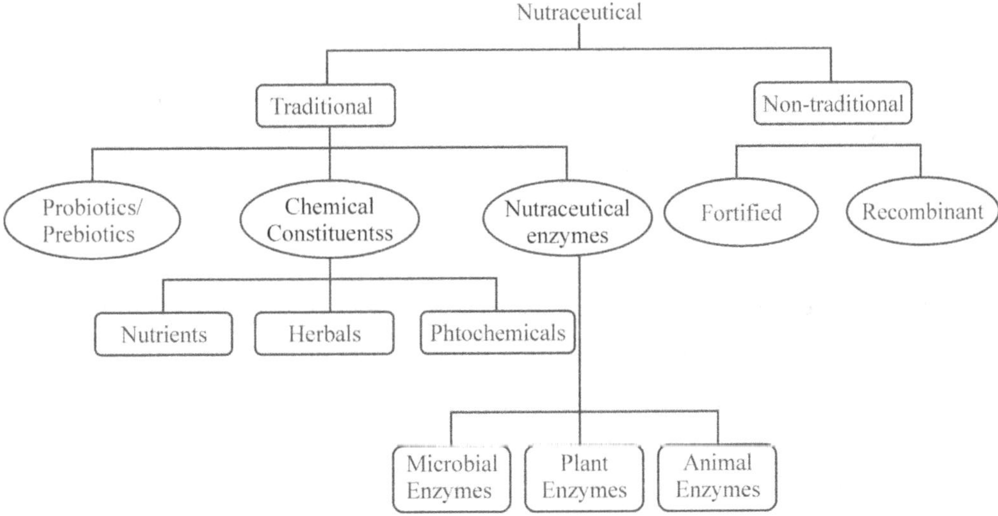

Fig. 43.1 Classification of Nutraceuticals

Traditional Nutraceuticals

Chemical constituents:

(a) *Nutrients:* Vitamins, minerals, fatty acids and amino acids

(b) *Herbals:* These include neutraceuticals showing promising role in improving acute and chronic diseases. E.g. salicin in Willow bark, lycopene in tomato, tannin in lavender, proantocynadin in cranberries, curcumin in Curcuma longa, resveratrol in grapes etc.

(c) ***Phytochemicals:*** These includes nutraceuticals which are categorised according to their chemical name and phytochemical properties. E.g. carotenoids, flavonoid polyphenolics, non-flavonoid polyphenolics, phenolic acids, isothiocyanates, catechins, lignans.

Probiotics/Prebiotics: They are the friendly bacteria which improve quality of intestinal microflora and gastrointestinal health. E.g. lactobacillus, Fructo-oligosaccharides.

Nutraceutical enzymes: Enzymes synthesized from microbes, plants and animal sources.

- Microbial enzymes: hemicellulose, catalase, amyloglucosidase, glucoamylase, invertase-sucrase, lactase-beta galactosidase
- Plant enzymes: hemicellulose, pectinase, β-amylase, bromelanin, biodiastase, glucoamylase.
- Animal enzymes: Oxbile, pancreolipase, trypsin, chymotrypsin, lysozyme and α-amylase.

Non-Traditional Nutraceuticals

Fortified: It includes fortified food from agricultural breeding or added nutrients. For example

- Prebiotic/probiotic fortified milk along-with bifidobacterium lactis
- Fortified banana having soybean ferritin gene

Recombinant: Food endowed with energy such as cheese, bread, alcohol, yogurt produced biotechnologically. For example

- Milk coagulated products from chymosin (*E.coli* K-12)
- Ascorbic acid of high level, carotenoids lutein and zeaxanthin from recombinant Gold Kiwi fruit
- Soybean ferritin gene from recombinant golden mustard
- Aminodeoxychorismate synthase from recombinant tomato
- Lactobacillus acidophilus American type culture collection from recombinant animal fermented soya.

Regulation of Nutraceuticals

The primary goal for the regulation of Nutraceuticals is to make sure the safety of consumer's health. These regulations will also help in introducing fair trade, harmonization, uniformity in practices, price control etc. In the past, in India several laws and regulations recommended diverse standards about food, labeling, food additives, food colors and contaminants.

International Regulatory Scenario

The international global food and nutrition policy related bodies include: World Health Organization (WHO), World Trade Organization (WTO), Codex Alimentarius (CODEX) and Food and Agriculture Organization (FAO).

In the United Nation, Dietary Supplement Health and Education Act (DSHEA) was passed in 1994 as a legislation which manufacture and market the nutraceuticals. Under this Act, before the marketing of any dietary ingredient, the manufacturer will be considered responsible regarding the safety of the product.

European Food and Safety Authority (EFSA) predominantly control food legislation in Europe.

In Canada and Australia, nutraceuticals are regulated more likely as drugs rather than as a food category.

China, government has set up China Health Care Association (CHCA) to supervise the nutraceutical industry.

Japan was among the first countries that faced the issue of regulating the food supplements and foodstuff by issuing the Foods for Specified Health Use (FOSHU) which was based on a voluntary request from stakeholders for approval. This legislation was originally set in 1991 but it became the Health Promotion Law in 1991. The Japanese government has also set up Consumer Affairs Agency (CAA) which is the Ministry of Health, Labor and Welfare (MHLW). It has the responsibility of implementing the laws to nutritional labeling and health claims approval in order to sustain the safety and standards of the nutritional foods.

Indian regulatory scenario: In India Nutraceuticals are generally categorized as functional foods and dietary supplements which is not incorporated in the Drugs and Cosmetic Act, 1940. For the regulation of nutraceuticals a number of acts have been passed and all these acts have been included under one roof. The Prime Minister's council decided on forming a single food regulatory authority in 1998 in order to make uniform licensing procedures, their process of registration, safety, sanitary and hygienic conditions. In 2006 in parliament passed Food safety and security (FSS) act. In 2008, food safety and standard authority of India (FSSAI) was constituted. Its main objective was to create a single reference guidelines for every nutrients related to food safety and values. India has notified the Food Safety and Standards Regulations, 2016 in the Gazette of India on 23 December 2016 (nutraceuticals, health supplements, food for special dietary use and medical purpose, functional and novel food). The regulations cover eight categories of food and is defined based on their contents and use. Further, FSSAI, vide its directions issued on 19 May 2017, has released the Food Safety and Standards (Fortification of Foods) Regulations, 2017. This regulation prescribes standards for fortification of oil, salt, milk, vanaspati, atta, maida and rice and has been made operationalized by FSSAI w.e.f 17 April 2017.

Nutraceuticals in Therapeutics

Use of Nutraceuticals in CNS Disorders

Group of neurological disorders that affects brain structure and function are known as CNS disorder. It may be as a result of metabolic disorder, any degenerative condition, brain tumour, stroke or as a result of infection. The two major similarities associated with all CNS disorder is oxidative stress and immune-mediated inflammation. Hence, the most appropriate approach in treating these CNS diseases is by using anti-oxidant molecules. These molecules will maintain and restore the normal physiological conditions of the brain from stressed situations. Natural nutraceuticals such as polyphenols, carotenoids, acetyl-L-carnitine, vitamin D, curcumin have been studied extensively having a potential therapeutic role in targeting multiple pathways in such disorders. Curcumin is a polyphenolic compound extracted from Curcuma longa, a south Asian herb. It has been demonstrated that oral administration of curcumin can enervate the deposition and oligomerisation of Aβ as well as the phosphorylation of tau protein in experimental animals. Hence improving the cognition and behavioral impairments. Some studies also depicted the preventive role of Vitamin E in AD and also showed improvement in cognitive functions by the consumption of alone Vitamin E or C.

Also, there is an increasing interest in the use of natural supplements for controlling the migraine headaches. Deficiency of Magnesium in the diet has been associated with migraine and studies have shown the use of magnesium in improving the symptoms of migraine. Some studies also exhibited its efficacious role of riboflavin in the reduction of headache attack frequency as it improves the energy metabolism. A couple of studies reported that alpha-linolenic acid plays a promising therapeutic effect in stroke by inhibition of glutamate excitotoxicity pathways and also enhancing the curative mechanisms.

Depression is also a very common problem affecting people of all ages and groups. It is also considered as affective or mood disorders to be a part of behavioral and mental problems. Owing much to the role of nutrients in the production of neurotransmitters affecting mood such as serotonin, there is growing evidence of the importance for the use of Omega-3 polyunsaturated fatty acids (n-3 PUFAs). Peet et al, observed that administration of Omega-3 fatty acid 2gm daily during 12 weeks had a significant effect on the clinical severity measured on PANSS scale. Studies also indicate a close association of Vitamin D deficiency and Schizophrenia but not in case of all patients suffering with the disease.

Nutraceuticals in Cardiovascular Diseases

Any congenital or acquired disease of the heart and blood vessels is known as cardiovascular disease. In developed countries cardiovascular diseases are most common health problem and cause of death. Most important of them are atherosclerosis, rheumatic heart disease, and vascular inflammation. These are characterized by risk factors such as impaired lipid and glycemic profile, obesity, increased plasma fibrinogen and coagulation factor, increased platelet activation, oxidative stress, inflammation, smoking, family history, ethnicity, age and unhealthy diets. Dysregulation of renin angiotensin system (RAAS) is involved in pathogenesis of cardiovascular diseases. Literature reports showed that low intake of dietary foods, vitamins and minerals increase incidence of cardiovascular diseases. Nutraceuticals in the form of vitamins, minerals, antioxidants, dietary fibres alongwith active lifestyle are recommended for cardiovascular diseases. Flavonoids present in wide variety of vegetables and fruits are available as flavones, flavanones and flavonols having an important role for curing CVD. These flavonoids inhibit angiotensin-converting enzymes, block cyclooxygenase enzymes and prevents platelet aggregation. These flavonoids also protect vascular system. Anthocyanins, tannins, carbolines, stilbines, dietary indoleamine and serotonin present in food materials are hypothesized to impose health benefits in CVDs. The rhizomes of Zingiber officinalis has antioxidant and anti-inflammatory properties and has been recommended for hypertension and palpitation. Phytosterols block uptake of dietary cholesterols via competing with them and facilitate their excretion. Omega-3 fatty acids present in fish lowers plasma lipid levels and cures CVD. Octacosanol present in whole grains and fruits of many plants control lipid levels.

Nutraceuticals in Skin Diseases

There is a saying that true beauty is the beauty from within. There is a relationship between nutrition, ageing and skin condition. One of the rapidly growing areas of nutraceutical industry is "nutricosmetic market". These are the supplements that help in maintaining the structure, health and function of the skin. There are various studies which have established a connection between specific nutrients and condition and health of the skin.

Skin ageing and age-related disorders have been related to the constant exposure of the skin to oxidative stress caused by numerous sources such as environmental pollutants, UV radiations and chemical oxidants. In order to prevent such adverse effects of the oxidative stress on the functioning and health of the skin anti-oxidants should be provided in sufficient amounts and composition in order to maintain the balance and avoid tissue damage.

In a placebo-controlled *in-vivo* study it was observed that the carotenoid-rich natural curly kale extract was able to prevent skin ageing and have the capacity to improve the extracellular matrix. In another study it was observed that 1,25D, DHA and curcumin were able to regulate certain genes that were involved in the pathogenesis of psoriasis.

Certain studies have also suggested the use of certain probiotics in the management of atopic dermatitis in adults over the age of 18 years. A number of micronutrients such as zinc and copper have been shown to play an integral part in the functioning of a healthy skin. Copper plays an important role in the maturation and structural integrity of both collagen and elastin. Zinc possesses anti-inflammatory properties and apart from this protects against UV radiations and also helps in wound healing. Although numerous nutraceuticals are available which promises to make the skin look younger and healthier but still there are certain factors which need to be considered while looking for the efficacy of any nutraceutical product.

Nutraceuticals in Eye Diseases

It has been shown that there is strong relation between good nutrition and healthy vision. There are various eye diseases such as Age-related macular degeneration, glaucoma, cataract, glaucoma and other retinal diseases such as diabetic retinopathy which can be a leading cause of blindness.

Studies suggested the consumption of vitamins with zinc slows the development of late AMD and vision loss. It has also been observed in some studies that use of certain anti-oxidants such as flavonoids, vitamins and carotenoids can be used to prevent the occurrence of cataract. Even some anti-glycating agents such as polyphenols and phenolic acids such as caffeic acids can be used as anti-cataract agents.

In a randomized, double-blind, placebo-controlled trial it was demonstrated that the supplementation with lutein can be a potential treatment for non-proliferative diabetic retinopathy (NPDR) for the improvement of visual functions.

Nutraceuticals as Immunomodulators

Immunity can be defined as a natural defense of our body towards any infectious disease. Immunomodulators are those agents which possesses those activities that can normalize or modulate the pathophysiological responses. Curcumin has been studied most considerably for its immunomodulatory properties. Some studies also suggested the role of resveratrol, Epigallocatechin-3-gallate, quercitin, colchicine, capsaicin, andrographolide and genistein as acting as potential immunomodulators. In a study a comparison was made between eleven most commonly used immunomodulators. Firstly it showed that only four of them which includes glucan, curcumin, Astragalus and Resveratrol stimulated phagocytosis. Next it was observed that resveratrol, curcumin, *Astragalus*, *Echinacea* and gingseng were able to induce cytotoxicity. The study also demonstrated that it was only resveratrol, curcumin, and glucan which significantly decreased the number of metastasis.

Nutraceuticals in Cancer

Cancer is a worldwide health problem which is growing rapidly because of increasing urbanization, lifestyle and changes in environmental conditions. Epidemiological data shows that lung, bronchus, breast, colorectal and prostate cancer are the most common forms. The prevalence of these cancers is more in western countries and in Asian countries its incidences are very low due to the inclusion of more of vegetable and fruit diet as compared to high fat/meat diet. So, many studies showed the effect of diet and environment on our cellular function and health. Many of the Phytochemicals have been studies for their curative properties in cancer. An effective Nutraceutical will be the one which will be nontoxic and will cause a great change in cancer dynamics. Hence it is better to use these nutraceuticals as a combination therapy. Epigallocatechin gallate (EGCG) is the main constituent of Green tea is obtained from the leaves of Camellia sinensis. It has been observed that it can inhibit NF-KB signaling. Some studies showed that green tea failed to decrease the levels of PSA in the blood in patients with prostate cancer. Hence it was shown that green tea and its extracts had very little or no anti-tumor activity when used alone.

It was first shown by some flavonoids that it possesses apoptotic activity in human lymphoid leukemic cells and human carcinoma cells. Lycopene and β-carotene found in tomato have the capacity of inducing apoptosis in prostate cancer cells and malignant lymphoblast cells. Garlic contains certain allylsulfur compounds which possesses significant anti-proliferative activity against human cancers.

Current therapies like chemotherapy, radiation and surgical treatment of cancer leads to severe side effects. Therefore there is an urgent need of providing an alternative therapy which can afford protective properties for treatment of cancer.

Along with preclinical studies large no. of nutraceuticals are investigated in clinical trials. Table 43.1 enlist the potential evidence of nutraceuticals in clinical trials in different disease conditions.

Table 43.1 Nutraceuticals in clinical trials

S. No.	Disease	Nutraceutical	Potential benefits
1.	Cardiovascular (CVS) diseases	Flavonoids (pulp of orange juice)	Blocks ACE. Also blocks COX and prevent platelet aggregation
		Hesperidin (citrus boflavonoid)	Used for the treatment of venous insufficiency and hemorrhoids
		Ginger	Potent anti-oxidant and possess anti-inflammatory activity. Also used in hypertension and palpitations. Protection against toxicity of synthetic drugs.
		Phytosterols	Reduction of morbidity and mortality of CVD
		Octacosanol	lowering activity

Table 43.1 *Contd...*

S. No.	Disease	Nutraceutical	Potential benefits
2.	Cancer	Daidzein, biochanin, isoflavones and genistein	Inhibition of cell growth in prostate cancer
		lycopene	Potent anti-oxidant
		β-carotene	Possess anti-oxidant activity
		Soyfoods, epigallocatechin gallate and curcumin	Possess cancer chemopreventive properties
		Saponins	Possess antimutagenic and antitumor activities
		Tannins	Scavenge harmful free radicals and detoxify carcinogens
		Ellagic acid	Act as anti-cancer agent
		Pectin	Prevention of metastasis of prostate cancer through inhibition of adherence of cancer cells to other cells in the body.
		Glucosinolates, indoles and isothiocyanates	Associated with lower risk of colorectal and lung cancer.
		Sulforaphane	Potent inducer of phase 2 enzymes. Acts as antioxidant and Stimulates the natural detoxifying enzymes.
		Curcumin	Possess antioxidative, anticarcinogenic, and anti-inflammatory properties
		Green tea, Vitamins D and E, selenium, lycopene, soy	Effective in preventing prostate cancer
3.	Eye disorders	n-3 fatty acids, lutein and zeaxanthin	Beneficial for age-related macular degeneration (AMD)
		Green tea, Allium spp., Vitamins C and E, polyphenols, carotenoids (mainly lycopene and ß-carotene), and coenzyme Q10.	Possess antioxidant properties and effective in AMD
		Astaxanthin	Protection from oxidation process and ultra violet light effects. Possess immune response and pigmentation, in aquatic animals. It helps in the protection of eyes and prevents macular degeneration. Protects heart from oxidative damage, and provides protection to the nervous system from degenerative diseases like AD and boosts immune system function
		Lutein and Zeaxanthin	Treatment of visual disorders

Table 43.1 *Contd...*

S. No.	Disease	Nutraceutical	Potential benefits
4.	CNS disorders	Curcumin	Leads to the suppression of increased in intracellular ROS and translocation of NF-κB. Inhibits the activation of NF-κB and prevented Aβ-induced cell death suggesting a possible role in AD
		Green tea flavonoid, epigallocatechin-3-gallate, curcumin and mustard oil glycoside	Inhibition of pro-inflammatory signalling via NF-κB or toll-like receptors and stabilizing the blood brain barrier in MS.
		Retinoic acid	Increase tolerance and decrease inflammation hence improving plasticity, regeneration, cognition and behaviour in patients with Multiple Sclerosis (MS)
		Vitamin D	Leads to alleviation of various inflammatory markers in patients with MS, PD and AD
		Vitamin E	Reduction of neuroinflammation and neuronal degeneration
		Soy isoflavones	Influence the brain cholinergic system and ameliorate age-related neuronal loss and cognition decline in male rats
		Resveratrol	Possesses antidepressant properties

Adverse effects of nutraceuticals: Although some dietary supplements have acceptable safety profile, but many of them are also associated with adverse events and drug interation. Alongwith this patients do not disclose use of supplements to the physicians, which results significant adverse drug –supplement interaction. Moreover most of the nutraceuticals are brought in the market without clinical trials. Intake of dietary supplements is generally safe but not totally without risk. An overview of major nutraceuticals used are summarized in table:

Adverse events associated with the use of nutraceuticals:

Nutraceuticals	Potential toxic effect associated with supplement
Fish oil and Omega-3 fatty acids	Hypervitaminosis if taken with vitamin supplements and exacerbate bleeding in patients taking warfarin
Protein powder	Excessive consumption can result ketoacidosis
• **Epigallocatechingallate**	Liver injury
• **Genisteinand daidzein**	Uterine hypertrophy, reproductive tract malformation
• **Isoflavones**	Increased risk of estrogen sensitive cancers, endometriosis

Contd...

Nutraceuticals	Potential toxic effect associated with supplement
Weight loss and Body building supplements	• **Ephedrine (weight loss):** Tremors, jitteriness, insomnia, increased perspiration • **1,3-dimethylamylamine (sports supplement) :** Tachycardia, nausea, vomiting • **OxyELITE (weight loss):** Liver diseases • **Body building supplemets adulterated with anabolic steroids:** Cardiomyopathy, altered serum lipids, acne, swollen breast tissue in men, hepatotoxicity
Botanical Supplements	• **Black cohosh:** Jaundice and liver failure in menopausal women • **Kava kava:** Liver toxicity • **Saw Palmetto:** Cholestatic hepatitis • **Valerian:** Jaundice • **Milk thistle:** Hemochromatosis • **Garlic and ginkgo biloba :** Bleeding diseases
Dietary supplements causes abuse and misuse of adolescents	• **Garciniacambogia:** Abdominal pain, agitation, hyperventilation, tachycardia • **Paulliniacupana:** Vomiting, agitation, tachycardia, hypertension, chest pain, dyspnea, headache, tremor • **Salvia divinorum:** Confusion, drowsiness, tachycardia, hallucinations, agitation, slurred speech, diaphoresis, mydriasis, nausea, tremor, vomiting • **Hypericumperforatum :** Nausea, agitation, bradycardia, chest pain, confusion, dizziness, drowsiness, headache, mydriasis.
Vitamins	Vitamin A at dose >5000 IU/day increases risk of hip fracture; show teratogenic effect at dose >1000-1500 IU/day; hair and skin changes, hepatotoxic effects. Beta Carotene At dose of >3000IU/day increase risk of lung cancer among smokers and people with asbestosis,yellowish of skin.Vitamin C at dose of >2000IU/day causes gastric upsets, diarrhoea. More than 2000IU/day Vitamin D intake results hypercalcemia and soft tissue calcification.Vitamin E Intake of >800IU/day results headache fatigue and blurred vision, nausea, vomiting, diarrhoea. Vitamin B6 >200 mg/day intake causes sensory neuropathy and ataxia. Niacin intake results Potential interaction with statins, gastrointestinal upsets, vasodilation, hyperglycemia

Labeling of nutraceuticals: Till date there is no strict criteria to label nutraceuticals, however most of the nutraceuticals claims that being a part of an overall healthy diet, they may reduce the risk of certain diseases. In 1993 FDA authorized seven health claims as a part of 1990 Nutrition Labeling and Education Act (NLEA). From 1993, FDA has authorized six more claims. There are some health related statements permitted on nutraceutical labels. a) Nutrient content claims express presence of specific nutrient content on label. b) Structure and function content claims effect of dietary components on structure and functions of the body. c) Dietary guidance claims health benefits of foods. d) Qualified health claims developing relationship between components in the diet and risk of disease as approved by FDA.

Challenges and opportunities: Nutraceuticals is a new field and is associated with a number of gaps in its understanding:

1. It is well established that protective effect of a food in any disease is not necessarily due to one single component, but may be due to few or many components. It results a marked archetype swing in pharmaceutical replica that is based on effectiveness of one agent and not multiple components.

2. Methods for handling and measurement of the phytochemicals are lacking, thus many of the phytochemicals under investigation are ignored.

3. Most of the time manufacturers want to write specific health benefits on their product labels, but these claims lack specific scientific background.

4. Regulatory government bodies are also challenged by new category of health products existing between medicines and food.

5. Numerous challenges have to be faced to launch a new product in to the market.

6. Presently consumption of dietary supplements is because of the fear of various side effects associated with prescription medications. It also includes its easy availability and safety to use.

Suggested Readings

1. Adefegha SA. Functional foods and nutraceuticals as dietary intervention in chronic diseases; novel prospective for health promotion and disease prevention. J Diet Suppl. 2017; 27: 1-33.

2. Arunabha Ray, Jagdish Joshi, Kavita Gulati. Regulatory Aspects of Nutraceuticals: An Indian Perspective. Nutraceuticals: efficacy, safety and toxicity. 941-946.

3. Bigford GE, Del Rossi G. Supplemental substances derived from foods as adjunctive therapeutic agents for treatment of neurodegenerative diseases and disorders. Adv Nutr. 2014; 5: 394-403.

4. Biggs JM, Morgan JA, Lardieri AB, Kishk OA, Klein-Schwartz W. Abuse and misuse of selected dietary supplements among adolescents: a look at poison center data. J Pediatr Pharmacol Ther 2017; 22: 385-392.

5. Blondeau N. The nutraceutical potential of omega-3 alpha-linolenic acid in reducing the consequences of stroke. Biochimie. 2016 Jan;120: 49-55

6. Deacon G, Kettle C, Hayes D, Dennis C, Tucci J. Omega 3 polyunsaturated fatty acids and the treatment of depression. Crit Rev Food Sci Nutr. 2017 Jan 2; 57(1): 212-223

7. Evans JR. Antioxidant vitamin and mineral supplements for slowing the progression of age-related macular degeneration. Cochrane Database Syst Rev. 2006 Apr 19; (2):CD000254. Review. Update in: Cochrane Database Syst Rev.2012; 11: CD000254

8. Huynh TP, Mann SN, Mandal NA. Botanical compounds: effects on major eye diseases. Evid Based Complement Alternat Med. 2013; 2013: 549174

9. Jantan I, Ahmad W, Bukhari SN. Plant-derived immunomodulators: an insight on their preclinical evaluation and clinical trials. Front Plant Sci. 2015 Aug 25; 6: 655

10. Karrys A, Rady I, Chamcheu RN, Sabir MS, Mallick S, Chamcheu JC, Jurutka PW, Haussler MR, Whitfield GK. Bioactive Dietary VDR Ligands Regulate Genes Encoding Biomarkers of Skin Repair That Are Associated with Risk for Psoriasis. Nutrients. 2018 Feb 4; 10(2)

11. Krause D, Roupas P. Dietary interventions as a neuroprotective therapy for the delay of the onset of cognitive decline in older adults: an umbrella review protocol. JBI Database System Rev Implement Rep. 2015; 13: 74-83.

12. Meinke MC, Nowbary CK, Schanzer S, Vollert H, Lademann J, Darvin ME. Influences of Orally Taken Carotenoid-Rich Curly Kale Extract on Collagen I/Elastin Index of the Skin. *Nutrients*. 2017; 9(7):775.

13. Ronis MJJ, Pedersen KB and Watt J. Adverse effects of nutraceuticals and dietary supplements. Annual review of pharmacology and toxicology. 2018; 58: 583-601.

14. Sadhukhan P, Saha S, Dutta S, Mahalanobish S, Sil PC. Nutraceuticals: An emerging therapeutic approach against the pathogenesis of Alzheimer's disease. Pharmacol Res. 2018; 129: 100-114.

15. Singh J, Sinha S. Classification, regulatory acts and applications of nutraceuticals for health. 2012; 2: 177-187.

16. Vernieri C, Nichetti F, Raimondi A, Pusceddu S, Platania M, Berrino F, de Braud F. Diet and supplements in cancer prevention and treatment: Clinical evidences and future perspectives. Crit Rev Oncol Hematol. 2018 Mar; 123: 57-73

17. Vetvicka V, Vetvickova J. Natural immunomodulators and their stimulation of immune reaction: true or false? Anticancer Res. 2014 May; 34(5): 2275-82.

CHAPTER 44

VIRTUAL CLINICAL TRIAL

Background

Virtual clinical trials (VCTs) are the boon for the predictive information data for a human trial due to the advancement in information technology. The data are based on disease parameters, pathways affected and molecular mechanisms associated with it. However, predictive systems pharmacology model based approach is bringing revolution to drug discovery industry. These models can be validated by comparing predicted and actual responses to therapy. This form of *"reverse"* methods can highly be informative and are being used as a predictive tool for hypothesis driven basic research.

These models can be used for virtual screening of both safety and efficacy of newer agents, which can specifically be useful in early phase drug development processes. Real clinical trials can sometimes be detrimental to participant's health, which can occur due to occurrence of side effects with no added clinical benefit. A real clinical trial takes time to complete and is quite expensive. Another issue is high failure rates of real life clinical trial.

In virtual clinical trial settings, these issues can be handled by application of different models, which can be carried forward to evaluate different aspects of the disease process, which is low cost to the developer. These strategies can reduce the number of failed clinical trials and help us choose the best candidate drug for further development.

There comes the importance of validated biomarkers which are associated with safety or efficacy of the drug, which can lead to cost effective and low-cost clinical trials and can reduce drug failure.

Mathematics and Medicine

Mathematics is being increasingly used in the field of medicine and thus a highly specialized field is coming up, which analyses relationship between bio-medical systems i.e., biomathematics. It incorporates medical, physiological, pathological and pharmacological data and thus incorporates diverse amount of information, which can be used to predict clinical consequences.

Luria and Delbruck are one of the pioneers in the field of biomathematics, which framed two mathematical models which embedded resistance mechanism as variable in the equation.

The revolution of use of biomathematics occurred in the field of cancer research. Effect of treatment on cancer growth was modelled mathematically as early as 1960s. The subsequent models tried to predict drug efficacy and toxicity using multi-scale mathematical models. Further development occurred which incorporated some important variables like "angiogenesis" and a new model of vascular tumour growth was formulated. Further development in these models enabled prediction of efficacy and toxicity of different agents, calculated cell death throughout therapy and helped in optimization of chemotherapy by framing strategies to increase efficacy and at the same time decreasing toxicity. These strategies are helpful to choose the most advantageous regimen from a particular set of regimens.

Some important models are mathematical model of granulopoiesis, developed by Wichmann HE et al, 1979. Another advanced model is mesenchymal chondrosarcoma model, which uses findings of *in-vitro* & *in-vivo* experiments, disease progression and PK-PD parameters for personalizing cancer chemotherapy in patients who are given angiogenesis inhibitors along with other chemotherapeutic agents. The predictions of this model was found good with 87% accuracy. Latest application of mathematics is seen in virtual clinical trials.

Virtual Clinical Trial

Despite increase in investment in pharma research and development, new entries to the market has decreased significantly over the years. So, we need a mechanism, which is more innovative, at the same time decrease drug development time and cost. Here comes the use of virtual research and development, which uses mathematics to model human body (virtual patients), which can mimic human body both normal physiological condition and pathological condition. Use of this virtual patients can dramatically reduce the new drug development time period, early prediction of new drug efficacy and safety and thus helping in go no go decision, optimal dose selection decreased number of failure in clinical trials and subsequent reduced cost of drug development.

Who is a Virtual Patient?

A virtual patient is basically a collection of mathematical models. The mathematical models are framed such that the model should be patient specific physiology and pathologic conditions using data from real population based experiments, physiological experiments, biopsies, lab parameters, genetic and kinetic experiments. By using simulation, a population of virtual patients or virtual cohort can be framed, which can be used for characterization of efficacy and safety of molecules. Gorelik B developed a new mathematical model to determine efficacy and safety of bevacizumab and docetaxel in patients with mesenchymal chondrosarcoma and the model was found to be 87.1% accurate.

Case Study: Sunitinib Malate and ISIS-5132

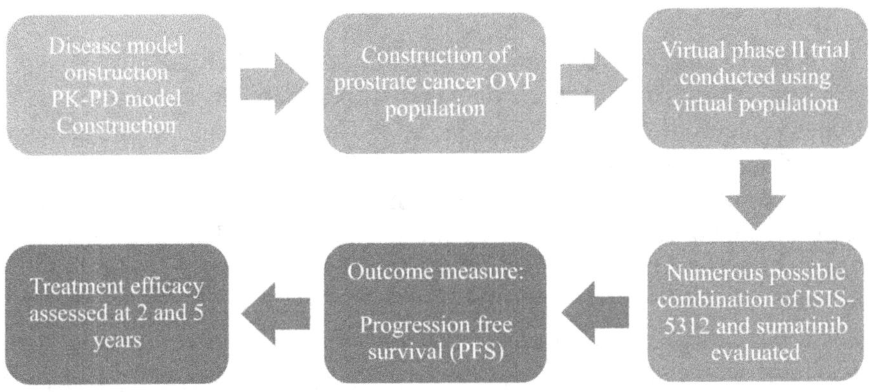

Flow chart 44.1 Case study: Virtual clinical study of ISIS-5312 and sunitinib maleate.

Kleiman M et al, 2009 used virtual clinical trial approach to rescue discontinued compounds in prostate cancer patient population. First they framed virtual patient population (OVP i.e. optimata virtual patients) and simulated the effect of various drug regimens in this population. OVP population was created by using integration of data from biological and physiological information (obtained from lab experiments and population based research) of lots of compounds and their combination, pharmacokinetics of the agents, their interactions, pharmacodynamic parameters (e.g. tumour growth, disease progression). These models allowed them to evaluate different compounds and their combinations in the OVP population. Results obtained from these virtual experiments were further evaluated in other independent sets of simulation experiments and predictive power of the same was explored for yet undiscovered different combinations. Kleiman M et al, in their study found that therapy of prostate cancer can be improved if ISIS – 5132 is combined with sunitinib malate, and in the OVP population, the use of the combination resulted in improved progression free interval at 5 years, compared to mono-therapy of each agents.

Case Study 2: The Virtual Anemia Trial (VAT)

In the VAT study, patients with anemia with different treatment algorithms were assessed with hemodialysis in an *in-silico* clinical trial. During the designing of RCTs, internal, external, and ecological validity was well focused and maintained which was further reported by Fuertinger DH, *et al*, 2018. In the virtual anemia trial, the authors explored the integrity of these validities in virtual trial context. In the VAT trial, Hemoglobin levels and subsequent anemia treatment were simulated at patient level over the course of a year and compared to real-life clinical data of 79,426 patients undergoing hemodialysis. In their study, they overcame the limitations of Monte Carlo simulations by applying advanced mathematical and computational techniques to create a large population of *in silico* representations ("AVATARS") of real patients and thus increasing the validity.

Virtual Trial in Academic Setting

As early as 1998, Weiner MG developed a "Health Services Research Workstation" for validating the results of formal clinical trials in that local population using virtual setting. Many such academic trials followed which included virtual clinical trial methodology e.g. "comparison of static versus dynamic PET imaging as a measurement of response to breast cancer therapy", virtual clinical trials for the "assessment and comparison of novel breast screening Modalities" etc. J Geoffrey Chase et al validated "glucose-insulin system model" was used to perform the virtual studies, taking insulin sensitivity as a critical marker. In their study conducted in Belgium, they first took data from 211 patients. Virtual patient population was created by using this data. The virtual patient population was validated by use of parameters like model fit & intra patient (forward) prediction errors. Self and cross-validation tests were used to further validate and evaluate the ability to predict clinical trial results.

Applications of Virtual Clinical Trial

Simulation experiments are currently very popular among researchers and development in computer science and mathematics is contributing in it more specifically development in the field of "in-silico" models and nonlinear mixed-effect PK-PD models. Proper use of these approaches allows simulation at "virtual patient" level. These virtual trial concept can be used in early drug development proof of concept studies, to identify basket groups in clinical trials, personalization of medicine, drug fails due to intolerable side effects, selection of best agent for most efficient drug combination, prediction of additive or synergistic interactions between different drug combinations etc. These trials can be used for optimizing early phase clinical trial design.

Conclusion

The concept of use of mathematical models in medicine is currently evolving, so is the concept of virtual clinical trial. This helps us to design, accomplish and obtain results of

VCTs very quickly which in real life are not feasible because of *ethical, economic or time constrain*. Thus, VCTs helps one to explore potential opportunities to use digital health tools in the field of clinical research which may prove to be a boon to mankind in future.

Suggested Readings

1. Agur Z. From the evolution of toxin resistance to virtual clinical trials: therole of mathematical models in oncology. Future Oncol. 2010 Jun; 6(6): 917-27.

2. Fuertinger DH, Topping A, Kappel F, Thijssen S, Kotanko P. The Virtual Anemia Trial: An Assessment of Model-Based In Silico Clinical Trials of Anemia Treatment Algorithms in Patients With Hemodialysis. CPT Pharmacometrics SystPharmacol. 2018 Jan 25.

3. Kleiman M, Sagi Y, Bloch N, Agur Z. Use of virtual patient populations forrescuing discontinued drug candidates and for reducing the number of patients in clinical trials. Altern Lab Anim. 2009 Sep; 37 Suppl 1: 39-45.

CHAPTER 45

METAGENOMICS

Introduction

Metagenomics is the main thirst area of the current scientific research scenario. The scope of metagenomics is developing very fast and covering vast area of research for the human well being. Initially, the term *"Metagenome"* was first time used in 1998 in its modern sagacity where it referred to all the microbial genomes collected in a soil sample and moreover also included those sequences of the organisms which cannot be cultured. Since that time, this term generally used to cover all the set of multiple genomes from environmental or clinical samples. A landmark study in 2004 by Ventor and his colleagues had explored not only microbial communities but taxonomic and sequence space also. This term was developed to counteract the main problem of microbiologists about the assessment of those microorganisms which cannot be cultured in the laboratory. The microbiologists now facing opportunities which are just akin to the reinvention of the microscope because metagenomics also leads to invention of new ways for examination of the world of microbes which is not only essential for every part of human life but also to run the entire world. This technique bypasses the processes of isolation and culturing of individual microbial communities. It helps in generating knowledge of microbial interactions which can be helpful to improve health, food security and production of energy for survival of human beings. It is the combination of powers of genomics, bioinformatics and systems biology simultaneously.

Metagenomics is defined as a set of both *research techniques* and a *research field*. The term *meta* corresponds to "transcendent" in Greek and this term overcomes the hurdles of genomic diversity and unculturability of most of the microbes. The meaning of

Meta can be sensed by two means, firstly transcending an entity organism to focus on the community genes and effect of genes on each other to work collectively. On the other hand, the second sense identifies the need for the development of computational approaches to understand the genetic composition of a community to be accurately sampled and characterized. Although it is a new science but it already has spread a lot of knowledge regarding the uncultured world of microbes due to involvement of fundamentally new ways of conducting microbiology experiments.

It is unique in its way due to fusion of far apart three areas of science i.e. microbiology, ecology and genomics. Therefore, its functioning also faces many obstacles both conceptually and technically. To spur this technology, the ultimate way is to work at multiple platforms with multiple expertises in many fields. The aim of the Global metagenomic initiative is to establish a number of large-scale projects and a larger number of middle and small-sized projects. The very first and initial step of all the genomic studies is the extraction of DNA.

Methodology

Sample Collection: Microbial diversity increases with the regions of sample collection. Sample should be collected for metagenomic analysis from desired or specific site (soil, water, plant and animal samples from community). The activity and growth pattern of a microorganism in a soil mainly depends upon the chemical, physical and biological properties. The selection of the method and the site of sampling are among the important points to be considered before starting the procedure. There are many sites for sampling such as soils, deep sediments and surface water of the sea, organs and tissues of humans and animals, acid mine, sludge, compost etc. The type of microorganisms generally depends upon the area of the sampling. In the sea, distribution of the microbes varies with the depth and the area of the sampling. The Global Ocean Sampling expedition is widely used for metagenomic aquatic sample collection. Various new methods are also being utilized like High throughput methods which will also help in increasing the accessed sample numbers (Table 45.1).

Table 45.1 Things to be considered during sampling in Metagenomic analysis

S. No.	Considerations during Analysis
1.	Scale including size of the habitat, sample of the habitat etc.
2.	Biological variations like sample to sample, site to site, subsample to subsample, flexibility of the community
3.	Experimental variability during processing of the sample, extracting of the DNA, during process of cloning, sample storage etc.
4.	Reproducibility of the results

Table 45.1 *Contd...*

S. No.	Considerations during Analysis
5.	Coordinates of the place and time
6.	Repository of the samples for future analysis
7.	Occurrence of singletons

Extraction of DNA

High quality of DNA is required to be extracted from environment samples for preparing a library to be used for metagenomics. The methods involved in DNA extraction mainly depend upon the size of the gene of interest as well as on screening strategies to be involved. Basically, there are two methods i.e. direct and indirect. In direct method, there is co-extraction of the sample with its contaminants and also less shearing of the DNA while in indirect method, there is no interference of detergents and enzymes for cultivation of the microbes. Samples are only treated with phenol and chloroform. This method is biased for not extracting ammonia and methane oxidizing bacteria from the soil particles. Physical methods including lysis-based extraction is an example of indirect extraction approach. The direct method of extraction results in higher recovery rate of DNA in comparison to the indirect methods which causes larger DNA fragments. Direct method also resulted in more impurities in extracted DNA.

There are various drawbacks of these methods of extraction such as almost 40% reduction in eukaryotic sequences by indirect method, presence of impurities in soil like humic acid, polysaccharides, polyphenols etc. also cause hindrance in application of PCRs and construction of metagenomic library. The methods for extraction of RNA are also found to be almost similar to DNA extraction methods. The main issues in RNA extraction is the instability of RNA leading to fast physical degradation and RNAase activity due to which a restricted protocol should be followed. Metagenomic samples should be freezed at -80°C and cellular RNA used to be isolated with sulphate salt solution. Metagenomic libraries of RNA after formation of cDNA can be constructed and identify the functional eukaryotic genes.

The quality of the isolated DNA is determined by measuring the absorbance at wavelength of 260 and 280 nm. It can also be done by visualizing the extracted community DNA on the agarose gel. The OD260/OD280 ratio should be between 1.6 to 1.9. (Figure 45.1.)

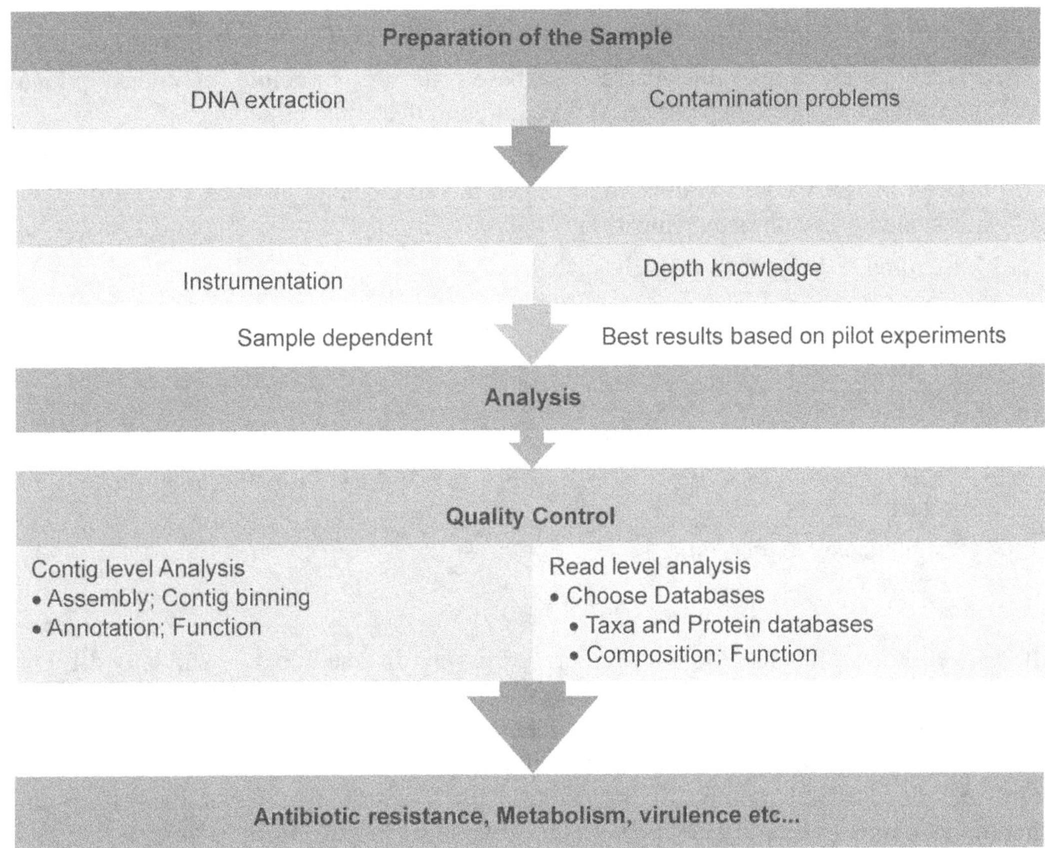

Fig. 45.1 Flowchart for the sample analysis for metagenomics

Enrichment Methods: There are different methods by which the number of clones can be increased in a metagenomic library. Most commonly used is Polymerase Chain Reaction (PCR) but main limitation of this technique is the dependence primers which are required to be designed only on the basis of existing sequences. It is also a lengthy procedure with additional steps for the assessment of full-length genes because gene specific PCRs used to amplify only a fragment of the structural gene. Various PCR based methods namely Tail PCR, cassette PCR, panhandle PCR, adapter ligation and pre-amplification inverse PCRs being time-consuming and lengthy are used very effectively to recover the new gene variants from genomic DNA extracted from the phenol and crude oil-degrading bacteria.

The other techniques like reverse transcriptase PCR are useful for studying not only a particular gene but for the phylogenetic group or metabolic pathway. So, the profiling of the functional microbial communities using RNA also proved to be more effective than DNA.

The following are some of the techniques used to enrich the genomic DNA

1. Differential expression analysis is based on the principle of transcriptional differences in gene expression. It is required to detect the target genes

2. Stable isotope probing (SIP) is based on the technique of labelling the microbial DNA or RNA with stable isotopes. Then the labeled and unlabeled DNA or RNA is separated by ultracentrifugation

3. 5-Bromo-2 deoxyuridine (BrdU) labeling

4. Culture enrichment technique

5. Suppressive substractive hybridization

6. Microarray method

7. Multiple displacement amplification: It is based upon the entire genome amplification by the use of Φ29 DNA polymerase and exonuclease resistant primers

8. Phage display expression

Preparation for Metagenomic DNA Libraries

It is a well-known fact that system of microbes is very diverse in nature and very difficult to explore it in uncultured system. It is very important to study the link of phylogenetic and functional relationships between microbes and environment. Metagenomic libraries used to act as a powerful tool to study the diversity and various advanced techniques has replaced the classical method of inserting a small sequence of fewer than 10kb and traditional cloning vectors. The large cloning vectors such as fosmids, cosmid, BACs (40-200 kb) etc. are used more efficiently in order to screen large number of clones which was not possible to screen with small size vectors and they used to miss the detection of large gene clusters or operons.

The most commonly used host strain is *E.coli* for selection of environment derived metagenomic DNA for many novel biocatalysts and small size molecules. Conversely, it has been found that *E.coli* did not express the entire DNA from the soil microorganisms. Moreover, a very less number of positive clones were obtained from a single set of screening i.e. only <0.01%. There are also various other host strains which are available for the discovery of secondary metabolites as well as new bioactive compounds. Examples include are *Pseudomonas putida*, *Pseudomonas aeruginosa*, *Rhizobium leguminosarum*, *Streptomyces lividans* etc.

Nowadays, the two systems namely 454/Roche and Illumina/Solexa are found to be extensively used for metagenomic samples. The emulsion polymerase chain reaction also known as ePCR has been applied by 454/Roche system to amplify the random DNA fragments especially attached to the microscopic beads. There are two very important aspects of metagenomic applications in this process i.e. firstly the production of artificial replicate sequences that are capable of impacting any estimates of gene abundance, secondly it is very much complicated to correlate the definite number of nucleotide positions with the light intensity produced during running of polymerase through a homopolymer.

Another system i.e. Illumina Solexa which works on the principle of immobilization of the random DNA fragments followed by solid surface PCR amplication is useful for the formation of clusters of identical DNA fragments. These DNA fragments are further sequenced by reversible terminators in a way of sequencing by synthesis process. It shows limited systematic errors in comparison to other datasets which showed higher error rate at the tail ends of the reads. A smaller version i.e. new Illumina MiSeq instrument could also be employed to test run the sequencing libraries. In the near future, there are many other additional sequencing technologies which may also be proved useful for the metagenomic applications like Applied Biosystems SOLid sequencer, Roche's system based on pyrosequencing, Ion Torrent (Ion Proton), Pacific Biosciences (PacBio), technology based on sequencing DNA nanoballs etc.

Process of Clone Screening from Metagenomic Libraries

1. **Sequence based analysis:** The analysis is based on the complete sequencing of clones having phylogenetic anchors like 16S rRNA gene and the archael DNA repair gene *radA*. It provides information regarding both functional and taxonomic group of the organisms from which the clones were obtained. Another alternative technique to identify the gene of interest is by random sequencing followed by screening of phylogenetic anchors in the flanking DNA. The expression of the cloned genes is not dependent on the foreign hosts in this sequence-based analysis. However, the disadvantage of this method is its non-selective analysis of full length genes as well as for individual clones with large inserts like cosmid, BAC libraries etc. Moreover, it is also very laborious.

2. **Function based analysis:** The technique is mainly used for screening those clones which expresses an exact function followed by screening. Therefore, it will help in identifying totally new class of genes with known functions and organisms phylogeny to which it belongs. Many novel antibiotics, its resistance genes, degradable enzymes, $Na^+(Li^+)/H^+$ transporters etc. can also be identified without sequence analysis. Sometimes these methods lead to low frequency of clones.

As an alternative to the *in-vitro* systems, a high throughput method has been developed by scientists which include both activity sensor and metagenomic DNA in a same cell like metabolite-related expression (METREX). The expression of a green fluorescent protein was identified by a quorum sensing inducer. The substrate-induced gene expression screening (SIGEX) method is another screening method for the isolation of catabolite genes from environmental metagenomic libraries.

Assembly: Assembly is defined as the process of assembling short read fragments into a longer genomic contigs. This technique is preferred when full length CDS are required for further sequencing characterization. The main aim of most of the assembly programs was to accumulate single clonal genomes and utilize them for complex pan genomic mixtures. The two most commonly employed strategies for the metagenomics samples are reference based assembly and de novo assembly.

Reference based assembly could be done easily with the help of software packages like Newbler, AMOS, MIRA etc. All these software packages utilized algorithms which are very user friendly and can easily be conducted on laptop sized machines. They are quiet memory efficient and very fast in completing the work in couple of hours only. The assembly is found to be fragmented when there is difference between the true genome of sample and reference like enormous insertion, deletion or polymorphisms.

The functioning of the De novo assembly classically required larger computational resources and is mainly created to handle huge amount of data. The de Bruijn assemblers Velvet or SOAP still require memory in hundreds of gigabytes per machine and run time is also very frequent in days. The assembly algorithms used to assume that the clonal genomes are less suitable for metagenomics due to significant variation in the strain and species of the microbial communities.

Many assemblers usually lead to repression of contigs formation for various heterogenous taxa. There is a need of a true gold standard and one should keep few points in mind before assembling metagenomics such as length of the sequencing reads, need of longer sequences for annotation and to confirm whether the dataset is assembled to reduce the requirements of data processing.

Binning: The process of sorting out DNA sequences into groups which represents an individual genome or genomes obtained from closely related organisms. Genome basically contains two types of information which is important for developing various types of algorithms.

1. **Compositional based binning algorithms:** Every genome have their conservative sequence and is reflected in its fragments. Normally, due to lack of enough information, this type of binning system is not reliable for the short reads.

2. **Similarity based binning software:** The similarity of the unknown DNA fragments with the reference gene in the database may be used to classify and bin the unknown sequence.

3. **Both composition and similarity binning are also used to develop some of the algorithms.**

Annotations

The annotations of the metagenomics can be done by employing following two different pathways.

1. If the size of the contigs is 30,000 bp or longer, then one should prefer to use the already existing pipeline for the genome annotations like RAST, IMG etc. for the reconstruction of the genomes.

2. The annotations can be executed on the whole community and it mainly relied on the short contigs or unassembled reads. The genomic annotation tools are not found to be very useful as compared to those which are entirely developed for metagenomics analysis.

The annotation of the metagenomic sequence data can be done in two ways: Feature prediction and functional annotation. The term Feature prediction is defined as the process of labeling the sequence either as genes or genomic elements. It emphasis on the detection of the features of interest of a particular gene whereas assigning of the function of a gene or taxonomc neighbours come under the characteristics of functional annotation.

A number of algorithms and tools like Frag Gene Scan, Meta Gene Annotator, Meta Gene Mark, Orphelia etc. were developed to specifically design to accurately identify and handle the predictions of the CDS. These tools function on the basis of using internal information to differentiate between coding and non-coding sequences. Mainly emphasis on the development of the short or the error prone sequences and the excellence of the training sets.

Frag Gene Scan (FGS): It is the most commonly used algorithm which extemporary models the sequencing errors and thus reducing the gene prediction error to 1-2%. It is almost 70% effective and the genes missing from this can easily be identified by BLAST. A number of non-protein coding genes like tRNAs, signalpeptides, CRISPRs etc. can be predicted by a number of tools.

The functional annotation used to represent a foremost challenge in front of most of the projects. Currently, upto 20 to 50% of the metagenomic sequences are able to be annotated and the importance and purpose of remaining genes still need to be annotated. As we know annotation can't be done *de novo*, but it is possible through mapping to gene or protein libraries with non-redundant databases. The sequences which are not able to be mapped to the known sequence space may be nominated as ORFans. These unknown fractions are found to be accountable for never ending genetic innovation in metagenomics.

MG-RAST: It is defined as a data repository or an analysis pipeline in a comparative genomics environment. It provides the automated quality control of the prediction of the features and functions of the short reads in a very accurate and efficient manner. The results of this repository can be expressed as professed profiles for the specific taxanomical or functional annotations. The data generated by the MG-RAST can easily be downloaded by the users and can be shared and published within the same portal. The data can be compared by using number of statistical tools and also helps in incorporating different types of metadata into the statistics. It has thousands of publicly accessible metagenomes.

IMG/M: It is also a known tool for providing standardized pipeline with very high sensitivity like hidden Markov model and BLASTX etc. The analysis done by this method is different from that of MG-RAST, it is based on an all versus all genes comparison. It assimilates all datasets into a single protein level abstraction. Both of them help in comparing the stored computational results and also enables the comparison between novel metagenomes and other rich datasets without the requirement of an end-user for reanalysis.

CAMERA: Although it provides more flexible annotation schemes, it is more complex and relies on the deep and confident understanding of the particular researchers about the interpretation and annoataion of the data. It helps in analyses and comparison of the data under same flow and also allows the publication of the data set simultaneously. CAMERA is also known to be the foremost to maintain the genomic Standards Consortium's Minimal Information checklists for metadata in their web interface.

MEGAN: It is also helpful in visualization of the annotations which are derived from based searches by BLAST in a functional and taxonomical dendrogram. It provides the collapsible network of data interpretation and which is very easy to analyze with the help of these dendrograms.

The summary of tools is given in Table 45.2.

Table 45.2 Different tools or databases commonly used for analysis in metagenomics

S. No.	Details	Tools/Databases
1.	A tool for Phylogenetic analysis	AMPHORA
2.	A tool for analysis and maintenance of sequence database	ARB
3.	Database for Non-redundant sequence data, Marine viromes, Hawai Ocean time series station ALOHA	CAMERA
4.	Database for alternate views of proteins, names and other information, reductant archival database	GenBank
5.	Automatic functional and phylogenetic analysis of the genome	RAST
6.	A tool for geographical and statistical analysis of data sets	MEGAN
7.	For worldwide metadata information of the projects related to genome and metagenome	GOLD
8.	For the nonreductant collection of genomic data and transcripts	RefSeq
9.	A tool for analysis of Marine metagenomics	Megx.net

Applications

Nowadays, metagenomics has been considered as a shot gun for detection and discovery of microbes in the samples (both clinical as well as environmental). This approach is also renamed as diagnostic metagenomics in the current scenario. The sequencing of clinical or environmental samples done by metagenomics would be considered/preferred as universal test to detect and diagnose any type of pathogens. It could also be useful for subtyping tests for routine/usual surveillance activities. It helps in recovering any information from a metagenome via creating library of their shotgun sequences. It is very difficult to study highly diverse habitats of earth with further complex nature of microbes and countless functions of the multiple genera. The metagenomics research can also be done for productive results in decentralized and small project settings. Now, there is extensive need for the projects that should involve multiple investigators to work collectively to enhance the advancement in the era of metagenomics.

It is unique in its part because it's a combination of branches which are apart from each other i.e. —microbiology, ecology, and genomics—that fuse to form this new science named "Metagenomics". This science could also offer us with various universal tests to detect pathogens, diagnose them clinically and subtyping tests as well for routine surveillance activities.

Food borne infections

In past times, it was very difficult to detect foodborne infections by culture techniques to perform the particular genotypes and phenotypes. Detecting the possible involvement of particular pathogens from different food items over time was another tedious task. The science of shotgun metagenomics had made every diagnosis possible in a rapid and accurate manner. It also helps in easy monitoring of trend of infections over time and detection of culprit food item in causing illness and outbreaks.

Viromics: The sequencing by metagenomics was surprisingly employed first time to detect human associated viruses not the bacteria's. This in turn was a challenge to culture the viruses. Since the last decade, numerous works was done in the field of viral metagenomics and the term *"viromics"* was investigated to use as a tool in diagnosing various cases of acute gastroenteritis. It was also considered as the proof of the concept study in clinical diagnostic settings. It helps in determining the etiological causal relation in development of gastroenteritis in a retrospective manner. This technique was proved to be useful in cases where the negative results were obtained by culture techniques in determining the disease causative agents.

Parasitic Metagenomics: The science of shotgun metagenomics in the diagnostic assays had made tremendous development starting from detection of encephalitis from CSF and serum specimens to the most advance techniques in a rapid manner for the detection of Leptospiraceae family. An accurate diagnosis of the Brucella species in the CSF specimens was also done by metagenomic analysis in brucellosis. Further, the techniques were developed and validated by CLIA-certified University of California, San Francisco clinical microbiology laboratory. It was also found that almost 8-11 plausible enteric pathogens particularly bacterial pathogens were detected by metagenomics and also those which were not detected by PCR etc. Parasitic metagenomics was also found to be effective in investigating *Cyclospora cayetanenisi* which is responsible for many food and waterborne infections worldwide.

Metagenomics Antimicrobial Resistance Gene Detection: The main limitation in determining antimicrobial resistance is the difficulty in culturing all the responsible pathogens and the resistome (resistance gene pool) that may be transferable to the pathogens. Therefore, the science of metagenomics is found to be capable of overcoming the challenges associated with conventional methods. Nowadays, both the functional as well as shotgun metagenomic sequencing have been used to interrogate the challenge of resistome. The metagenomic reads are compared with the database comprising of catalog of resistant genes like CARD, MEGARes, ARDB, Resfams etc. Moreover, in the reverse scenario, the metagenomics read can also be accumulated into contigs and then compared with a functional annotation database. With this way, a large number of resistant genes had been detected in the gastrointestinal tract.

Functional metagenomics technique is capable of discovering numerous highly divergent and novel antimicrobial resistant genes. This technique was used to involve cloning of total community of genomic DNA into an expression vector and transformation of them into a susceptible host such as *E. coli*. These methods can be useful in large scale for both clinical as well as public health laboratories for rapidly and accurately diagnosing outbreaks in microbial infections.

Challenges faced by Metagenomics

As met genomics provides a rapid and accurate means of detecting various worldwide infections, it should now be moved to the forefront of the diagnostic laboratories in the coming future. Various proof of concept studies, surveys, real-time accomplishment of the projects regarding public health surveillances and world outbreaks, will undoubtedly promote the acceptance of this metagenomic methodologies in the public and medical health care centres at a large scale.

Following are the various challenges faced by metagenomics in begging its position in the diagnostic world:

1. Issue of historical or epidemiological data as the reference
2. Standardization of the technique to all foodborne pathogens
3. Multidisciplinary approach is required to run the system smoothly
4. Regular audits and quality control system is required to assure the smooth conduct of the system

5. Training and knowledge of the technical as well as qualified personnel

6. Various bioinformatic techniques like algorithms, pielines, softwares etc. are required to be developed, validated and standardized

7. Requirement of curative sequence databases to proper patient diagnosis

8. Procurement of regulatory approval to implement this technique in food safety and public health laboratories

9. Protection of patient privacy regarding its genome is an issue of ethical concern

10. The knowledge of their metagenomes to the patients may also lead to uncertain implications of self diagnosing

11. Asses to the patent DNA can pose unwarranted legal implications

12. Patent infringement

13. It also helps in detecting the fraud in species, mislabeling of food products, incorrect claims etc. which may also lead to increased scrutiny.

14. Undesirable outcomes due to detection of antimicrobial resistant genes lead to ban of various subtherapeutic food use in animals.

To avoid the hurdles, the regular audits and quality control system is required to assure the smooth conduct of the system. Guidelines should be prepared and approved by the world-wide authorities for validation and standardization of the techniques.

Suggested Readings

1. Coughlan LM, Cotter PD, Hill C, Alvarez-Ordonez A. Biotechnological applications of functional metagenomics in the food and pharmaceutical industries. Frontiers in Microbiology 2015; 6: 672-94.

2. Forbes JD, Knox NC, Ronholm J, Pagotto F and Reimer A. Metagenomics: The Next Culture-Independent Game Changer. Front. Microbiol. 2017; 8: 1069-89.

3. Mulcahy-O'Grady H and Workentine ML. The Challenge and Potential of Metagenomics in the Clinic. Front. Immunol. 2016; 7: 29.

CHAPTER 46

THERAPEUTIC USE EXEMPTION

In this era of sports where the spirit of healthy competition has lost completely and where the difference of millisecond can decide between gold and a silver medal, doping has increased considerably in every area of sport. Due to this the athletes are willing to sacrifice their integrity and future for having that one moment of pride. Sports Illustrated issue of 1997 showed a report when aspiring US Olympians were asked, if they would go for doping in order to win and not get caught, 98% said "Yes." Then, when asked, "Would you take the same banned substance if it would get you the gold medal for 5 consecutive years, then leading to death?", 50% still said "Yes." This shows the mentality of the athletes in the current era that they would go to any length to win and the spirit of sport is of no concern.

The origin of using drugs in sport goes back to the very creation of sports itself. The origin of doping is still a matter of debate. It is thought that an African tribe, the Kaffirs gave the name "dop" to a beverage which was consumed as a stimulant drink in religious ceremonies. Painting of the Chinese Emperor Shen-Nung from 2737 BC became the first document related to the use of doping agents, which showed the emperor with leaves of "machuang" (Ephedra). Drugs enhancing performance have been used from the very beginning of Olympics as well. Doping is not an unique phenomena to modern athletic competition. Various mushrooms, plants, herbs have been used by the athlete's in ancient Olympic games in Greece and Rome. Diet modifications was also used widely for enhancing the performance. Apart from dietary supplements, magical potions which were derived from various vegetables and animal realms were being abused for improving performance in sport in the ancient Olympics. The term doping also came into existence in around late 1800s when a potion comprising of opium was being abused in horses.

According to WADA, doping is said to be present if one of the following rules are violated:

- Presence of prohibited substances or its metabolites in athletes sample
- Attempting the use of banned substance or method
- Refusing to provide the sample without proper justification after the notification from the concerned authorities
- Tampering or attempt to tamper with any part of doping control
- Possession of banned substances and methods
- Administration or attempting to administer a prohibited substance or method to any athlete or even assisting, encouraging or covering up for any violation of the anti-doping rules

In 1964 Tokyo became the first Olympiad to conduct a trial of drug testing and various foreign substances were found in several athletes which led to formation of banned substances list which is being updated regularly. A substance or method is included in WADA list for banned substances only if it meets certain criteria –

- Evidence that the substance or method can help in increasing the performance of the athlete
- Evidence that the substance or method can potentially cause risk to the health of the athletes
- Use of the substance or method leads to violation of spirit of the sport.

The International Olympic Committee did not start testing for doping until 1968 after a Danish cyclist KnudEnemark Jensen died following a cycle crash in 1960 Olympics and later it was found that the athlete had consumed Amphetamine. Before that many of the known cases of athletes are present who consumed performance enhancing substances in order to get advantage over their respective opponents.English cyclist Arthur Linton was alleged to have overdosed on "trimethyl" (compound containing either caffeine or ether) and died in 1886 during a 600-km race. Very well known athletes like Maria Sharapova, Tyson Gay, Maria Luisa Calle Williams, Lance Armstrong were all involved in doping scandals. When Ben Johnson's gold medal was taken back along with all his records in 1988 Olympics and in World Championships in 1987, the world became aware of doping.

In 2011 World Championships, more than 30 % of the athletes admitted to use banned substances during their careers but more than 40% of the athletes had used them but only 0.5% of them were caught. This is the main problem that only some amount of violations are being caught. So the athletes which are being caught are only the tip of the iceberg whereas the problem lies much deeper.

In 2013, out of 115 nations, Russia was the worst offender with more than 200 positive tests for banned substances. India with 91 positive tests was third in the list. India is far from becoming a leading medal nation, but it ranked third in 3 consecutive years from 2013-2015 in doping violation figures released by WADA. In 2014, India had 96 positive samples with athletics contributing highest. India is only behind Russia with 148 positive samples and Italy with 123 positive samples.To the nation's shame, in 2015 again India stood third in the list with number of positive samples increasing from 96 to 117 with weightlifting contributing highest number of positive samples followed by athletics. In 2016, India maintained their poor record of being in top 10 list of Anti-Doping violations with sixth position with 69 positive samples.

The prohibited substances which are used mostly in sports are –

- Anabolic Steroids – they are among the most popular performance enhancing drugs. It is used to increase the muscle mass and strength.
- Stimulants – such as Amphetamines improve mood, alertness and the reaction time.
- Diuretics – can help in reducing weight and can dilute the concentration of other drugs in the urine.
- Erythropoietin – increases the RBC production which improves oxygen availability to tissues
- HGH – Human Growth Hormone increases the muscle mass which in turn increases the performance
- Beta blockers – lower the blood pressure and heart rate and make people less jittery. They are banned in sports which require steady hands such as archery, shooting etc.

Diseases are a part and parcel of life and can happen to any person and the athletes are no exception. It doesn't mean that the athletes can't take part in their respective sports. For many athletes, making a career in sports is not safe without the use of drugs and it can be demonstrated best by the case of American sailor Kevin Hall. He had to lose his testicles because of cancer and he needed testosterone injections for maintaining his health. In simple terms, TUE is a process which was established by WADA to allow the athletes to apply for exemption to use prohibited substancesdescribed in the "International Standard for Therapeutic Use Exemptions." The TUE process clearly defines the mechanism by which the athlete can get approval for the usage of a prohibited substance or method. But it is only allowed where that use is indicated to be mandatoryfor the appropriate treatment of a documented clinical condition. Prof Ken Fitch, a leading anti-doping expert and past member of Medical Commission of the International Olympic

Commission laid the foundation in late 1980s of a process to grant athletes permission for using prohibited substances and methods but only if the justification is present for their usage. He is the the forerunner of the modern TUE. He linked the prohibited substances to the clinical conditions where these substances would be needed.

Earlier the plan for "medical dispensation" which was introduced by IOC was the requirement of written, clinical explanation for the consumption of these substances. In some scenarios it can also be collected retroactively and often there was no demand placed upon the attending doctor to make advance notice to a sporting body. The disadvantages which comes with this approach are self-explanatory which has lead to more stringent and consistent rules and regulations.

TUE: The International Standard

It defines, describes, and delineates the procedure that must be followed for ensuring athlete's right to get proper medical treatment within the context of sport and the anti-doping rules.

It describes:

- All the conditions that mustbe satisfied in order for a TUE to be granted
- The duties upon the various anti-doping agencies for ensuring clean implementation of TUE
- Procedures that must be followed by an athlete while applying for TUE
- Roles and responsibilitiesof a TUE Exemption Committee (TUEC)
- Process for appealing to the decision

Athletes play at different levels (international, national, state) so it also specifies the organisation for which the application should be addressed. The sporting administrations of the various countries should be familiar with this International Standard.

Therapeutic use Exemption Committee

Therapeutic use exemption committee operates at various levels, one at the national level in the National Anti-doping Agency of the particular country, then there is International Federation (IF) and Major Event Organisation (MEO). It must consist of three clinicians experienced in treating athletes and having sufficient information regarding sports medicine. The physicians must be quite experienced in treating sports related injuries. For ensuring impartial attitude, the members of the committee must declare no conflict of interest and all the details should be confidential. The decision for TUE must be independent without any influence and the spirit of sport should be maintained. TUEC is responsible for reviewing the applications for TUE before the permission is granted. All TUEC's have the power to seek expert opinion additionally for more accuracy in their judgement. They can also ask for more relevant data from the athlete or the clinician for TUE. The responsibility of making decisions should reside with the clinicians and not the administrative department as the decision is based on medical grounds.

Applications for TUE

Application by the athlete for TUE depends upon which level of competition he/she is going to take part as it can be at national level or international level. TUE granted by the NADA is only valid in the domestic competitions and not in international events, for it to be valid even in international events the TUE must be applied in IF or MEO which then evaluate the application and come to a decision. The submission of the applicatons are the sole responsibility of the athletes however it must be duly signed by the treating clinician. Unfortunately many times the applications are not complete which leads to unnecessary delay in the process.

The deadline before which the application should be submitted depends whether the substance is banned in or out of the competition. If the substance is banned In-competition then the application must be submitted 30 days before the participation in the event as the TUEC have 21 days to come to a decision. The substances which are banned both in and out of the competition, then the athlete has to apply for TUE as soon as the condition is diagnosed and which requires the use of the banned substance or method. Some of the conditions may require emergency interventions and which may lead to the use of such substances or methods which are prohibited for athletes. For such conditions the International Standard permits retroactive TUE application. It is only based on emergency grounds where the athlete did not have sufficient time or oppurtunity to file for TUE. But it is not guaranteed that the application will be accepted as was the case of Samir Nasri who is a professional footballer in Spanish League. During his holiday in USA, he fell ill and was diagnosed with dehydration and was given IV infusion of Nacl. He applied for TUE afterwards but the application was rejected as there was no medical justification as to why oral rehydration was not considered and it was not considered as an emergency.

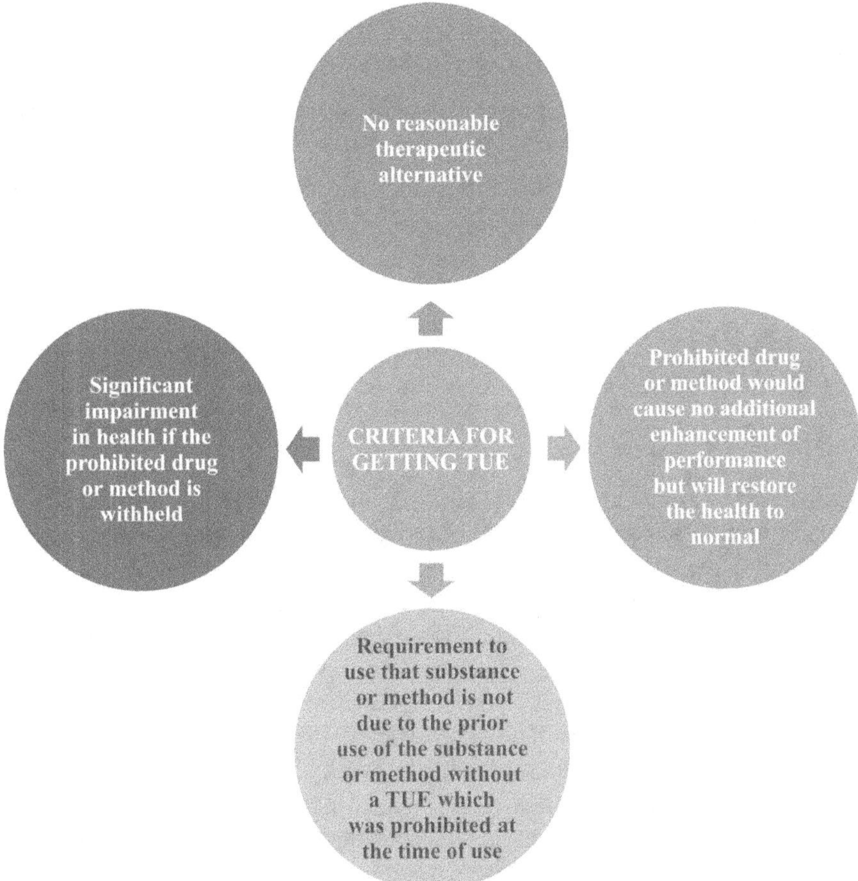

What Happens when the Athlete is Granted a TUE ?

TUE's permits the use of a specific dose and route of administration by the athlete. The TUE are valid only for a period of time after which they get expired and have to be renewed. The athletes must adhere to guidelines outlined in the application. When the IF or NADA grants TUE to an athlete, the application goes to WADA which then reviews it and can reverse their decision if it does not met the International Standard for TUE.

Appeal of Decision given by TUEC

The International Standard has specified that athlete as well as sporting bodies can appeal against the decision. If the TUE is refused by the IF, then WADA has the authority for reviewing the decision as per article 8.1 of the International Standard.

The process is:

- Reviewing request must be sent to WADA within 21 days of the decision given by the TUE granting authority.

- If the case is accepted then the athlete will have to pay fees of 500 US dollars to WADA.

- The documents reviewed previously will again be reviewed by WADA and it may ask for other relevant data which may be linked to the case.

- WADA will give its decision within the time frame which depends upon case to case basis

- Refusal of TUE will stand until WADA gives the decision, so the athlete cannot use the banned substances during that time.

- The decision given by WADA can again be appealedto the Court of Arbitration for Sport (CAS).

TUE for Paralympians

Paralympians are often the source of inspiration, motivation and they are even described as heroic. Paralympics has also started gaining world attention along with that the athletes taking part in it have also started becoming famous. As Paralympics has also grown competitive, some the athletes have started to use performance-enhancing substances. So, most paralympians inspire but some cheat. If they are caught doping, they also receive the same penalty as the Olympians. The testing however is more complicated for Paralympians especially for athletes who urinate through catheters, so doping control officers have to be more trained. The International Paralympic Committee recognises TUE's from as many Anti-Doping organisations as possible. For these organisations certain substances will be automatically recognised as TUE except for some substances which will be reviewed by the International Paralympic Committee Medical board. These substances are:

S0. Non-Approved Substances

S1: Anabolic Agents

S2: Peptide Hormones, Growth Factors, Related Substances and Mimetics

S.8 Cannabinoids, Meldonium Prohibited Methods: M1, M2 and M3.

P.1 Beta-Blockers in World Shooting Para Sport only

Challenges of TUE

Controversially there has been increase in use of testosterone and androgenic precursors in males having low testosterone levels. These applications demanding TUE have increased considerably but it requires critical observation from TUEC.

Diagnosis of adrenal suppression secondary to the use of systemic glucocorticoids is also a controversial issue and remains a challenge for TUEC when the application is made for the use of a combination of glucocorticoids and DHEA.

Another challenging issue is the use of androgens and other hormones in transgendered athletes. It is quite uncommon but still it is an issue for TUEC and requires scrutiny.

The consumption of medical marijuana has emerged in certain jurisdictions produces a challenge for the TUEC. This issue is more relevant for the athletes participating in Paralympics as this substance is mainly used for treating pain and spasticity. Their administration has increased in the clinical set-up but standardizing of dose and product is minimal.

There has been increase in TUE applications for attention deficit hyperactivity disorder (ADHD). The treatment of this condition involves amphetamines or other stimulants which is a big issue in granting TUE. A successful application for ADHD requires the athlete to be diagnosed with this condition according to DSM-V criteria. Famous Olympic champions data have been leaked who had a TUE for this disorder which led to a huge debate over the world about the authenticity of TUE.

WADA stated that between 2014 and 2016 the number of exemptions granted to athlete's increased by 48%. It is a necessary compromise which is on a rise. The international standards are well developed, but still have several limitations to address.

As the medical conditions are not static but dynamic so the process should consider athletes going for frequent check-ups by independent medical board which will provide detailed report about the athlete which must remain confidential. So that the medical treatment which is ongoing without any medical ground should be stopped.

To restore the integrity of TUE process, an independent TUE system is required. Applications for a particular condition must be looked over by one independent board. The fight against doping is not an easy fight just as monitoring of TUE is not easy. So it would require a lot of commitment from the personnel looking over this process. Anti-Doping organization along with the TUEC aim to protect the spirit of sport and provide every athlete to compete against evenly matched opponent without any unfair advantage

Suggested Readings

1. Baron DA, Martin DM, Abol Magd S. Doping in sports and its spread to at-risk populations: an international review. World psychiatry : official journal of the World Psychiatric Association (WPA). 2007; 6(2): 118-23.

2. Conti AA. Doping in sports in ancient and recent times. Medicina nei secoli. 2010; 22(1-3): 181-90.

3. Gerrard D, Pipe A. Therapeutic Use Exemptions. Medicine and sport science. 2017; 62: 55-67.

4. Malve HO. Sports Pharmacology: A Medical Pharmacologist's Perspective. Journal of pharmacy & bioallied sciences. 2018; 10(3): 126-36.

5. NADA. Therpeutic Use Exemptions [Available from: https://www.nadaindia.org/en/therapeuticuseexemptionstue.

6. Pitsiladis Y, Wang G, Lacoste A, Schneider C, Smith AD, Di Gianfrancesco A, et al. Make Sport Great Again: The Use and Abuse of the Therapeutic Use Exemptions Process. Current sports medicine reports. 2017; 16(3): 123-5.

7. WADA. THERAPEUTIC USE EXEMPTION [Available from: https://www.wada-ama.org/en/questions-answers/therapeutic-use-exemption-tue.

CHAPTER 47

SYSTEMS PHARMACOLOGY

"Systems pharmacology is not synonymous to systemic pharmacology."

Introduction

Systemic pharmacology is a branch of medicine involving the study of mode of action of drug on different systems like cardiovascular system, central nervous system etc. comprising the entire body. It also deals with pharmacokinetics, pharmacodynamics, uses and adverse effects of a drug on living systems.

Systems pharmacology is a developing field of pharmacology which involves the application of the fundamentals of systems biology to the field of pharmacology. It helps us to know how drugs influence the human body as a single complex biological system. Systems pharmacology as defined by the National Institutes of Health (NIH) white paper is "an approach to translational medicine that combines computational and experimental methods to elucidate, validate and apply new pharmacological concepts to the development and use of small molecule and biologic drugs with the aim of determining mechanisms of action of new and existing drugs in preclinical and animal models and in patients." According to systems pharmacology the effect of a drug is not only the consequence of a single specific drug-protein interaction but a network of interactions which may include chemical-protein, protein–protein and various signalling pathways. In biological systems, there exists different signaling networks and they are not unidirectional, there is extensive clustering of these signals. Hence, any single perturbation in the regulatory network , like an increase in protein level or rate of a biochemical reaction, may not definitely result in a diseased state; whereas signaling networks responsible for the disease state need to be disturbed persistently at multiple points. Systems pharmacology by using bioinformatics and statistical techniques helps to integrate and interpret these networks.

Since most of the current drug-discoveries are focused towards complex diseases, one needs to understand the underlying pathophysiology at systems level. This would help in the designing of novel drugs with favourable outcomes. Although technological limitations in drug discovery have been overcome to a great extent, still there exist challenges like lack of identification of appropriate targets for various diseases involving complex pathophysiology. This is because knowledge about the role of biological systems implicated in human pathophysiology is yet to be explored. However the integration of systems-based experimental and computational approaches have made it easier to overcome this problem to a great extent.

A Network-Based view of Drug Action

The concepts from graph theory is the branch of mathematics which mainly focuses on learning about networks, is extensively being used in acquiring knowledge about regulatory functions of cells, tissues and organs. In biological systems, its not just one drug and one target interaction but a network of interactions. Networks on capturing these interactions are believed to impart frameworks to know how regulation occurs from the interactivity between various cellular constituents. So there exists multiple large regulatory networks in biological system. By identifying these networks, one can have a mechanistic understanding about how the systems organize themselves for a particular regulatory function to occur. Dysregulation of these networks occur in a pathophysiological state. Such approaches which are mainly network-based are useful in various combination regimens in disease states like cancer.

An Overview of Bioinformatics

Bioinformatics is an interdisciplinary domain of science, that combines biology, mathematics, computer science and statistics. It aids in developing different methodologies and software tools for a better understanding and interpretation biological data. It is used in identification of particular genes likely to cause a disease and single nucleotide polymorphisms (SNPs). The main aim of such identification is to throw light on the genetic basis of a disease, unique adaptations and difference between populations. It also helps in simulation and modeling of DNA, RNA, proteins as well as biomolecular interactions. Therefore, the field of bioinformatics although started in mid 1990s has rapidly grown with the advent of Human Genome Project and by expeditious advancement in the field of DNA sequencing technology.

Mechanisms of Disease: Analyzing through Regulatory Networks

To have a better knowledge of drug action, a systems level approach is essential. One should also have thorough knowledge about pathophysiology of complex diseases. This can be accomplished by integration of physiological, biochemical and genomic datasets which inturn needs variety of computational approaches. Thus by putting in order the high-dimensional biological datasets, significant information can be extracted by making use network analysis of cellular systems.

A network is described as a series of entities which are connected to each another on the grounds of a pre defined criterion. These entities are called as nodes, that constitutes genes, proteins, drugs and disease. Each interaction between 2 nodes becomes an "edge". Nodes are also used to define the condition of a system. These stipulations can be figured out using Boolean dynamics, wherein every node has a probability to be present in two states either inactive or active. With involvement of multiple nodes and edges, these network models become increasingly complicated and computational tools become essential. Network analyses aids us to explain the relationship between developing functions and topology at molecular, tissue, organ, and organism level and connections between them. With the need to analyse through a systems-level perspective, molecular aspect of disease as well as its network view is needed to gain knowledge about a particular physiological function. Experimental and computational approaches are considered as foundation of systems pharmacology.

Network Analysis - Establishing Novel Drug Targets and Drug Development

Drug discovery is a challenging, time consuming and a tedious process. It costs billions of dollars to bring a drug into market. Most of the compounds fail at later stages of clinical trial. The cost of drug discovery is huge and rapidly rising, hence drug failure at a later stage causes substantial rise in pharmaceutical expenses. To successfully overcome this expensive winding up of production of drugs, the pharmaceutical industries are now interested to adopt computational methods in drug discovery process. Models have the potential in providing new intuition into basic principles of biology that would further help in a better understanding of nature of diseases. Currently, physiologically based pharmacokinetics models (PBPK) are used along with traditional pharmacokinetic, pharmacodynamic and statistical pharmacometric models. The physiological based approach divides the body into different anatomical sections/compartments which are connected to each other through the body fluid systems. This approach also provides insight into interspecies variability, specific organ metabolism/transport. Pharmacometric models are sketched to estimate the biological variability in patients from which clinical trial outcomes are predicted. This may help in reducing the expenses of late stage attrition of drug development process.

Structural Considerations During Drug Discovery

Effectiveness of a drug in general depends on the extent a phenotype is controlled by the target and the affinity for binding between the drug and its targets. Affinity is expressed in terms of druggability which is a term utilized in drug discovery to elucidate a biological target that is known to or speculated to bind to a drug/target with high affinity. Binding of drug to its target should alter the function of the target thereby producing a therapeutic effect in the patient. Computational methodologies are utilized for identification of new chemical structure and for optimization of lead compounds against certain targets. Incase of traditional drug discovery approaches, a drug is designed towards a single specific biological target whereas modern drug discovery includes polypharmacology, in which a drug is not designed to bind only to a single target but with many targets with considerable affinity to establish a productive treatment. This principle is applied in disorders of central nervous system and cancers.

Computational Methodologies in Drug Discovery

Computer aided drug discovery (CADD) has greatly reduced the time duration and cost of research and drug development. Such technologies can bring down the number of lead compounds which would otherwise be screened during experimental evaluation. Apart from reducing time and cost, CADD also ensures that lead compound which enters preclinical studies is probably the supreme compound, predicts effectiveness and possible adverse effects. Hence it behaves as a "virtual shortcut" in the process of drug discovery.

Computer aided drug discovery methods are broadly grouped into:

- Structure based drug discovery (SBDD)
- Ligand based drug discovery (LBDD)

Incase of SBDD, one needs to know the three dimensional conformation of disease associated drug target. If target information is not known, computational methods like homology modeling are used to predict the structure. When the target information cannot be obtained by SBDD, LBDD acts as an alternative. This method depends on the data regarding known active binders of the target. Therefore, computational methodologies make it possible to classify drugs based on their conformation and proteins to which they attach. Adopting such methodologies helps us to make prophecises about curative outcomes of drugs for complex diseases and off-target effects.

Pharmacogenomics – An Efficient Model for Systems Pharmacology

Pharmacogenomics is the study of how genes affect a person's response to drugs. As the name suggests it is a combination of both pharmacology and genomics. Advancement in pharmacogenomics has enabled to develop a safe and an effective medication, wherein the dose can be adjusted according to an individual's genetic constitution. Tailoring the dosage of a medication keeping in mind individual's genetic constitution is known as personalized medicine. To know how systems biology works, one needs to have a knowledge about the relationship between pharmacogenomics and systems pharmacology. It is observed that when an individual consumes a drug, there occurs substantial intra -individual and inter- individual variations. Age, underlying disease, sex, adherence to prescribed medication and genetic polymorphism are causes for such variations. It is important to understand influence of inherent variability apart from drug interactions with their targets as well as off-targets, with enzymes involved in metabolism. Discovering the genetic variants responsible for variation will permit physicians to impart personalized therapy which is the eventual target of pharmacogenomics. Example is prediction of dosage of warfarin based on the inherent variation. Warfarin is an anticoagulant with narrow therapeutic index, thus even a minor variation in its plasma concentrations may lead to dose dependent adverse drug reactions or therapeutic failure. There occurs a wide inter individual variation in warfain dose which is needed to attain target concentration. The VKORC1 and CYP2C9 genotypes play an important role in warfarin dosing.VKORC1 is an enzyme which plays an important role in vitamin K recycling and CYP2C9 an isoform of cytochrome P450 controls the metabolism of warfarin. A dose curtailment is also advocated for individuals who carry 2 copies of the variant VKORC1 A allele(VKORC1,c.-1639G>A/A). CYP2C9 variants, CYP2C9*2 and*3 require low dose of warfarin. Sometimes these genetic variants fail to be detected, with increased warfarin concentrations in blood there is a greater risk of haemorrhage. So, in patients with these polymorphisms, the dose of warfarin should be adjusted accordingly inorder to reduce the risk of haemorrhage. With the advent of pharmacogenomics, these genetic variants can be identified well in advance thereby preventing increased risk of bleeding which otherwise would prove to be fatal.

Apart from macromolecular structure, genetic and epigenetic variabilities, various biomolecular targets, and influence of surrounding environment play an important role in molecular interactions to occur but till date not much information is available, hence it has to be explored in systems pharmacology. Inorder to overcome these deficits, a three dimensional structural view of biological system is a must. This macromolecular structure acts as a connecting link between chemical and genomic space, thereby helps to find an association between drug and their targets, biological pathways. Recent advancement in experimental as well as computational methodologies has greatly uncovered entire human genome. But still there occurs difficulty in developing a well predictive statistical model. The reason is that state of a disease is not constant during therapy. Disease state might unfold to different forms during the course of treatment, a process known as adapatation. So the major setback is that when sufficient data are gathered to give a detailed account of state of disease and an efficient model is designed, the course of disease might have evolved to a different state. Hence it might not resemble with the model designed. Further, an issue arises that what amount of information is required to design a precise model for complex disease taking into considerations like genetic and epigenetic mechanisms. Another question arises about functioning of a model if a person possesses a novel mutation. Hence, along with mathematical based pharmacokinetics and pharmacodynamics approaches it is also important to combine physiochemical-based macromolecular structure models, pharmacogenomics as well as systems pharmacology. This helps in development of better predictive models to optimize therapy as well decrease undesirable side effects.

Applications of Systems Pharmacology

- Drug discovery process
- Has drastically reduced time and expenses that occur during drug development.
- Focuses on targeting strategies, thus helps in target identification.
- Possible explanations for drug interacting with on target and off targets and resulting effects can be elucidated.
- Can predict uses and adverse drug reactions well in advance thereby leading to optimization of therapy with decreased number of hospitalizations due to untoward effects.
- By throwing light on both systems biology as well as pharmacology, helps in better understanding of pathophysiology of a disease and pharmacological intervention needed to target the underlying defect.
- QSP models are used in validation of targets and discovery of possible treatment responsive biomarkers. Such models are being developed for neurodengenerative disorders like alzheimers disease and for treatment of cancers where multiple targeting becomes essential.
- With the emerging scope for pharmacogenomics along with systems pharmacology, genetic polymorphisms are detected and dose can be titrated accordingly. This has lead to the trend of personalized medicine.

Barriers to Systems Pharmacology – Solution to Overcome?

Systems Pharmacology is a multidicplinary field which requires novel ideas, computational technologies, advancement of –omics like proteomics, genomics etc. This requires involvement of different group of population. This population comprises of academicians, industrialists and a molecular biologists. Every group has a major role in this field, lack of any one would shut off the network .Hence it is important to educate these groups and make them aware of importance of their integration with each other. Novel ideas and discoveries can be made only with collaboration between these groups.

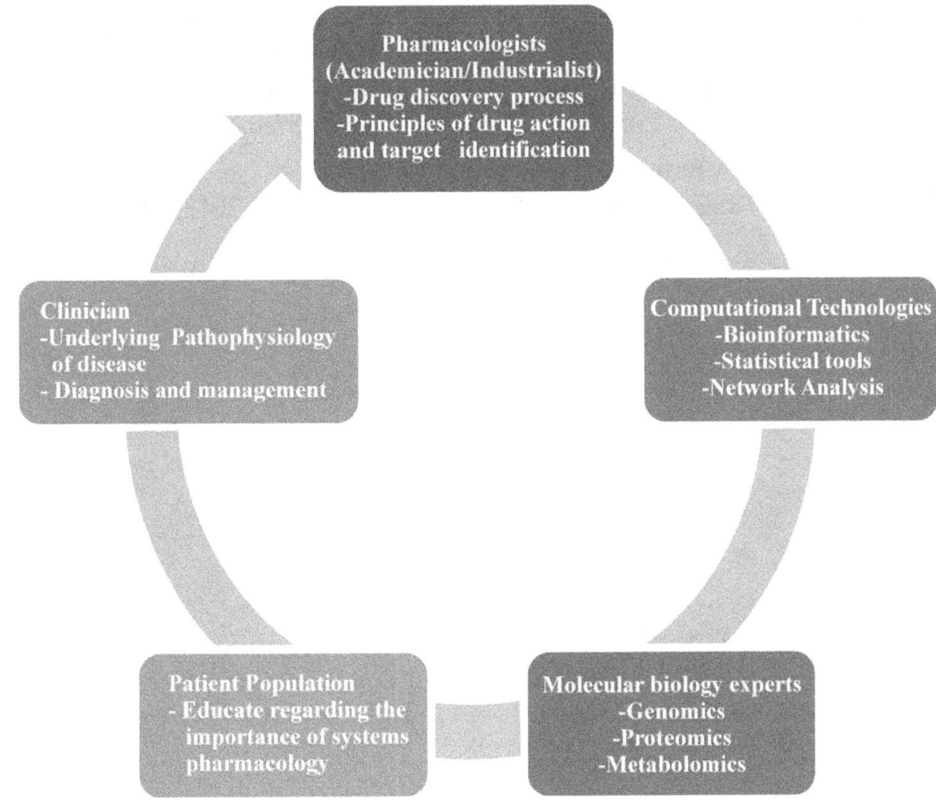

Conclusion

Systems pharmacology is still a developing field , which combines both experimental as well as computational technologies to know how drugs influence human beings as a sole complex biologic system. This is further supported with the evolution of translational medicine and computational technologies.

Suggested Readings

1. Berger SI, Iyengar R. Network analyses in systems pharmacology. 2009; 25(19): 2466-72.

2. Boran ADW, Iyengar R. Systems Pharmacology. Mt Sinai J Medoicine. 2010; 77(4): 333-44.

3. Leelananda SP, Lindert S. Computational methods in drug discovery. 2016; 2694-718.

4. Sorger PK, Allerheiligen SRB, Abernethy DR, Altman RB, Brouwer KLR, Califano A, et al. Quantitative and Systems Pharmacology in the Post-genomic Era□: New

Approaches to Discovering Drugs and Understanding Therapeutic Mechanisms An NIH White Paper by the QSP Workshop Group – October , 2011. 2011; 0-47.

5. Xie L, Ge X, Tan H, Xie L, Zhang Y, Hart T, et al. Towards Structural Systems Pharmacology to Study Complex Diseases and Personalized Medicine. 2014; 10(5).

6. Zhao S, Iyengar R. Systems Pharmacology: Network Analysis to Identify Multiscale Mechanisms of Drug Action. Annu Rev Pharmacol Toxicol. 2012; 52: 505-21.

CHAPTER 48

DRUGS AND RADIATION: INTERACTION TO THERAPY

Introduction

The use of combined modality treatment, chemotherapy and radiotherapy, during the cancer treatment has become one of the standard treatment strategies. The use of radiotherapy as a cancer treatment modality is over 100 year old and the discovery of 5-fluoruracil in 1950's lead to the combined therapy. The use of combined therapy has shown to improve the survival rates in the randomized clinical trials as compared to either chemotherapy or radiotherapy alone in the advanced stages of head and neck, lungs, liver, breast, pancreas and esophagus. To obtain overall effective therapeutic strategy during cancer treatment, it is assumed that greater cell death in tumors rather than the normal surrounding tissues is of prime importance. The rationale for use of chemotherapeutic drugs during radiation treatment includes the efficacy of chemotherapeutic drugs and others being improving the radiation effects. During these processes there may or may not be an interaction between the drugs and radiation treatment. The overall therapeutic effect will improve if the drugs can eradicate the secondary tumors or subclinical metastases and radiation eradicates the primary tumor. The overall goal of the combined chemoradiotherapy is to increase the patient survival by gaining the control over local tumor and eliminating metastasis, while preserving the tissue/organ integrity and function. The overall positive therapeutic efficacy could be achieved using many strategies such as (a) spatial cooperation, (b) independent toxicity, (c) enhancement of tumor response and (d) protecting normal tissues. The major mechanistic contributing factors that play vital roles during improving the tumor response with the combined chemoradiotherapy include (a) enhancing the radiation damage by the DNA incorporating drugs, (b) cell repair inhibition, (c) elimination of radio-resistant and hypoxic cells, (d) inhibition of repopulated tumor cells.

Chemotherapeutic Drugs

The various classes of chemotherapeutic drugs include alkylating agents (chlorambucil, cyclophosphamide, thiotepa, and busulfan), antimetabolities (purine antagonists, pyrimidine antagonists, and folate antagonists), plant alkaloids (Taxanes, actinomycin D, vinorelbine, doxorubicin, mitomycin), platinum derivatives (cisplatin, carboplating and oxaliplatin) and antitumor antibiotics (Doxorubicin, mitoxantrone, and bleomycin).

Radiotherapy

Two months after the discovery of X-rays in 1896, the first ever patient was treated with radiation. Radiotherapy could be used either for curing cancer or reducing the symptoms of it. Radiotherapy could be delivered either externally or internally. The use of external radiation source delivers the radiation using a linear accelerator called as External Beam Radiotherapy (EBRT) and for the internal radiotherapy or brachytherapy purpose a radioactive source is placed inside the patient. The types of external radiation therapy include proton beam therapy, neutron beam therapy and stereotactic radiotherapy. The different types of brachytherapy include intracavity, interstitial and tumor surface. The use of these two types of radiotherapy depends on the type of tumor, its size and location. However, there are some disadvantages in using EBRT which include the high dose delivery to the skin, increasing depth reduces the dose and high bone absorption dose. The disadvantages of brachytherapy include its unsuitability for treatment of large tumors, lymph nodes and require special skills for accurate positioning of the radiation source.

Mechanisms of Chemotherapeutic Drugs and Radiation Interactions

Enhancing initial radiation damage: Halogenated pyrimidines (5-FU) which bind to DNA makes them more susceptible for radiation induced DNA damage. 5-FU slows down the nuclei acid synthesis by inhibiting thymidylate synthase which inturn depletes the nucleotide triphosphates which are required for cell cycle progression, leads to DNA fragmentation and ultimately leads to apoptosis. 5-FU usually affects the S-phase of the cell cycle, which is considered as the radioresistant phase, by binding to DNA/RNA and enhances the radiation induced-DNA damage. Due to the short half-life and quick metabolite formation of 5-FU, continuous and optimal dosage is required during radiotherapy for continuous thymidylate synthase inhibition. Another enzyme thymidine phosphorylase has the ability to convert Capecitabine, an oral drug, into 5-FU is also used for the cancer treatment along with radiotherapy. Temozolomide, cytotoxic alkylating agent, used to treat gliomas has the ability to cross blood brain barrier and causes DNA damage by methylating the guanine O-6 position leading to p53-activated DNA damage mechanism. During the radiotherapy O-6 methylguanine DNA-methyltransferase gets radiosensitized and inturn inhibits the p53 mediated DNA repair enzyme. Cisplatin forms the intra and inter-strand cross-links with DNA by binding to their nucleophilic sites which enhances the radiation induced DNA damage. This mechanism could well be used in both the cases of adequate oxygen rich cells and hypoxic cells. The other mechanism by which the radiation induced damage could be enhanced by drugs is by interfering with the cellular repair mechanisms. Generally, cells have the ability to repair from the lethal and sub-lethal doses of radiation. Some of the drugs that interfere with cellular repair mechanisms include cisplatin, pyrimidines and nucleoside analogs (fludarabine, gemicitabine) (Table 48.1).

Cell cycle effects: Cell cycle plays a vital role in damage and repair mechanisms of an organism. The deregulated cell cycle leading to high proliferation of the cells leads to cancer. It is a complex molecular signaling pathway involving various stages such as Go or resting stage, G1 or gap phase, S or synthesis phase, G2 or second gap phase and M or mitosis phase. Like in cancer cells, the proliferating cells will be more resistant towards radiation damage at S stage and sensitive in the G2 and M phase of the cell cycle. The different phases of the cell cycle have various roles and the overall cytotoxic effects of either radiation or drugs or both depend on the phase of the cell cycle. Therefore the therapeutic strategy could be developed into two ways based on the sensitivity and resistant nature of the cells undergoing cell cycle. The chemotherapeutic drugs could be used to either arrest the cells in the radiosensitive phase or eliminate the radio resistant S-phase cells. The use of nucleoside analogs, fludarabine and gemicitabine, eliminates the radio resistant S-phase cells and improves the overall chemoradiotherapeutic effect. Taxanes, paclitaxel and docetaxel, block the proliferating cancer cells in the G2/M phase, by inhibiting tubul in depolymerization and improve their microtubule assembly and stability, thus making them more sensitive towards radiation damage.

Table 48.1 Effect of drug – radiation interactions on the cellular functions and mechanisms

Drugs	Function		
	Cell kinetics	**Mechanisms**	
		Cell cycle	
Methotrexate, hydroxyurea, gemcitabine, docetaxel, 5-FU, Cisplatin, Carboplatin		G1/S-phase elimination (radioresistant)	
Paclitaxel, docetaxel, mitomycin, vinorelbine, Irinotecan		G2/M phase arrest (radiosensitive)	
Oxaliplatin		G0 phase	
Methotrexate, hydroxyurea, cisplatin, etoposide, campothecin, doxorubicin, BCNU, CCNU, fludarabine		Cell repair	

Table 48.1 *Contd...*

Most chemotherapeutic agents combined with concurrent radiotherapy		Cell proliferation/ repopulation	
	Cell Physiology		
Mitomycin-C, tirapazamine		Hypoxic cells (elimination)	
Most chemotherapeutic agents		Increasing oxygenation	

Hypoxia: Hypoxia, low oxygen area, in tumors exist and are 2–3 times more radioresistant regions than the well-oxygenated tissue regions. It is considered that hypoxic tumors also exhibit aggressive growth behavior and present poor prognosis. The factors which influence the chemotherapeutic effect to have high efficacy with radiotherapy include 1) eliminating well oxygenated tumor cells, 2) removing hypoxic cells and 3) sensitizing hypoxic cells to radiation. Few reports have shown that improving the tumor oxygenation, measured by intratumoral PO_2, by administering the chemotherapeutic drugs like taxol and paclitaxel has enhanced the radiosensitivity. On the other hand drugs such as tirapazamine, mitomycin, nitroimidazole and nimorazole kill the hypoxic cells and improve theradiosensitization thereby overall increasing the survival rates. Tirapazamine, a hypoxic cytotoxic agent, in the hypoxic conditions has the ability to donate electrons generating oxygen free radicals. The radicals damage the DNA by extracting proton from the deoxyribose ring. Under the normoxic conditions the oxygen free radicals generated bind to molecular oxygen and reduces the cytotoxic effect.

Clinical Studies

There are 3 different ways of using the chemotherapy along with the radiation therapy. If the chemotherapy is given before, during or after radiation therapy it is called as neoadjuvant (induction), concurrent or adjuvant therapy.

Neoadjuvant (Induction) therapy

This strategy was developed clinically to address the enhanced toxicity issues manifested during the combine chemoradiotherapy. Therefore, the major goal of this type of chemotherapeutic strategy in the clinical settings is to address and achieve two major objectives: (a) to remove the most possible remaining tumor cells i.e., micrometastases. This would reduce the clonogenic cell number in the tumor and improves the radiotherapy regime for tumor control and (b) to reduce the tumor size that is to be irradiated. This will enhance the efficacy of radiotherapy due to the small tumor size and at the same time reduces the surrounding normal tissue damage.

Clinical studies in NSCLC have shown that chemotherapeutic drugs followed by radiotherapy have reduced the distant metastases rate. However, there was no improvement in the local control rate as show in head and neck cancer, cervical cancer, esophageal cancer, thereby showing improvements in the survival rates. However, there was no effect of chemotherapy on other tumor studies and have accounted this due to the enhanced repopulation of tumor cells. Other reason could be that during radiotherapy process there could be tumor cell proliferation enhancement due to the oxygenation enrichment of tumor microenvironment. In few cases of NSCLC the duration between treatment with gemcitabine and cisplatin followed by radiotherapy, enhanced tumor cell proliferation could be observed with recurrence of doubling the tumor volume between 8 – 171 days. Studies in esophageal cancer cases treated with and without cisplatin having significant differences of Ki-67 labeling indexes of 47% and 67% have shown resistance towards chemoradiotherapy. This could also be accounted for enhanced levels of radioresistance cells where chemotherapy has no effect and resistance towards quiescent tumor cells.

Concurrent Therapy

The objective of this treatment is the concurrent use of chemotherapy-radiation interaction to have maximum anti-tumor effect with reduced side effects. During the alternate treatment of chemotherapy followed by radiation treatment without any treatment gap the cancer cell cycle and reoxygenation mechanisms are perturbed without having any toxic effects on the surrounding normal cells. Such treatment strategy has been performed in the NSCLC, head and neck cancer, nasopharyngeal cancer, esophageal cancer, cervical and anal cancers. This treatment strategy has been used as a standard treatment regime. However, trials have also shown that acute toxicities was also observed including hematological and gastrointestinal toxicities. Later systematic studies have shown that concurrent CT could not be used in cases of poor bone marrow function, poor renal function etc. Studies have also shown that maximum radiosensitization in esophageal cancer could also be achieved with cisplatin/5-FU with daily or weekly administration of chemotherapy combined with radiation treatment have better results as compared to full-dose chemotherapy and radiation treatment.

Drug-Targeted Radiotherapy

Not only the use of drug therapy, a new advancement includes the targeted drug along with radiotherapy in the new modality shaping up for therapeutic strategy. Here, the use of monoclonal antibody along with the drug treatment during radiotherapy is the new upcoming. Some examples of the approved targeted drugs includes the use of Erbitux®, a monoclonal antibody cetuximab, for the advanced head and neck squamous cell cancer and others at various stages of clinical development such as trastuzumab,panitumumab, erlotinib, cilengitide and bevacizumab. Approximately, 40 or more of the US-FDA and/or EMA-approved targeted drugs are listed in Table 48.2. These approved drugs have the potential to increase the sensitivity of the tumor cells along with the radiation treatment. Most of the approved targeted drugs act through the inhibition of EGFR or VEGFR mediated pathway which play clinically and physiologically relevant roles during the cancer treatment.

Cetuximab, an EGFR inhibitor, in combination with radiotherapy of a five year study on the squamous cell head and neck (SCCHN) cancer patients has shown an overall survival rates from 29 to 49 months. Recently, it has also been resolved that the SCCHN patients who are not eligible for Cetuximab and cisplatin combination therapy could go with Cetuximab and radiotherapy as a standard treatment. The other advantage includes overcoming the side effects often encountered in patients with SCCHN who are given standard treatment with platinum drugs and radiotherapy which include radiation-induced mucositis and chemotherapy mediated renal and hematopoietic side effects. The most probable mechanisms of radiosensitization include inhibition of cellular repopulation, inhibition of DNA repair machinery, slowing down of tumor angiogenesis, increasing the radiation induced apoptosis and attenuation of radiation-induced EGFR nuclear import.

Table 48.2 Targeted drugs in cancer (US-FDA approved).
(www.centerwatch.com/drug-information/fda-approvals/)

S. No.	Drugs	Mechanism – primary target
1	Aflibercept	VEGF-A, PlGF
2	Axitinib	VEGFR-1 to 3, PDGFR, KIT
3	Abiraterone acetate	Androgen biosynthesis inhibitor
4	Bevacizumab	VEGF
5	Bortezomib	Proteasome inhibitor
6	Brentuximabvedotin	CD30
7	Bosutinib	Bcr-Abl
8	Brentuximabvedotin	CD30
9	Cabozantinib	Pan-tyrosine kinase inhibitor
10	Carfilzomib	Proteasome inhibitor
11	Catumaxomab	CD3, EpCAM
12	Cetuximab	EGFR type I
13	Crizotinib	ALK and ROS 1
14	Dasatinib	BCR-ABL, SRC family)
15	Degarelix	GnRH receptor
16	Denosumab	RANKL
17	Enzalutamide	Androgen receptor
18	Gemtuzumabozogamicin	CD 33 antigen
19	Erlotinib	EGFR type I
20	Everolimus	mTOR pathway
21	Gefitinib	EGFR
22	Imatinib	Bcr-Abl, PDGF, KIT
23	Imatinib	CTLA-4
24	Ipilimumab	EGFR type I/II
25	Lapatinibditosylate	Mechanism unclear

Table 48.2 *Contd...*

S. No.	Drugs	Mechanism – primary target
26	Nilotinib	Bcr-Abl, PDGF-R, KIT
27	Ofatumumab	CD 20
28	Panitumumab	EGFR type I
29	Pazopanib	VEGFR-1 to 3, PDGFR-a/b, KIT
30	Ponatinib	Dual Abl/Src protein inhibitor
31	Pertuzumab	HER2
32	Pralatrexate	Dihdrofolate reductase
33	Regorafenib	VEGFR, TIE2, PDGFR, RET, KIT, RAF
34	Rituximab	CD 20
35	Sorafenib	Raf, KIT, FLT-3, VEGFR-2,3, PDGFR-B
36	Sunitinib	PDGFR, VEGFR 1 to 3, KIT, FLT, CSF-1R
37	Temsirolismus	mTOR
38	Trametinib	MEK
39	Trastuzumab	EGFR type II
40	Vandetanib	VEGFR, EGFR, RET
41	Vorinostat	HDAC inhibitor
42	Vemurafenib	Activated BRAFV600E gene
43	Vismodegib	Hedgehog pathway

Suggested Readings

1. Blackstock AW *et al.* (2005) Initial pulmonary toxicityevaluation of chemoradiotherapy (CRT) utilizing 74 Gy3-dimensional (3-D) thoracic radiation in stage III non-small cell lung cancer (NSCLC): a Cancer andLeukemia Group B (CALGB) randomized phase II trial[abstract #7060]. Presented at the 2005 ASCO annualmeeting, Orlando, FL.

2. Bonner JA *et al.* (2000) Enhanced apoptosis withcombination C225/ radiation treatment serves as theimpetus for clinical investigation in head and neckcancers. *J ClinOncol* **18 (Suppl):** 47S-53S.

3. Bonner JA, Harari PM, Giralt J et al. Radiotherapy plus cetuximab for locoregionally advanced head and neck cancer: 5-year survival data from a phase 3 randomised trial, and relation between cetuximab-induced rash and survival. Lancet Oncol.11, 21-28 (2010).

4. Brown JM (1993) SR 4233 (tirapazamine): a newanticancer drug exploiting hypoxia in solid tumours.*Br J Cancer* **67:** 1163-1170.

5. Chevalier TL, Arriagada R, Quoix E, et al. (1991) Radiotherapyalone versus combined chemotherapy and radiotherapy innonresectable non-small-cell lung cancer: first analysis of arandomized trial in 353 patients. J Natl Cancer Inst 83: 417-423.

6. Dittmann KH *et al.* (2001) Characterization of the aminoacids essential for the photo- and radioprotectiveeffects of a Bowman-Birk protease inhibitor-derivednonapeptide.*Protein Eng* **14:** 157-160.

7. El Sharouni SY, Kal HB, Battermann JJ (2003) Acceleratedregrowthof non-small cell lung tumours after induction chemotherapy.Br J Cancer 89: 2184-2189.

8. Green JA, Kirwan JM, Tierney JF, et al. (2001) Survival andrecurrence after concomitant chemotherapy and radiotherapy forcancer of the uterine cervix: a systematic review and metaanalysis. Lancet 358: 781-786.

9. Gregoire V, Hunter N, Brock WA, et al. (1996) Improvement in the therapeutic ratio of radiotherapy for a murine sarcoma by indomethacin plus fludarabine. Radiat Res 146: 548-553.

10. Hatlevoll R, Hagen S, Hansen HS, et al. (1992) Bleomycin/cisplatin as neoadjuvant chemotherapy before radical radiotherapyin localized, inoperable carcinoma of the esophagus. A prospectiverandomized multicentre study: the second Scandinavian trial inesophageal cancer. RadiotherOncol 24: 114-116.

11. Hermisson M *et al.* (2006) O6-methylguanineDNA methyltransferase and p53 status predicttemozolomide sensitivity in human malignant gliomacells. *J Neurochem* **96:** 766-776.

12. Horii N, Nishimura Y, Okuno Y, et al. (2001) Impact ofneoadjuvant chemotherapy on Ki-67 and PCNA labeling indicesfor esophageal squamous cell carcinomas. Int J RadiatOncolBiolPhys 49: 527-532.

13. Lawrence TS *et al.* (1997) Fluoropyrimidine-radiationinteractions in cells andtumors.*SeminRadiatOncol* **7:** 260-266.

14. McGinn CJ and Lawrence TS (2001) Recentadvances in the use of radiosensitizing nucleosides.*SeminRadiatOncol***11:** 270–280.

15. McGinn CJ, Shewach DS, Lawrence TS: Radiosensitizing nucleosides. J Natl Cancer Inst 88: 1193-1203, 1996.

16. Milas L *et al.* (2000) *In vivo* enhancement of tumorradioresponse by C225 antiepidermal growth factorreceptor antibody.*Clin Cancer Res* **6:** 701-708.

17. Milas L, Cox JD (2003) Principles of combining radiation therapy and chemotherapy. In: Cox JD, Ang KK (eds) Radiation oncology, rationale, technique, results. Mosby, St. Louis, pp 108-124.

18. Milas L, Hunter N, Mason KA, et al. (1995) Tumor reoxygenation as a mechanism of taxol-induced enhancement of tumor radioresponse. ActaOncol 34: 409-412.

19. Milross CG, Mason KA, Hunter NR, et al. (1997) Enhanced radioresponse of paclitaxel-sensitive and -resistant tumours in vivo. Eur J Cancer 33: 1299-1308.

20. Nishimura Y, Suzuki M, Nakamatsu K, et al. (2002) Prospectivetrial of concurrent chemoradiotherapy with protracted infusion of5-fluorouracil and cisplatin for T4 esophageal cancer with orwithout fistula. Int J RadiatOncolBiol Phys 53: 134-139.

21. Pignon JP, Bourhis J, Domenge C, Designe L (2000) Chemotherapyadded to locoregional treatment for head and neck squamous-cell carcinoma: three meta-analyses of updated individualdata. Lancet 355: 949-955.

22. Pignon JP, Bourhis J, Domenge C, Designe L (2000) Chemotherapyadded to locoregional treatment for head and neck squamous-cell carcinoma: three meta-analyses of updated individualdata. Lancet 355: 949-955.

23. Pritchard RS, Anthony SP (1996) Chemotherapy plus radiotherapycompared with radiotherapy alone in the treatment of locally advanced, unresectable, non-small-cell lung cancer: a metaanalysis.Ann Intern Med 125: 723-729.

24. Sai H, Mitsumori M, Yamauchi C, et al. (2004) Concurrentchemoradiotherapy for esophageal cancer: comparison betweenintermittent standard-dose cisplatin with 5-fluorouracil and dailylow-dose cisplatin with continuous infusion of 5-fluorouracil. Int JClinOncol 9: 149-153.

25. Specenier P, Vermorken JB. Cetuximab: itsunique place in head and neck cancer treatment. Biologics 7, 77-90 (2013).

26. Suzuki M, Nakamatsu K, Kanamori S, et al. (2003) Additive effects of radiation and docetaxel on murine SCCVII tumors in vivo: special reference to changes in the cell cycle. Radiat Res 159: 799-804.

27. Tannock IF (1996) Treatment of cancer with radiation and drugs. J ClinOncol 14: 3156-3174.

28. Vincenzi B, Zoccoli A, Pantano F,Venditti O, Galluzzo S. Cetuximab: frombench to bedside. Curr. Cancer Drug Targets10(1), 80-95 (2010).

29. Vokes EE, Weichselbaum RR (1990) Concomitant chemoradiotherapy: rationale and clinical experience in patients with solid tumors. J ClinOncol 8: 911-934.

30. Vokes EE, Weichselbaum RR (1990) Concomitant chemoradiotherapy:rationale and clinical experience in patients withsolid tumors. J ClinOncol 8: 911-934.

31. Wick W *et al.* (2002) Prevention of irradiation-inducedglioma cell invasion bytemozolomide involvescaspase 3 activity and cleavage of focal adhesionkinase. *Cancer Res* **62:** 1915-1919.

FORENSIC PHARMACOLOGY

Intoduction

Pharmacology is defined as the science of drugs or any chemical entity that is incorported in chemical processes of living things for the benefit of the recipients. It includes the study of substances that bind to regulatory molecules and activate or inhibit normal body processes. Pharmacology deals with research and experimentation of new chemicals in a laboratory with the recent advancement in solving crimincal cases and drug abuse in legal systems as well as civil cases, sports medicine and doping. All of these range in "forensic pharmacology". It describes toxicity of substance abuse, doping and adverse drug reactions in dead persons in criminal justice system.

What is Forensic Pharmacology?

Forensic pharmacology bridges the interface of pharmacology and toxicology with medical and behavioral sciences in criminal justice system.It interpretates the effects of the drug, use or abuse and its duration of action for the medicolegal process. Based on victim's clinical history and laboratory findings, experts can help in legal matters.

Forensic Pharmacology and Forensic Toxicology

There is fine line between pharmacology and toxicology. One can study all aspects of drug/substance, including cellular and molecular mechanism of the drug/substance on biological sample in Pharmacology.While toxicology refers only to the study of toxicity and adverse effects of the therapeutic agents or other chemicals on biological organisms. Both of them depend on dose dependent tests to analyse the effect from no effect to toxic effects. Forensic pharmacology discusses the effect of the all substances ranges in therapeutic agents, drugs with no medical value, absued drugs, "street" and "designer" drugsin medico-legal cases in establishing the relation between individual's behavior, illness, cause of death, disease or injury with the drug/substance. A pharmacologist is a scientist who conducts research experiments and tests drugs to study their effects on animals and humans. He/she useshis/her expertise to resolve litigations and drug regulatory process in criminal justice system on the basis of pharmacokinetics, physiological and cellular mode of action of the drugs on victims.

Envolvement of Forensic Pharmacovigilance

Pharmacovigilance experts plays an important role during the criminal proceedings, where the identifying authorities found the involvement of drugs in a case, i.e. the death cases which has overdose toxicity of drugs like sedatives, the suicidal tendencies that left mystery behind which may or may not be the use of antidepressants etc. These abnormal drug levels are precisely assess by TDM associated the form of adverse finding with the normal behavior of such drugs.

Adverse drug reactions (ADR) have been collected by pharmacovigilance applications. But when we found the presence of pharmaceuticals compounds or products in the environment, the concerning detection, understanding, assessment, and prevention of adverse effects comes under ecopharmacovigilance. It helps in finding the ecological abnormalities which affects the flora and fauna also. It may help in the development of pharmacovigilance sciences which protects our surrounding and the environmental.

Why we need Forensic Pharmacologist?

Today's world is totally into television and some serials like Crime Petrol, Forensic files, Law & Order and Cold Cases; they have shown importance of forensic pharmacologists along with advanced forensic laboratory techniques in courtroom procedures. Now responsible authorities and common public are more relay on expert pharmacologist in these types of cases. Their role is more into administrative level (via analyzing patents, scientific frauds and testing), clinical evaluators (via analyzing use of drugs in drug induced violence, ADRs, substance abuse and date rape drug) and distributive level (adulteration or contamination of drugs and use of counterfeit drugs). They can testify as an expert witness in legal matters via analyzing drug interaction, drug abuse, overdose and ADR of medicines in victim. Analyzing all above parameters in dead people is little tricky, therefore a forensic pharmacologist must possess special skills, experience, knowledge and training to give honest opinions in courtrooms.

Scope of Forensic Pharmacology

Mostly civil and criminal cases come under the forensic law involving the use of drugs and different chemicals. The forensic pharmacologist is highly specific of his expertise, skill, and work. Forensic pharmacologist is well trained and rich with the knowledge of drug interactions, pharmacodynamics, pharmacokinetics and adverse drug reactions.

There are few scenarios where forensic pharmacologist can be useful include: Drug Abuse, road traffic accidents, assault, doping, criminal cases, murder, rape, forensic pharmacovigilance, off-label drug use, Environmental toxicology and ecotoxicology etc.

Drug abuse was quite commonly has been seen among Indian males aged 12–60 years. In recent update with this context, the panel comprises of senior ministry officials as well as members of AIIMS' National Drug Dependence Treatment Centre (NDDTC) is near to finish an exhaustive survey for drug abuse by 2018. When we go through the data in last few years we have found that in 2004, the Indian Ministry of Social Justice and Empowerment (IMSJE) has conducted a national survey. These facts revealed the most common abuse was in the use of tobacco (55.8%), alcohol (21.4%), cannabis (3.0%), opiate (0.7%) and sedatives (0.1%). It also has been found that the drugs interfere with the mind of individual. These affect the behavior and thought process of a person to commit the crime, which results in assault, road transport accidents, rape, suicide and murder. Medico-legal implications have been intensified by their actions and addiction liability.

Forensic pharmacology is the field that deals with the study to identify the "drugs of abuse" and their derivatives. These abusive drugs have different categories like:

- Central nervous system (CNS) stimulants i.e. marijuana, tobacco, heroin, cocaine, amphetamine and its derivatives,
- CNS depressants i.e. uploads, benzodiazepines, and alcohol,
- Cannabinoids,
- Inhalants i.e. chloroform,
- Dissociative anesthetics i.e. ketamine
- Anabolic steroids
- Hallucinogens such as, phencyclidine, mescaline and lysergic acid diethylamide.

In 1930's the ergogenic performance enhancing agents i.e. androgens has been identified. These ergogenic drugs include anabolic steroids, growth hormone, diuretics, sympathomimetic agents, narcotic analgesics, amphetamines, oral peptide hormones, beta blockers, erythropoietin, cocaine and caffeine. World Anti-Doping Agency (WADA) has precise regulations and guidelines on the use of ergogenic drugs. National Anti-Doping

Agency (NADA) has initiated a vision of "dope free" sport in India. It is responsible for coordinating, promoting and monitoring the doping control program in sports.

There are many cases where a forensic pharmacologist can provide a testimonial such as use of drug or poison as a weapon, mental impairment caused due to the effect of a medication, or the use of a specific drug as the reason for criminal aggression.

The forensic pharmacologist can properly elucidate the level, concentration of alcohol products in the blood. He can also help to clarify the synergistic/antagonistic effect of alcohol along with drug interactions on alcohol absorption or metabolism. Pharmacokinetics is an application to examine and measure the level of alcohol in blood at supposed crime period. The blood samples of a person has been also used to determine signs of toxicity, high/low/borderline doses, lack of therapeutic effect, or a suspected case of poor adherence. He can also identify any type of alterations in postmortem and ante-mortem blood levels because he closely monitor the narrow therapeutic range of different drugs such as, lithium, theophylline, digoxin.

The science that deals with adverse effects or any other drug related problems is known as pharmacovigilance. Forensic pharmacologist work on detection, warning, management, and advice of drugs and its adverse reactions that can reduce the harm and benefit in clinical practice which ultimately helps in improving patient safety in therapeutics. In forensic cases, establishing the effects of the drugs leading to crime is an important medical discipline to develop. Different counterfeit medicines, adulteration, contamination or other substandard medicinal products are identified by application of standard procedure of pharmacovigilance in the form of adverse drug reactions (ADR) and confirm any injury/death. It differs from Pharmacovigilance as it considers the medico-legal implications as well.

Forensic pharmacologist also plays a significant role in civil cases, which involve review of insurance claims. Forensic pharmacologist can evaluate the use of "off-label" and unlabeled use of drugs after testifies the appropriateness and urgency.

Our modern time is ongoing with the industrialization and urbanization processes. We are using certain dosages or durations of time of several different chemicals, currently inhale, ingest, or absorb which at can lead to subsequent morbidities or mortalities. A forensic pharmacologist can play an important role in resolving the medico legal issues in the surrounding. He also help in spreading the awareness about the good/bad drugs, their evaluation, diagnosis of particular problem, treatment, and also the prevention measures of toxic exposures if any.

Question to be asked in Forensic Pharmacology

In all medico-legal cases, courts expect the analyst to know the advanced techniques to be used to achieve particular result and limitations that could affect that result. The scientific and legal validity of the drug evidence must be defensible to be effective in medico-legal cases. Therefore, forensic pharmacologist should be up to date with latest laboratory techniques, scientific question of the courtroom and government policies & rules to be used in criminal justice system. Their expertise can be very helpful in solving following problems:

- Whether the drug is involved in behavior, illness, injury or death in particular case?
- What amount of drug should be considered as overdose that cases death or aggressive nature?
- How to determine the appropriate tests to determine presence and quantity of the drugs?
- How to measure dose responsiveness, adverse reactions, and individual susceptibility and medication errors in samples?

Testing Process (type of samples, analytical techniques, precaution)

To detect and interpret the drugs/ substances in forensic samples, the forensic pharmacologists should have several analytical techniques, expertise and experience for medico-legal systems. The qualitative and quantitative analysis depends upon following parameters:

- **Sensitivity:** In terms of forensic pharmacology, sensitivity refers for the 'reliability' of the test to detect drug/chemical in question.
- **Specificity:** In terms of forensic pharmacology, specificity refers for detection of 'exact' drug/ chemical in question and not mistakenly identifies other compound.
- **Timing of sample collection:** Different samples can be collected at different time points for accurate results. Detail mentioned in table 1.
- **Source of sample collection:** Samples should be collected as earliest as possible and store at suitable condition with proper labeling. Urine and blood can be collected in both living and postmortem samples, while vitreous humor, gastric contents, bile, CSF, tissue, liver, brain, lungs and kidney can be used in postmortem samples (TIAFT – The International Association of Forensic Toxicologists).

S. No.	Source of Sample	Amount	Time points	Method to collect the sample

Before Testing Process

Before starting the testing procedure on forensic samples, forensic pharmacologist should know the following aspects:

- Proper legal status of the case.
- Knowledge of relevant pharmacological properties.
- Selection of optimal analytical techniques.
- Laboratory should be accreditated and reliable.
- The forensic scientists must have several analytic techniques available for screening and confirming the compound that completely depends upon the sample in use.

Analytical Techniques

Forensic pharmacology aims to assist in detection and interpretation of drugs for medico-legal cases. After proper collection, packaging of the samples and screening tests, forensic pharmacologist basically uses immunoassays and chromatography techniques to analyze and confirm the drug of interest. Different category of drugs has different protocol to analyze the test drugs. The results also depend upon type of sample, time of sample collection and expertise of forensic pharmacology. There are basically two test batteries to analyze forensic substance, Screening tests and Confirmatory tests.

Screening test: Screening test or Presumptive tests (e.g. color tests) can narrow down the class of the drug/chemicals in question. For the correct results and detect correct class of the drug/substance, pharmacologist/analyst should know:

- The exact age of test kits or reagents- it should not be in use after its expiry date.
- How the resulting color should be measured?
- Whole test procedure filmed and photographed properly.
- Take the precautions- avoid cross contamination.

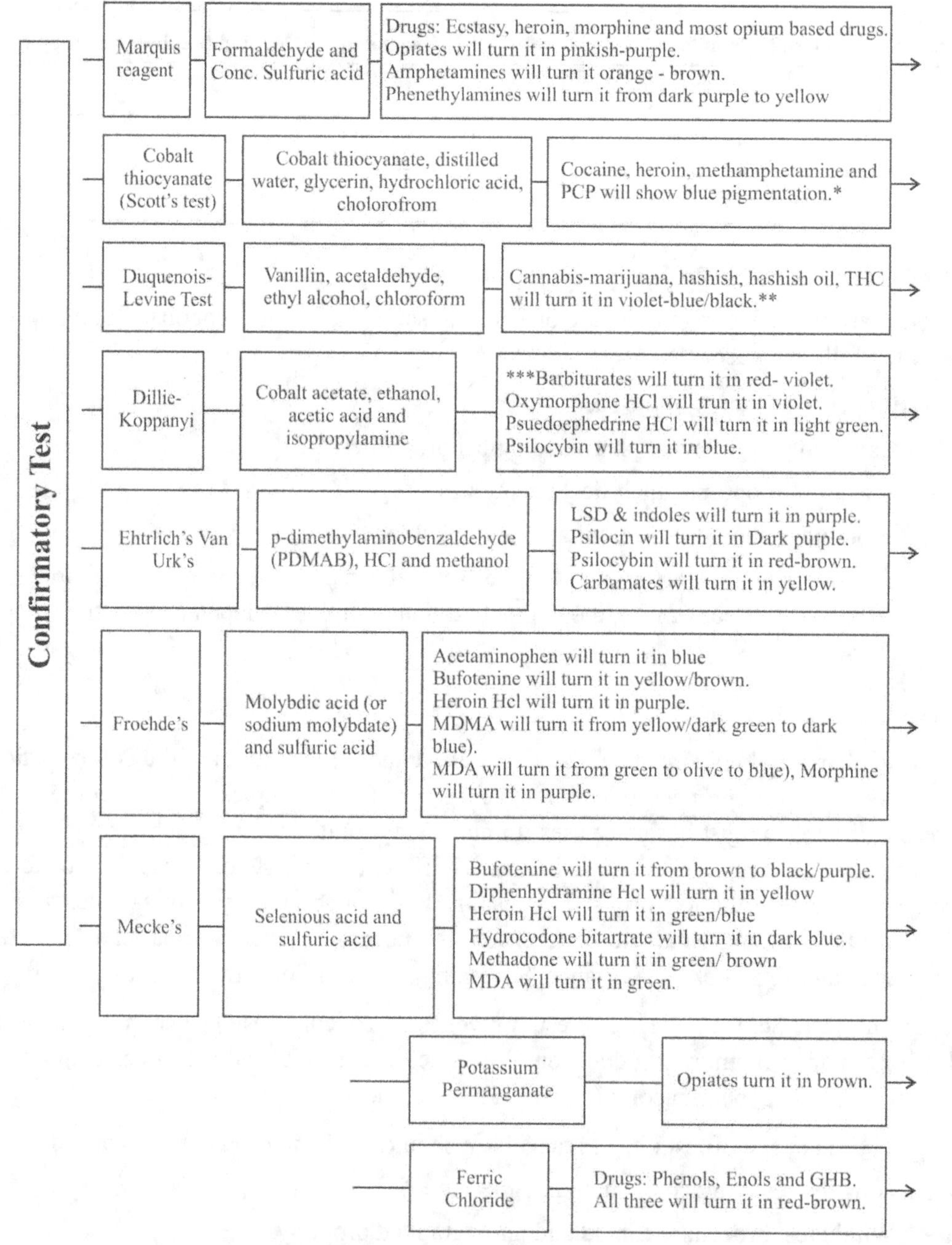

* Produce a false positive in the presence of Demerol or other non-controlled substances.
**False positives may occur in the presence of Advil, Nuprin, aspirin, and some brands of coffee.
***Upon addition of the Isopropylamine reagent, the barbiturate will turn the Koppanyi paper red-violet.

Fig. 49.1 List of screening test or presumptive tests in forensic pharmacology.

Other than these tests, immunoassays are considered important as initial screening methods but it also requires confirmatory test to identify exact class of the test compound/drug.

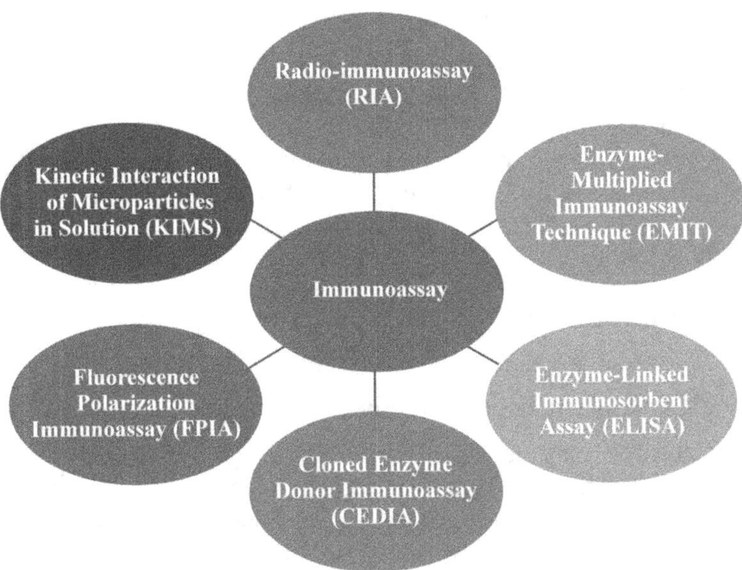

Fig. 49.2 Type of Immunoassays used in forensic pharmacology.

Confirmatory tests: Sometimes some over the counter cold medications or few substances may give false positive results because of their structural or chemical similarity with illegal substances. Therefore confirmatory tests, like Gas chromatography (GC), Mass spectroscopy, HPLC, etc should be performed alone or in combination. These tests are very specific, definitive, and reliable and considered as 'gold standard' in test drug identification. Another branch of forensic sciences, forensic drug chemistry deals with molecular interaction and bonding of the drug/ substances to be tested. The confirmatory testing requires:

- Multistep process to separate the individual compounds.
- Determine the chemical characteristics of the test compounds.
- Federal level cases require amount and purity of the test compounds.

GC-MS (Gas Chromatography-Mass Spectrometry):

This analytical technique allows detection and analysis of tiny amount of the test chemical in link to help in medico-legal cases. GC is an analytical technique in which sample is vaporized in gas chromatogram and analyzed in detector after its transport through various chambers/column of different temperature. This variability in temperature separates the test compound based on its volatility and chromatogram of different compounds is generated as different peaks. Analyst may use retention time (time taken by test molecule to move through entire machine and be detected by detector) to differentiate among different compounds but many different compounds may have similar retention time in same chromatogram.

Therefore, mass spectrometer play vital role to determine the exact molecular weight and distinguish the test compound based on mass-to-charge (m/z) ratio (Tsai and Lin, 2005).Separated ionized test samples are further separated because of molecular weight in electromagnetic field of mass analyzer. The analyst may manipulate the flow rate, temperature or type of gas used etc to obtain desired test drug/compound.

Characteristics

- Very specific and sensitive.
- High resolution and low background interference.
- Refine forensic drug database search via interfacing with computer.

Coupling of GC and MS may increases specificity and sensitivity of the forensic drug analysis and determine the accurate molecule's identity. Same peak of different compounds at same retention time can be distinguished via using mass spectrum. It eliminates incorrect identity and narrow down the potential identities to one test compound.

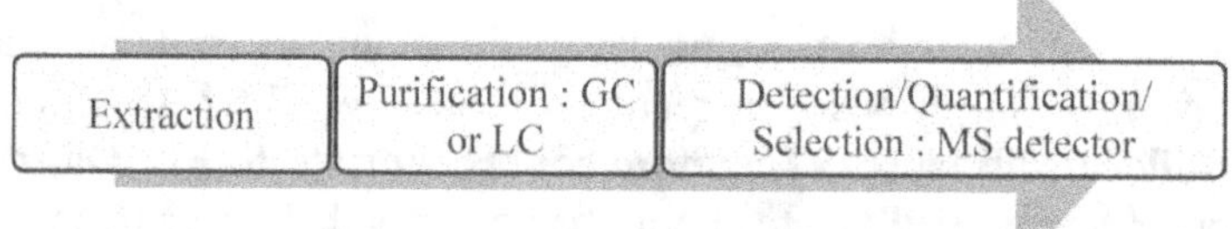

The GC-MS can separate and analyze only volatile or heat stable compounds/drugs that is main concern with drugs and its metabolites. LC-MS can overcome this situation by using electro spray ionization (ESI) in MS, but high cost and inability to use inter-laboratory spectra for test compound/drug identification restricts the use of LC-MS in daily forensic drug analysis. Electron ionization (EI), electro spray ionization (ESI), atmospheric pressure chemical ionization (APCI), matrix assisted laser deportation ionization (MALDI), fast atom bombardment (FAB) and most recently discovered direct analysis in real time (DART) are the most commonly used ionization method for forensic drug analysis. Few more limitations and troubleshooting are mentioned in table below,

Limitations and Troubleshooting in GC-MS in forensic drug analysis

S. No.	Limitations	Troubleshoot
1	A mass spectrometer (MS) cannot identify compounds in mixed sample.	Sample need to separate using GC or LC prior to running in mass spectrum.

Contd...

S. No.	Limitations	Troubleshoot
2	The enantiomers (same molecular weight but different chemical structure) cannot be differentiated by MS. e.g. pseudoephedrine and ephedrine.	Subsequent FTIR testing can help in distinguish the enantiomers.
3	Methamphetamine stereoisomers cannot be differentiated by GC-MS as they both create same peaks on GC-MS.	L- Methamphetamine is illegal, therefore analyst need to quantify each stereoisomers (by means of percentages) in the sample
4	MS destroy the sample during testing process.	DART is fast, non-destructive testing process and quantify the sample in no time.

Precautions

- Analyst need to maintain and calibrate the machine time to time.
- Analyst need to take care of reagents and follow the SOP to perform the experiment.
- Results should not be interpreted only on the basis of computer generated comparison to library of standard, analyst's individualized interpretation of the analyst may also help.
- Only GC or only MS results are not sufficient to identify correct test compound/ drug. Both chromatogram and spectrum should be interpreted together for final identification.

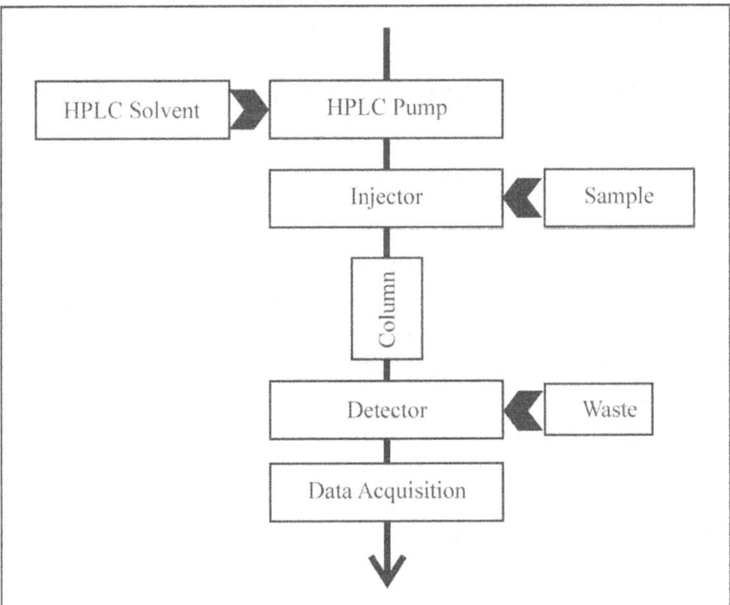

Fig. 49.3 Workflow of HPLC in forensic drug analysis.

High Performance Liquid Chromatography (HPLC)

Unlikely to GC, in which mobile phase is an inert gas, HPLC can have combination of several different solvents as mobile phase. This increases flexibility and range of applications of HPLC in forensic drug analysis. High performance liquid chromatography (HPLC) is basically a highly improved form of column liquid chromatography. Instead of a solvent being allowed to drip through a column under gravity, it is forced through under high pressures of up to 400 atmospheres. That makes it much faster.

All chromatographic separations, including HPLC operate under the same basic principle; separation of a sample into its constituent parts because of the difference in the relative affinities of different molecules for the mobile phase and the stationary phase used in the separation. Instead of having different detectors in HPLC (e.g. refractive index detector (RI), UV/VIS detectors and UV/VIS spectrophotometers, photodiode array detector (PDA), MS), UV/VIS detector and MS are most common used detectors in wide range of compounds of forensic interest with excellent accuracy and sensitivity.

Characteristics

- Non-Specific.
- Qualitative and quantitative measurements.
- Analyze high molecular weight compound/drug.

Fourier Transform Infrared Spectroscopy (FTIR)

The Infrared spectroscopy is the most recent and important analytical Category A technique of available to today's scientists for drug identification in medico-legal cases. This technique identify the test compound/drug on the basis of vibration frequency of atom/molecules.

Conclusion: Need of Improvement in Forensic Pharmacology in Indian Scenario

The concept of forensic pharmacologist is very helpful in finding abnormal drugs effect in patients with overdose, toxicity of any drug or ADRs related to drug use and even very important to help in detection of doping, accidental use of ergogenic drugs by athletes in blood or urine samples. Additionally, they can also advise on the drug interactions and use of drugs for therapeutic purposes in athletes.

Suggested Readings

1. Anderson PD, O'Donnell JT. The forensic pharmacists. In: O'Donnell JT, editor. Drug Injury: Liability, Analysis and Prevention. 3rd ed. Tucson, AZ: Lawyers and Judges Publishing Company; 2012. pp. 761-70.

2. Anderson PD, O'Donnell JT. The forensic pharmacists. In: O'Donnell JT, editor. Drug Injury: Liability, Analysis andPrevention. 3rd ed. Tucson, AZ: Lawyers and Judges Publishing Company; 2012. pp. 761-70.

3. Anderson PD. Forensic aspects of drug interactions part II. Forensic Exam. 1999; 8: 137-67.

4. Anderson PD. The broad field of forensic pharmacy. J Pharm Pract. 2012; 25: 7-12.

5. Anderson PD. The broad field of forensic pharmacy. J Pharm Pract. 2012; 25: 7-12.

6. Beynon CM, McVeigh C, McVeigh J, Leavey C, Bellis MA. The involvement of drugs and alcohol in drug-facilitated sexualassault: A systematic review of the evidence. Trauma Violence Abuse. 2008; 9: 178-88.

7. Body D, Edwards IR, Hartigan Go K, Healy D, Herxheimer A, Labadie J. Is there a need for forensic pharmacovigilance as aspecialty? Int J Risk Saf Med. 2011; 23: 31-42.

8. Edwards IR, Body D. Forensic pharmacovigilance. Int J Risk Saf Med. 2012; 24: 1-2.

9. Favretto D, Pascali JP, Tagliaro F. New challenges and innovation in forensic toxicology: Focus on the New PsychoactiveSubstances. J Chromatogr A. 2013; 1287: 84-95.

10. Ferner RE, editor. Forensic Pharmacology: Medicines, Mayhem and Malpractices. Oxford, New York: Oxford UniversityPress; 1996. Effect of drugs on behavior; pp. 73-8.

11. Ferner RE, editor. Forensic Pharmacology: Medicines, Mayhem and Malpractices. Oxford, New York: Oxford UniversityPress; 1996. Effect of drugs on the victims of crime; pp. 79-89.

12. Ferner RE. Toxicological evidence in forensic pharmacology. International Journal of Risk & Safety in Medicine. 2012 Jan 1; 24(1): 13-21.

13. Handelsman DJ, Gooren LJ. Hormones and sport: Physiology, pharmacology and forensic science. Asian J Androl.2008; 10: 348-50.

14. Harper L, Powell J, Pijl EM. An overview of forensic drug testing methods and their suitability for harm reduction point-of-care services. Harm reduction journal. 2017 Dec; 14(1): 52.

15. Imobersted A. The role of pharmacist in evaluating drug use in drivers: The drug evaluation and classification program. JPharm Pract. 2000; 13: 202-9.

16. Kielholz P, Battegay R. Behandlung depressiver Zustandsbilder, unter spezieller Berücksichtigung von Tofranil, einem neuen Antidepressivum. Schweiz Med Wochenschr 1958; 88: 763e7.)

17. Knopp WD, Wang TW, Bach BR., Jr Ergogenic drugs in sports. Clin Sports Med. 1997; 16: 375-92.

18. Labadie J. Forensic pharmacovigilance and substandard or counterfeit drugs. Int J Risk Saf Med. 2012; 24: 37-9.

19. Malve HO. Forensic pharmacology: An important and evolving subspecialty needs recognition in India. Journal of pharmacy & bioallied sciences. 2016 Apr; 8(2):92.

20. Medhi B, Sewal RK. Ecopharmacovigilance: an issue urgently to be addressed. Indian J Pharmacol 2012; 44(5): 547e9.)

21. Modi JP. History of forensic medicine. In: Kannan K, Mathiharan K, editors. Modi – A Textbook of Medical Jurisprudence and Toxicology. 16th ed. New Delhi: LexisNexis Butterworths Wadhwa; 2011. pp. 1-18.

22. Mukherjee JB. Toxicology. In: Karmakar RN, editor. Forensic Medicine and Toxicology. 2nd ed. Kolkata: Academic Publishers; 2007. pp. 49-50.

23. Parikh CK. Parikh's Textbook of Medical Jurisprudence, Forensic Medicine and Toxicology for Classrooms and Courtrooms. 6th ed. Sec. 1. New Delhi: CBS Publisher and Distributor; 2012. Introduction; pp. 1-16.

24. Patel G. Postmortem drug levels: Innocent bystander or guilty as charged. J Pharm Pract. 2012; 25: 37-40.

25. Pounder DJ. The nightmare of postmortem drug changes. In: Wecht CH, editor. Legal Medicine. Salem, New Hampshire: Butterworth Legal Publishers; 1994. pp. 163-91.

26. Rakesh K. Sewal, Vikas K. Saini, Bikash Medhi. Forensic pharmacovigilance: Newer dimension of pharmacovigilance. Journal of Forensic and Legal Medicine 34 (2015) 113e118.

27. Schulz M, Schmoldt A. Therapeutic and toxic blood concentrations of more than 500 drugs. Pharmazie. 1997; 52: 895-911.

28. Trestrail JH. 2nd ed. New York: Humana Press; 2007. Criminal Poisoning: Investigational Guide for Law Enforcement, Toxicologists, Forensic Scientists and Attorneys; pp. 47-60.

29. Tsai JSC, Lin GL. Drug-testing technologies and applications. In: Wong RC, Tse HY, editors. Drug-testing technologies and applications. Totowa: Humana Press; 2005. p. 29-69.

30. Wick J. Forensic pharmacy: can you prove it?. The Consultant Pharmacist®. 2013 Jul 1; 28(7): 418-24.

31. Zedeck BE, Zedeck MS. Introduction: The role of the forensic pharmacologist, In: Kobilinsky L, editor. Inside Forensic Science - Forensic Pharmacology. 6th ed. New York: Chelsea House publishers; 2007. p. 1-12.

32. Zedeck BE, Zedeck MS. Introduction: The role of the forensic pharmacologist. In: Kobilinsky L, editor. Inside ForensicScience: Forensic Pharmacology. 1st ed. New York: Infobase Publishing; 2007. pp. 1-11.

33. Zedeck BE, Zedeck MS. Introduction: The role of the forensic pharmacologist. In: Kobilinsky L, editor. Inside Forensic Science: Forensic Pharmacology. 1st ed. New York: Infobase Publishing; 2007. pp. 1-11.

CHAPTER 50

DRUG REPOSITIONING

Introduction

Pharmaceutical growth and productivity are measured by how much input (investment) has been done and how much outcome (new drugs and financial profits) has earned. For the past decade there is dramatic decrease in the productivity and outcome while the investments are increasing enormously of the pharmaceuticals. This decreased productivity problem has coupled with many factors -global pressure related to increased costs in development process, increased competition cause of generics, highly conserved regulatory policies and insufficient bombarding innovations. As a result pharmaceutical industries are more focusing towards finding new targets and indications for existing drugs rather than *de novo* drug discovery.

"Drug repositioning" or "drug repurposing", defined as the method of establishing new therapeutic use for "drug candidates" already in the market (i.e. existing drugs) and also known as drug rescuing, drug re-tasking, drug recycling, therapeutic Switching, drug re-profiling or drug repurposing. As compared to the traditional system of drug development, drug repositioning offers reduced cost and timeframes of developing and launching a drug into the market by omitting/bypassing the need of various stages of drug development (i.e.*in-vitro* screening, preclinical trials, pharmacokinetic & toxicological profile studies and even phase I clinical trials as the drug has already approved into the market) (Figure 50.1). Sometimes drugs are shown to be safe in phase I trials but fails as an effective therapy in phase II and phase III trials (i.e. besides safe, fails to be effective in medical condition they are meant for). In this scenario drug repositioning can be adopted as a salvageable approach for such drugs to be thrown out of the market. Also it reduces uncertainty associated with safety concerns, pharmacokinetics and toxicology concerned with new drug candidates. Pharmaceutical industries are inclined more towards scanning of pharmacopoeia so as to find repositioning of existing drug candidates.

One of the remarkable examples in history of drug repositioning is thalidomide revival as immunosuppressant drug. In 1957, Thalidomide was introduced into the market as sedative and was given pregnant females for morning sickness in Germany and England. In 1962, it had been revealed that its use in pregnancy caused damaged to the limbs of 10,000 newborns (Thalidomide Disaster). After this disaster, law has been introduced known as the 'Arzneimittelgesetz', in Germany according to which it had been made compulsory to pharmaceutical industries to provide the proof of safety before it comes into the market. Another example big success of drug repurposing is sildenafil (*Viagra*); drug which was initially developed for angina but later repurposed for treatment of erectile dysfunctioning.

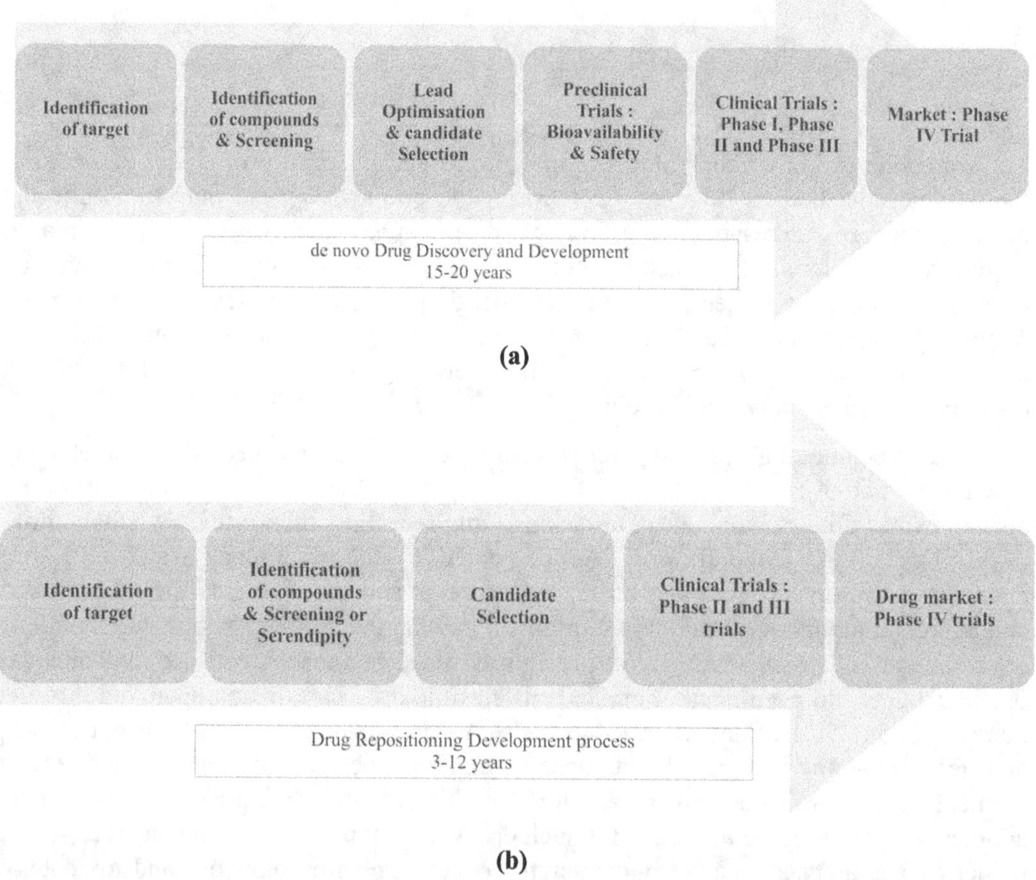

Fig. 50.1 Drug development process to market: A) *de novo* Drug discovery and Development Process and B) Drug Repositioning Development Process.

Off-label Drug Use

Off-label drug use refers to make the use of approved drug for unapproved therapeutic condition i.e. use for which the prior approval has not been obtained from regulatory authorities. It may also involve the use of drug using different dosage, formulation, contraindication, route of administration and patient group/age. It provides clinicians kind of freedom to think and apply new therapeutic use of existed drug which in turn poses certain benefits like that of innovations in existing clinical treatments and practices. Also it provides add-on treatments to orphan diseases. Drug gets approval for its market in a specific therapeutic condition only after getting confirmatory positive results in safety and efficacy studies done preclinical as well as clinical. During initial years of drug development it is not possible for pharma company to identify all potential uses of a drug/agent under investigation. Also, it is not feasible to identify all possible dosage forms, routes of administration and for all age groups involving pediatrics, pregnant and lactating mothers. This makes off-label drug use a common practice across world. Bavdekar and Gogtay reviewed off-label drug usesvaried from 10.8 to 66.0% among different European countries and its prevalence was found to be more in premature, neonates and infants. Although new indication may be added to existed drug's use but it involves huge cost for conducting clinical trials and application to NDA (new drug application). The maximum rates of uses of off-label were mainly for anticonvulsants (74%), followed by antipsychotics (60%), and antibiotics (41%). Alsooff-label is usually use for numerous biologics (such as epoetinalfa [Procrit] and bevacizumab [Avastin]). Concomitantly, off-label use has also negative consequences. Like, it challenges the expectations of safety as well as efficacy that needs to be completely evaluated, increases overall health care costsand its uses may discourage evidence-based practice.

Off-label uses follow the FDA Modernization Act of 1997 for marketing. This legislation also enormously eased restrictions imposed on drug promotions. Aparts, current FDA policy also impede the direct promotion for unapproved uses of products.

Approaches to Drug Repositioning

For drug repositioning, two basic strategies can be adopted namely: "activity-based screening strategies" and "computational based strategies".

1. **Activity-based screening strategies**

   (a) ***Existing Drug's Data Bank***: One of the common first-line approach for finding drug repurposing to use data banks or libraries of existing and approved drug/drug candidate/chemical moieties. At present various clinical library databases are being used commercially: "Evotec by National Institutes of Health (NIH) Clinical Collections", "Microsource compounds database (Spectrum collection)", "National Institute of Neurological Disorders and

Stroke custom collection (NINDS) collection II", "Sigma Aldrich", "Tocris" and "Enzo Life Sciences etc."

(b) ***Phenotypic Screening and Target Oriented Approach***: "Phenotypic drug discovery (PDD)" involves evaluating drug candidate for its phenotypic effect using cell cultures or tissues or whole/intact organism. While in target based approach, compound is evaluated for its binding capacity to specific protein target using in-vitro assays.

2. **Computational Based Approaches:** On account of ability to screen large number of compounds (virtually), computational based analysis is more powerful and systematic tool that is being used to predict and find new targets in drug repositioning. Drug-drug or drug-disease interactions or connectivity forms the fundamentals of this approach. There are different computational methods available for finding "drug-disease connections".

(a) ***Transcriptomic-based   or   Signature-based   Drug   Repositioning***: "Connectivity mapping" (also referred as CMap) forms the basis of this approach. Disease associated gene expressions are determined using microarray technique in order to get "disease signatures": expression/pattern of set of genes, upregulated or downregulated in that particular disease; obtained from omics data. These are referred to as disease-signatures. These disease-signatures are matched with corresponding drug-signatures and new purpose of drug can be elucidated. New indication needs to be validated further using *in vivo* experiments. One of the examples is topiramate, which was introduced as an epileptic drug, has found to be effective in inflammatory bowel disease. In order to validate this new indication, in vivo studies were done to evaluate topiramate efficacy as anti-inflammatory drug in colitis using experimental colitis model in rodents. Some of freely accessible databases are: NCBI-GEO (http://www.ncbi.nlm.nih.gov/geo/), SRA [LM2] (http://www.ncbi.nlm.nih.gov/Traces/sra/), CMAP and CCLE. This method has advantage that it relies on molecular based mechanisms as explained by changes in gene expressions.

(b) ***Genome-Wide Association Studies***: "Genome-wide association studies" (GWAS) provides an influential strategy in elucidating new targets for drug repositioning. In past few years, GWAS has provided unmatchable knowledge related to gene variations associated with complex trait diseases like that of neurodegenerative conditions i.e. Alzheimer's Disease (AD). On the basis of GWAS, analysis can be done in order to find that variations in gene subset that be can considered as drug target for drug repositioning.

Regulatory Pathways for Approval of Drug Repositioning

In US for regulatory approval of drugs, FDA has mentioned three regulatory pathways. Among which 505(b)(2) is being used for regulatory approval of drug repurposing. Regardless of therapeutic condition or use of drug, it has to be submitted via section 505(b)(2).[9] For 505(b)(2) approval; drug manufacturer has to find out novel/different route of administration or dosage or formulation or indication as compared to already existed knowledge (route of administration/use/formulation/dosage)use of the drug.

In Europe, a parallel approval pathway is regulated by the European Medical Agency (EMA) under Article 10 of Directive 2001/83/EC. Nonetheless, contrary to section 505(b)(2) of the FDA, which permits the employ of non-proprietary studies that have formerly attained a outrage standard of safety and quality for supporting any part of an application, Article 10 mainly concerns with the drugs that needs studies customised to the differences from reference listed drugs—it does not provide a legal basis for the use of non-proprietary studies.Also, Article 10 cannot be employ for molecular entities which is entirely new as, by definition, only changes from the reference listed drug apply. EMA takes on average of 6 months more as compared to the FDA to approve new indications for a drug.

Classical Examples Of Drug Repositioning

		Mechanism of Action	Original Therapeutic Indication	New Therapeutic Indication
A.	**Anti-depressants & Neurological Disorders**			
	Atomoxetine	Serotonin and norepinephrine inhibitor (SNRI)	Parkinson's disease	Attention Deficit hyperactivity Disorder (ADHD)
	Bupropion	Noradrenaline and dopamine reuptake inhibitor	Depression	Smoking cessation
	Chlorpromazine	Dopamine receptor blocker	Anti-emetic/ antihistamine	Non-sedating tranquillizer
	Dapoxetine	Selective serotonin reuptake inhibitor (SSRI)	Analgesia and depression	Premature ejaculation
	Duloxetine	Serotonin and norepinephrine inhibitor (SNRI)	Depression	Urinary incontinence
	Fluoxetine	Selective serotonin reuptake inhibitor (SSRI)	Depression	Premenstrual dysphoria
	Galantamine	Acetylcholinesterase Inhibitor	Polio, paralysis and anesthesia	Alzheimer's disease

Contd...

	Mechanism of Action	Original Therapeutic Indication	New Therapeutic Indication
Lidocaine	Sodium Channel blocker	Local anaesthesia	Oral Corticosteroid Dependent Asthma
Milnacipran	Serotonin and norepinephrine inhibitor (SNRI)	Depression	Fibromyalgia syndrome
Ropinirole	Dopamine-2 agonist	Hypertension	Parkinson's disease and Idiopathic restless leg syndrome
Sibutramine	Serotonin and norepinephrine inhibitor (SNRI)	Depression	Obesity
Tofisopam	Unclear	Anxiety-related conditions	Irritable bowel syndrome
Topiramate	Sodium Channel blocker, GABA stimulation, Kainate/AMPA antagonist	Anti-epileptic	Anti-Obesity
B.	**Drugs other than Neurological Disorders**		
Amantadine	Non-competitive NMDA receptor antagonist	Influenza	Parkinson's disease
Amphotericin	Binds irreversibly to ergosterol, resulting in disruption of membrane integrity and ultimately cell death.	Fungal infections	Leishmaniasis
Bosentan Monohydrate	Endothelin receptor antagonists	Treatment of congestive heart failure (intended)	Pulmonary Arterial Hypertension (PAH)
Botulinum Toxin A	Block the release of the neurotransmitter acetylcholine	Blepharospasm, cervical dystonia	Axillary hyperhidrosis
Bromocriptine	Dopamine D2-receptors agonist	Parkinson's disease	Diabetes mellitus
Colchicine	Inhibits microtubule polymerizations	Gout	Recurrent pericarditis
Celecoxib	Cyclooxygenase-2 inhibitor	Rheumatoid arthritis, Osteoarthritis	Familial adenomatous polyposis (FAP), breast cancer
Crizotinib	Inhibitor of receptor tyrosine kinase	Anaplastic large-cell lymphoma	Non-small cell lung cancer (NSCLC)
Eflornithine	Ornithine decarboxylase Inhibitor	Anti-microbial	Unwanted facial hair reduction in women

Contd...

		Mechanism of Action	Original Therapeutic Indication	New Therapeutic Indication
	Etanercept	Specifically to tumor necrosis factor (TNF)	Rheumatoid arthritis	Asthma
	Finasteride	5-α-reductase inhibitor	Benign prostatic hyperplasia	Hair loss
	Gabapentin	Binds to presynaptic NMDA receptors. activate the adenosine A1 receptor.	Epilepsy	Neuropathic pain
	Hydroxychloroquine	Not Clear	Antiparasitic	Anti-arthritic systemic lupus erythematosus
	Imatinib	A protein-tyrosine kinase inhibitor that inhibits the Bcr-Abl tyrosine kinase	Chronic myeloid leukemia (CML)	Gastrointestinal stromal tumor (GIST)
	Imidapril	Angiotensin-converting enzyme (ACE) inhibitor	Hypertension	Cancer cachexia
	Leflunomide	Selective inhibitor of de novo pyrimidine synthesis	Rheumatoid arthritis	Prostate cancer
	Lumigan	Prostaglandin analogue	Glaucoma	Hypotrichosis simplex
	Mecamylamine	Nicotinic Receptor Antagonist	Essential hypertension	Attention deficit hyperactivity disorder (ADHD)
	Metformin	Inhibits mitochondrial complex I activity	Diabetes mellitus	Breast, adenocarcinoma, prostate,colorectal cancer
	Methotrexate	Inhibition of folic acid reductase	Cancer	Psoriasis, rheumatoid arthritis
	Mifepristone	Glucocorticoidtype II Receptor Inhibitor	Termination of pregnancy	Psychotic major depression
	Miltefosine	Inhibits cytochrome-c oxidase, inhibitsphosphatidylcholine biosynthesis and inhibits Akt.	Cancer	Visceral Leishmaniasis
	Minoxidil	β-adrenergic receptor blocker	Hypertension	Hair loss
	Paclitaxel	Promotes tubulin polymerization and causing micro-tubule disruption	Cancer	Restenosis
	Phentolamine	α-Adrenergic receptor antagonist	Hypertension	Impaired night vision

Contd…

		Mechanism of Action	Original Therapeutic Indication	New Therapeutic Indication
	Plerixafor	Inhibits the CXCR4 chemokine receptors on CD34+ cells	Human immunodeficiency virus (HIV) (intended)	Mobilization of hematopoietic stem cell
	Propranolol	Competes with sympathomimetic neurotransmitters such as catecholamines for binding at beta(1)-adrenergic receptors	Hypertension	Migraine prophylaxis
	Raloxifene	Selective estrogen receptor modulator (SERM)	Breast and prostate cancer	Osteoporosis
	Retinoic acid	Binds to the retinoic acid receptor (RAR	Acne	Acute promyelocytic leukemia
	Rituximab	Activation of immune effector mechanisms	Non-Hodgkin's lymphoma (NHL)	Rheumatoid arthritis
	Sildenafil	Phosphodiesterase-5 (PDE5) inhibitor	Angina	Male erectile dysfunction
	Statins	Act by competitively inhibiting HMG-CoA reductase	Myocardial infarction	cancer, leukemia
	Sunitinib	Multi-targeted receptor tyrosine kinase (RTK) inhibitor	GIST, renal cell carcinoma	Pancreatic tumors/Gastrointestinal Tumor
	Thalidomide	TNF-α inhibition	Sedation, nausea and insomnia	Erythema Nodosum Laprosum (ENL) in leprosy and as chemotherapeutic agent in multiple myeloma
	Vesnarinone	Inhibits phosphodiesterase	Cardioprotective	Oral cancer, leukemia, lymphoma
	Wortmannin	Selective inhibitor for phosphoinositide 3-kinases (PI3Ks)	Antifungal	Leukemia
	Zidovudine	Reverse transcriptase Inhibitor (RTI)	Cancer	HIV/AIDS

Suggested Readings

1. Ashburn TT, Thor KB. Drug repositioning: identifying and developing new uses for existing drugs. Nat Rev Drug Discov. 2004; 3(8): 673-83.

2. Bavdekar SB, Gogtay NJ. Unlicensed and off-label drug use in children. J Postgrad Med. 2005; 51(4): 249-52.

3. Dubus E, Ijjaali I, Barberan O, Petitet F. Drug repositioning using in silico compound profiling. Future Med Chem. 2009; 1(9): 1723-36.

4. Dudley JT, Sirota M, Shenoy M, Pai RK, Roedder S, Chiang AP, et al. Computational repositioning of the anticonvulsant topiramate for inflammatory bowel disease. SciTranslMed. 2011; 3(96): 96ra76.

5. Gazarian M, Kelly M, McPhee JR, Graudins LV, Ward RL, Campbell TJ. Off-label use of medicines: consensus recommendations for evaluating appropriateness. Med J Aust. 2006; 185(10): 544-8.

6. Gupta SK, Nayak RP. Off-label use of medicine: Perspective of physicians, patients, pharmaceutical companies and regulatory authorities. J PharmacolPharmacother. 2014; 5(2): 88-92.

7. Harrold JM, Ramanathan M, Mager DE. Network-based approaches in drug discovery and early development. ClinPharmacolTher. 2013; 94(6): 651-8.

8. Hernandez JJ, Pryszlak M, Smith L, Yanchus C, Kurji N, Shahani VM, et al. Giving Drugs a Second Chance: Overcoming Regulatory and Financial Hurdles in Repurposing Approved Drugs As Cancer Therapeutics. Front Oncol. 2017 7: 273.

9. Hurle MR, Yang L, Xie Q, Rajpal DK. Computational drug repositioning: from data to therapeutics. Clinical [Internet]. 2013; Available from: http://onlinelibrary.wiley.com/doi/10.1038/clpt.2013.1/full

10. Iorio F, Rittman T, Ge H, Menden M, Saez-Rodriguez J. Transcriptional data: a new gateway to drug repositioning? Drug Discov Today. 2013; 18(7-8): 350-7.

11. Jin G, Wong STC. Toward better drug repositioning: prioritizing and integrating existing methods into efficient pipelines. Drug Discov Today. 2014; 19(5): 637-44.

12. Kim T-W. Drug repositioning approaches for the discovery of new therapeutics for Alzheimer's disease. Neurotherapeutics. 2015; 12(1): 132-42.

13. Lamb J, Crawford ED, Peck D, Modell JW, Blat IC, Wrobel MJ, et al. The Connectivity Map: using gene-expression signatures to connect small molecules, genes, and disease. Science. 2006; 313(5795): 1929-35.

14. Lamb J. The Connectivity Map: a new tool for biomedical research. Nat Rev Cancer. 2007; 7(1): 54-60.

15. Li YY, Jones S. Drug repositioning for personalized medicine. Genome Med [Internet]. 2012; Available from: https://genomemedicine.biomedcentral.com/articles/10.1186/gm326

16. Oberoi SS. Regulating off-label drug use in India: The arena for concern. PerspectClin Res. 2015; 6(3): 129-33.

17. Padhy BM, Gupta YK. Drug repositioning: Re-investigating existing drugs for new therapeutic indications. J Postgrad Med. 2011; 57(2):153-60.

18. Pammolli F, Magazzini L, Riccaboni M. The productivity crisis in pharmaceutical R&D. Nat Rev Drug Discov. 2011; 10(6): 428-38.

19. Sanseau P, Agarwal P, Barnes MR, Pastinen T, Richards JB, Cardon LR, et al. Use of genome-wide association studies for drug repositioning. Nat Biotechnol. 2012 10; 30(4): 317-20.

20. Scannell JW, Blanckley A, Boldon H, Warrington B. Diagnosing the decline in pharmaceutical R&D efficiency. Nat Rev Drug Discov. 2012; 11(3): 191-200.

21. Schulze U, Baedeker M, Chen YT, Greber D. R&D productivity: on the comeback trail. Nat Rev Drug Discov. 2014; 13(5): 331-2.

22. Stafford RS. Regulating off-label drug use—rethinking the role of the FDA. N Engl J Med. 2008; 358(14): 1427-9.

23. Stephens T, Brynner R. Dark remedy: the impact of thalidomide and its revival as a vital medicine. 2009; Available from: https:// www. researchgate. net/profile/Martin_Schulz/publication/24953236_Dark_Remedy_The_Impact_of _Thalidomide_and_its_Revival_as_a_Vital_Medicine/links/09e4150daf66a6b86a 000000/Dark-Remedy-The-Impact-of-Thalidomide-and-its-Revival-as-a-Vital-Medicine.pdf

24. Xue H1, Li J1, Xie H1, Wang Y. Review of Drug Repositioning Approaches and Resources. Int J Biol Sci. 2018; 14(10): 1232-1244.

INDEX